# Middle Range Theories

## Application to Nursing Research and Practice

### Fifth Edition

**SANDRA J. PETERSON, PhD, RN**
Professor Emerita
Bethel University
St. Paul, Minnesota
Accreditation Partner
NurseTim, Inc.
Waconia, Minnesota

**TIMOTHY S. BREDOW, PhD, RN, NP-C**
Professor Emerita
Bethel University
St. Paul, Minnesota

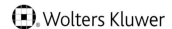. Wolters Kluwer

Philadelphia • Baltimore • New York • London
Buenos Aires • Hong Kong • Sydney • Tokyo

**Not authorised for sale in United States, Canada, Australia, New Zealand, Puerto Rico, and U.S. Virgin Islands.**

*Vice President and Publisher*: Julie K. Stegman
*Executive Editor/Acquisitions Editor*: Mark Foss
*Director of Product Development*: Jennifer K. Forestieri
*Associate Development Editor*: Rebecca J. Rist
*Editorial Coordinator*: Blair Jackson
*Marketing Manager*: Brittany Clements
*Editorial Assistant*: Kate Campbell
*Design Coordinator*: Joseph Clark
*Art Director, Illustration*: Jennifer Clements
*Production Project Manager*: Kim Cox
*Manufacturing Coordinator*: Karin Duffield
*Prepress Vendor*: SPi Global

Fifth edition

**Library of Congress Cataloging-in-Publication Data**
Names: Peterson, Sandra J., editor. | Bredow, Timothy S., editor.
Title: Middle range theories : application to nursing research and practice / [edited by] Sandra J. Peterson, Timothy S. Bredow.
Description: Fifth edition. | Philadelphia : Wolters Kluwer, [2020] | Includes bibliographical references and index. | Summary: "Middle Range Theory: Application to Nursing Research and Practice, Fifth Edition is a premier resource for Nursing Theory courses and for nursing students completing a research or practice project as part of their degree requirements. Authors Sandra Peterson and Tim Bredow review the processes used to initiate a project. They offer expert guidance on how to select an appropriate middle range theory for a project"—Provided by publisher.
Identifiers: LCCN 2019029633 | ISBN 9781975108311 (paperback)
Subjects: MESH: Nursing Theory | Nursing Research
Classification: LCC RT81.5 | NLM WY 86 | DDC 610.73072—dc23
LC record available at https://lccn.loc.gov/2019029633

CCS1219

*I am grateful for the opportunity to once again be involved in the development of this book. I appreciate my colleague and partner in this project, all the amazing nurse scholars who contributed, and the Wolters Kluwer staff who managed this publication journey. I also want to express my thanks to every nurse who reads the book and experiences a greater understanding of nursing theories, of their contribution to nursing's body of knowledge, and of their value to their nursing practice.*

*But most of all, I am so thankful for my family: husband (Ray), 102-year-old mother and nurse (Margaret Cairns), son (Christopher), daughter-in-law (Alisa), grandchildren (Liam and Jane), and last but not least (sorry for the cliché) daughter (Beth) and husband (Lars). They bring joy to my life.*

**Sandra J. Peterson**

*I would like to dedicate this fifth edition to my family who provides me with the love and support to complete a project such as this: KTJB, A, B, C, Tiff, Ben, and also little Kata, Pepper, Penelope, Finley, Madilyn, and Anne Jo. I echo the appreciation of Sandy to all nurse contributors to their specific chapters and to all my students with the hope that in using this text, they will more fully understand the relationships between theory, research, and evidence-based practice.*

**Timothy S. Bredow**

# Contributors to the Fifth Edition

**Timothy S. Bredow, PhD, RN, NP-C**
Professor Emerita
Bethel University
St. Paul, Minnesota

**Lisa Burkhart, PhD, RN, ANEF**
Associate Professor
Marcella Niehoff School of Nursing
Loyola University Chicago
Maywood, Illinois
Research Health Scientist
Center of Innovation for Complex Chronic Healthcare
Hines VA
Hines, Illinois
*Contributor to the fourth edition*

**Diane O. Chlebowy, PhD, RN**
Associate Professor
School of Nursing
University of Louisville
Louisville, Kentucky

**Connie Lynn Clark, PhD, RN**
Professor
Bethel University
St. Paul, Minnesota

**Cecelia L. Crawford, DNP, RN, FAAN**
Director of Evidence-Based Nursing Practice
Southern California Patient Care Services
Kaiser Permanente
Pasadena, California

**Kennith Culp, PhD, RN, FAAN, FGSA**
Professor
College of Nursing
University of Iowa
Iowa City, Iowa

**Georgene Gaskill Eakes, EdD, RN**
Director, Clinical Education
Vidant Medical Center
Greenville, North Carolina
*Contributor to the fourth and third editions*

**Marion Good, PhD, FAAN**
Professor Emerita
Frances Payne Bolton School of Nursing
Lakewood, Ohio

**Joan E. Haase, PhD, RN, FAAN**
Holmquist Professor in Pediatric Oncology Nursing
Science of Nursing Care Department
Indiana University School of Nursing
Indianapolis, Indiana
Full Member
Cancer and Prevention Control
IU Simon Cancer Center
Indianapolis, Indiana
*Contributor to the fourth and third editions*

**Sonya R. Hardin, PhD, CCRN, NP-C, FAAN**
Dean and Professor
School of Nursing
University of Louisville
Louisville, Kentucky
*Contributor to the fourth edition*

**Nancy S. Hogan, RN, PhD, FAAN**
Professor Emerita
Loyola University Chicago
Maywood, Illinois
*Contributor to the fourth edition*

**Eun-Ok Im, RN, PhD, FAAN**
Professor and Dean
Duke University
North Carolina

**Trine Klette, PhD**
Associate Professor
Diakonova University College
Oslo, Norway
*Contributor to third edition*

**Elizabeth R. Lenz, PhD, RN**
Professor Emeritus and Academy Professor
College of Nursing
The Ohio State University
Columbus, Ohio
*Contributor to the fourth and third editions*

**Marjorie C. McCullagh, PhD, RN, FAAOHN, FAAN**
Professor
School of Nursing
University of Michigan
Ann Arbor, Michigan
*Contributor to the fourth and third editions*

**Sandra J. Peterson, PhD, RN**
Professor Emerita
Bethel University
St. Paul, Minnesota
Accreditation Partner
NurseTim, Inc.
Waconia, Minnesota

**Celeste R. Phillips, PhD, RN**
Assistant Professor
School of Nursing
Indiana University
Indianapolis, Indiana
*Contributor to the fourth edition*

**Mertie L. Potter, DNP, PMHNP-BC, PMHCNS-BC**
Professor Emerita
Nursing
MGH Institute of Health Professions
Boston, Massachusetts
Nurse Practitioner
Merrimack Valley Counseling Association
Nashua, New Hampshire
*Contributor to the fourth and third editions*

**Barbara Resnick, PhD, CRNP, FAAN, FAANP**
Professor
School of Nursing
University of Maryland
Baltimore, Maryland
*Contributor to the fourth and third editions*

**Kristin E. Sandau, PhD, RN, CNE, FAHA, FAAN**
Professor of Nursing
Bethel University
St. Paul, Minnesota

**Marjorie A. Schaffer, PhD**
Professor Emerita
Nursing
Bethel University
St. Paul, Minnesota
*Contributor to the fourth and third editions*

**Danuta M. Wojnar, PhD, RN, FAAN**
Professor and Associate Dean for Academic Affairs
RWJF Executive Fellow
J. Bushman Endowed Chair in Nursing
Seattle University College of Nursing
Seattle, Washington
*Contributor to the fourth and third editions*

## Contributors to Previous Editions

**Laurel Ash, DNP, CNP, RN**
Assistant Professor
College of St. Scholastica
Duluth, Minnesota

**Audrey Gift, PhD, RN, FAAN**
Professor Emeritus
College of Nursing
Michigan State University
East Lansing, Michigan

**Marion Good, PhD, FAAN**
Professor Emerita
Frances Payne Bolton School of Nursing
Lakewood, Ohio

**Brian Goodroad, DNP, APRN, C-NP**
Associate Professor
Metropolitan State University
St. Paul, Minnesota

**Barbara Hoglund, EdD, MSN, RN, FNP-C**
Associate Professor of Nursing
Bethel University
St. Paul, Minnesota

**Trine Klette, PhD**
Associate Professor
Diakonova University College
Oslo, Norway

**Katherine Kolcaba, RN, MSN, PhD**
Associate Professor
Ursuline College
The University of Akron
Akron, Ohio

**Elizabeth R. Lenz, PhD, RN**
Professor Emeritus
College of Nursing
The Ohio State University
Columbus, Ohio

**Renee Milligan, MD**
Term Professor
School of Nursing
George Mason University
Fairfax, Virginia

**Linda C. Pugh, PhD, RNC, CNE, FAAN**
Director, Graduate Programs in Nursing
York College of Pennsylvania
York, Pennsylvania

**Ellen D. Schultz, PhD, RN, CHTP, AHN-BC**
Professor of Nursing
Metropolitan State University
St. Paul, Minnesota

**Marjorie Webb, PhD(c), DNP, APRN, C-NP**
Associate Professor
Metropolitan State University
St. Paul, Minnesota

# Preface

Middle range theories have understandably emerged as the focus of knowledge development in nursing. There is a growing acknowledgment that middle range theories make an important contribution to the advancement of nursing practice.

There is a dynamic relationship between theory, research, and practice. Research is a source of theory development, and theory is a source of research questions. Theory is used to improve practice, and practice is used to generate, test, and refine theories. Basically, it is by testing the theories through research that the evidence for practice is generated. In the fourth edition, the title changed to *Middle Range Theories Application to Nursing Research and Practice* to better reflect this dynamic relationship with increased emphasis on applications of middle range theories to practice. We continue to hope that this edition can serve as a resource for nurse scholars and practitioners, making middle range theories more accessible and useful. The ultimate goal is the advancement of nursing as a profession and improving the quality of its practice.

With the increase in the number of middle range theories being developed, determining which to include in this edition is always a challenge. As for the previous editions, we reviewed published research and practice applications of theories. We also solicited input from practitioners. The goal was to identify those theories, though in the middle range of abstraction, are not particularly narrow in their possible applications.

## Organization

### PART I

Part 1 is devoted to an overview of the state of nursing's body of knowledge and the processes by which it is evaluated.

Chapter 1 introduces the interrelationship between nursing theory, research, and practice. In addition to a brief discussion of epistemology with a summary of Carper's conceptualization of nurses' ways of knowing, the majority of the chapter addresses the hierarchy of nursing knowledge. The emphasis, of course, is on the place of middle range theory within that hierarchy (i.e., paradigm, philosophy, conceptual framework, and theories). For each component of the hierarchy, the chapter includes a description of its nature, review of its development, a discussion of its contributions to nursing knowledge, consideration of controversies related to its nature or use, and examples of nurse scholars' work. The section devoted to middle range theories includes an expanded and updated table with multiple examples of middle range theories referenced. Also included is an expanded discussion of practice or situation-specific theories with a table that provides recent examples of this level of theory development.

Chapter 2 emphasizes the analysis and evaluation of middle range theories, including issues to consider in the selection of a middle range nursing theory for research purposes. This chapter also describes a brief evaluative process for theory analysis. Using this evaluation process, readers can compare and contrast their conclusions about the theory as presented in the chapter with those of a nurse scholar who has also used this evaluation process. The theory analysis exercises related to each chapter are available in the Student Resources located on https://thepoint.lww.com/Peterson5e.

A new chapter has been added to introduce project management, and how middle range theory can provide direction to the project. The chapter describes the process and provides tools to be used to assist in the completion of a successful project.

### PARTS II TO V

Parts II to V are devoted to specific middle range theories. The selected theories are labeled by their developers or by nurse scholars as middle range theories and are ones frequently cited in published nursing research or practice applications. Many of the chapters contain unique nursing theories; some are borrowed from related disciplines but are, nonetheless, useful to nursing. All theories in the text, however, have the intrinsic capability to be applied to nursing research and practice. They address a wide range of phenomena that allow the researcher to consider a variety of nursing research questions and uses in practice. The theories have been organized by categories to reflect a general focus of research questions or practice applications. The categories are not presented as absolute but more as a guide to direct the user of the book to the theories that might be most relevant to their issue of interest.

- Physiological—Pain: Balance of Analgesia and Side Effects, Unpleasant Symptoms
- Psychological—Self-efficacy, Chronic Sorrow, Spiritual Care in Nursing Practice
- Social—Social Support, Caring, Interpersonal Relations, Attachment
- Integrative—Comfort, Heath-Related Quality of Life, Health Promotion, Deliberative Nursing Process, Resilience, Planned Change, AACN Synergy Model

## Special Features

Each theory chapter provides the nurse researcher with a variety of tools. Key features include the following:

- **Definitions of Key Terms** appear at the beginning of each chapter to define concepts and aid the reader's understanding of the theory.
- **Using Middle Range Theories in Research** boxes provide examples of how the theory has been used in published research. These have been updated and reformatted, using an outline based on the research process.
- **Using Middle Range Theories in Practice** boxes provide examples of theories applied to a specific clinical practice situation. They too have been reformatted so that the clinical issue and the use of the theory as a foundation for nursing intervention are clearly identified.
- **Using Middle Range Theories in Projects** boxes provide examples of actual projects completed by students in graduate programs or nurses in clinical practice.
- **Critical Thinking Exercises** at the end of each chapter engage readers in analysis of the theory and its application to practice.

## Teaching and Learning Resources

To facilitate mastery of this text's content, a comprehensive teaching and learning package has been developed to assist faculty and students.

## RESOURCES FOR INSTRUCTORS

Tools to assist you with teaching your course are available upon adoption of this text on thePoint® at https://thePoint.lww.com/Peterson5e.

- An **Image Bank** provides you with digital images of the charts, graphs, and figures in this textbook that can be added to PowerPoint presentations, provided as a standalone resource, or incorporated into other instructional materials.
- **Ebook** access is provided to the instructor so that they are able to refer to the text at any time. The ebook also provides its own functionality of notetaking, highlighting, reading aloud, etc., to facilitate convenience to the instructor.

## RESOURCES FOR STUDENTS

An exciting set of resources is available on thePoint® to help students review material and become even more familiar with vital concepts. Students can access all these resources at https://thePoint.lww.com/Peterson5e using the codes printed in the front of their textbooks.

- **Analysis of Theory Learning Exercises** are provided for each chapter to facilitate students in arriving at their own conclusions about the theory. They are presented with a nurse scholar's evaluation to compare against their own analysis. By analyzing the particular theory with the detail suggested in Chapter 2, students can become more intimately involved with the theory and are more likely to develop an understanding through deeper evaluation of its constructs. This allows students to grapple with the theory and more fully appreciate its application to nursing research while building a solid foundation to support evidence-based practices in nursing.
- **Web Resources** provide links to pertinent Web sites to aid students in their own research.
- **Journal articles**, related to each chapter, help further understanding of concepts and their applications.

# Acknowledgments

There is a sense of accomplishment that accompanies the completion of a project such as this text. We would have never been able to experience that rather pleasant sensation without the significant involvement of many others. The quality of the scholarship of the chapter authors will be evident to all those who read the text. Their willingness to invest themselves in this project, consistently providing what was needed in a timely fashion, is much appreciated. Those who completed the Analysis of Theory, that is available on thePoint®, have added what we believe will be a useful resource to readers, enabling them to clarify their understanding of the theories.

The staff at Wolters Kluwer was invaluable. Christina C. Burns, Senior Acquisitions Editor, and Mark Foss, Acquisitions Editor, who continued to see this book as a contribution to the body of nursing literature. Rebecca "Beck" Rist, Associate Development Editor, expertly coordinated the project. We would also like to thank Blair Jackson and Tim Rinehart, Editorial Coordinators; Kim Cox, Production Manager; Joseph Clark, Design Coordinator; and the myriad other parties who aid in shepherding this project to completion. And finally, we are profoundly grateful for the forbearance of our family and friends (especially husband, Ray Peterson, and wife, Kate Bredow). They helped us have "lives" beyond the scope of completing this book.

# Contents

# Introduction to the Nature of Nursing Knowledge

Sandra J. Peterson

## *Definition of Key Terms*

| | |
|---|---|
| **Concept** | Symbolic representation of a phenomenon or set of phenomena |
| **Conceptual model** | "Set of abstract and general concepts and the propositions" (Fawcett, 1997, pp. 13–14) that represents a phenomenon of interest |
| **Deduction** | Reasoning from the general or universal to the particular or specific |
| **Discipline** | A field or branch of knowledge that involves research |
| **Domain** | Related components or items that reflect the unified subject matter of a discipline |
| **Empiricism** | A philosophical theory of knowledge acquisition through experience, observation, and experiment |
| **Ethics** | A branch of philosophy concerned with moral principles |
| **Epistemology** | A branch of philosophy concerned with the sources of knowledge of truth and the methods used to acquire it |
| **Induction** | Reasoning from the individual or particular to the general or universal |
| **Logic** | A branch of philosophy concerned with sound reasoning and validity of thought |
| **Logical positivism** | Philosophical perspective that espouses logic, objectivity, falseness/truth, observable and operationally defined concepts, and prediction |
| **Metaparadigm** | Global concepts specific to a discipline that are philosophically neutral and stable |
| **Metaphysics** | A branch of philosophy concerned with the study of ultimate cause and underlying nature of that which exists |
| **Metatheory** | A philosophical theory about theories, concerned with "logical and methodological foundations of a discipline" (Beckstrand, 1986, p. 503). Examines "how theory affects and is affected by research and practice within nursing, and philosophy and politics outside nursing" (McKenna, 1997, p. 92). |
| **Ontology** | Examination of the nature of being or reality |
| **Paradigm** | A worldview, a common philosophical orientation, that serves to define the nature of a discipline |
| **Phenomenon** | A designation of an aspect of reality |
| **Philosophy** | (a) A set of beliefs or values; (b) science concerned with the study of reality and the nature of being. Composed of but not limited to aesthetics, epistemology, ethics, logic, and metaphysics |

*(Definition of Key Terms continued on next page)*

## *Definition of Key Terms* (Continued)

| | |
|---|---|
| **Science** | A systematized body of knowledge that has as its main purpose the discovery of "truths about the world" (Jacox, 1974, p. 4), confirmed through empirical investigation |
| **Theory** | "Set of interrelated concepts, based on assumption, woven together through a set of propositional statements" (Fitzpatrick, 1997, p. 37) used to provide a perspective on reality |

Nurses are fundamentally knowledge workers (Porter-O'Grady, 2003). Because "nurses rely on extensive clinical information and highly specialized knowledge to implement and evaluate the processes and outcomes of their clinical decision making" (Snyder-Halpern, Corcoran-Perry, & Narayan, 2001, Nurses as Knowledge Workers, para. 1), this title seems quite appropriate. What then is knowledge? What are its sources? How is the quality of the knowledge determined? How can knowledge be translated into practical applications that improve patient outcomes? Answering these questions serves to advance the discipline of nursing and improve the way it is practiced.

Attempts to answer the question of what constitutes the nature of knowledge have been primarily the domain of the branch of philosophy referred to as epistemology. Traditionally, knowledge has been defined as a belief that was justified as true with absolute certainty. This definition requires that for knowledge to exist, it must be believed; if not believed, something cannot be known. It also must be true; if not true even if well justified and believed, it cannot be considered knowledge. Finally, there must be sound reasons for the belief; if there are no sound reasons for a belief, it would be more a probable opinion or lucky guess than knowledge. There is not universal agreement about the nature of a sound reason or adequate evidence for a belief.

There are multiple epistemological theories to describe the nature of knowledge and explain its sources or how something can be known. Examples of epistemological theories include idealism, pragmatism, rationalism, and relativism. The theory of empiricism, most closely associated with natural science, considers knowledge to be a result of human experience. Ideas and theories can then be tested against reality and accepted or rejected on the basis of how well they are congruent with observable facts. This falls within the domain of research.

Theory, research, and practice are inextricably linked in the ways nursing knowledge is developed and used. "In 2001, the Institute of Medicine challenged all health care professionals to decrease variation in practice through adoption of interventions based on best evidence to improve patients' outcomes" (Flynn Makic, Rauen, Watson, & Will Poteet, 2014, p. 1). Theory and research are sources of the evidence that improve the quality of nursing care, as noted in the 2012 American Association of Critical-Care Nurses Levels of Evidence. In their hierarchy, the synthesis and analysis of multiple research studies were identified as the highest level of experimental evidence; theories were identified at a lower level but directly useful as recommendations (Peterson et al., 2014). The relationship between theory, research, and practice is actually a reciprocal one as illustrated in Figure 1.1. For instance, as noted in the figure, the practice environment is not only where theory and research are used but also a source of research questions and data to answer those questions as well as the source of many nursing theories. Though the relationship among the three is considered reciprocal, theory and research should ultimately serve the needs of practice.

Though most discussions of evidence focus on empirical knowledge, there are other ways to conceptualize the knowledge base needed to practice nursing. Carper (1978) has proposed four distinct patterns that she called ways of knowing: (a) empirics, the science of nursing; (b) aesthetics, the art of nursing; (c) personal knowing, the intra- and interpersonal nature of nursing; and (d) ethics, the moral component of nursing. These patterns expand the notion of what constitutes the knowledge nurses need to practice.

Empirical knowing is positivistic science, which means that it is logically determined and based on observable phenomenon. It is knowledge that is systematically organized into general laws and theories that serve to describe, explain, and/or predict the phenomena of interest to nursing (Carper, 1978). The sources of empirical knowledge are research and theory and model development. Nurse scholars have suggested that what constitutes

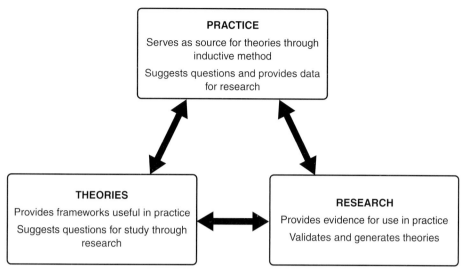

**Figure 1.1**    Reciprocal relationships among theory, research, and practice.

research and model development should include "more individualistic empirical strategies, such as phenomenology" (Porter, 2010, p. 4).

There is no coherent conceptual structure that is generally accepted as nursing's scientific paradigm, which can lead to the possibility of a confusing and sometimes conflicting knowledge base. For the practicing nurse, empirical knowledge must always be interpreted within the context of specific clinical situations.

Aesthetic knowing is a process of "perceiving or grasping the nature of a clinical situation; interpreting this information in order to understand its meaning for those involved, while envisioning desired outcomes in order to respond with appropriate skilled action; and subsequently reflecting on whether the outcomes were effectively achieved" (Johns, 1995, Aesthetics, para. 1).

Aesthetic knowing comes from the nurse's ability to grasp and interpret the meaning of a situation. It makes use of the nurse's intuition and empathy. This type of knowing also involves the nurse's skills in imagining a desired and practical outcome in the actual situation and responding based on an interpretation of the whole situation, analyzing the interrelationships of its various aspects. This phenomenon encompasses the whole knowledge continuum, integrated in a way that results in the "art-act" that is nursing practice (Bender & Elias, 2017, p. 26).

Traditionally aesthetic knowing has been considered a way of knowing that cannot be articulated nor transferred to others. But with an expanded conceptualization of empirics to include qualitative methods of inquiry, this perspective is considered no longer accurate.

Personal knowing is knowledge of the concrete, individual self; it is not knowledge about the self. It involves encountering and actualizing the self in a way that enables the nurse to transcend the notion of other individuals as objects, but instead, the nurse engages with others in authentic personal relationships. The type of knowing and the nature of these relationships result in an increasing willingness to accept ambiguity, vagueness, and discrepancy in oneself and others. Personal knowing is the basis of the therapeutic use of self in the nurse–patient relationship. Reflection is the primary means by which personal knowing occurs. It involves three interrelated factors:

1. The perception of the self's feelings and prejudices within the situation
2. The management of the self's feelings and prejudices in order to respond appropriately (to the other)
3. Managing anxiety and sustaining the self (Johns, 1995, The personal way of knowing, para. 2)

Like aesthetic knowing, personal knowing cannot be described; it can only be actualized. In order to escape the problem of self-delusion, there is a need for individual reflection that is informed by the responses of others. But data about self from others can also be problematic in that it can be misperceived. In addition, personal knowing presents the nurse with a dilemma; personal knowledge needs to be integrated or reconciled with the professional responsibility of the nurse to manipulate the environment in order to work toward a desired health outcome (Carper, 1978, p. 19). Personal knowing, of all the ways of knowing, is the most difficult to teach and to master (White, 2004, p. 253).

Ethical knowing is knowledge of what is right or wrong and the commitment to act on the basis of that knowledge. It involves "judgments of moral value in relation to motives, intentions and traits of character" (Carper, 1978, p. 20) and focuses on obligations, on what ought to be done related to those judgments.

Sources of ethical knowledge include the nursing's ethical codes and professional standards. It is also important for the nurse to have an understanding of different philosophical positions as to what is considered good and what is identified as an obligation. Consideration of the philosophical positions can also create confusion since ethical theories of what is good and what constitutes an obligation can conflict. For instance, the teleological perceptive considers what is good on the basis of its production of the greatest good for the greatest number (consequentialism), whereas the deontological perspective identifies good not by the consequences of actions but by the nature of the actions themselves.

Each of the ways of knowing represents a necessary but incomplete representation of the discipline of nursing. There is also an inherent interrelationship between the four patterns. For instance, aesthetic knowing would require empirical knowledge in order to envision what the desired and practical outcomes in a situation might be and what would constitute valid means of helping to bring about that desired outcome. Although Carper acknowledged that the patterns were interdependent, she has been criticized for failing to integrate the patterns and not specifying exactly how they are related (Risjord, 2010). With an acknowledgment of the contributions of all the ways of knowing to the practice of nursing, this book focuses on empirical knowing in the broadest sense, on nursing theories, especially those that are considered middle range.

Two claims can be made about the state of empirical knowledge in nursing—it exists in varying degrees of abstraction, and it is characterized by a lack of consistency in the use of its language. Fawcett (2005b) refers to a structural "holarchy" of contemporary nursing knowledge to establish the relationships between the various components that constitute nursing's body of knowledge. In her early writings, Fawcett identified four components arranged from most abstract to most concrete in the following order: philosophy/paradigm, conceptual model, and theories. Recently, she added a fifth and most concrete component, empirical indicator, which refers to "a very concrete and specific real world proxy or substitute for a middle-range theory concept; an actual instrument, experimental condition, or procedure that is used

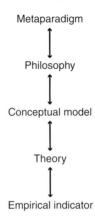

**Figure 1.2** Holarchy of nursing knowledge.

to observe or measure a middle-range theory concept" (p. 36). Figure 1.2 provides a representation of this holarchy.

The types of theories available to nurses also exist on a continuum from most abstract to most concrete, with grand theories identified as most abstract, practice- or situation-specific theories as most concrete, and middle range theories in the logical middle. There are few components in the holarchy or hierarchy that appear consistently in the literature with a single label. The terms conceptual models, conceptual frameworks, and theories are sometimes used interchangeably. The terms grand theory, macro theory, and general theory all refer to the same level of theory development. The literature also provides examples of the terms conceptual model and middle range theory used as equivalent terms.

This chapter addresses each component of the conceptual hierarchy or continuum, with special emphasis on middle range theories. The nature of the component, its development, its contributions to nursing's body of knowledge, and the debates engaged in by nurses in relation to the component are considered.

## Philosophy

In the nursing literature, the term philosophy is used in two ways, as a unique discipline and as a set of beliefs of a separate discipline, for example, nursing. As a discipline, it is often defined by its main branches: metaphysics, epistemology, ethics, logic, and aesthetics. Philosophy is primarily concerned with the nature of being, the meaning and purpose of life, and the theory and limits of knowledge, whereas science is more concerned with causality (Silva, 1997). Philosophy is considered unorganized and noninvestigative, more dependent on common experience, in contrast to science, which is considered investigative and dependent on special experience (Simmons, 1992, pp. 16–17).

For a discipline, philosophies represent its beliefs and values and its mind-set or worldview. They function "to communicate what the members of a discipline believe to be true in relation to the phenomena of interest to that discipline, what they believe about how the knowledge about those phenomena should be developed and what they value with regard to their actions and practices" (Fawcett, 2005a, p. 34). Like other disciplines, nursing has reflected and is reflecting the modern and postmodern, and some would include neomodern thinking or worldview of its time.

## DEVELOPMENT

Philosophies emerge as a reflection on the issues of interest to philosophers, primarily logic, ethics, aesthetics, metaphysics, and epistemology. In the 20th and 21st centuries, these reflections or philosophies have been often characterized as either modern or postmodern perspectives. Although modernism and postmodernism do not represent singular philosophies but, rather, a collection of philosophies (Burbules, n.d., para. 2), each possesses commonly occurring themes that can serve as points of contrast.

The most basic comparison between the schools of thinking is in their perspectives on metanarratives, defined as efforts to offer "general and encompassing accounts of truth, value, and reality" (Burbules, n.d., para. 5). In modernism, the metanarratives are a primary concern. In postmodernism, metanarratives are dismissed. This dismissal is not necessarily rejection or denial but instead doubt and uncertainty about what metanarratives have to offer. These schools of thought also differ in their view of the nature of problems. In modern thinking, problems are to be solved. In postmodern thinking, they are to be deconstructed, requiring a disassembling of the metanarratives that are entangled in values and beliefs that fail to reveal reality or liberate the oppressed (Reed, 1995), Historical Background: Modernism and Postmodernism, para. 3).

Reed (1995) also identifies distinctions in epistemology: modernism, concerned with the truth of findings, and postmodernism, concerned with the usefulness of findings. She also suggests a neomodernism perspective, which rejects modernism's logical positivism and postmodernism's radical relativism and lack of coherent vision to focus instead on a plurality of realistic visions of a possible future (Bisk, n.d.). Reed's neomodern perspective for nursing embraces the metanarratives of health and the processes of healing but integrates them with the postmodern assumptions that knowledge is value laden and that context is critical in order to achieve the desired future.

A schema proposed by Lerner (1986), which considered the nature of human development, is useful in categorizing nursing philosophies. Three worldviews of most interest are

1. Mechanistic, in which the machine is the metaphor for the human being. The whole is equal to the sum of the parts, and the goal is a return to equilibrium.
2. Organistic, in which a biologic organism composed of complex interrelated parts is the basic metaphor. The organism is active in a passive environment. Change is probable, goal directed, and developmental.
3. Developmental–contextual, in which historical events are the metaphor. The individual is immersed in a dynamic context. Change in the person and the environment is ongoing, irreversible, innovative, and developmental. Chaos and conflict are an energy source for change (Reed, 1995).

## USES

Kikuchi (1992) claims that "without an understanding of philosophy in nursing there can be no science of nursing" (p. 45). The branches of philosophy suggest a set of questions with relevance to nursing. For instance, ethical nursing questions would be concerned with what is good to do and to seek to attain nursing's goals (Kikuchi, 1992). Epistemological questions would focus on the structure, scope, and reliability of nursing's knowledge, and ontological questions would relate to the meaning of nurses' and clients' realities (Silva, Sorrell, & Sorrell, 1995). But these important questions are ones that are best addressed through philosophical inquiry. Philosophy makes a significant contribution to nursing's theories, research, and practice as demonstrated in Table 1.1.

The contribution philosophy makes to theory cannot be overestimated. "... All nursing theory or research derives from or leads to philosophy" (Phillips, 1992, p. 49). The conceptual clarification specified by the philosopher of science helps the theorist generate better theories, and the speculation engaged in by the philosopher of science can also suggest the theories of the future (Smart, 1968, p. 17). Analysis of a theory reveals the underlying assumptions and worldview (philosophy). By considering these philosophical

**Table 1.1    Contributions of Philosophy to Nursing**

| | Theory | Research | Practice |
|---|---|---|---|
| Logic | Concepts should be consistent and logically built on each other to form a rational explanation of the phenomenon (internal consistency) | Logic is required in the use of the research process, with a logical progression from problem identification and hypotheses to methods and finally to data analyses and conclusions (Silva, 1997). | Nurses use a problem-solving approach in caring for patients. This is sometimes referred to as the nursing process. |
| Epistemology | The theory should make a unique contribution to nursing's body of knowledge (significance) | The quality of research is judged not only by the nature of the evidence obtained but with the methods used to obtain it. | Nurses base their care on sound evidence of best practices. |
| Metaphysics | The theory's assumptions ought to represent the real world (reality convergence) | Cause and effect is an important consideration in many research studies, for example, random controlled trials. | Nurses have a sound rationale for their actions, knowing not only what to do but why they are doing it. |
| Ethics | The theory should advance an approach that results in a "substantive contribution to the betterment of humankind" (Cody, 1999, p. 13) (Beneficence) | There are ethical considerations in relation to research problems, research methods, and dissemination of research findings. | Nurses in practice promote the autonomy of patients, to promote their welfare (beneficence) and to do them no harm (nonmaleficence). |

statements, nurses can determine the fit between the values and beliefs expressed through the theory and their own. This enables researchers and practitioners to select theories that are philosophically congruent with their own perspectives on nursing. Therefore, philosophy plays a critical role in the formulation of questions important to nursing, the consideration of research methods, and the development of theories and their analysis and use in practice.

## CONTROVERSY

The controversy about nursing philosophy centers on the belief systems that exist within the discipline of nursing and the relative value of unity or diversity in nursing thought. Roach (1992) argues that philosophical inquiry in nursing is the pursuit of universal, transcendent principles and suggests metaphysics as the basis for nursing's unity. Others refer to this search for a coherent philosophical foundation in nursing as a pursuit of unity in diversity of thought (Newman, 2002; Phillips, 1992). A search for the unitary nature of phenomena of concern to nursing has led to the recognition of a number of core beliefs:

- A holistic view of persons (Phillips, 1992; Roach, 1992)
- A commitment to caring as an expression of the human mode of being (Newman, Sime, & Corcoran-Perry, 1996; Roach, 1992)
- A perspective on education that acknowledges the unity of mind–body–spirit and

recognition of the universe of knowledge that is necessary to achieve and makes a contribution to human understanding (Roach, 1992)
- A view of humans in relationship, with awareness of ethical–moral bonds (Roach, 1992)

Though diversity may result in confusion and lack of clarity in nursing's theory development and research agenda, others believe that a philosophy that represents the worldview of all nurse scientists would be diluted to the point of becoming meaningless and useless (Landreneau, 2002). Diversity of philosophies may be viewed as a more accurate representation of reality, a perspective consistent with postmodern thinking, and may have the potential of stimulating greater creativity and variety in the development of nursing models and theories.

## Metaparadigm and Paradigms

The terms metaparadigm and paradigm are frequently found in the nursing literature. A metaparadigm is considered the most abstract set of concepts of the discipline and serves to determine what constitutes its unique domain. Similar to philosophies, paradigms are an abstract means of expressing and organizing a discipline's knowledge. The metaparadigm of a discipline is considered global, philosophically neutral, and fairly stable.

Paradigms are distinguished from a metaparadigm in that they are considered discipline specific, philosophical, and mutable. "Under the umbrella of the metaparadigm, there are supposed to be several paradigms" (Risjord, 2010, p. 100).

## METAPARADIGM

Metaparadigm is defined as the global concepts specific to a discipline and the global propositions that define and relate the concepts (Fawcett, 2000, p. 4). A metaparadigm transcends all specific philosophical or paradigmatic orientations and serves to unify them. There are four requirements for the metaparadigm of any discipline: (a) a domain distinctive from other disciplines, (b) inclusive of all phenomena of interest to the discipline in a parsimonious way, (c) perspective neutral, and (d) international in scope and substance (Fawcett, 1996, p. 94).

The metaparadigm is composed of several domains, often referred to as a typology. These domains are a classification system to identify the constructs or phenomena that are the focus of nursing. Several nursing metaparadigms have been suggested. For instance, Kim (2000) suggested a four-domain typology consisting of client, client–nurse, practice, and environment. The client domain is concerned with only those phenomena that pertain to the client. The client–nurse domain focuses on the phenomena that emerge from nurse–client interactions. The practice domain refers to what nurses do as a professional. The environment domain is composed of physical, social, and symbolic components of the client's external world, both past and present.

The four-domain typology most frequently cited in nursing literature includes man/person, health, society/environment, and nursing (Fawcett, 1978; Yura & Torres, 1975). The metaparadigm described by Fawcett is also composed of four nonrelational and four relational propositions. The nonrelational propositions provide the definitions of the four domains and the relational propositions describe the linkages between the domains. For instance, in nonrelational propositions, person would be defined not only as an individual but also as families, communities, and other groups and nursing would be defined as the discipline and actions taken by nursing on behalf of and with the person in consideration with the outcomes of those actions. In a relational proposition, the concern would be with how the domains interact with each other. For instance, nursing would be concerned with the health of persons, recognizing that they are in continuous interaction with their environments (Fawcett, 2000, pp. 5–6).

### Development

A metaparadigm is not so much constructed as it is identified. This identification process occurs through the analysis of the recurring themes of nursing's theories (Sarter, 1988). This analysis is philosophical in nature and allows for recognition of the "common and coherent philosophical orientation" (p. 52) of the discipline of nursing.

### Uses

Metaparadigms, or in Kim's (1983) words, a typology, are "boundary-maintaining devices" (p. 19) and as such help delineate nursing's frame of reference. The primary purpose then is to provide a means of focusing on that which is inherently nursing and marginalizing that which is not. This enables nurse practitioners, theorists, and researchers to concentrate their energies on the business of nursing. In addition, the metaparadigm is used for the purpose of analysis, a framework for comparing the perspectives of various nursing theorists (Fawcett, 2000; Kim, 1983). For instance, Fitzpatrick and Whall noted that Levine defined health as wholeness, whereas Johnson found health to be a moving state of equilibrium.

### Controversy

By definition, a discipline possesses only one metaparadigm. The controversy involves what that metaparadigm should be. Fawcett (2005a, 2005b) critiqued nine other paradigms using the criteria of distinctiveness, inclusiveness, neutrality, and internationality. The paradigms suggested by Newman; Conway; Kim; Meleis; King; Newman, Sime, and Corcoran-Perry; Malloch, Martinez, Nelson, Predeger, Speakman, Stienbinder, and Tracy; Parse; and Leininger/Watson all failed to meet one or more of the stated criteria. Fawcett's most common criticism was failure of the paradigms to meet the criterion of inclusion. For example, Kim (1983) did not address health; King (1984) eliminated environment and nursing; and Newman and associates (1996) failed to include environment. Obviously, nursing is still in search of a commonly shared metaparadigm, and further philosophical analysis is required to arrive at this metaparadigm.

The metaparadigm proposed by Fawcett has also received criticism. It was faulted for using outdated language (Fawcett, 2003), being oriented to a particular paradigm (Fawcett, 2003), providing a limited perspective of the domains (Malone, 2005), and reflecting a cultural bias (Kao, Reeder, Hsu, & Cheng, 2006). Leininger criticized use of the term person as being too individualistic, and Fawcett now proposes using the term persons (Fawcett, 2003, p. 273).

Malone (2005) found the conceptualization of the domain, environment, to be underdeveloped; she believed greater emphasis is needed on the policy environment. This view was further elaborated by Bender and Feldman (2015). They believe that there is a "lack of conceptual and proportional link between nursing practice and the environment" (p. 107). They argue that the work environment of nurses clearly influences the ways nursing care is delivered. The relational statements therefore need to be expanded to establish this linkage.

The Western orientation of the metaparadigm is also criticized. In light of the fact that nursing is a global enterprise, this criticism seems warranted. Kao et al. (2006) provided definitions of each of the four domains from the perspective of Chinese philosophies. For instance, the concept *person* can be defined in part as a social being engaged in ethical relationships, relationships governed by certain rules (p. 93). Alimohammadi, Taleghani, Mohammadi, and Abarian (2014) provided an Islamic perspective on the definitions of persons, emphasizing the nature of person as a coherent being, unified with the universe. Fawcett (1996) believes that the nursing metaparadigm that she proposed is the final conceptualization for the discipline, though likely to change. "Indeed, it is anticipated that modifications in the metaparadigm concepts and propositions will be offered as the discipline of nursing evolves" (p. 95). Recent nursing literature reveals only limited consideration of the discipline's metaparadigm.

## PARADIGMS

Kuhn introduced the term paradigm and stimulated interest in its use as a method of defining and analyzing the nature of a discipline. He also acknowledged the existence of multiple and conflicting definitions of the term (Kuhn, 1977, p. 294). Kuhn (1996) included the following as the components of paradigms or, as he later referred to them, disciplinary matrices: (a) symbolic generalizations; the laws accepted by a scientific community and the language used to express them; (b) shared commitments to beliefs in particular models; shared beliefs about and commitment to the prevailing theories of the discipline and the motivation and methods used to create and test them; (c) values; shared values that serve to identify what is significant or meaningful to the scientific community; and (d) exemplars; the specific problems to be solved and the methods used to solve them.

Guba (1990) suggested a means of differentiating paradigms. Paradigms can be distinguished by the answers to three questions:

1. *Ontological*: What is the nature of the "knowable"? Or, what is the nature of "reality"?
2. *Epistemological*: What is the nature of the relationship between the knower (the inquirer) and the known (or knowable)?
3. *Methodological*: How should the inquirer go about finding out knowledge (p. 18)?

The components identified by Kuhn and the answers to the questions posed by Guba express the nature of existing paradigms. Before a paradigm is identified, the facts generated by the discipline and the methods used to generate them are disorganized. The discipline is considered to be in a preparadigm stage of development.

### Development

Paradigms emerge when they are recognized as a dominant way of thinking about the discipline by its scientific community. Kuhn (1996) refers to the emergence of a new paradigm as a revolution in which the new paradigm replaces an older one. Shapere (1980) criticized the notion of revolution, noting that scientific advances can be cumulative in that later sciences build on what existed earlier. This is a more evolutionary perspective on paradigm development. Integration has also been proposed as a form of paradigm development. This form of paradigm development describes a pattern in progress that is created "through accommodation, refinement, and collaboration between thoughts, ideas, and individuals" (Meleis, 1997, p. 80). Meleis believes paradigm development in nursing is characterized by this approach.

There are multiple paradigms and systems of classifying the paradigms used to express the worldview of the discipline of nursing. Three commonly cited paradigms are those of Parse (1987), Fawcett (1995), and Newman (1996). Of these three, the most frequently cited in the nursing literature is Parse's. Each focuses on different constructs or domains of nursing's metaparadigm: Parse on the relationship between persons and their environments, Fawcett (2013) on persons (more recently referred to as human beings), and Newman, Sime, and Corcoran-Perry on caring and health. Table 1.2 summarizes these paradigms.

There are a number of similarities in the paradigms proposed by Parse, Newman et al., and Fawcett. The totality, particulate–deterministic, and reaction paradigms share features in common as do the simultaneity, unitary, and simultaneous action paradigms.

| Table 1.2 | Examples of Nursing's Paradigmatic Schemes |
| --- | --- |
| **Author** | **Categorization of Perspectives** |
| Parse (1987) | • *Totality.* Man is a total, summative organism, composed of biopsychosocial–spiritual features. The environment is a source of external and internal stimuli to which man must adapt in order to maintain balance and achieve goals.<br>• *Simultaneity.* Man is a unitary being in continuous and reciprocal interrelationships with the environment. Health is an unfolding phenomenon. |
| Newman et al. (1996) | • *Particulate–deterministic.* Phenomena are specific, reducible, measurable entities. Relationships between and within entities are causal and linear. Change, as a result of prior conditions, can be predicted and controlled.<br>• *Interactive–integrative.* Phenomena include experiences and subjective data. Multiple interrelationships that are contextual and reciprocal exist between phenomena. Change is a function of multiple prior conditions and probabilistic relationships.<br>• *Unitary–transformative.* A phenomenon is a unitary, self-organizing field and is identified through pattern recognition and interaction with the larger whole. Change is unidirectional and unpredictable. |
| Fawcett (1995) | • *Reaction.* Person is viewed as composed of discrete biological, psychological, sociological, and spiritual aspects, who responds in a reactive manner to environmental stimuli. Change occurs when survival is challenged.<br>• *Reciprocal interaction.* Person is holistic, interactive being. Interactions with the environment are reciprocal. Change occurs as a result of multiple factors at varying rates throughout life and can only be estimated, not predicted.<br>• *Simultaneous action.* Person is viewed as a holistic, self-organized field. Person–environment interactions are mutual and rhythmical processes. Change is unpredictable and evolutionary. |

*Note*: These philosophical schemes are also referred to as paradigms.

There are a number of other classifications of paradigms identified in the literature to describe actual or preferred perspectives of nursing. Many seem to be a renaming of or very similar to the conceptualizations of previously identified paradigms, particularly Parse's totality and simultaneity. For instance, Monti and Tingen (1999) suggest empiricism and interpretative; Guiliano, Tyer-Viola, and Lopez (2005) identify received view and perceived view; Weaver and Olson (2006) propose positivism/postpositivism and interpretive; and Pilkington and Mitchell (1999, 2003) refer to natural science and human science.

## Uses

One function of a paradigm is to identify the boundary or limits of the subject matter of concern to a discipline (Kim, 1989). A paradigm also provides a summary of the intellectual and social purposes of the discipline. It provides the "perspective with which essential phenomena of concern are conceptualized" (Kim, 1997, p. 32). A paradigm is considered to represent a worldview, "a coherent and common philosophical orientation" (Sarter, 1988, p. 52).

Therefore, paradigms can provide the frames of reference for the construction of nursing theory and the use of nursing and nonnursing theories in nursing research. "The paradigm determines the way in which scientists make sense of the world.

Therefore, without it, there is nothing about which to construct theories" (Antiognoli-Toland, 1999, p. 39). Multiple theories generally emerge from a single paradigm.

Paradigms also are important to nursing researchers. Researchers need to be assured that what is being studied will contribute to the body of nursing knowledge. Paradigms more specifically suggest the types of research questions that need to be addressed and appropriate methods used to answer the questions (Guiliano et al., 2005). Thus, nursing paradigms function as a means for nurse theorists and researchers to determine the congruence of their work in both focus and methods with the discipline of nursing, as expressed through a particular worldview.

## Controversy

The topic of nursing paradigms is much debated by nurse scholars with differing opinions articulated about which paradigm best serves the discipline's needs in regard to knowledge development. This debate has not always been viewed as particularly constructive. "The paradigm debates have done more to create divisiveness with theoretical nursing than to clearly define our unique mission and facilitate effective communication among nurses" (Thorne et al., 1998, A Unifying Definition, para. 1). The nursing literature reveals four major positions: (a) emergence of a singular dominant paradigm; (b) integration of the most predominant paradigms, that is, totality and simultaneity; (c) the coexistence of multiple paradigms; and (d) avoidance of the issue.

Kikuchi and Simmons (1996) arguing from the perspective of the logic of truth, which holds that "two contradictory positions cannot both be true—one must be true and the other false" (p. 8), seem to support the necessity of a single dominant paradigm for the discipline of nursing. It has been argued that a predominant paradigm demonstrates the legitimacy of the science of a discipline. When Parse (1987) labeled and described the totality and simultaneity paradigms, she acknowledged the existence of a dominant paradigm and suggested the emergence of a new and preferred perspective for nursing. She noted that the simultaneity paradigm was gaining "recognition among scientists" and was "beginning to have an impact on research and practice competitive with the totality paradigm" (p. 135). Her use of the term "competition" initiated a debate over a preferred paradigm for nursing that is ongoing. The case for a single dominant paradigm is articulated by Leddy (2000); citing Kim, she concluded that multiple paradigms, instead of leading to coherence and patterning, actually result in "chaos, fragmentation, and arbitrariness" (p. 229).

Others support the existence of a single dominant paradigm, but one that has not yet been identified. "The dialog is not to determine which [existing] paradigm is, finally, to win out. Rather it is to take us to another level at which all of these paradigms will be replaced by yet another paradigm whose outlines we can see now but dimly, if at all" (Guba, 1990, p. 27). Some nurse scholars have suggested new paradigms. For instance, Georges (2003) recommends a paradigm that claims social justice as the central teleology of the discipline's scholarship, one that is critical of dominant practices, and embraces diversity and the contextual nature of phenomena.

A variation on the position that nursing is best served by a single paradigm is the recommendation made by some nurse scholars that a paradigm integrating both the totality and simultaneity paradigms become the dominant perspective of the discipline. Rawnsley believes that "constructing new paradigms to complement totality and simultaneity is one way of respecting the contributions of colleagues without compromising philosophical integrity" (Rawnsley, 2003, p. 11). Several nurse scholars have suggested this approach, and Winters and Ballou (2004) identified integration as a trend that values not only the traditional scientific worldview but also the phenomenological and philosophical worldviews (p. 535).

Arguing for "a less extreme and more integrated reference point for nursing's theory and practice," Thorne and her coauthors proposed a unifying definition of nursing (Thorne et al., 1998, p. 1257), with human health and illness processes as the core. Nursing practice is facilitating, supporting, and assisting individuals, families, communities, and/or societies to enhance, maintain, and recover health and to reduce and ameliorate the effects of illness. Nursing's relational practice and science are directed toward the explicit outcome of health-related quality of life within the immediate and larger environmental contexts (Thorne et al., 1998, A Unifying Definition, p. 1265).

Rawnsley (2003) conceptualized two paradigms that she believed promoted an inclusive nursing science, the heuristic paradigm and the complementarity paradigm. The focus of the heuristic paradigm is a valuing of the process of discovery and of the complementarity paradigm a valuing of inclusiveness. Roy is also a proponent of an integrative paradigm, which she refers to as unity in diversity (Guiliano et al., 2005, p. 246). She believes in the existence of universal truths and that knowledge generated from multiple perspectives can and should be unified to serve the needs of nursing practice.

Willis, Grace, and Roy (2008) also proposed a unifying paradigm that focuses on facilitating humanization, meaning, choice, quality of life, and healing in living and dying. They based their paradigm on a 2-year inquiry process to identify a central focus for the discipline. They claimed a number of assumptions as a basis for their inquiry. Among the 11 proposed assumptions were that nursing requires a central unifying focus and that this focus will not change over time (p. E29).

Risjord (2010) has entered the discussion by proposing an integrative, unitary paradigm that acknowledges the significance of both science and values in nursing. He suggests "nursing standpoint" derived from the feminist philosophers' "standpoint epistemology" as the perspective that best represents the nature of nursing. Fundamental to this perspective is the notion that nurses are required to understand both the patient's and the physician's perspectives on the health of the patient. Within this paradigm, there is a commitment to develop the knowledge of the nurse who occupies this special social role and to value the patient's autonomy and well-being and the unique nursing role (pp. 71–72).

The third position in this debate is that nursing science is best served by a multiparadigm perspective. As noted by Pilkington and Mitchell (2003), other disciplines exist with multiple and distinctively different paradigms (pp. 107–108), and Barrett (1992) claims uniformity of perspective is neither possible nor desirable (p. 156). Other nurse scholars express similar views. Whitehead (2005) claims "that the *real reality* is that there is not single reality or truth in nursing practice and subsequently no one method [for acquiring knowledge] prevails over the next." Fawcett (2003) also acknowledges the contributions of both the totality and simultaneity paradigms (p. 273). Those who support the multiple paradigm perspective have concluded that the complexity of the knowledge base that nurses need to practice requires paradigmatic plurality. "The existence of multiple paradigms in nursing science indicates a strong and flourishing science… because they encourage creativity, stimulate debate and the exchange of ideas, provide diversity of views, promote productivity, and keep open avenues of inquiry" (Monti & Tingen, 1999, p. 75).

Though not as common as the other positions, some nurse scholars are suggesting that the paradigm debate be suspended. Thorne et al. (1998) claim that "paradigm discourse inhibits rather than fosters productive knowledge development within the discipline (p. 124)," certainly a serious indictment. They identify the dichotomies in perspectives (old versus new) that become the focus of discussions on paradigms as unhelpful in knowledge development. Kikuchi (2003) suggests a rejection of worldviews, that is, paradigms, in favor of a philosophy of moderate realism with its emphasis on probable, not absolute, truths and on a belief that reality exists independent of the human mind.

This approach to nursing knowledge development is viewed as a public enterprise, one in which (a) questions are posed that all scholars can answer, (b) questions are answered in a piecemeal fashion, (c) there is both agreement and disagreement regarding the answers proposed, (d) disagreements are resolved using a accepted standards, and (e) scholarly work is cooperative so that the cumulative knowledge can better answer the questions. This avoidance of the paradigm dilemma may be a trend. Cody and Mitchell (2002) noted that there were decreasing numbers of publications addressing the fundamental philosophical issues of nursing, that is, ontology and epistemology. By definition, paradigms cannot be discussed without consideration of questions of ontology and epistemology.

The paradigm debate remains unresolved. Without the emergence of a single dominant paradigm, nursing is left with multiple paradigms that are either competing or complementary or with the need to develop an integrated paradigm that dialectically combines the perspectives of the multiple paradigms. With this state of paradigm confusion, it would be helpful for nurse theorists to identify the paradigmatic perspective from which the theory is developed and nurse researchers to identify the paradigmatic perspective from which the research questions were posed and the research methods chosen.

## Conceptual Models

Conceptual models are a "set of interrelated concepts that symbolically represent and convey a mental image of a phenomen[on]" (Fawcett & Alligood, 2005, p. 228). Adam (1992) claims that they are the cornerstone of nursing's development (p. 61). Conceptual models are considered less abstract and more explicit and specific than philosophies but more abstract and less explicit and specific than theories. The term conceptual model has been used interchangeably, accompanied by some controversy, with conceptual framework, theoretical framework, conceptual system (King, 1997), philosophy (Adam, 1992), disciplinary matrix, paradigm, theory (Dickhoff & James, 1968; Fitzpatrick & Whall, 2005; Meleis, 1997, 2018), and macro theory (Adam, 1992).

Beginning in the 1960s, conceptual models emerged as nursing attempted to distinguish itself from other disciplines, especially medicine (Kikuchi, 1992; Schlotfeldt, 1992). Since the 1960s, nursing models have been developed, proposed, analyzed, critiqued, and refined. Table 1.3 provides examples of the work of nurse scientists during that time period that have been labeled as conceptual models.

In recent nursing literature, the term conceptual model seems to be occurring with increasing frequency and with a focus on less global and more specific phenomenon. The following are examples of this understanding of conceptual models:

- Older persons seeking nursing care (Boggatz & Dassen, 2011)
- Effective nurse-to-nurse communication (Carrington, 2012)
- Nurse turnover (Battistelli, Portoghese, Galletta, & Pohl, 2013)
- Quality of life for children with cancer (Anthony et al., 2014).
- Deliberative collaboration to support patients (Elwyn et al., 2014)
- Relational nurse continuity using health information technology (Stifter et al., 2015)
- Palliative care nursing (Kirkpatrick, Cantrell, & Smeltzer, 2017)
- Pediatric cardiac intensive care unit parental stress (Lisanti, Golfenshtein, & Medhoff-Cooper, 2017)

| Table 1.3 | Conceptual Models |
|---|---|
| **Model** | **Selected Sources** |
| Johnson's Behavioral System Model | Johnson, D. E. (1959). The nature and science of nursing. *Nursing Outlook, 7*, 291–294.<br>Johnson, D. E. (1990). The behavioral system model for nursing. In M. E. Parker (Ed.), *Nursing theories in practice* (pp. 23–32). New York, NY: National League for Nursing. |
| King's General Systems Framework | King, I. M. (1968). A conceptual frame of reference for nursing. *Nursing Research, 17*, 27–31.<br>King, I. M. (1981). *A theory for nursing: Systems, concepts, process.* New York, NY: Wiley. |
| Neuman's System Model | Neuman, B. (1982). *The Neuman systems model: Application to nursing education and practice.* Norwalk, CT: Appleton-Century-Crofts.<br>Neuman, B. (1995). *The Neuman systems model* (3rd ed.). Norwalk, CT: Appleton & Lange.<br>Neuman, B. (1996). The Neuman systems model in research and practice. *Nursing Science Quarterly, 9*(1), 67–70. |
| Rogers' Science of Human Beings | Rogers, M. E. (1980). Nursing: A science of unitary man. In J. P. Reihl & C. Roy (Eds.), *Conceptual models for nursing practice* (2nd ed., pp. 207–216). New York, NY: Appleton-Century-Crofts.<br>Rogers, M. E. (1994). The science of unitary human beings: Current perspectives. *Nursing Science Quarterly, 7*, 33–35. |
| Roy's Adaptation Model | Roy, C. (1971). Adaptation: A conceptual framework for nursing. *Nursing Outlook, 18*(3), 42–45.<br>Roy, C., & Andrews, H. A. (1999). *The Roy adaptation model: The definitive statement.* Norwalk, CT: Appleton & Lange. |

These models seemed designed more to "… orient research and practice by guiding the selection of problems and making phenomena salient" (Risjord, 2010, p. 173).

## DEVELOPMENT

Conceptual models are typically developed through the three stages of conceptualization: formulation, model formalization, and validation (Young, Taylor, & Renpenning, 2001, p. 11). The process can be empirical or intuitive, deductive or inductive. Empirically, nurse scholars make observations from practice; intuitively, they develop insights. Deductively, they combine ideas from a variety of areas of inquiry, particularly other theories (e.g., general systems), and inductively, they generalize from specific situations or observations (e.g., qualitative research, content/concept analysis). Conceptual nursing models reflect assumptions, beliefs, and values and, according to Adam (1992), are composed of six units, with commonly occurring philosophical perspectives. The following list summarizes the units and philosophical perspectives with examples from Johnson's Behavioral System Model:

1. *Goal of nursing, generally idealistic, pragmatic, and humanistic*; for instance, "fostering effective and efficient behavioral functioning" (Johnson, 1990, p. 24).
2. *Conceptualizations of the client, usually existential and humanistic and almost certainly holistic*; as evidenced by Johnson's eight behavioral subsystems (Grubbs, 1974).
3. *Social role of nurse, often humanistic and idealistic*; for example, nursing is viewed as a service that makes a unique contribution to the health and well-being of individuals—specifically, nurses act to "provide a distinctive service to society" (Grubbs, 1974, p. 160) and "to seek the highest possible level of behavioral functioning [for the patient]" (Grubbs, 1974, p. 161).
4. *Source of difficulty, primarily pragmatic, because it identifies the scope of nursing's responsibility*; for instance, behavioral disequilibrium and unpredictability, indicating a malfunction in the behavioral system (Grubbs, 1974).
5. *Intervention, typically humanistic, idealistic, and pragmatic*; for example, restrict (e.g., set limits on dysfunctional behavior), defend (e.g., use isolation techniques), inhibit (e.g., teach new skills), and facilitate (e.g., provide adequate nutrition) (Grubbs, 1974).
6. *Desired consequences, also typically humanistic, idealistic, and pragmatic*; as evidenced by Johnson's goal of system balance and stability (Grubbs, 1974; Johnson, 1990).

Though Johnson's Behavioral System Model was used as one example of how these components are addressed in a conceptual model, all the conceptual models found in Table 1.4 consider these six components, each from its unique perspective.

## USES

The development of conceptual models is essential to the professional identity of nursing. The conceptual models delineate the goals and scope of nursing and provide frameworks for considering the outcomes of nursing. In general, they can direct

| Table 1.4 | Examples of Grand Theories With Sources of Information |
|---|---|
| **Theory** | **Primary Sources of Information** |
| King's Theory of Goal Attainment | King, I. M. (1981). *A theory of goal attainment: Systems, concepts, process.* New York, NY: Wiley.<br>King, I. M. (1996). The theory of goal attainment in research and practice. *Nursing Science Quarterly, 9,* 61.<br>King, I. M. (1997). King's theory of goal attainment in practice. *Nursing Science Quarterly, 10,* 180–185. |
| Leininger's Theory of Culture Care and Universality | Leininger, M. M. (1978). *Transcultural nursing: Concepts, theories, and practices.* New York, NY: Wiley.<br>Leininger, M. M. (1988). Leininger's theory of nursing: Cultural care diversity and universality. *Nursing Science Quarterly, 1,* 152–160.<br>Leininger, M. M. (1995). *Transcultural nursing: Concepts, theories, research, and practice.* Columbus, OH: McGraw Hill College Custom Series. |
| Newman's Theory of Health as Expanding Consciousness | Newman, M. A. (1990). Newman's theory of health as praxis. *Nursing Science Quarterly, 3,* 37–41.<br>Newman, M. A. (1994). *Health as expanding consciousness* (2nd ed.). Boston, MA: Jones & Bartlett.<br>Newman, M. A. (1997). Evolution of a theory of health as expanding consciousness. *Nursing Science Quarterly, 10,* 22–25. |
| Orem's Self-Care Deficit Theory | Orem, D. E. (1983). *The self-care deficit theory of nursing.* New York, NY: Wiley.<br>Orem, D. E. (1987). *Orem's general theory of nursing.* Philadelphia, PA: Saunders.<br>Orem, D. E. (2000). *Nursing: Concepts of practice* (6th ed.). New York, NY: McGraw Hill. |
| Parse's Theory of Human Becoming | Parse, R. R. (1981). *Man-living-health: A theory of nursing.* New York, NY: Wiley.<br>Parse, R. R. (1987). *Nursing science: Major paradigms, theories, and critiques.* Philadelphia, PA: Saunders.<br>Parse, R. R. (1992). Human becoming: Parse's theory of nursing. *Nursing Science Quarterly, 5,* 35–42.<br>Parse, R. R. (1998). *The human becoming school of thought.* Thousand Oaks, CA: Sage. |

a professional discipline's theory development, practice, education, and research.

Conceptual models can give birth to nursing theories. Because, by definition, conceptual models are considered more abstract and less specific than theories, several can develop from a single conceptual model. For instance, several grand theories were derived from Rogers' conceptual model, the Science of Unitary Human Beings. The Theory of Power as Knowing Participation in Change (Barrett, 1986) is one example of a theory with its origins in Rogers' conceptual model.

The relationship between nursing's conceptual models and practice is a reciprocal one. Conceptual models can provide a structure for nursing practice, and practice experiences can provide evidence of the credibility of the model (Kahn & Fawcett, 1995). Fawcett (2014) argues for their inclusion in quality improvement (QI) projects. "When applied to a QI project, a conceptual model of nursing provides an explicit nursing specific rationale and selection of one or more concepts of the model provided the needed guidance for identification of the specific phenomenon the quality of which is to be improved" (Fawcett, 2014, pp. 336–337). This recommendation would be appropriate for many of the projects that Doctor of Nursing Practice (DNP) students complete during their courses of study.

In practice, the models have most often been used as a framework for implementation of the nursing process (Archibald, 2000, Nursing Models, para. 2) Assessment based on a conceptual model tends to be more comprehensive, focused, and spe-

cific (Hardy, 1986). Historically, because of their level of abstraction, models tended to be less effective in prescribing specific nursing interventions. Instead, the conceptual models suggested general areas of nursing action. The unique focus of each conceptual model also implies criteria for determining when problems have been solved, thus aiding the process of evaluation.

Because recently developed conceptual models are more focused on a specific phenomenon, they could be used prescriptively in practice. For instance, in their model, Benoit and Mion (2012) suggest risk factors for the development of pressure ulcers in critically ill patients, and Giovannetti et al. (2013) in their model identify performance measures for people with multiple chronic conditions.

Conceptual models can also guide research. "Research is nursing research only if it examines phenomena of special interest to nursing, that is, phenomena that are indicated by one or the other of the conceptual models for nursing" (Adam, 1992, p. 59). Since conceptual models of nursing represent foci of scientific inquiry, they can identify questions for research. For instance, in King's General Systems Framework, what factors interfere with goal attainment? (Kameoda & Sugimori, 1993). It is important to note that avenues of questioning suggested by conceptual models are not the same as those of empirical testing, which less abstract theories undergo. Models also serve to guide the review of literature that identifies the state of nursing science on the topic of interest (Fawcett, 2013).

The more recently developed conceptual models are generating specific hypotheses that are tested in research. For instance, research by Gobbens, Van Assen, Luijkx, and Schols (2012) tested the hypothesis that the effects of disease are mediated by frailty. This hypothesis was derived from the integral model of frailty.

## CONTROVERSY

There are some controversies about the use and usefulness of conceptual models. Although conceptual models from the 1960s through 1980s were criticized as being too abstract to be tested or validated (Adam, 1992; Downs, 1982), they can and should be evaluated. Evaluation of conceptual models has revealed some general limitations. They have been criticized for:

- Their level of abstraction, limiting their usefulness
- Rigidity and inflexibility, which inhibit change
- The subjectivity of perspective, which may not be shared by professional colleagues or clients
- The use of a unique language or jargon, requiring specialized education or resulting in confusing communication
- Potential to be used in inappropriate situations and for incorrect purposes (Adam, 1992; Hardy, 1986; Littlejohn, 2002; Tierney, 1998; Young et al., 2001)
- Not necessary for theory development (Rodman, 1980)

Controversy about the use of conceptual models in relation to theory development is complicated by lack of consistency in labeling the work of nurse scientists. Fawcett's (2005a) position is that conceptual models are more abstract and global and less specific than theories. Kramer (1997) identifies conceptual models as a type of theory but claims not all theories are conceptual models. Meleis (1997, 2018) concludes that most of the differences between the two are semantic and noted that the nurse scientists themselves referred to their work using a variety of terms. For instance, Rogers called her conceptualization of nursing a science (Science of Unitary Human Beings); Erickson referred to her work as both a theory and a paradigm (Modeling and Role Modeling: A Theory and Paradigm); and Watson identified her thinking as both philosophy and theory (Watson's Philosophy and Theory of Human Caring). Although there is some confusion about the term and some limitations regarding their use, conceptual models have proved valuable for the advancement of nursing research, the development of theories, and practice applications.

# Theory: General Issues

Similar to conceptual models, theories are composed of concepts and propositions. In a theory, the concepts are traditionally defined more specifically and the propositions are more narrowly focused. Though theory and paradigm are sometime used interchangeably, theories differ from both paradigms and philosophies in that they represent what is rather than what should be (Babbie, 1995, pp. 37, 47). A theoretical body of knowledge is considered an essential characteristic of all professions (Johnson, 1974). Therefore, theories serve to further specify the uniqueness or distinctiveness of a profession. "Theories have in fact distinguished nursing from other caring professions by fixing professional boundaries" (Rutty, 1998, Theory, para. 2). The definition of theory by Kerlinger is classic and comprehensive. "Kerlinger (1973) defines theory as follows: A theory is a set of interrelated constructs (concepts, definitions, and propositions) that present a systematic view of phenomena by specifying relations among variables, with the purpose of explaining and predicting phenomena" (King, 1978, p. 11). In addition to explanation and prediction of phenomena, Glaser and Straus (1967) identify other uses of theory. They believe theories by definition should also be able to further advance theory development; guide practice by providing understanding and the possibility of controlling some situations; offer a perspective on behavior, a means of interpreting data; and provide an approach or style for the research of a specific area of human behavior. Theories should be inherently useful.

In addition to considering the development and uses of nursing theories, it is important to address their classifications. Theories can be classified in a number of ways: by their purposes, sources, and levels. The three major levels of nursing are grand, middle range, and practice, with middle range theory of special interest as it grows in importance in nursing research and practice. As with philosophies, metaparadigms, paradigms, and conceptual models, there are a number of controversies surrounding nursing theories.

## DEVELOPMENT

The development of a theory involves both content and process. Theories are composed of concepts and their relationships and are constructed through a variety of processes. The history of theory development in nursing helps provide a context for understanding the ongoing work of nurse scientists in the advancement of nursing's body of knowledge.

## Components

A variety of terms are used to describe concepts and propositions, the two basic elements of a theory. The terms concept, construct, descriptor, and unit are often used interchangeably, with concept being the most common. Definitions of the concepts can be considered an aspect of the basic element, concept, or as a separate and additional component of a theory. Statements of relationships or propositions refer to the same notion. Also, some scientists include axioms and postulates as other components of a theory. Though they are relational statements, axioms or postulates are considered unique in that they are the assertions assumed to be true that lay the groundwork for the propositions (Babbie, 1995, p. 48).

**Concepts.** Concepts are considered the basic building blocks of theory. Kim (2000, p. 15) defines concepts as "a symbolic statement describing a phenomenon or a class of phenomena." In other words, a concept is a mental representation of a phenomenon, an idea or construct of an object or action (Walker & Avant, 2011, p. 59). Although there are several more complicated classifications of concepts, basically they can be classified on a continuum of abstractness, which some label primitive, abstract, and concrete (Meleis, 1997, 2018) and others global, middle range, and empirical (Moody, 1990). They can also be categorized as property or process concepts (Kim, 2000).

Primitive concepts are those that have a culturally shared meaning (Walker & Avant, 2011, p. 59) or are those that are introduced as new in the theory (Meleis, 1997, p. 252). For instance, in culturally derived concepts, a color is usually primitive because it cannot be defined except by giving examples of another color different from the original color. Grass and apples would be examples of green and sky, and coal would be examples of not green. As an original concept in a new theory, role supplementation in the theory of "Role Insufficiency and Role Supplementation" would be an example of a theory-specific primitive concept (Meleis, 1997, p. 252).

Concrete concepts are those that exist in a spatial–temporal reality. They can be defined in terms of primitive concepts. Grass, *leaves*, apples, sky, and coal would all be examples of concrete concepts. In nursing, touch used by the nurse would be considered a concrete concept. Abstract concepts can be defined by primitive or concrete concepts but are not limited by time or space. "They refer to general cases" (Kim, 2000, p. 16). Communication could be identified as an abstract concept that would be of interest to nursing. Theories can include both concrete and abstract concepts.

For theories using abstract concepts, operational definitions of those concepts are an important inclusion because the definitions enable the theory to be more easily tested empirically through research. An operational definition "assigns[s] explicit meaning to that [abstract] concept" (Duldt & Giffin, 1985, p. 95). Operational definitions can be (a) experimental, providing specific details necessary to manipulate the concept; (b) measurable, describing the means by which the concept can be measured; (c) administrative, including particular information on how to obtain data about the concept; and (d) evaluative, establishing the criteria for operationalizing the concept and the means of determining the degree to which the criteria are met.

The classification of concepts as property or process is significant because it promotes understanding of the concept as defined by the theorist. Property concepts are those that deal with the state of things, and process concepts are those that relate to the way things happen. Stage of grief would be a property concept, whereas grieving as the means by which an individual deals with loss would be a process concept. A concept can be considered both a property and process concept, such as communication. In general, theories contain both types of concepts. "The classification system of concepts into property and process types is useful in an analytic sense" (Kim, 2000, p. 18). It provides a clearer sense of the nature of the concepts included in the theory and thus a better understanding of the theory itself.

**Propositions.** Propositions, defined as statements of the relationships between two or more concepts, provide a theory "with the powers of description, explanation or prediction" (Meleis, 1997, p. 252). Propositional statements can be considered either relational or nonrelational. Relational statements can be either correlational or causal. Nonrelational statements include descriptions of the properties and dimensions of the concept in the definition of the term proposition (Meleis, 1997, 2018).

In propositional statements that are correlational, the assertion is that two or more concepts exist together or are associated. The associations can be positive, negative, or neutral. Orem's Self-Care Deficit Nursing Theory provides examples of positive and neutral correlational statements. The nurse affects the movement from the "'present state of affairs' to 'a desirable future state of affairs' by using the 'nursing means' the nurse selects" (Orem, 2001, p. 151) is an example of a positive correlational statement. "Engagement in self-care or dependent-care is affected by persons' valuation of self care measures with respect to life, development, heath, and well-being" (Orem, 2001, p. 146) is an example of a more neutral or directionless correlational statement.

Causal propositional statements establish cause-and-effect relationships. Examples of causal statements are found in Parse's Man-Living-Health Theory of Nursing. "In a nurse–family process, by synchronizing rhythms, the members uncover the opportunities and limitations created by the decisions made in choosing irreplaceable ways of being together. The choices of new ways of being together mobilize transcendence" (Parse, 1987, p. 170). Causal statements are more difficult to establish than are correlational statements and therefore more rare.

"Nonrelational statements provide assertions of the existence of concepts or definitions of concepts of a theory and thus help explain the nature of the theory" (Parse, 1987, p. 167). An example of a nonrelational existence proposition would be Parse's statement that the practice methodology of her theory is composed of three dimensions: illuminating meaning, synchronizing rhythms, and mobilizing transcendence. Parse also provides nonrelational definitional propositions, for example, "health is Man's unfolding. It is Man's lived experiences, a non linear entity that cannot be qualified by terms as good, bad, more, or less" (Parse, 1987, p. 160).

The nature of the elements of the theory relates to the purposes for which the theory can be used. Theories with only nonrelational propositional statements serve to describe, whereas theories with relational propositional statements have the potential to explain (correlational statements) and predict (causal statements).

### Process

Walker and Avant (2011) describe strategies of theory development that involve analysis, synthesis, and derivation, which can be applied to concepts, statements, and/or theories. Analysis involves examination of the structural and functional components of a concept, relational statement, and/or theory. This process provides a means to clarify, refine, and hone existing theoretical knowledge (p. 64). Synthesis is used to combine pieces of information, often observations from research, for the purpose of identifying or defining a new concept, relational statement, or theory (p. 63). Derivation involves transposing and modifying a concept, relational statement, or theory from one discipline to another, providing a more meaningful context for nursing (p. 63). Walker and Avant (2011) describe in detail these processes in their book, *Strategies for Theory Construction in Nursing.*

Lenz, Suppe, Gift, Pugh, and Milligan (1995) used these processes as they collaborated on the development of the middle range theory of unpleasant symptoms. For instance, the researchers used existing literature for concept analysis, examining attributes, characteristics, and dimensions of the concept of dyspnea. The literature review also served as a basis of concept derivation, resulting in the identification of pain as an analog of dyspnea. And through synthesis of the literature and the researchers' own experiences, they conceptualized dyspnea as having five components: sensation, perception, distress, response, and reporting.

### Sources

The content of a theory comes from other theories, practice, or research or a combination of two or more of these sources. Theories from other disciplines are one source of nursing theory content. Informed by their clinical practices, psychiatric and pediatric nursing, respectively, Peplau made use of psychoanalytic theory and Johnson made use of systems theory. Nursing theories and conceptual models often give rise to middle range theory. For instance, from Orem's Self-Care Deficit Theory came the Theory of Dependent-Care Deficit, Theory of Self-Care, and Theory of Nursing Systems (Alligood & Tomey, 2005, p. 53).

"Some theories are driven by clinical practice situations and are inductively developed" (Meleis, 1997, p. 230). This grounded theory approach uses observations and analysis of similarities and differences of observed phenomena to develop concepts and establish their relationships. Emancipatory nursing praxis, a **theory** of social justice in nursing (Walter, 2017) is an example of a middle range theory that was developed using this approach.

Research is often cited as the most common and acceptable source for theory development, frequently leading to the development of a middle range theory. "Theories evolve from replicated and confirmed research findings" (Meleis, 1997, p. 231, 2018). This is considered an empirical quantitative approach and involves (a) identifying a phenomenon, listing all its characteristics; (b) measuring these characteristics in a variety of settings; (c) analyzing the results to determine if patterns exist; and (d) formalizing these patterns as theoretical statements (Reynolds, 1971, p. 140). Johnson and Rice's (1974) theory of sensory and distress components of pain was developed using this approach.

Qualitative research is often referred to as theory generating, with grounded theory and phenomenology often used by nurse scientists to develop theories. Fagerhaugh's (1974) theory of pain expression and control is an example of theory developed through qualitative research. Metasynthesis is emerging as an approach for developing theory, especially middle range theory (Annells, 2005; Walsh & Downe, 2005). This method addresses the criticism that theory development from qualitative research relies on a small number of homogeneous participants (Estabrooks, Field, & Morse, 1994). Metasynthesis involves aggregation of qualitative data, employing four processes—"comprehending, synthesizing, theorizing, and recontextualizing" (Estabrooks et al., 1994, p. 505)—with greatest emphasis on theorizing and recontextualizing. "Dynamics of Hope in Adults Living with HIV/AIDS: A Substantive Theory," was developed using metasynthesis (Kylma, 2005). McKenna (1997) noted similarities between the quantitative and qualitative approaches: both use inductive methods, and both generally result in the development of middle range theories.

### History

Nursing theory development can trace its roots to the work of Florence Nightingale (Alligood & Tomey, 2005; Dunphy, 2001; Fitzpatrick & Whall, 2005; Meleis, 1997, 2018), with her concern for the relationship between health and environment and the nurse's role in that relationship. Hildegard Peplau is credited with being the first contemporary nurse theorist (McKenna, 1997). Other theorists of the 1950s (1955; Johnson, 1959; McKenna, 1997, p. 95; Orem, 1959) were influenced by Peplau's conceptualization of interpersonal relationships in nursing. Others were influenced by their involvement at Columbia University's Teachers' College and the practical-oriented philosophy of John Dewey, who served on its staff. From Teachers' College in the 1950s, Abdellah, King, Wiedenbach, and Rogers emerged as nurse theorists (Meleis, 1997, 2018). Not all of the work of these nurse scientists would be considered theory by today's definition. The theoretical work that did take place in the 1950s focused on what nurses did, not why or how they did it, and the conceptual frameworks developed at this time were more often used as a basis for the development of curricula than as a guide for practice. The 1950s also saw the introduction of the journal *Nursing Research*, which provided a forum for the development of nursing theories and their testing.

In addition to continuing development of individual nursing theories, the 1960s brought a more national and coordinated approach to theory development. Federal financial support became available in 1962 to nurses pursuing doctoral education; the American Nurses Association stated in 1965 that theory development was a significant goal for the profession; and in 1967, Case Western Reserve University sponsored a national nursing symposium, a third of which was devoted to nursing theory. The theorists associated with this decade include "Abdellah et al. (1960), Orlando (1961), Wiedenbach (1964), Levine (1966), Travelbee (1966), and King (1968)" (McKenna, 1997, pp. 95–96). Theorists, particularly Wiedenbach and Orlando, began to consider not only what nurses did but what effect it had on patients. Debate, stimulated by the metatheorists, focused on the issue of the types of theories that nursing should develop rather than the content of theories.

Although nursing theorists continued to develop and publish their work, Rogers (1970), Paterson (1972), Riehl (1974), Adam (1975), Patterson and Zderad (1976), Leininger (1978), Watson (1979), Newman (1979), McKenna (1997, p. 97), and Roy (2014), the questions posed by metatheorists dominated the decade of the 1970s (Meleis, 1997, 2018). Efforts were made to determine what is meant by theory, to identify the structural components of theories, and to clarify the methods of analysis and critique of theory. The previously developed theories were criticized for a failure to include explicated propositions and for their lack of empirical testing (McKenna, 1997, p. 97). The development and use of nursing theories were advanced by (a) the adoption by the National League for Nursing of an accreditation criterion requiring a theory base to nursing curricula, (b) the formation of two groups (Nursing Theories Conference Group and Nursing Theory Think Tank) that considered application of theory to practice, and (c) the publication of *Advances in Nursing Science*, a journal dedicated to the development of nursing science.

Alligood and Tomey (2005) refer to the 1980s as the Theory Era, even though few new nursing theories emerged. "Only three new nursing theories were published in the 1980s: the work of Parse (1981), Fitzpatrick (1982), Erickson, Tomlin, and Swain (1983), and McKenna (1997, p. 97)." Fawcett's (1984, 1989) explication of a metaparadigm for nursing allowed for the comparative content analysis of theories, and her delineation of the levels of abstraction of nursing knowledge helped nurse scientists and practitioners make the distinctions between grand, middle range, and practice theories. Her work also clarified how nursing grand theory can be derived from nursing conceptual models and how middle range theory can be derived from grand theory. The importance of nursing theory to the profession was well established, and the shift by the end of this decade was away from theory development toward theory use (Alligood & Tomey, 2005, p. 9). There was both an increased interest in the relationship between theory and practice and an increased emphasis on the relationship between theory and research.

The decade of the 1990s was hallmarked by the development of the middle range and practice theories. These theories are less abstract and therefore more directly applicable to practice and more easily tested empirically by research. Interest in nursing theory was evidenced by the publication of *Nursing Science Quarterly*, edited by Parse, focusing on theory development and testing and by the increasing number of European-based nursing theory conferences.

Six trends emerged during the decade of 2001 to 2011 (Im & Chang, 2012). From three data bases, using search criteria to identify articles that included content on nursing theory, Im and Chang reviewed 17,549 abstracts and identified 2,317 relevant articles. From the analysis of these articles, they identified the following trends: (a) *specific focuses*, theory work was more about the specific concepts of existing theories, rather than the development of new ones; (b) *coexistence of theories*, all levels of abstraction and various methods of theory development were included; (c) *linkage of theory to research*, research was used for theory development and theories served as frameworks of research studies; (d) *international collaboration*, theories developed by American theorists were applied to international settings and publications often had American coauthors; (e) *application to practice*, there was an emphasis on development of prescriptive theories to guide practice; and (f) *selective evolution*, further development or refinement of theories primarily focused on only four grand theories, that is, Roy's adaptation, Orem's self-care, Neuman's systems, and Rogers' unitary human beings. These trends suggest an encouraging future for theory development and theory use in research and practice.

There is also the possibility that in the early 21st century, there will be less emphasis on nursing theory. Parse (2016) criticized the recommendations from the Council for the Advancement of Nursing Science's recommendations regarding PhD education in nursing and its emphasis on content and research in omics, that is, biology the molecular level. Science would be then be developed in areas such as genomics, ergonomics, and metabolomics (Conley et al., 2015). These areas of scientific interest are not nursing science and would not advance the discipline's unique body of knowledge (Parse, 2016).

## USES

Nurse scientists have worked on the development of nursing theory as part of the process of establishing nursing as a profession with a unique body of knowledge. Nursing theories provide nurses with the language of nursing, a means of communicating the nature of the discipline within and outside the profession. In addition, as a component of nursing knowledge considered less abstract than conceptual frameworks, nursing theories generate more specific research questions and provide greater guidance to nursing practice.

Nursing theories provide nursing-specific identifications, definitions, and interrelationships of concepts. This allows the profession to distinguish itself from the medical and behavioral sciences. For example, in nursing, we speak of unitary human beings, self-care, and the centrality of caring. Through analysis of theories, nursing's metaparadigm emerges, providing us with a common and basic frame of reference for communicating about nursing.

The relationship between nursing theory and research is symbiotic. Research provides for both theory generating and theory testing. Qualitative research seeks to identify and define phenomena of interest to nursing, thus serving as a theory-generating tool. By contrast, quantitative research is a means by which the propositions of theories can be substantiated, thus functioning as a theory-testing tool. Theories then serve as a framework for relating the data generated by research, resulting in a more coherent nursing body of knowledge than a collection of isolated facts.

In addition, the greater clarification of concepts and their relationships that nursing theories provide allows researchers to formulate more specific and nursing-relevant research questions. The evidence that is generated through the study of these questions, because of the level of specificity and relevance, in turn is more directly applicable to nursing practice. Parse (1999) challenges nurses "to conduct research to ensure that the practice of nursing serves people in a unique way" (Recommendations, para. 1). It is through nursing theories that the profession identifies its unique service to people. The testing of nursing theories also leads to theory-guided evidence-based practice. "Evidence itself refers to evidence about theories. Similarly, theory determines what counts as evidence" (Fawcett, Watson, Neuman, Walker, & Fitzpatrick, 2001). Thus, theory as it guides research has the potential to provide the evidence that makes nursing practice more efficient and more effective.

The relationship between practice and theory is reciprocal though not always acknowledged as so. In fact, the term theory–practice gap is a reflection of a number of factors that influence this phenomenon: (a) the belief that theory is not necessary for practice, (b) nurse educators' failure to prepare new graduates to practice from a theory base, (c) the busyness of nurses in practice that does not allow time for nurses to reflect on what they are doing from a theoretical perspective, (d) and nurse leaders' and administrators' lack of vision and support for theory-based practice, provided by nurse leaders and administrators. Others claim that the gap is not exactly a reality and that "nurses perhaps unknowingly apply nursing theory in their daily practice" (Jacobson, 2017, p. 1).

The use of theory is what ideally provides "the basis for understanding nursing reality in practice" (El Hussein & Osuji, 2017, p. 21) and is seen as empowering (Jacobson, 2017):

> The value of theory development and use within the discipline of nursing cannot be over emphasized. This is because when nurses deliberately use theories to inform their practices, "they can facilitate processes that significantly benefit patients, nurses, the health care system, and the broader environment" (El Hussein & Osuji, 2017, p. 22).

Practice is a fundamental source for theory building. For instance, grounded theory research, involving field studies, is used to "discover theoretical explanations about a particular phenomenon" (Peter, 2017, p. 102). The theory of caregiver attentiveness in hospital care (Klaver & Baart, 2016) is an example of a theory generated by this approach. Phenomenological research, which focuses on the lived experience of individuals, also serves as an approach to theory development. A theory of ethical caring, knowing–doing–valuing as systems of cocreations (Renosa, 2016), was developed from phenomenological research that used semistructured interviews, field notes, and the aesthetic expressions of the participants. The goal was to determine the characteristics of a culture of caring, particularly for nursing researchers.

## CLASSIFICATIONS

Theories differ in their purposes, sources, and, most importantly, levels of abstraction and scope. These differences lead to classifications. The basic purposes of theory are description, explanation, prediction, and/or control. The sources of theory in nursing include those developed by nurse scientists (unique) and those that are used in nursing but come from other disciplines (borrowed). The terms "theory of nursing" and "theory in nursing" are often used to distinguish between these two sources, respectively.

### Abstraction and Scope

There are multiple terms used to classify the various levels or scope of nursing theories. The broad-scope theories are referred to as "macro," "holistic," "molar," "general," "situation," and, most commonly, "grand." Narrow-scope theories are called "middle range," "circumscribed," or "situation/factor." Theories narrowest in scope are labeled "micro," "molecular," "atomistic," "narrow range," "phenomena," "prescriptive," "factor," "situation specific," or "practice" (Babbie, 1995; George, 1995; Parker, 2006; Rinehart, 1978). The most common labels for the levels of nursing theory are grand, middle range, and micro, practice, or most recently situation specific. The level is determined primarily by the theory's degree of abstraction. Examination of the level of abstraction of the "purpose, concept, and definitional components of the theory" (Kramer, 1997, p. 65) allows for the identification of the level of the theory.

### Purposes

Though theories are designed to describe, explain, predict, and/or control, some nurse scientists claim that only theories that enable nurses to control outcomes are legitimate for a practice discipline (Dickhoff & James, 1968). Descriptive theories are limited to naming and classifying characteristics of the phenomenon of interest, which identify what is happening. Peplau's Theory of Interpersonal Relationships has been labeled a descriptive theory.

Explanatory theories expand the knowledge base by delineating the relationships between characteristics of the phenomenon, clarifying why it is happening. Watson's Theory of Human Caring is considered an explanatory theory. But predictive theories provide the conditions that can result in a preferred outcome, determining how it can intentionally happen. Orlando's Theory of the Deliberative Nursing Process is an example of a predictive theory. Theories whose purpose is to control, often referred to as prescriptive theories, guide action to create an intended result. The three ingredients for this type of theory are content of goal, primary prescription for activity to achieve goal, and list of additional recommendations of activity (Dickhoff & James, 1968, p. 201).

The existence of descriptive and explanatory theories is a necessary precursor to the development of predictive and prescriptive theories. "Predictive theory presupposes the prior existence of more elementary types of theories" (Dickhoff & James, 1968, p. 200). The relationship between the purposes of a theory has been conceptualized in some instances as a hierarchy:

1. Factor-isolating theories (descriptive)
2. Factor-relating theories (descriptive/ explanatory)
3. Situation-relating theories (explanatory/ predictive)
4. Situation-producing theories (prescriptive) (Dickhoff & James, 1968, pp. 200–201)

## Sources

The source of theory refers to the discipline from which it developed. The possibilities include theories unique to nursing, theories borrowed from other disciplines, and theories from other disciplines adapted for nursing. A borrowed theory is one in which the knowledge "is developed in the main by other disciplines and is drawn upon by nursing" (Johnson, 1986, p. 118). The distinctions between these three sources are difficult to make since "the man-made, more-or less arbitrary divisions between the sciences are neither firm nor constant" (Johnson, 1986, p. 117).

Given that the differences between the sources of theory may be less than perfectly precise, unique theory can be defined "as that knowledge derived from the observation of phenomena and the asking of questions unlike those which characterized other disciplines" (Johnson, 1986, p. 118). Many argue that nursing's identity as a profession and, ultimately, its ability to improve nursing practice are dependent on the existence of nursing theories unique to the discipline. According to Cody (1999), borrowed theories "do not contribute to the distinct core knowledge of nursing science, nor can practice guided by these theories be distinguished as uniquely nursing practice" (p. 12). Wald and Leonard (1964), who are also proponents of this position, claimed that to become an independent discipline, nursing is required to develop its own theories rather than borrow theories or apply principles from other disciplines. They expressed concern about nursing's reliance on these borrowed theories.

As recently as 2001, the literature reveals an ongoing reliance on theories from fields other than nursing. Fawcett and Bourbonniere (2001) found that of 90 research studies published in two clinical journals, *Geriatric Nursing* and *Nurse Practitioner*, and two research journals, *Nursing Research* and *Research in Nursing and Health*, only 9 (10%) used nursing conceptual models or theories (p. 314). The borrowed theories or models used in these studies came from psychology, sociology, medicine, dentistry, physiology, biology, education, decision sciences, economics, ethics, epidemiology, management sciences, marketing, and communications.

A survey of 46 studies published by *Nursing Research* in 2017 revealed only 14 (<31%) with an identified theory or model. Though the nature of many of the research questions or hypotheses did not obviously lend themselves to a nursing theory or conceptual model, only four of the studies provided a theoretical nursing framework for their research. Borrowed theories remain the norm for the research published in this nursing research journal. In past decades, the practice of borrowing theories seemed to be the result of a belief in the superiority of theories "imported" from other disciplines (Meleis, 1997, 2018). This perspective was reinforced by nurses whose advanced degrees were in fields other than nursing. Theories from sociology, psychology, education, ecology, physiology, and others were and still are borrowed. The argument for borrowed theories seems to be that theorists and practitioners should not place boundaries on any knowledge that might be useful to nursing because "knowledge does not innately 'belong' to any field of science" (Johnson, 1986, p. 117). "… borrowing theories presents no threat to the discipline of nursing. A theory is appropriately used by nurse scholars insofar as it helps solve nursing problems" (Risjord, 2010, p. 39) and identifies an appropriate linkage between nursing and the other discipline.

Borrowing theories from other disciplines is sometimes referred to as theory adoption and involves the unchanged use of a theory developed from a field other than nursing. The use of unmodified theories from physiology, for instance, acid–base balance, is an example of a completely borrowed theory. Though the need for adopted borrowed theories does exist, there is concern about their prevalence. The preferred approach for the use of borrowed theories seems to be to adapt them to a distinctively nursing perspective.

As noted previously, nurses adapt borrowed theories. Adaptation refers to altering the content or structure of a theory that was initially developed for application to a discipline other than nursing. Borrowing and altering theory is seen as necessary "to acquire a means of explanation and prediction about some phenomena that is currently poorly understood, or for which there is no present means to study it, or for which there is no theory at all" (Walker & Avant, 1995, p. 172). The debate about the value of borrowed theories continues. Fawcett and Bourbonniere (2001) identify premises necessary for a healthy future for the nursing profession. They claim that "the discipline of nursing can survive only if we celebrate our own heritage and utilize nursing knowledge" (p. 311). This premise and the future it suggests are challenged by the ongoing dependence of nurses on perspectives of nursing that are grounded in the knowledge of other disciplines. The solution they suggest is to end nursing's "romance" with borrowed theories. Few would argue that nursing needs to attend to the ongoing development of its unique body of knowledge, perhaps not for the sole purpose of divorcing itself from other disciplines but for creating a body of knowledge that could be shared across disciplines. Thus, nursing theory could be borrowed.

## CONTROVERSY

There are recurring themes in the criticisms of nursing theories: the issue of consistency in labeling, the appropriateness of the sources of the theories used by nurses, the creation of a theoretical hierarchy, and the often cited theory–practice gap. The lack of definitional clarity between what is labeled a conceptual model and what is considered a theory is further complicated by confusion over identification of the level of the theory, that is, grand, middle range, or practice/situation specific. Nurse scientists have not consistently classified the level of the developed theory in the work they publish. This issue is further addressed in the discussion of the middle-range level of theory development. In addition, there is some disagreement over the appropriate source of theories to be used by nurses, borrowed or unique. As noted in the section on classification of theories by source, the debate focuses onto what degree nurses can use theories from other disciplines and still advance nursing's unique body of knowledge. Risjord (2010) is the primary critic of the notion of a hierarchy of levels of nursing knowledge. He claims that

> … the idea that theory must fit within a hierarchy of levels distorts the way in which theories work together to provide scientific understanding. Much scientific progress has been achieved when theories from different domains are integrated. (p. 116)

The response to that criticism is that different levels of abstraction can exist within a discipline without assuming a particular process of development. What is considered the most significant issue is a perceived and persistent "schism between efforts to create a discipline [the work of nurse theorists]… and the pragmatics of work and workforce" (Litchfield & Jónsdóttir, 2008, p. 81). The debate is whether nursing's theories are relevant or irrelevant to practice (Risjord).

## Grand Theory

Grand theories, as the most abstract of the three identified levels, attempt "to create a view of the whole of nursing" (Liehr & Smith, 1999, Juxtaposition with Grand Nursing theory, para. 1). They address the nature, mission, and goals of nursing care (Meleis, 1997, 2018) in a general fashion and are created through the observations and/or insights of the theorist. The development of grand theories served to differentiate the discipline of nursing from the medical model, stimulated the expansion of nursing knowledge (McKenna, 1997),

and provided a general "structure for the organization of nursing knowledge" (Orem, 2001, p. 139). Orem also claimed that the unstructured nature of grand or general theories allows for a wide range of knowledge available to practitioners and scholars within a nursing-specific frame of reference. McKenna (1997) outlined the benefits of grand theories to include (a) a guide for practice as an alternative to practicing solely by tradition or intuition, (b) a framework for education by suggesting a focus and a structure for curricula, and (c) an aid to the professionalization of nursing by providing a basis of practice.

More than 50 grand theories have been identified (McKenna, 1997, p. 93), although that number may vary based on the label assigned to the work. Because of their level of abstraction, there has been some difficulty in distinguishing between grand theories, philosophies, and conceptual models. Examples of nursing theories that have been designated as grand include Leininger's Theory of Culture Care Diversity and Universality, Newman's Theory of Health as Expanding Consciousness, and Parse's Theory of Human Becoming (Fawcett, 2005a; Fawcett & Bourbonniere, 2001; Parker, 2006). Parker (2006) also identifies Orem's Self-Care Deficit, Rogers' Science of Human Beings, and Roy's Adaptation Model as theories, whereas Fawcett (2005a) and Alligood and Tomey (2005) label these nursing scientists' work as conceptual models. Orem (2001) refers to her work as a general theory. Table 1.4 provides sources of information about specific grand theories.

The level of abstraction makes it difficult to test grand theories empirically. In fact, Donnelly (2001), citing the work of Lundh, Soder, and Waerness (1988), claimed that because the theories were abstract and normative "rather than facilitating research development [they] actually made research development in nursing 'more difficult'" (p. 337). This conclusion is supported in part by the findings of Moody et al. (1988) that in nursing practice research published from 1977 to 1986, fewer than 13% of the 720 studies identified were linked to one of the grand theories.

Grand theories seem better able to serve as a basis for the development of the more specific theories of the middle and practice/situation-specific range, which can undergo empirical testing. For instance, the middle range theory, "A Theory of Sentient Evolution," was derived from Rogers' Science of Unitary Human Beings (Parker, 1989). In addition, grand theories have fulfilled the important functions of distinguishing nursing from other helping professions and providing legitimization to its science. But because of their success in fulfilling these functions, grand theories have become less necessary and the focus of theory development has changed to the middle range theories (Suppe, 1996a).

## Middle Range Theory

Compared to grand theories, middle range theories are less abstract. Merton (1968), whose work served to promote the development of middle range theories, described them as lying between "the minor but necessary working hypotheses that evolve in abundance during day to day research and the all-inclusive systematic efforts to develop a unified theory…" (p. 39). Consistent with Merton's conceptualization, nurse authors have described middle range theories in comparison to grand theories as

- Narrower in scope (Fawcett, 2005a; Liehr & Smith, 1999; McKenna, 1997; Meleis, 1997, 2018; Parker, 2006; Walker & Avant, 1995)
- Concerned with less abstract, more specific phenomena (Fawcett, 2005a; Meleis, 1997, 2018)
- Composed of fewer concepts and propositions (Fawcett, 2005a; McKenna, 1997; Walker & Avant, 1995)
- Representative of a limited or partial view of nursing reality (Jacox, 1974; Liehr & Smith, 1999; Young et al., 2001)
- More appropriate for empirical testing (Liehr & Smith, 1999; McKenna, 1997; Meleis, 1997, 2018; Parker, 2006; Walker & Avant, 1995)
- More applicable directly to practice for explanation and implementation (McKenna, 1997; Walker & Avant, 1995; Young et al., 2001)

The attributes of middle range theories make them attractive to nurses who wish to engage in theory-based research and practice.

The appeal of these theories to nurse researchers and practitioners is demonstrated by their proliferation. In the 1980s, theory development in the middle range became of greater interest to nurse scientists with proliferation of these theories in the subsequent years (Lenz, 1996). Table 1.5 provides a partial listing of theories used by nurses in research and/or practice that have been considered to be middle range. Included in the table are middle range theories in various stages of development and testing classified by their primary focus. Most theorists identify their theory by a patient problem (e.g., acute pain and chronic stress), but some identify by the action or characteristic of the nurse (e.g., empathy and humor) or the desired outcome

of an action (e.g., hope and maternal role attainment). Typically, a middle range theory would not identify a specific population or disease experience (Liehr & Smith, 2017).

## DEVELOPMENT OF MIDDLE RANGE THEORY

Liehr and Smith (1999) outlined the relationships between the intellectual processes and the sources of content related to the development of middle range theories, which included

- Inductive theory, building theory through research
- Deductive theory, building from grand nursing theories
- Combining existing nursing and nonnursing theories
- Synthesizing theories from published research findings
- Developing theories from clinical practice guidelines (Approaches for Generating Middle Range Theory, para. 1).

In developing a middle range theory for nursing, the data that are used for theory building would obviously come from the practice setting.

Qualitative research, particularly phenomenological and grounded theory studies, has served as a source of middle range theory development. Ten qualitative studies conducted through the Nursing Consortium for Research on Chronic Sorrow provided a foundation for the development of the middle range theory of chronic sorrow (Eakes, Burke, & Hainsworth, 1998). The research findings of these and of other studies underwent concept analysis as part of the process of developing this theory. A major source of middle range theory development is the qualitative research produced by nursing's PhD students and presented in their doctoral dissertations.

Several conceptual models and grand theories have served as the foundation for the development of middle range theories. Seiloff and Frey's (2007) book, *Middle Range Theory Development Using King's Conceptual System*, describes King's conceptual system and theory of goal attainment as a source for middle range theory development. A number of other grand theories have provided a foundation for further theory development.

One of the more ambitious projects involved the use of RAM (Roy, 2014). The Roy Adaptation Association Executive Board developed what they described as an alternative process for developing middle range theories for practice, one that involved analysis of 126 quantitative studies and 40 qualitative studies, which were organized around major propositional statements of the RAM. From

**Table 1.5    Examples of Middle Range Theories**

| Theory | Reference |
|---|---|
| **Physiologic** | |
| Acute pain | Good, M. A. (1998). A middle range theory of acute pain management: Use in research. *Nursing Outlook, 46*, 120–124. |
| Chronotherapeutic intervention for postsurgical pain | Auvil-Novak, S. E. (1997). A mid-range theory of chronotherapeutic intervention of postsurgical pain. *Nursing Research, 46*, 66–71. |
| Dyspnea | Gift, A. G. (1992). Dyspnea. *Northern Clinics of North America, 25*, 955–965. |
| Perimenopausal process | Quinn, A. A. (1991). A theoretical model of the perimenopausal process. *Journal of Nurse-Midwifery, 36*(1), 25–29. |
| Pressure ulcers and other dependent-related lesions | Garcia-Fernandez, F. P., Agreda, J. J., Verdú, J., & Pancorbo-Hidlago, P. L. (2014). A new theoretical model for the development of pressures ulcers and other dependent-related lesions. *Journal of Nursing Scholarship, 46*(1), 28–38. doi: 10.3928/00989134-20161109-07 |
| Sensing presence and sensing space | Orticio, L. P. (2007). Sensing presence and sensing space: A middle range theory of nursing. *Insight: The Journal of American Society of Ophthalmic Registered Nurses, 32*(4), 7–11. |
| Symptom self-management | Hoffman, A. J. (2013). Enhancing self-efficacy for optimized outcomes through the theory of self-management. *Cancer Nursing, 36*(1), 16–26. doi: 10.1097/NCC.0b013e31824a730a |
| Weight management | Pickett, S., Peters, R. M., & Jarosz, P. A. (2014). Toward a middle–range theory of weight management. *Nursing Science Quarterly, 27*(3), 242–247. doi: 10.1177/0894318414534486 |
| **Cognitive** | |
| Cognitive authority | Hunt, K. J., & May, C. R. (2017). Managing expectations: Cognitive authority and experience control in complex healthcare processes. *BMC Health Services Research, 17*, 1–13. doi: 10.1186/s12913-017-2366-1 |
| Facilitated sensemaking | Davidson, J. E. (2010). Facilitated sensemaking a strategy and new middle range theory to support families of intensive care unit patients. *Critical Care Nurse, 30*(6), 28–39. |
| Health belief[a] | Champion, V. L. (1985). Use of the health belief model in determining frequency of breast self-examination. *Research in Nursing & Health, 8*, 373–379. |
| Nursing intellectual capital | Covell, C. L. (2008). The middle range theory of nursing intellectual capital. *Journal of Advanced Nursing, 63*, 94–103. |
| Planned behavior | Ajzen I. (1991). The theory of planned behavior. *Organizational Behavior and Human Decision Processes, 50*, 179–211. |
| Risk perception | Siaki, L. A., Loescher, L. J., & Trego, L. L. (2013). Synthesis strategy: Building a culturally sensitive mid-range theory of risk perception using literary, quantitative, and qualitative methods. *Journal of Advanced Nursing, 69*(3), 726–737. |
| Self-care of chronic illness | Riegel, B., Jaarsma, T., & Strömberg, A. (2012). A middle-range theory of self-care of chronic illness. *Advances in Nursing Science, 35*(3), 194–204. |
| Social learning theory[a] | Bandura, A. (1986). *Social foundations of thought and action: A social cognitive theory*. Englewood Cliffs, NJ: Prentice-Hall. |
| Story theory | Smith, M. J., & Liehr, P. (2005). Story theory: Advancing nursing practice scholarship. *Holistic Nursing Practice, 19*(6), 272–276. |
| **Emotional** | |
| Adaptive spirituality | Dobratz, M. C. (2016). Building a middle-range theory of adaptive spirituality. *Nursing Science Quarterly, 29*(2), 146–153, 146–153. doi: 10.1177/0894318416630090 |
| Awaiting diagnosis | Morse, J. M., Pooler, C., Vann-Ward, T., Maddox, L. J., Olausson, J. M., Roche-Dean, M.,…, Martz, K. (2014). Awaiting diagnosis of breast cancer: Strategies for enduring and preserving self. *Oncology Nursing Forum, 41*(4), 350–359. doi: 10.1188/14/ONF.350-359 |
| Caregiver stress | Tsai, P. (2003). A middle range theory of caregiver stress. *Nursing Science Quarterly, 16*(2), 137–145. doi: 10.1177/0894318403251789 |
| Carrying on | Knobf, M. T. (2013). Being prepared: Essential to self-care and quality of life for the person with cancer. *Clinical Journal of Oncology Nursing, 17*(3), 255–260. doi: 10.1188/13.CJON.255-261 |
| Chronic stress | Peters, R. M. (2006). The relationship of racism, chronic stress emotions, and blood pressure. *Journal of Nursing Scholarship, 38*, 234–240. |

*(Continued)*

**Table 1.5   Examples of Middle Range Theories** (Continued)

| Theory | Reference |
| --- | --- |
| **Emotional (*Continued*)** | |
| Empathy | Olson, J., & Hanchett, E. (1997). Nurse-expressed empathy, patient outcomes, and development of a middle range theory. *Image: Journal of Nursing Scholarship, 29*, 71–76. |
| Fulfillment | Kylma, J., & Vehvilainen-Julkunen, K. (1995). Hope in nursing research: A meta-analysis of the ontological and epistemological foundations of research on hope. *Journal of Advanced Nursing, 25*(2), 364–371. |
| Grief | Chapman, K. J., & Pepler, C. (1998). Coping, hope and anticipatory grief in family members with palliative home care. *Cancer Nursing, 21*(4), 226–234. |
| Hope | Morse, J. M., & Doberneck, B. (1995). Delineating the concept of hope. *Image: Journal of Nursing Scholarship, 27*(4), 277–285. |
| Postpartum depression | Beck, C. T. (1993). The lived experience of postpartum depression: A substantive theory of postpartum depression. *Nursing Research, 42*, 42–48. |
| Successful aging | McCarthy, V. L. (2011). A new look at successful aging: Exploring a mid-range nursing theory among older adults in a low-income retirement community. *Journal of Theory Construction & Testing, 15*(1), 17–23. |
| Uncertainty in illness | Mishel, M. H. (1991). Reconceptualization of the uncertainty in illness theory. *Image: Journal of Nursing Scholarship, 2*, 256–261. |
| **Social** | |
| Bureaucratic caring | Ray, M. (1989). The theory of bureaucratic caring for nursing practice in the organizational culture. *Nursing Administration Quarterly, 13*(2), 31–42. |
| Caregiver attentiveness | Klaver, K., & Baart, A. (2016). Managing socio-institutional enclosure: A grounded theory of caregivers' attentiveness in hospital care. *European Journal of Oncology Nursing, 22*, 95–102. doi: 10.1016/j.ejon.2016.04.002 |
| Caring through relation and dialogue | Sanford, R. C. (2000). Caring through relation and dialogue: A nursing perspective for patient education. *Advances in Nursing Science, 22*(3), 1–15. |
| Coercion in the development of behavior[a] | Patterson, G. R. (1982). *Coercive family process.* Eugene, OR: Castalia. |
| Cultural marginality | Southwick, M., & Polaschek, N. (2014). Reconstructing marginality: A new model of cultural diversity in nursing. *Journal of Nursing Education, 53*(5), 249–255. doi: 10.3928/01484834-20140415-01 |
| Department (group power) | Sieloff, C. L., & Dunn, K. (2008). Factor validation of an instrument measuring group power. *Journal of Nursing Measurement, 16*(2), 113–124. |
| Entry into nursing home as a status passage | Chenitz, W. C. (1983). Entry into a nursing home as status passage: A theory to guide nursing practice. *Geriatric Nursing, 4*, 92–97. |
| Family vigilance | Carr, J. M. (2014). A middle range theory of family vigilance. *Medsurg Nursing: Official Journal of the Academy of Medical-Surgical Nurses, 23*(4), 251–255. |
| Home care | Smith, C. E., Pace, K., Kochinda, C., Kleinbeck, S., Koehler, J., & Popkess-Vawter, S. (2002). Caregiver effectiveness model evolution to a midrange theory of home care: A process for critique and replication. *Advances in Nursing Science, 25*(1), 50–64. |
| Humor | McCreaddie, M., & Wiggins, S. (2009). Reconciling the good patient personal with problematic and non-problematic humor: A grounded theory. *International Journal of Nursing Studies, 46*, 1079–1091. |
| Maternal role attainment | Mercer, R. T. (1986). *First time motherhood: Experiences from teens to forties.* New York, NY: Springer. |
| Motivation–facilitation | Phillippi, J. C., & Roman, M. W. (2013). The motivation-facilitation theory of prenatal care access. *Journal of Midwifery & Women's Health, 58*(5), 509–515. doi: 10.1111/jmwh.12041 |
| Negotiating partnerships | Powell-Cope, G. M. (1994). Family caregivers of people with AIDS: Negotiating partnerships with professional health care providers. *Nursing Research, 43*, 324–330. |
| Nonviolent social transformation | Perry, D. J. (2015). Transcendent pluralism: A middle-range theory of nonviolent social transformation through human and ecological dignity. *Advances in Nursing Science, 38*(4), 317–329. doi: 10.1097/ANS.000000000000086 |
| Nursing presence | McMahon, M. A., & Christopher, K. A. (2011). Toward a mid-range theory of nursing presence. *Nursing Forum, 46*(2), 71–82. |

**Table 1.5    Examples of Middle Range Theories** (Continued)

| Theory | Reference |
| --- | --- |
| **Social** (*Continued*) | |
| Nursing services delivery | Meyer, R. M., & O'Brien-Pallas, L. L. (2010). Nursing services delivery theory: An open system approach. *Journal of Advanced Nursing, 66*(12), 2828–2838. |
| Patient advocacy | Bu, X., & Jezewski M. A. (2007). Developing a mid-range theory of patient advocacy through concept analysis. *Journal of Advanced Nursing, 57*(1), 101–110. |
| Quality of family caregiving | Phillips, L. R., & Rempusheski, V. F. (1986). Caring for the frail elderly at home: Toward a theoretical explanation of the dynamics of poor quality family caregiving. *Advances in Nursing Science, 8*(4), 62–84. |
| Self-transcendence | Reed, P. (1991). Toward a nursing theory of self-transcendence: Deductive reformulation using developmental theories. *Advances in Nursing Science, 12*, 64–74. |
| Social justice in nursing | Walter, R. R. (2017). Emancipatory nursing practice: A theory of social justice in nursing. *Advances in Nursing Science, 40*(3), 225–243. doi: 10.1097/ANS.0000000000000157 |
| Spiritual empathy | Chism, L. A., & Magnan, M. A. (2009). The relationship of nursing students' spiritual care perspectives to their expressions of spiritual empathy. *Journal of Nursing Education, 48*, 597–605. |
| Superlink system | Chen, H., & Boore, J. R. P. (2007). Establishing a super-link system: Spinal cord injury rehabilitation nursing. *Journal of Advanced Nursing, 57*, 639–648. |
| Waiting theory model | Trimm, D. R., & Sanford, J. T. (2010). The process of family waiting during surgery. *Journal of Family Nursing, 16*, 435–461. doi: 10.1177/1074840710385691 |
| **Integrative** | |
| Adapting to diabetes mellitus | Whittemore, R., & Roy, C. (2002). Adapting to diabetes mellitus: A theory synthesis. *Nursing Science Quarterly, 15*, 311–317. |
| Adolescent vulnerability to risk behaviors | Cazzell, M. (2008). Linking theory, evidence, and practice in assessment of adolescent inhalant use. *Journal of Addictions Nursing, 19*(1), 17–25. |
| Career persistence | Hodges, H. F., Troyan, P. J., & Keeley, A. C. (2010). Career persistence in baccalaureate-prepared acute care nurses. *Journal of Nursing Scholarship, 42*, 83–91. |
| Client experience | Holland, B. E., Gray, J., & Pierce, T. G. (2011). The client experience model: Synthesis and application to African Americans with multiple sclerosis. *Journal of Theory Construction & Testing, 15*(2), 36–40. |
| Crisis for individuals with severe mental illness | Ball, J. S., Links, P. S., Strike, C., & Boydell, K. M. (2005). "It's overwhelming… everything seems to be too much:" A theory of crisis for individuals with severe persistent mental illness. *Psychiatric Rehabilitation Journal, 29*(1), 10–17. |
| Empowered holistic nursing education | Love, K. (2014). A midrange theory of empowered holistic nursing education: A pedagogy for a student-centered classroom. *Creative Nursing, 20*(1), 47–58. |
| Experiencing transitions | Meleis, A. I., Sawyer, L. M., Im, E., Messias, D. K., & Schumacher, K. (2000). Experiencing transitions: An emerging middle range theory. *Advances in Nursing Science, 23*(1), 12–28. |
| Facilitated sensemaking | Davidson, J. E. (2010). Facilitated sensemaking a strategy and new middle-range theory to support families of intensive care unit patients. *Critical Care Nurse, 30*(6), 28–39. |
| Illness constellation | Morse, J. M., & Johnson, H. K. (1991). *In the illness experience: Dimensions of suffering.* Newbury Park, CA: Sage. |
| Interaction model of client behavior | Cox, C. L. (1982). An interaction model of client behavior: Theoretical prescription for nursing. *Advances in Nursing Science, 5*(1), 41–56. |
| Music, mood, and movement | Murrock, C. J., & Higgins, P. A. (2009). The theory of music, mood, and movement to improve health outcomes. *Journal of Advanced Nursing, 65*, 2249–2257. |
| Nursing time | Jones, T. L. (2010). A holistic framework for nursing time: Implications for theory, practice, and research. *Nursing Forum, 45*(3), 185–196. |
| Self-care management for vulnerable populations | Dorsey, C. J., & Murdaugh, C. L. (2003). Theory of self management for vulnerable populations. *Journal of Theory Construction & Testing, 7*(2), 43–49. |
| Simulations as teaching strategies | Jeffries, P. R. (2005). A framework for designing, implementing and evaluating simulations used as teaching strategies in nursing. *Nursing Education Perspectives, 26*(2), 96–103. |
| Symptom management | Linder, L. (2010). Analysis of the UCSF Symptom Management Theory: Implications for pediatric oncology nursing. *Journal of Pediatric Oncology Nursing, 6*, 316–324. doi: 10.1177/1043454210368532 |

[a]Theories used in nursing research that are not nursing-developed theories.

this analysis and synthesis of the grouped studies, there emerged five middle range theories: (a) coping; (b) adapting to life events; (c) adapting to loss; (d) adapting to chronic health conditions, a lifelong process and common journey; and (e) the adapting to family. This approach provides a way of avoiding the proliferation of middle range theories lacking in coherence. It makes use of a grand theory and the body of research related to the theory as a means of developing middle range theories with clear application to practice.

Other examples of middle range theories derived directly and specifically from nursing's major conceptual models and grand theories are found in Table 1.6. For example, middle range theories have been developed from Johnson's Behavioral System Model, Levine's Conservation Principles, Rogers' Science of Unitary Beings, and RAM (Alligood & Tomey, 2005).

Theories from nursing have been combined with those from other disciplines to create middle range theories. Mercer used Rubin's work on maternal role attainment (i.e., attachment and role identity during pregnancy and early infancy) and integrated role and developmental theories from the field of psychology to arrive at her Theory of Maternal Role Attainment. She also conducted a number of research studies on the subject, the findings of which were reflected in the theory.

Published research findings have been cited as the most common source for constructing middle range theories of nursing (Lenz, 1998). The development of Online Social Support Theory is an example of this approach (LaCoursiere, 2001). Synthesized research findings from various patient populations (e.g., patients diagnosed with cancer or cardiovascular illness) that reflected the perspectives of those involved with the use of online social support (i.e., patient, caregiver, and nurse) served as a foundation for LaCoursiere's theory.

Clinical practice and clinical practice guidelines are sources of middle range theory development. Peplau is credited with introducing the use of clinical data in the development of her theory, the Theory of Interpersonal Relations. She based her understanding of the stages of the nurse–patient relationship on the observations of interactions between student nurses and psychiatric patients. The clinical practice guidelines established by the Agency for Health Care Policy and Research for the management of acute pain were used by Good and Moore as an example of this approach to middle range theory development. The result was the theory of a balance between analgesia and side effects in the management of pain.

It is important to note that most of the nurses involved in the development of middle range theories used more than one approach. As part of arriving at the creation of the middle range theory, often findings from previous research studies were reviewed and analyzed, conceptual models and theories were considered, and additional research was conducted that targeted the phenomenon of most interest.

## USES OF MIDDLE RANGE THEORY

Middle range theory has been found to be useful in both research and practice. "Theory can serve a heuristic function to stimulate and provide the rationale for studies, as well as help guide the selection of research questions and variables" (Lenz, 1998, p. 26). Middle range theories also can assist practice by facilitating understanding of client's behavior, suggesting interventions, and providing possible explanations for the degree of effectiveness of the interventions.

In their published work, researches need to clearly identify and describe the theory that provided the framework for the research, including how the theory was used. This then provides a means, by which other studies using the same theory can be used to build the body of scientific knowledge, thus advancing best practices in nursing. There are no recent studies of the use of middle range theory in research. Through the 1990s, it was most often middle range theories from other disciplines (Lenz, 1998) that were used. This was particularly evident when comparing how frequently middle range theories and grand theories of nursing

| Table 1.6 | Middle Range Theories Derived From Conceptual Models |
|---|---|
| **Conceptual Model** | **Middle Range Theory** |
| Johnson's Behavioral System Model | Theory of a Restorative Subsystem<br>Theory of Sustenal Imperatives |
| Levine's Conservation Principles | Theory of Redundancy<br>Theory of Therapeutic Intention |
| Rogers' Science of Unitary Human Beings | Theory of Perception of Dissonant Pattern<br>Theory of Health Empowerment (Shearer, 2009) |
| Roy's Adaptation Model | Theory of the Physiologic Mode<br>Theory of the Self-Concept Mode<br>Theory of the Interdependence Mode<br>Theory of the Role Function Mode |

Source with exception of Shearer, 2009: Alligood, M. R., & Tomey, A. M. (2002). *Nursing theory: Utilization & application* (pp. 46–54). St. Louis, MO: Mosby. With permission from Elsevier Science.

are cited in the nursing research literature. Of 173 studies included in nursing research from January 1994 through June 1997, only 79 (45.7%) identified any theory. Of the 79 studies that identified a theory, 25 were nursing theories and 54 were middle range theories borrowed from other disciplines, most frequently from psychology. Of the 25 using nursing theories, middle range accounted for most of the nursing theories used in the studies, 22 of the 25 (Lenz, 1998, p. 27).

Though middle range theory has great potential for guiding nursing practice, the nursing literature suggests that the potential has not been fully realized. Many authors note a gap between theory and practice. There is a lack of useful information on middle-range theories available to practicing nurses (Lenz, 1998). Nurse theorists need to address the last factor by producing literature describing their theories in understandable terms, identifying the theories' implications for practice, and placing that information in practice-oriented journals. Hospitals need to make use of nursing theory as a means of delivering the best possible patient care. The Magnet Status has supported this endeavor by requiring a professional model of care as one of the components of the Magnet Model®. Frequently, hospitals adopt a specific theory; for instance, Cedars-Sinai Medical Center in Los Angeles integrated Orem's Self-Care Deficit Theory into their shared governance model to improve patient safety (Swanson & Tidwell, 2011). In addition, it is hoped that advance practice nurses, who are increasing in number, will provide the leadership necessary to better integrate nursing theory into practice for the purpose of improving the quality of patient care and outcomes.

## CONTROVERSY SURROUNDING MIDDLE RANGE THEORY

The identification of middle range theories is not unambiguous. For instance, Chenitz, primary author of *Entry into a Nursing Home as Status Passage*, labeled it practice theory, whereas others considered it middle range theory (Liehr & Smith, 1999, Analysis of the Middle Range Theory Foundation, para. 2). "The question about what constitutes theory at the middle range is not a black and white issue for which a precise and clear definition can be offered. Middle range theory holds to a given level of abstraction. It is not too broad nor too narrow, but somewhere in the middle" (Liehr & Smith, 1999, Analysis of the Middle Range Theory Foundation, para. 3). To reduce confusion, nurse theorists are encouraged to clearly identify their work as middle range and provide a name that represents its conceptual components (Liehr & Smith, 1999; Sanford, 2000).

The imprecision of what constitutes a middle range theory is only one of several criticisms of middle range theory. In addition to lack of definitional clarity, middle range theory has been criticized for relying on a positivistic idea of testability to distinguish itself from grand theories. Suppe (1996b) suggests an alternative approach to considering the testability of middle range theory. He rejects the widely accepted notion of theories as a set of propositions and proposes the idea that theories are "state-transitions systems modeling the behaviors of real world systems within the theory's scope" (Suppe, 1996b, p. 10). By his designations, operational concepts become descriptors; the values of these concepts become state specifications; and the propositions become specifications of state–transition relations (Suppe, 1996b, p. 11). The purpose of testing using this understanding of the nature of theories is delineating the scope of the middle range theory rather than subjecting a hypothesis to statistical analysis or qualitative data to coding. The basic research question is for what systems does the theory work and for what systems does it not, a question of scope. He claims this type of research question is well suited to the testing of middle range theories.

Since Merton (1968) first promoted the notion of middle range theories, they have been criticized as being intellectually unambitious. Critics argue that their scope and suggested methods of inquiry are too limited. Merton countered that middle range theory was addressing just the questions that the discipline of sociology was asking and that middle range theories can undergo the same systematic empirical testing that both more and less abstract theories can (pp. 63–64).

Another criticism of middle range theories is that their increasing numbers can lead to fragmentation of nursing's knowledge base into unrelated and distinct theories, theories not linked to the philosophical underpinnings of the discipline (Cody, 1999). Merton acknowledged that risk and proposed consolidating theories to create groups of like theories at the middle range (Whall, 1996). Nurse scientists have addressed this issue. The identification of a metaparadigm is an attempt to create some conceptual cohesion for nursing's knowledge base. In addition, there has been an intentional effort to relate middle range theories to nursing's conceptual models, grand theories, and taxonomies. For instance, the middle range theory of Therapeutic Intention is clearly linked to Levine's Conservation Principles. Nurse scientists have proposed anchoring middle range theories to nursing's taxonomies of (a) diagnoses, North American Nursing Diagnosis Association (NANDA); (b) interventions, Nursing Interventions Classification

(NIC); and (c) outcomes, Nursing Outcomes Classification (NOC) (Blegan & Tripp-Reimer, 1997) and have identified a structure to accomplish that linkage (Tripp-Reimer, Woodworth, McCloskey, & Bulechek, 1996). Others consider these taxonomies as types of middle range theories rather than frameworks for categorizing the theories because they consist of concepts, definitions of concepts, propositional statements, and assumptions (Whall, 1996). As taxonomies, these middle range theories could not be considered unrelated and fragmented aspects of nursing's knowledge base. Nurse scientists continue to recommend persistence in efforts to "create an association between the proposed theory and a disciplinary perspective in nursing" (Liehr & Smith, 1999).

Nurse researchers have been denounced for making use of middle range theories from disciplines other than nursing. This was certainly true of nursing research published from the mid-1970s to the mid-1980s. During this period, more than half of the studies made use of theories or models from disciplines other than nursing (Moody et al., 1988). The increasing number of nursing middle range theories is reversing that trend. Liehr and Smith (1999) found 22 middle range nursing theories published in the decade from 1988 to 1999 through a CINAHL search. These theories met a number of criteria, including identification by the author that the theory was of the middle range. The criticism that nurse researchers use middle range theories from disciplines other than nursing is also being addressed by a call to continue to develop theories in the midlevel of scope and abstractness. "Situating middle range theory at the forefront for practice and research is critical to epistemologic and ontologic growth in nursing" (Sanford, 2000, Recommendation 5, para. 1).

## Practice Theory/Micro Theory/ Situation-Specific Theory

The literature includes a confusing variety of terms to refer to the level of theory that is considered less abstract, more specific, and narrower in scope than middle range theory. *Practice theory* has been the most commonly used term (Jones, 2001; McKenna, 1997; Walker & Avant, 1995). Suppe (1996b), Kramer (1997), and Parker (2006) referred to both practice and micro theory. The term *micro theory* was also used by Kim (2000), Duldt and Giffin (1985), and Chinn and Kramer (1999, 2005) and by George (1995) and Young et al. (2001), who both cited Chinn and Kramer. The most recently introduced term is *situation-specific theory* (Im, 2005; Im & Meleis, 1999; Meleis & Im, 2001).

Im and Meleis (1999) argue for this level of theory development, claiming that grand and middle range theories fail to address "the diversities, complexities, and contextual complexities… for which its members [nurses in practice] have been striving" (para. 5). They assert that the grand and middle range theories consist of a wide range of generalizations and universalizations that fail to provided adequate guidance in determining the nursing care for the increasing diverse clients in complex health care systems.

There are a number of features that distinguish these theories from either grand or middle range theories. They exhibit "(a) a lower level of abstraction, (b) reflection of specific nursing phenomena, (c) context, (d) readily accessible connection to nursing research and practice, (e) reflection of diversities in nursing phenomena, and (f) limitation of generalization" (Im & Meleis, 1999, Properties of situation-specific theories, para. 1). A somewhat unique quality of situation-specific theories is their emphasis on sociopolitical, cultural, and historical contexts.

Several authors have provided a list of the necessary components of a *practice theory*. Dickhoff and James (1968) referred to this goal-oriented theory as "situation-producing" and identified its essential elements as "(a) goal-content specified as aim for activity; (b) prescriptions for activity to realize the goal-content; and (c) a survey list to serve as a supplement to present prescription and preparation for future prescription for activity toward the goal-content" (p. 201).

Jones (2001) interprets these elements to include the use of nursing diagnosis and outcomes classification systems as components of practice theory. Walker and Avant (1995) and Kramer (1997) referred to these three components in their definitions of practice theory, and both suggested additional considerations. Walker and Avant claim that without a basis in situation-relating (predictive) theories, it would require a liberal definition of theory to identify practice or situation-producing theory as theory. They suggest that it would be more legitimate to refer to practice theory as nursing practices (pp. 12–13). Kramer identifies a similar issue, the importance of connecting practice theory to the more encompassing knowledge structures of nursing as identified by metatheory. To the traditional understanding of practice theory, she adds theory about nursing practice (e.g., administrative and educational theories). This is not a commonly occurring use.

*Micro theory*, a term sometimes identified as interchangeable with practice theory, is included in the writings of Kim (2000), Suppe (1996b), and Chinn and Kramer (2005). Kim's (1983) definition of micro theory as a set of "theoretical statements, usually hypotheses, that deal with narrowly defined phenomena" (p. 13) suggests a research-based theory. Suppe (1996b) also identifies hypothesis testing as a primary feature of micro theories and claims that this feature provides the primary distinction between micro theory and middle range theory, both of which could be considered practice theories (pp. 12–13). According to Suppe, the term micro theory is found with increasing frequency in the literature to refer to theories that are too limited in scope to be considered middle range. He provided a hypothetical example of a micro theory of pain management for a hospitalized patient with acute postamputation pain, who was treated with PCA morphine, with possible Valium potentiation, which focused on pain intensity and addiction outcomes (Suppe, 1996b, p. 12). Kim (1983) provided examples of what she labeled as micro theories, for example, maternal attachment, pressure sores, wound healing, and positioning. Other examples of this level of theory development found in the literature include alcoholism recovery in lesbian women (Hall, 1990), quality of care (Nielson, 1992), milieu therapy for short-stay units (LeCuyer, 1992), caring for patients with chronic skin disease (Kirkevold, 1993), therapeutic touch (Green, 1998), exercise as self-care (Ulbrich, 1999), and ecological view of protection (Shearer, 2002).

Im (2005) proposes *situation-specific* as the preferred term for this most specific classification of nursing theory, and Meleis (2016) notes that "support for their use has been increasing" (p. 397). Referring to Jacox, who defined practice theories as those that identify actions that a nurse takes to produce a desired change in a patient's condition, she suggests that all situation-specific theories are practice theories, as are many middle range theories, and some grand theories (pp. 138–139). Situation-specific theories are then defined as "theories that focus on specific nursing phenomena that reflect nursing practice, and are limited to specific populations or to particular fields of practice" (pp. 137–138). Im and Meleis (1999) use the term situation specific to refer to that level of nursing theory that focuses on specific nursing phenomena with direct application to nursing practice. As noted earlier, a somewhat unique quality of situation-specific theories is their emphasis on sociopolitical, cultural, and historical contexts, demonstrated by the theory of menopausal transition of Korean immigrant women described by Im and Meleis.

## DEVELOPMENT OF PRACTICE THEORY

Practice theory can trace its origins to the work of metatheorists Dickhoff and James (1968). Their position, similar to that of Jacox, is that because nursing is a profession, and its theory must have an action orientation that can shape reality to create a desired goal. "The major contention here is that theory exists finally for the sake of practice" (p. 199).

Like other levels of theory, practice theories as situation producing are derived from middle range and grand theories, review of the literature, practice experiences, research, and collaborative efforts. Im (2005) describes an integrative approach, which involves exploring these sources but also includes checking assumptions about theory development, theorizing, and sharing and validating the theory.

Middle range theories can be the source of developing prescriptions directed at a specified goal (McKenna, 1997; Parker, 2006; Walker & Avant, 1995), and if not specifically derived from these middle range theories, at the very least, practice theories should identify how the concepts from both levels of theory are interrelated. Meleis' transition theory (2010) is an example of a middle range theory that has served as a source of multiple practice/situation-specific theories, for instance, the situation-specific theory of well-being in refugee women experiencing cultural transition (Baird, 2012).

Qualitative research, particularly, grounded theory, is often the source of situation-specific theory. The goal of this approach is to explain at a conceptual level a phenomenon (often a process or interaction) developed through an inductive reasoning that is "grounded" in data. The Theoretical Model for Parent–Child Transfer of Asthma Responsibility (Buford, 2004) is an example of this type of theory development.

Analysis of existing research is also an important source of practice theories. Walker and Avant (2011) note the contributions of the Conduct and Utilization of Research in Nursing Project in the formulation of practice theories. This project, initiated in 1975, identified a need for change in practice and summarized the relevant research to arrive at research-based principles for nursing interventions. There were 10 practice theories or protocols that were considered during the project. Examples of the protocols that were developed include (a) lactose-free diet; (b) sensation information, distress; (c) intravenous cannula change regimen; and (d) prevention of decubiti by means of small shifts of body weight (Haller, Reynolds, & Horsley, 1979, p. 47).

## EXAMPLES

In current literature for this level of theory development, the term *situation specific* is found more frequently than is either *practice* or *micro* theory. Table 1.7 provides examples of these theories. Several have used a middle range theory as a foundation of the situation-specific theory, for instance, Meleis' transition theory, and others have used a grounded theory approach.

**Table 1.7    Examples of Situation-Specific Theories**

| Focus | Population | Reference |
|---|---|---|
| Aftercare | Survivors of human trafficking in shelters with limited resources | Curran, R. L., Naidoo, J. R., & Mchunu, G. (2017). A theory for aftercare of human trafficking survivors for nursing practice in low resource settings. *Applied Nursing Research, 35*, 82–85. doi: 10.1016/j.apnr.2017.03.002 |
| Critical caring for protection | Migrant and seasonal workers | Shearer, J. E. (2017). Critical caring theory of protection for migrants and seasonal farmworkers. *Public Health Nursing, 34*(4), 370–379. doi: 10.1111/phn.12304 |
| Self-care | Individuals with heart failure | Riegel, B., Vaughan, D., & Faulkner, K. M. (2016). The situation-specific theory of heart failure self-care. *Journal of Cardiovascular Nursing, 31*(3), 226–235. doi: 10.1097/JCN.0000000000000244 |
| Suffering | Men who were maltreated in childhood | Willis, D. G., DeSanto-Madeya, S., & Fawcett, J. (2015). Moving beyond dwelling in suffering: A situation specific theory of men's healing from childhood maltreatment. *Nursing Science Quarterly, 28*(1). 57–63. doi: 10.1177/0894318414558606 |
| Quality of life | Korean adults with type 2 diabetes | Song, R., Ahn, S., & Oh, H. (2013). A structural equation model of quality of life in adults with type 2 diabetes in Korea. *Applied Nursing Research, 26*(3), 116–120. doi: 10.1016/j.apnr.2013.04.001 |
| Crisis emergencies | Individuals with severe, persistent mental illness in emergency departments | Brennaman, L. (2012). Crisis emergencies for individuals with severe, persistent mental illnesses: A situation-specific theory. *Archives of Psychiatric Nursing, 26*(4), 251–260. doi: 10.1016/j.apnu.2011.11.001 |
| Well-being during cultural transitions | Refugee women | Baird, M. B. (2012). Well-being in refugee women experiencing cultural transition. *Advances in Nursing Science, 35*(3), 249–263. doi: 10.1097/ANS.0b013e31826260c0 |
| Crisis emergencies in emergency rooms | Individuals with severe, persistent mental illness | Brennen, L. (2012). Crisis emergencies for individuals with severe, persistent mental illness: A situation-specific nursing theory. *Archives of Psychiatric Nursing, 44*(4), 251–260. doi: 10.1016/j.apnu.2011.11.001 |
| Health promotion behaviors | Korean Americans at risk or diagnosed with hepatitis B viral infection | Lee, H., Fawcett, J., Yang, J., & Hann, H. (2012). Correlates of hepatitis B virus health-related behaviors of Korean Americans: A situation-specific nursing theory. *Journal of Nursing Scholarship, 44*(4), 315–322. doi: 10.1111/j.1547-5069.2012.01468.x |
| Factors that influence participation in physical activity | Women in midlife | Im, E., Stuifbergen, A. K., & Walker, L. (2010). A situation-specific theory of midlife women's attitudes toward physical activity (MAPA). *Nursing Outlook, 58*(1), 52–58. doi: 10.1016/j.outlook.2009.07.001 |
| Pain | Asian Americans diagnosed with cancer | Im, E. (2008). The situation-specific theory of pain experience for Asian American cancer patients. *Advances in Nursing Science, 31*(4), 319–331. doi: 10.1097/01.ANS.0000341412.02177.77 |
| Self-care | Individuals with heart failure | Riegel, B., & Dickson, V. V. (2008). A situation-specific theory of heart failure self-care. *Journal of Cardiovascular Nursing, 23*(3), 190–196. doi: 10.1097/01.JCN.0000305091.35259.85 |
| Family caregiver perspectives | Adults transitioning to adult day care services | Bull, M. J., & McShane, R. E. (2008). Seeking what's best during the transition to adult day health services. *Qualitative Health Research, 18*(5), 597–605. doi: 10.1177/1049732308315174 |
| Transition responses | Migrant farmworker women | Clingerman, E. (2007). A situation-specific theory of migration transition for migrant farmworker women. *Research and Theory for Nursing Practice, 21*(4), 220–235. |
| Empowerment | School nurses | Broussard, L. (2007). Empowerment in school nursing practice: A grounded theory approach. *Journal of School Nursing, 23*(6), 322–328. |
| Breast-feeding experience for mother and infant | Families of infants | Nelson, A. M. (2006). Toward a situation-specific theory of breastfeeding. *Research and Theory for Nursing Practice, 20*(1), 9–27. |

| Table 1.7 | Examples of Situation-Specific Theories (Continued) | |
| --- | --- | --- |
| **Focus** | **Population** | **Reference** |
| Pain | Caucasians diagnosed with pain | Im, E. (2006). A situation-specific theory of Caucasian cancer patients' pain experience. *Advances in Nursing Science, 29*(3), 232–244. |
| Family health | Families of children hospitalized with a chronic condition | Hopia, H., Paavilainen, E., & Åstedt-Kurki P. (2004). Promoting health for families of children with chronic conditions. *Journal of Advanced Nursing, 48*(6), 575–583. |
| Quality of life | Children with cancer | Anthony, S. J., Selkirk, E., Sung, L., Klassen, R. J., Dix, D., Scheinemann, K., & Klassen, A. F. (2014). Considering quality of life for children with cancer: A systematic review of patient-reported outcome measures and the development of a conceptual model. *Quality of Life Research, 23*(3), 771–789. |

## CONTROVERSY SURROUNDING PRACTICE THEORY

In addition to the debate on the term to use in referring to this level of theory, the controversies about practice theory center on whether it further fragments nursing knowledge, whether it is a theory, and, finally if so, whether it is needed. Similar to Cody's (1999) critique of middle range theories, practice theories often fail to identify links to an existing school of thought, that is, extant grand and middle range theories. These linkages provide for cohesion in the development of nursing science. When efforts are made to establish these relationships, "the resulting practice theory [is elevated] above simple dictates or imperatives for practice" (Walker & Avant, 2011, p. 9). Unfortunately, this occurrence is not routine.

The question of what constitutes a theory is disputable, particularly as it relates to practice theory. Walker (1986) suggests that, based on a definition of practice theory as sets of principles or directives, the terms policy, procedure, or principles of practice might be more appropriate. Her conclusion is based on an understanding of theory as a "systematic description and explanation" (p. 28). Walker's position seems consistent with the increasingly popular phenomena of research utilization and evidence-based practice.

Beckstrand's (1986) contention is that practice theory is unnecessary. She claims that "all the theoretical knowledge relevant to practice can be discovered within existing systems of knowledge such as metatheory, philosophy, science, and ethics." Collins and Fielder (1986) respond to Beckstrand's conclusion by emphasizing the unique issues that nursing theories must address. They assert that Beckstrand's position does not consider the nurse's responsibility for caring for the client as a "particular" individual. Nursing still has a need for "a nursing theory that will set out the kinds of nursing practice and the particular set of moral ideals that nursing practice seeks to bring about" (Collins & Fielder, 1986, p. 510). The increasing number of practice theories or their semantic equivalent identified in the literature since the 1990s seems to be supporting, if not a need, at least an interest in this level of theory development.

## Summary

■ Nurses are inherently knowledge workers with knowledge taking a variety of forms.

■ Theory, research, and practice are inextricably linked in the way nursing knowledge is developed and used.

■ Nursing knowledge exists to define the nature of the profession but more importantly to serve the needs of those in practice.

■ A metaparadigm identifies the concepts of most significance to a discipline and thus provides a means of distinguishing one discipline from another. For nursing, the four most frequently cited domains of nursing's metaparadigm are person, health, society/environment, and nursing.

■ Nursing knowledge exists on a continuum of abstraction with philosophy/paradigm the most abstract and conceptual models and theories becoming progressively more concrete.

■ Nursing theories also exist on a continuum with grand theories the most abstract, practice or situation-specific theories the most concrete, and middle range theories in the obvious middle.

■ A theory consists of concepts and propositions that serve to describe, explain, predict, and/or control in relation to a defined phenomenon.

■ Theories can be developed using several processes: analysis, synthesis, and derivation. The sources from which theories are developed include research, practice, and other theories, both nursing and those borrowed from other disciplines.

■ Because middle range theories are general enough to be used across populations and settings but yet focus on a specific clinical phenomenon of interest to nurses, they can be applied to practice and validated through research.

■ The development of nursing knowledge is an ongoing process, though debates continue on the direction this development should take, for instance: (a) Should there be diversity or unity in the paradigmatic perspective of nursing? (b) Can borrowed theories legitimately contribute to nursing's body of knowledge? (c) Without a specific link to nursing's grand theories, is the development of middle range theories further fragmenting the profession's body of knowledge?

## CRITICAL THINKING EXERCISES

1. In the debate on nursing paradigms, which of the currently proposed considerations— emergence of a single paradigm, coexistence of complementary paradigms, or creation of an integrated paradigm from the two most prominent paradigms—seems to best serve the advancement of nursing knowledge? What would be the implications of the chosen perspective on paradigms for the development of nursing knowledge?

2. Make a case for the ongoing development and use of nursing grand theories. Conversely, make a case for the obsolescence of nursing grand theories for today's practice and research.

3. Identify a research topic or develop a research question. Refer to Table 1.6, *Examples of Middle Range Theories*. Which middle range theory might be applicable to the research topic or question? If none seems appropriate, why might that be?

## REFERENCES

Adam, E. (1992). Contemporary conceptualization of nursing: Philosophy or science? In J. F. Kikuchi & H. Simmons (Eds.), *Philosophic inquiry in nursing* (pp. 55–63). London, UK: Sage.

Alimohammadi, N., Taleghani, F., Mohammadi, E., & Abarian, R. (2014). The nursing metaparadigm concept of human being in Islamic thought. *Nursing Inquiry, 21*(2), 121–129. doi: 10.1111/nin.12040

Alligood, M. R., & Tomey, A. M. (2005). *Nursing theory: Utilization and application* (3rd ed.). St. Louis, MO: Mosby.

Annells, M. (2005). Guest editorial: A qualitative quandary: Alternative representations and meta-synthesis. *Journal of Clinical Nursing, 14*(5), 535–536.

Anthony, S. J., Selkirk, E., Sung, L., Klassen, R. J., Dix, D., Scheinemann, K., & Klassen, A. F. (2014). Considering quality of life for children with cancer: A systematic review of patient-reported outcome measures and the development of a conceptual model. *Quality of Life Research, 23*(3), 771–789.

Antiognoli-Toland, P. L. (1999). Kuhn and Reigel: The nature of scientific revolutions and theory construction. *Journal of Theory Construction & Testing, 3*(2), 38–41.

Archibald, G. (2000). A postmodern nursing model. *Nursing Standard, 14*(34), 40–42.

Babbie, E. (1995). *The practice of social research* (7th ed.). Belmont, CA: Wadsworth.

Baird, M. B. (2012). Well-being in refugee women experiencing cultural transition. *Advances in Nursing Science, 35*(3), 236–248. doi: 10.1097/ANS.0b013e31829260c0

Barrett, E. A. M. (1986). Investigation of the principle of helicy: The relationship of human filed motion and power. In V. Mailinski (Ed.), *Explorations on Martha Rogers' science of unitary human beings* (pp. 173–184). Norwalk, CT: Appleton-Century-Crofts.

Barrett, E. A. M. (1992). Diversity reigns. *Nursing Science Quarterly, 5*(4), 155–157.

Battistelli, A., Portoghese, I., Galletta, M., & Pohl, S. (2013). Beyond the tradition: Test of an integrative conceptual model on nurse turnover. *International Nursing Review, 60*(1), 103–111.

Beckstrand, J. (1986). A critique of several conceptions of practice theory in nursing. In L. H. Nicholl (Ed.), *Perspectives on nursing theory* (pp. 494–504). Boston, MA: Little, Brown and Company.

Bender, M., & Elias, D. (2017). Reorienting esthetic knowing as an appropriate "object" of scientific inquiry to advance understanding of a critical pattern of nursing knowledge in practice. *Advances in Nursing Science, 40*(1), 24–36. doi: 10.1097/ANS.0000000000000160

Bender, M., & Feldman, M. S. (2015). A practice theory approach to understanding the interdependency of nursing practice and the environment: Implications for nurse-led care delivery models. *Advances in Nursing Science, 38*(2), 96–108. doi: 10.1097/ANS.0000000000000068

Benoit, R., & Mion, L. (2012). Risk factors for pressure ulcer development in critically ill patients: A conceptual model to guide research. *Research in Nursing & Health, 35*(4), 340–362. doi: 10.1002/nur.21481

Bisk, T. (n.d.). Utopianism come to age: From post-modernism to neo-modernism. Retrieved August 16, 2006 from http://www.wfs.org/bisk.htm

Blegan, M. A., & Tripp-Reimer, T. (1997). Implications of nursing taxonomies for middle-range theory development. *Advances in Nursing Science, 19*(3), 37. Retrieved December 14, 1999 from Health Reference Center–Academic database.

Boggatz, T., & Dassen, T. (2011). Why older persons seek nursing care: Toward a conceptual model. *Nursing Inquiry, 18*(3), 216–225. doi: 10.1111/j.1440-1800.2011.00563.x

Buford, T. A. (2004). Transfer of asthma management responsibility from parents to their school-age children. *Journal of Pediatric Nursing, 19*(1), 3–12.

Burbules, N. C. (n.d.). Postmodern doubt and philosophy of education. Retrieved June 6, 2002 from University of Illinois at Urbana-Champaign Web site http://www.eduiuc.edu/EPS/PES-Yearbook/95_docs/burbules.html

Carper, B. A. (1978). Fundamental patterns of knowing. *Advances in Nursing Science, 1*(2), 13–24.

Carrington, J. M. (2012). Development of a conceptual framework to guide a program of research exploring nurse-to-nurse communication. *Computers Informatics Nursing, 30*(6), 293–299.

Chinn, P. L., & Kramer, M. K. (1999). *Theory and nursing: Integrated nursing knowledge* (5th ed.). St. Louis, MO: Mosby.

Chinn, P. L., & Kramer, M. K. (2005). *Theory and nursing: Integrated nursing knowledge* (6th ed.). St. Louis, MO: Mosby.

Cody, W. K. (1999). Middle-range theories: Do they foster the development of nursing science? *Nursing Science Quarterly, 12*(1), 9–14.

Cody, W. K., & Mitchell, G. J. (2002). Nursing knowledge and human science revisited: Practical and political considerations. *Nursing Science Quarterly, 15*(1), 4–13.

Collins, R. C., & Fielder, J. H. (1986). Beckstrand's concept of practice theory: A critique. In L. H. Nicholl (Ed.), *Perspectives on nursing theory* (pp. 505–511). Boston, MA: Little, Brown and Company

Conley, Y. P., Heitkemper, M., McCarthy, D., Anderson, C. M., Corwin, E. J., Daack-Hirsch, S.,…, Voss, J. (2015). Educating future nursing scientists: Recommendations for integrating omics content in PhD programs. *Nursing Outlook, 63*, 417–427. doi: 10.1016/j.outlook.2015.06.006

Dickhoff, J., & James, P. (1968). A theory of theories: A position paper. *Nursing Research, 17*(3), 197–203.

Donnelly, E. (2001). An assessment of nursing theories as guides to scientific inquiry. In N. L. Chaska (Ed.), *The nursing profession: Tomorrow and beyond* (pp.331–344). Thousand Oaks, CA: Sage.

Downs, F. S. (1982). A theoretical question. *Nursing Research, 3*, 259.

Duldt, B. W., & Giffin, K. (1985). *Theoretical perspectives for nursing*. Boston, MA: Little, Brown and Company.

Dunphy, L. H. (2001). Florence Nightingale care actualized: A legacy for nursing. In M. E. Parker (Ed.), *Nursing theories and nursing practice* (pp. 31–53). Philadelphia, PA: F.A. Davis Company.

Eakes, G. G., Burke, M. L., & Hainsworth, M. A. (1998). Middle-range theory of chronic sorrow. *Image: Journal of Nursing Scholarship, 30*(2), 179–184.

El Hussein, M. T., & Osuji, J. (2017). Bridging the theory-practice dichotomy in nursing: The role of nurse educators. *Journal of Nursing Education and Practice, 7*(3), 20–24.

Elwyn, G., Lloyd, A., May, C., van der Weijden, T., Stiggelbout, A., Edwards, A.,…, Epstein, R. (2014). Collaborative deliberation: a model for patient care. *Patient Education and Counseling, 97*(2), 158–164. doi: 10.1016/jpec.2014.07.027

Estabrooks, C. A., Field, P. A., & Morse, J. M. (1994). Aggregating qualitative findings: An approach to theory development. *Qualitative Health Research, 4*(4), 503–511.

Fagerhaugh, S. Y. (1974). Pain expression and control on a burn care unit. *Nursing Outlook, 22*, 645–650.

Fawcett, J. (1978). The "what" of theory development. In National League for Nursing (Ed.), *Theory development: What, why, how?* (pp. 106–122). New York, NY: National League for Nursing.

Fawcett, J. (1984). *Analysis and evaluation of conceptual models of nursing*. Philadelphia, PA: F.A. Davis.

Fawcett, J. (1989). *Analysis and evaluation of conceptual models of nursing* (2nd ed.). Philadelphia, PA: F.A. Davis.

Fawcett, J. (1995). *Analysis and evaluation of contemporary nursing knowledge: Nursing models and theories* (3rd ed.). Philadelphia, PA: F.A. Davis.

Fawcett, J. (1996). On the requirements for a metaparadigm: An invitation to dialogue. *Nursing Science Quarterly, 9*(3), 94–97.

Fawcett, J. (1997). The structural hierarchy of nursing knowledge: Components and their definitions. In I. M. King & J. Fawcett (Eds.), *The language of nursing theory and meta theory* (pp. 11–17). Indianapolis, IN: Sigma Theta Tau.

Fawcett, J. (2000). *Analysis and evaluation of contemporary nursing knowledge: Nursing models and theories* (3rd ed., pp. 5–6). Philadelphia, PA: F.A. Davis Company.

Fawcett, J. (2003). Critiquing contemporary nursing knowledge: A dialogue. *Nursing Science Quarterly, 16*(3), 273–276.

Fawcett, J. (2005a). *Contemporary nursing knowledge: Analysis and evaluation of nursing models and theories* (2nd ed.). Philadelphia, PA: F.A. Davis Company.

Fawcett, J. (2005b). Middle range nursing theories are necessary for the advancement of the discipline. *Aquichan, 5*(1), 32–43.

Fawcett, J. (2013). Thoughts about conceptual models, theories, and literature reviews. *Nursing Science Quarterly, 26*(3), 285–288. doi: 10.1177/089431841348156

Fawcett, J. (2014). Thoughts about conceptual models, theories, and quality improvement projects. *Nursing Science Quarterly, 27*(4), 336–339. doi: 10.1177/089431841454611

Fawcett, J., & Alligood, M. R. (2005). Influences on advancement of nursing knowledge. *Nursing Science Quarterly, 18*(3), 227–232.

Fawcett, J., & Bourbonniere, M. G. (2001). Utilization of nursing knowledge and the future of the discipline. In N. L. Chaska (Ed.), *The nursing profession: Tomorrow and beyond* (pp. 311–320). Thousand Oaks, CA: Sage.

Fawcett, J., Watson, J., Neuman, B., Walker, P. H., & Fitzpatrick, J. J. (2001). On nursing theory and evidence. *Journal of Nursing Scholarship, 33*(2), 115–119.

Fitzpatrick, J. J. (1997). Nursing theory and metatheory. In I. M. King & J. Fawcett (Eds.), *The language of theory and metatheory* (pp. 37–39). Indianapolis, IN: Sigma Theta Tau.

Fitzpatrick, J. J., & Whall, A. L. (2005). *Conceptual models of nursing: Analysis and Application* (4th ed.). Bowie, MD: Robert J. Brady.

Flynn Makic, M. B., Rauen, C., Watson, R., & Will Poteet, A. (2014). Examining the evidence to guide practice: Changing practice habits. *Critical Care Nurse, 34*(2), 28–46.

George, J. B. (1995). *Nursing theories: The base for professional nursing practice* (4th ed.). Norwalk, CT: Appleton & Lange.

Georges, J. M. (2003). An emerging discourse: Toward epistemic diversity in nursing. *Advances in Nursing Science, 26*(1), 44–52.

Giovannetti, E. R., Dy, S., Leff, B., Weston, C., Adams, K., Valuck, T. B.,…, Boyd, C. M. (2013). Performance measurement for people with multiple chronic conditions: Conceptual model. *American Journal of Managed Care, 19*(10), e359–e366.

Glaser, B. G., & Straus, A. L. (1967). *The discovery of grounded theory: Strategies for qualitative research*. Chicago, IL: Aldine.

Gobbens, R. J., Van Assen, M. A., Luijkx, K. G., & Schols, J. M. (2012). Testing an integral conceptual model of frailty. *Journal of Advanced Nursing, 68*(9), 2047–2060.

Green, C. A. (1998). Critically exploring the use of Rogers' nursing theory of unitary beings as a framework to underpin therapeutic touch practice. *European Nurse, 3*(3), 158–169.

Grubbs, J. (1974). An interpretation of the Johnson behavioral system model for nursing practice. In J. P. Riehl & C. Roy (Eds.), *Conceptual models for nursing practice* (pp. 160–206). New York, NY: Appleton-Century-Crofts.

Guiliano, K. K., Tyer-Viloa, L., & Lopex, R. P. (2005). Unity of knowledge in the advancement of nursing knowledge. *Nursing Science Quarterly, 18*(3), 242–248.

Guba, E. G. (1990). *The paradigm dialog*. Newbury Park, CA: Sage.

Hall, J. M. (1990). Alcoholism recovery of lesbian women: A theory in development. *Scholarly Inquiry for Nursing Practice, 4*(2), 109–122.

Haller, K. B., Reynolds, M. A., & Horsley, J. A. (1979). Developing research-based innovation protocols: Process, criteria, and issues. *Research in Nursing and Health, 2*, 45–51.

Hardy, L. K. (1986). Janforum: Identifying the place of theoretical frameworks in an evolving discipline. *Journal of Advanced Nursing, 11*, 103–107.

Im, E. O. (2005). Development of situation-specific theories: An integrative approach. *Advances in Nursing Science, 28*(2), 137–151.

Im, E. O., & Chang, S. J. (2012). Current trends in nursing theory. *Journal of Nursing Scholarship, 44*(2), 156–164. doi: 10.1111/1547-5069.2012.01440x

Im, E. O., & Meleis, A. (1999). Situation-specific theories: Philosophical roots, properties, and approach. *Advances in Nursing Science, 22*(2), 11–24. Retrieved June 3, 2002 from CINAHL/OVID database.

Jacobson, S. (2017). Building bridges from theory to practice: Nursing theory for clinical practice. *MedSurg Matters, 26*(3), 1, 14, 15.

Jacox, A. (1974). Theory construction in nursing: An overview. *Nursing Research, 23*(1), 4–13.

Johns, J. (1995). Framing learning through reflection within Carper's fundamental ways of knowing in nursing. *Journal of Advanced Nursing, 22*(2), 226–234.

Johnson, D. E. (1959). The nature of a science of nursing. *Nursing Outlook, 7*(50), 291–294.

Johnson, D. E. (1974). Development of theory: A requisite for nursing as a primary health profession. *Nursing Research, 23*(5), 372–377.

Johnson, D. E. (1986). Theory in nursing: Borrowed and unique. In L. H. Nicholl (Ed.), *Perspectives on nursing theory* (pp. 117–121). Boston, MA: Little, Brown and Company.

Johnson, D. E. (1990). The behavioral system model for nursing. In M. E. Parker (Ed.), *Nursing theories in practice* (pp. 23–32). New York, NY: National League for Nursing.

Johnson, J. E., & Rice, V. H. (1974). Sensory and distress components of pain. *Nursing Research, 23*, 203–209.

Jones, D. A. (2001). Linking nursing language and knowledge development. In N. L. Chaska (Ed.), *The nursing profession: Tomorrow and beyond* (pp. 373–386). Thousand Oaks, CA: Sage.

Kahn, S., & Fawcett, J. (1995). Critiquing the dialogue: A response to Draper's critique of Fawcett's "Conceptual models and nursing practice: The reciprocal relationship." *Journal of Advanced Nursing, 22*(1), 188–192.

Kameoda, T., & Sugimori, M. (1993, June). Application of King's goal attainment theory in Japanese clinical setting. Paper presented at the meeting of Sigma Theta Tau International's Sixth International Nursing Research Congress, Madrid, Spain.

Kao, H. S., Reeder, F. M., Hsu, M., & Cheng, S. (2006). A Chinese view of the western metaparadigm. *Journal of Holistic Nursing, 24*(2), 92–101.

Kikuchi, J. F. (1992). Nursing questions that science cannot answer. In J. F. Kikuchi & H. Simmons (Eds.), *Philosophic inquiry in nursing* (pp. 26–37). Newbury Park, CA: Sage.

Kikuchi, J. F. (2003). Nursing knowledge and the problem of worldviews. *Research and Theory for Nursing Practice, 17*, 7–17.

Kikuchi, J. F., & Simmons, H. (1996). The whole truth and progress in nursing knowledge development. In J. F. Kikuchi, H. Simmons, & D. Romyn (Eds.), *Truth in nursing inquiry* (pp. 5–18). Newbury Park, CA: Sage.

Kim, H. S. (1983). *The nature of theoretical thinking in nursing.* Norwalk, CT: Appleton-Century-Crofts.

Kim, H. S. (1989). Theoretical thinking in nursing: Problems and perspectives. *Recent Advances in Nursing, 24*, 106–122.

Kim, H. S. (1997). Terminology in structuring and developing nursing knowledge. In I. M. King & J. Fawcett (Eds.), *The language of nursing theory and meta theory* (pp. 27–35). Indianapolis, IN: Sigma Theta Tau.

Kim, H. S. (2000). *The nature of theoretical thinking in nursing* (2nd ed.). New York, NY: Springer.

King, I. M. (1968). A conceptual frame of reference for nursing. *Nursing Research, 17*(1), 27–30.

King, I. M. (1984). Philosophy of nursing education: A national survey. *Western Journal of Nursing Research, 6*, 387–406.

King, I. M. (1997). Knowledge development for nursing: A process. In I. M. King & J. Fawcett (Eds.), *The language of nursing theory and meta theory* (pp. 19–25). Indianapolis, IN: Sigma Theta Tau.

Kirkevold, M. (1993). Toward a practice theory of caring for patients with chronic skin disease. *Scholarly Inquiry for Nursing Practice, 7*(1), 37–57.

Kirkpatrick, A. J., Cantrell, M. A., & Smeltzer, S. C. (2017). A concept analysis of palliative care nursing: Advancing nursing theory. *Advances in Nursing Science, 40*(4), 356–369. doi: 10.1097/ANS.0000000000000187

Klaver, K., & Baart, A. (2016). Managing socio-institutional enclosure: A grounded theory of caregivers' attentiveness in hospital care. *European Journal of Oncology Nursing, 22*, 95–102. doi: 10.1016/j.ejon.2016.04.002

Kramer, M. K. (1997). Terminology in theory: Definitions and comments. In I. M. King & J. Fawcett (Eds.), *The language of nursing theory and meta theory* (pp. 61–71). Indianapolis, IN: Sigma Theta Tau.

Kuhn, T. S. (1977). *The essential tension.* Chicago, IL: Chicago University Press.

Kuhn, T. S. (1996). *The structure of scientific revolutions* (3rd ed.). Chicago, IL: Chicago University Press.

Kylma, J. (2005). Dynamics of hope in adults living with HIV/AIDS: A substantive theory. *Journal of Advanced Nursing, 52*(6), 620–630.

LaCoursiere, S. P. (2001). A theory of online social support. *Advances in Nursing Science, 24*(1), 60–77.

Landreneau, K. J. (2002). Response to: "The nature of philosophy of science, theory and knowledge relating to nursing and professionalism." *Journal of Advanced Nursing, 38*(3), 283–285. Retrieved November 6, 2002 from CINAHL/OVID database.

LeCuyer, E. A. (1992). Milieu therapy for short stay units: A transformed practice theory. *Archives of Psychiatric Nursing, 6*(2), 108–116.

Leddy, S. K. (2000). Toward a complementary perspective on worldviews. *Nursing Science Quarterly, 13*(3), 225–233.

Leininger, M. (1978). *Transcultural nursing concepts, theories and practices.* New York, NY: Wiley.

Lenz, E. R. (1996). Role of middle range theory for research and practice. Paper presented at the Proceedings of the Sixth Rosemary Ellis Scholars' Retreat, Frances Payne Bolton School of Nursing, Case Western Reserve University, Cleveland, OH.

Lenz, E. R. (1998). Role of middle range theory for nursing research and practice. Part 1. Nursing research. *Nursing Leadership Forum, 3*(1), 24–33.

Lenz, E. R., Suppe, F., Gift, A. G., Pugh, L. C., & Milligan, R. A. (1995). Collaborative development of middle-range theories: Toward a theory of unpleasant symptoms. *Advances in Nursing Science, 17*(3), 1–13.

Lerner, R. M. (1986). *Concepts and theories of human development* (2nd ed.). New York, NY: Random House.

Liehr, P., & Smith, M. J. (1999). Middle range theory: Spinning research and practice to create knowledge for the new millennium. *Advances in Nursing Science, 21*(4), 81–91. Retrieved June 11, 2002 from CINAHL/OVID database.

Liehr, P., & Smith, M. J. (2017). Middle range theory: A perspective on development and use. *Advances in Nursing Science, 40*(1), 51–63. doi: 1097/ANS.0000000000000162

Lisanti, A. J., Golfenshtein, N., & Medhoff-Cooper, B. (2017). The pediatric cardiac intensive care unit stress model refinement using directed content analysis. *Advances in Nursing Science, 40*(4), 319–336. doi: 10.1097.ANS.0000000000000184

Litchfield, M. C., & Jónsdóttir, H. (2008). A practice discipline that's here and now. *Advances in Nursing Science, 31*(1), 79–91. doi: 10.1097/01/ANS.0000311531.58317.46

Littlejohn, C. (2002). Are nursing models to blame for low morale? *Nursing Standard, 16*(17), 39–41.

Malone, R. E. (2005). Assessing the policy environment. *Policy, Politics & Nursing Practice, 6*(2), 135–143.

McKenna, H. (1997). *Nursing theories and models.* London, UK: Routledge.

Meleis, A. I. (1997). *Theoretical nursing: Development and progress* (3rd ed.). Philadelphia, PA: Lippincott-Raven.

Meleis, A. I. (2010). *Transition theory: Middle range and situation-specific theories in nursing practice.* New York, NY: Springer.

Meleis, A. I. (2016). *Transition theory: Middle-range and situation specific theories in nursing research and practice.* New York, NY: Springer.

Meleis, A. I. (2018). *Theoretical nursing: Development and progress* (6th ed.). Philadelphia, PA: Wolters Kluwer Heath.

Meleis, A. I., & Im, E. (2001). From fragmentation to integration in the discipline of nursing: Situation-specific theories. In N. L. Chaska (Ed.), *The nursing profession: Tomorrow and beyond* (pp. 881–891). Thousand Oaks, CA: Sage.

Merton, R. K. (1968). *On social theory and social structure.* New York, NY: Free Press.

Monti, E. J., & Tingen, M. S. (1999). Multiple paradigms in nursing. *Advances in Nursing Science, 21*(4), 64–80.

Moody, L. E. (1990). *Advancing nursing science through research* (Vol. 1). Newbury Park, CA: Sage.

Moody, L. E., Wilson, N. E., Smyth, K., Schwartz, R., Tittle, M., & Van Cott, M. L. (1988). Analysis of a decade of nursing practice research: 1977–1986. *Nursing Research, 37*(6), 374–379.

Newman, M. (1996). Prevailing paradigms in nursing. In J. W. Kenney (Ed.), *Philosophical and theoretical perspectives for advanced nursing practice* (pp. 302–307). Boston, MA: Jones and Bartlett.

Newman, M. A. (2002). The pattern that connects. *Advances in Nursing Science, 24*(3), 1–7.

Newman, M. A., Sime, A. M., & Corcoran-Perry, S. A. (1996). The focus of the discipline of nursing. In J. W. Kenney (Ed.), *Philosophical and theoretical perspectives for advanced nursing practice* (pp. 297–301). Boston, MA: Jones and Bartlett.

Nielson, P. A. (1992). Quality of care: Discovering a modified practice theory. *Journal of Nursing Care Quality, 6*(2), 63–76.

Orem, D. E. (1959). *Guides for developing curricula for the education of practical nurses.* Washington, DC: Government Printing Office.

Orem, D. E. (2001). *Nursing: Concepts of practice* (6th ed.). St. Louis, MO: Mosby.

Parker, K. P. (1989). The theory of sentience evolution: A practice-level theory of sleeping, waking, and beyond waking patterns based on the science of unitary human beings. *Rogerian Nursing Science News, 2*(1), 4–6.

Parker, M. E. (2006). *Nursing theories and nursing practice* (2nd ed.). Philadelphia, PA: F.A. Davis Company.

Parse, R. R. (1987). *Nursing science: Major paradigms, theories, and critiques.* Philadelphia, PA: W. B. Saunders.

Parse, R. R. (1999). Nursing science: The transformation of practice. *Journal of Advanced Nursing, 30*(6), 1383–1387. Retrieved November 6, 2002 from Ovid/CINAHL database.

Parse, R. R. (2016). Where have all the nursing theories gone? *Nursing Science Quarterly, 29*(2), 101–102. doi: 10.1177/0894318416636392

Paterson, J. G., & Zderad, L. T. (1976). *Humanistic nursing.* New York, NY: Wiley & Sons.

Peter, E. (2017). Language of research (part 12)—Research methodologies: Grounded theory. *Wounds UK, 13*(1), 102–103.

Peterson, M. H., Barnason, S., Donnelly, B., Hill, K., Miley, H., Riggs, L., & Whiteman, K. (2014). Choosing the best evidence to guide clinical practice: Application of AACN levels of evidence. *Critical Care Nurse, 34*(2), 58–68.

Phillips, J. R. (1992). The aim of philosophical inquiry in nursing: Unity or diversity of thought. In J. F. Kikuchi & H. Simmons (Eds.), *Philosophic inquiry in nursing* (pp. 45–50). Newbury Park, CA: Sage.

Pilkington, F. B., & Mitchell, G. J. (1999). A dialogue on the comparability of research paradigms—And other theoretical things. *Nursing Science Quarterly, 12*(4), 283–289.

Pilkington, F. B., & Mitchell, G. J. (2003). Mistakes across paradigms. *Nursing Science Quarterly, 16*(2), 102–108.

Porter, S. (2010). Fundamental patterns of knowing in nursing: The challenge of evidence-based practice. *Advances in Nursing Science, 33*(1), 3–14.

Porter-O'Grady, T. (2003). Nurses as knowledge workers. *Creative Nursing, 9*(2), 6–9.

Rawnsley, M. M. (2003). Dimensions of scholarship and the advancement of nursing science: Articulating a vision. *Nursing Science Quarterly, 16*(1), 5–15.

Reed, P. G. (1995). A treatise on nursing knowledge development for the 21st century: Beyond postmodernism. *Advances in Nursing Science, 17*(3), 70–84. Retrieved June 3, 2002 from CINAHL/OVID database.

Renosa, M. D. C. (2016). Knowing-doing-valuing as systems of cocreations: A germinal theory on ethical caring. *International Journal of Human Caring, 20*(2), 60–75.

Reynolds, P. D. (1971). *A primer for theory construction.* Indianapolis, IN: Bobbs-Merrill.

Rinehart, J. M. (1978). The "how" of theory development in nursing. In National League for Nursing (Ed.), *Theory development: What, why, how?* (pp. 67–74). New York, NY: National League for Nursing.

Risjord, M. (2010). *Nursing knowledge: Science, practice, and philosophy.* West Sussex, UK: Wiley-Blackwell.

Roach, M. S. (1992). The aim of philosophical inquiry in nursing: Unity or diversity of thought. In J. F. Kikuchi & H. Simmons (Eds.), *Philosophic inquiry in nursing* (pp. 38–44). Newbury Park, CA: Sage.

Rodman, H. (1980). Are conceptual frameworks necessary for theory building? The case of family sociology. *The Sociological Quarterly, 21,* 429–441.

Rutty, J. E. (1998). The nature of philosophy of science, theory and knowledge relating to nursing and professionalism. *Journal of Advanced Nursing, 28*(2), 243–250. Retrieved July 16, 2002 from Ovid/CINAHL database.

Sanford, R. C. (2000). Caring through relation and dialogue: A nursing perspective for patient education. *Advances in Nursing Science, 22*(3), 1–15. Retrieved April 15, 2002 from CINAHL/OVID database.

Sarter, B. (1988). Philosophical sources of nursing theory. *Nursing Science Quarterly, 1*(2), 52–59.

Schlotfeldt, R. M. (1992). Answering nursing's philosophical questions: Whose responsibility is it? In J. F. Kikuchi & H. Simmons (Eds.), *Philosophic inquiry in nursing* (pp. 97–104). Newbury Park, CA: Sage.

Seiloff, C. L., & Frey, M. A. (2007). *Middle range theory development using king's conceptual system.* New York, NY: Springer.

Shapere, D. (1980). The structure of scientific revolutions. In G. Gutting (Ed.), *Paradigms and revolutions* (pp. 27–38). Notre Dame, IN: University of Notre Dame Press.

Shearer, J. E. (2002). The concept of protection: A dimensional analysis and critique of a theory of protection. *Advances in Nursing Science, 25*(1), 65–78.

Shearer, N. B. (2009). Health empowerment theory as a guide to practice. *Geriatric Nursing, 30*(2). 4–10. doi: 10.1016/j.gerinurse.2009.02.003

Silva, M. C. (1997). Philosophy, science, theory, interrelationships and implications for nursing research. *Image: Journal of Nursing Scholarship, 29*(3), 210–213. Retrieved June 7, 2002 from CINAHL/OVID database.

Silva, M. C., Sorrell, J. M., & Sorrell, C. D. (1995). From Carper's ways of knowing to ways of being: An ontological philosophical shift. *Advances in Nursing Science, 18*(1), 1–13.

Simmons, H. (1992). Philosophic and scientific inquiry: The interface. In J. F. Kikuchi & H. Simmons (Eds.), *Philosophic inquiry in nursing* (pp. 9–25). Newbury Park, CA: Sage.

Smart, J. J. C. (1968). *Between science and philosophy.* New York, NY: Random House.

Snyder-Halpern, R., Corcoran-Perry, S., & Narayan, S. (2001). Developing clinical practice environments supporting the knowledge work of nurses. *Computers in Nursing, 19*(1), 17–23.

Stifter, J., Yingwei, Y., Lopez, K. D., Khokhar, A., Wilkie, D. J., & Keenan, G. M. (2015). Proposing a new conceptual model and exemplar measure using health information: Technology to examine the impact of relational nurse continuity on hospital-acquired pressure ulcers. *Advances in Nursing Science, 38*(3), 241–251. doi: 10.1097/ANS.000000000000081

Suppe, F. (1996a). Middle-range theory: Nursing theory and knowledge development. Paper presented at the Proceedings of the Sixth Rosemary Ellis Scholars' Retreat, Frances Payne Bolton School of Nursing, Case Western Reserve University, Cleveland, OH.

Suppe, F. (1996b). Middle-range theories: Historical and contemporary perspectives. (Available from Institute for Advanced Study, Indiana University, Poplars 335, Bloomington, IN 47405).

Swanson, J. W., & Tidwell, C. A. (2011). Improving the culture of patient safety through the Magnet journey. *Online Journal of Issues in Nursing, 16*(3). Retrieved from http://www.nursingworld.org/MainMenuCategories/ANAMarketplace/ANAPeriodicals/OJIN/TableofContents/Vol-16-2011/No3

Thorne, S., Canam, C., Dahinten, S., Hall, W., Henderson, A., & Kirkham, S. R. (1998). Nursing's metaparadigm concepts: Disimpacting the debates. *Journal of Advanced Nursing, 27*(6), 1257–1268.

Tierney, A. J. (1998). Nursing models: Extant or extinct? *Journal of Advanced Nursing, 28*(1), 77–85. Retrieved June 3, 2002 from CINAHL/OVID database.

Tripp-Reimer, T., Woodworth, G., McCloskey, J. C., & Bulechek, G. (1996). The dimensional structure of nursing interventions. *Nursing Research, 45*(1), 10–17.

Ulbrich, S. L. (1999). Nursing practice theory of exercise as self-care. *Image: the Journal of Nursing Scholarship, 31*(1), 65–70. Retrieved August 1, 2002 from CINAHL/OVID database.

Wald, F. S., & Leonard, R. C. (1964). Towards development of nursing practice theory. *Nursing Research, 13*, 309–313.

Walker, L. O. (1986). Toward a clearer understanding of the concept of nursing theory. In L. H. Nicholl (Ed.), *Perspectives on nursing theory* (pp. 26–38). Boston, MA: Little, Brown and Company.

Walker, L. O., & Avant, K. C. (1995). *Strategies for theory construction in nursing* (3rd ed.). Norwalk, CT: Appleton & Lange.

Walker, L. O., & Avant, K. C. (2011). *Strategies for theory construction in nursing* (5th ed.). Boston, MA: Prentice Hall.

Walsh, D., & Downe, S. (2005). Meta-synthesis method for qualitative research: A literature review. *Journal of Advanced Nursing, 50*(2), 204–211.

Walter, R. R. (2017). Emancipatory nursing practice: A theory of social justice in nursing. *Advances in Nursing Science, 40*(3), 225-243. doi: 10.1097/ANS.0000000000000157

Weaver, K., & Olson, J. K. (2006). Understanding paradigms used for nursing research. *Journal of Advanced Nursing, 53*(4), 459–468.

Whall, A. L. (1996, May). Overview of middle-range theory. Paper presented at the Proceedings of the Sixth Rosemary Ellis Scholars' Retreat, Frances Payne Bolton School of Nursing, Case Western Reserve University, Cleveland, OH.

White, J. (2004). Patterns of knowing: Review critique, and update. In P. G. Reed, N. C. Shearer, & L. H. Nicholl (Eds.), *Perspectives in nursing theory* (6th ed., pp. 247–258). Philadelphia, PA: Lippincott Williams & Wilkins.

Whitehead, D. (2005). Guest editorial: Empirical or tacit knowledge as a basis for theory development. *Journal of Clinical Nursing, 14*(2), 143–144.

Willis, D. G., Grace, P. J., & Roy, C. (2008). A central unifying focus for the discipline: Facilitating humanization, meaning, choice, quality of life, and healing in living and dying. *Advances in Nursing Science, 31*(1), E28–E40. doi: 10.1097/01/ANS.0000311534.04059.d9

Winters, J., & Ballou, K. A. (2004). The idea of nursing science. *Journal of Advanced Nursing, 45*(5), 533–535.

Young, A., Taylor, S. G., & Renpenning, K. (2001). *Connections: Nursing research, theory, and practice*. St. Louis, MO: Mosby.

Yura, H., & Torres, G. (1975). Today's conceptual frameworks within baccalaureate nursing programs. In National League for Nursing (Ed.), *Faculty-curriculum development part III: Conceptual frameworks—Its meaning and functioning* (pp. 17 30). New York, NY: National League for Nursing.

# 2

# Analysis, Evaluation, and Selection of a Middle Range Nursing Theory

Timothy S. Bredow and Eun-Ok Im

## Definition of Key Terms

| | |
|---|---|
| **Adequacy** | Determines how completely the theory addresses the topics it claims to address. Establishes if there are holes or gaps that need to be filled in by other work or further refinement of the theory. Addresses if the theory accounts for the subject matter under consideration |
| **Clarity** | Addresses if the theory clearly states the main components to be considered. Determines if it is easily understood by the reader |
| **Complexity** | Reviews how many concepts are involved as key components in the theory. Decides how complicated the description of the theory is, and if it can be understood without lengthy descriptions and explanations; considers the number of variables being addressed and exists on a continuum from parsimony—limited number of variables to complex—extensive number of variables |
| **Consistency** | Addresses whether the theory maintains the definitions of the key concepts throughout the explanation of the theory. Determines if it has congruent use of terms, interpretations, principles, and methods throughout |
| **Discrimination** | Addresses whether the hypothesis generated by the theory led to research results that could not be arrived at using some other nursing theory. Determines how unique the theory is to the area of nursing that it addresses. Decides if it has precise and clear boundaries and definitive parameters of the subject matter |
| **External criticism** | Considers the fit between the theory and criteria external to the theory, such as the social environment and the prevailing views on the nursing metaparadigm. Criticism here is dependent on individual preference. It depends on reasonableness and perceptions of the evaluator. |
| **Internal criticism** | Deals with the criteria concerning the inner workings (internal dimensions) of the theory and how the theory's components fit with each other |
| **Logical development** | Resolves the following questions: Does the theory logically follow a line of thought of previous work that has been shown to be true or does it launch out into unproven territory with its assumptions and premises? Do the conclusions proceed in a logical fashion? Are the arguments well supported? |
| **Nursing metaparadigm** | Global concepts that identify the phenomena of nursing, including person, environment, health, and nursing (Fawcett, 1995) |
| **Pragmatic** | Determines if the theory can be operationalized in real-life settings |
| **Reality convergence** | Determines if the theory's underlying assumptions ring true. Decides if the theory's assumptions represent the real world, and if it represents the real world of nursing. Does the theory reflect the real world as understood by the reader? |
| **Scope** | Determines how broad or narrow is the range of phenomena that this theory covers. Does it stay in a narrow range of scope to keep it a middle range theory? (Narrower implies more applicable to practice; wider implies more global and all-encompassing.) |

*(Definition of Key Terms continued on next page)*

## *Definition of Key Terms* (Continued)

| | |
|---|---|
| **Significance** | Will the result of the research that is conducted because of the hypotheses generated by the theory have any impact on the way nurses carry out nursing interventions in the real world, or does it merely describe what nurses do? Does the theory address essential, not irrelevant, issues to the discipline? |
| **Theory analysis** | Systematic examination of exactly what was written by the theory author(s) |
| **Theory evaluation** | The identification of component parts of a theory and the judgment of them against a set of predetermined criteria |
| **Theory testing** | Testing of a theory through empirical investigations, which includes tests of utility, tests of nonnursing propositions, tests of concepts, and tests of propositions |
| **Utility** | Determines if the theory can be used to generate hypotheses that are researchable by nurses |

Middle range nursing theories can help nurses, undergraduates, and graduate nursing students alike meet and accomplish their goals of carrying out nursing research or competent reviews of the literature for sound evidence-based practice projects. When nursing theories are analyzed and evaluated in a thorough, systematic fashion, it is easier to determine which middle range nursing theory will provide the proper guidance and direction for the research or project under consideration. This chapter should help student, research, and staff nurses deal with the problem of how to analyze, evaluate, and choose a middle range nursing theory for their PhD and DNP research, Masters level assignments, and evidence-based nursing projects.

Theory analysis is the systematic examination of what was personally written over time by the theory author(s) about the theory. When performing a middle range theory analysis, the component parts are identified and the relationships of these components to each other and to the whole theory are examined. This analysis can provide the nurse a thorough understanding about the theory. Theory evaluation is the identification of the theory's same components and judging them against a set of predetermined criteria or through empirical investigations (e.g., research projects). The criteria used for judging theories are not standardized within the field of nursing but, rather, have evolved over time and are different depending on who is presenting the evaluation. Also, theory evaluation through empirical investigations in nursing has not involved any standardized process yet. Nonetheless, a thorough evaluation of a middle range theory will help the nurse researchers determine the robustness of a theory of their interest and the goodness of fit for application to their particular research or project.

Over the years, nursing theorists have emerged with different theoretical positions and theories proposing how various nursing concepts and the nursing metaparadigm are uniquely linked. Most of these theorists have constructed theories of nursing that could be termed grand theories, while later theorists have constructed middle range nursing theories. There are now more than 50 different grand nursing theories (McKenna, 1997) and several dozen middle range nursing theories for nursing researchers to choose from.

## Historical Background

Historically, nursing theorists worked hard to explain the nature of nursing, carving out a differentiated scientific field to call their own. At the same time, nursing researchers wanted nursing theory to be constructed to aid the generation of testable research hypotheses and also have the ability to affect the practice of nursing. As nursing theory developed and progressed through different stages of maturity, so did the evaluation process of what constitutes sound nursing theory.

In the past, nurses had Nightingale's environmental model, the medical model, and borrowed theories to use as a basis for nursing research. Through the 1960s, 1970s, and 1980s, several different grand nursing theories and some middle range theories were developed for nurses to use as a basis for their research. In the 1990s and beyond, many more middle range theories have emerged with an increasing number of situation-specific theories derived from middle range theories (Im, 2014; Im & Meleis, 1999; Meleis, 2010, 2011), allowing nurses to move away from using the Nightingale model, the medical model, borrowed theories, and grand nursing theories. When compared to grand theories, middle range theories contain fewer concepts, with relationships that are adaptable and concrete enough to be tested. Middle range theories have a particular substantive focus and consider only a limited aspect of reality. For example, Orem's Self-Care Deficit grand nursing theory would consider patients who are unable to carry out the activities of daily living and provide nursing care necessary to aid them back to a level of living where they were able to provide self-care. The middle range theory of unpleasant symptoms would use this same situation and consider the actual unpleasant symptom that was causing the problem for the patient. It would address the patient's symptom as a consideration for a multidimensional approach to health care symptom management. Kolcaba states that "for these reasons middle range theories are particularly cogent as nursing science addresses the challenges of the 21st century" (Kolcaba, 2001, p. 86). The use of many different middle range nursing theories for research purposes became a relatively new and exciting possibility for nurses during the 1990s. Now, researchers are expanding the knowledge base of nursing by enhancement of nursing's frameworks and theories (Parse, 2001). Because of this evolutionary process of theory building, nurses need to understand the historical roots for the analysis and evaluation of middle range nursing theories. In addition, understanding the process of analysis and evaluation provides insight to the evaluator about the strengths and weaknesses of the individual theory itself, as well as its possible use and application to nursing research and practice.

Meleis (1997, p. 245) states that "nurses have always evaluated theories." She provides the reasons why evaluation of theory is an essential component of nursing research:

- To decide which theory is more appropriate to use as a framework for research
- To identify effective theories for guiding a research project
- To compare and contrast different explanations of the same phenomenon
- To identify epistemological approaches of a discipline through attention to the sociocultural context of the theorist and the theory
- To assess the ontological beliefs and schools of thought in a discipline
- To define research priorities (Meleis, 1997)

Indeed, theories have always been evaluated throughout nursing history. From 1960s to 1980s, nursing scholars focused on theory analysis (critique) through proposing various sets of theory evaluation criteria. In the beginning stage of theory evaluation in nursing, evaluation criteria were mainly adopted from two major disciplines—sociology and psychology (Duffy & Muhlenkamp,

1974; Ellis, 1968; Johnson, 1974). Then, due to disciplinary differences between nursing and these two disciplines, other sets of evaluation criteria that were unique to nursing began to emerge. From the 1960s and 1970s, nursing-specific evaluation criteria were proposed by Johnson (1974), Ellis (1968), Hardy (1974), and Duffy and Muhlenkamp (1974). Even in the 1980s, these efforts to propose theory evaluation criteria that were unique to nursing continued. Examples of these efforts are Chinn and Jacobs (1987)'s initial five criteria for theory evaluation and Parse's proposed criteria for critiquing theory (Parse, 1987). In 1990s, additional sets of theory evaluation criteria were suggested, which included Barnum's (1994) criteria for both internal and external criticism. During the same period, Meleis also suggested a model of theory evaluation that was philosophically based on a historical view of science. In 2000s, the efforts to further develop the evaluation criteria and refine the already proposed evaluation criteria were made. In 2010, Chinn and Kramer (2010) refined the initial five criteria for theory evaluation by Chinn and Jacobs and proposed a set of questions for the evaluation of integrated knowledge. In 2005, Parse (2005) further developed her initial criteria for critiquing theory and proposed evaluation criteria for middle range theories and for grand theories. In 2005, Fawcett (2005a, 2005b) also suggested two sets of criteria including an analytical and evaluative framework for conceptual models and the other for theories. Then, later, she proposed different evaluation criteria for grand theories and for middle range theories Fawcett (2005a, 2005b). and further developed the criteria in 2012.

From the mid 1980s, nursing scholars have changed their focus in theory evaluation from theory analysis (critique) using the evaluation criteria to theory testing through empirical investigations. Around the same time, criticism on theory evaluation in nursing emerged due to advances in nursing research, specifically on theory testing through empirical investigations. For example, Silva (1986) reported her analysis of 62 theory testing studies and classified them as minimal (24 studies), insufficient (29 studies), and adequate (9 studies) use of models for theory testing. Then, Moody et al. (1988) critiqued that only 3% of the papers published in six research journals actually tested theory, concepts, or hypotheses/propositions. Subsequently, Acton, Irvin, and Hopkins (1991) conducted a literature review on theory testing research and developed 15 criteria that would be essential to evaluate theory-testing research. However, these criteria for theory testing research have rarely been used in nursing.

# Theory Analysis/Critique

## EARLY THEORY ANALYSIS/CRITIQUE UNTIL 1980s

The analysis of nursing theory has evolved over time as nurses have proposed increasingly sophisticated methods for reviewing and analyzing nursing theory. Three "early approaches" to theory analysis by Duffy and Muhlenkamp, Hardy, and Chinn and Jacobs will be discussed followed by a discussion of "recent approaches" by Barnum, Meleis, and Fawcett.

Duffy and Muhlenkamp (1974) wrote that nursing theory should be examined using four distinct questions. They suggested looking at the origin of the problem, the methods used in the pursuit of knowledge, the subject matter, and the kind of outcomes of testing generated by this theory.

These four questions when used alone to examine a nursing theory provided a fairly good evaluation of the theory; however, additional evaluation questions were proposed when the theory was used for research. Their additional questions for analyzing a nursing theory for nursing research included the following:

- Does it generate a testable hypothesis, and is it complete in terms of subject matter and perspective?
- Are the biases or values underlying the theory made explicit?
- Are the relationships among the propositions made explicit, and are they parsimonious?

With all of these questions in hand, a nurse could do what was thought, at the time, to be a thorough and complete assessment of any particular nursing theory to be used for nursing research.

During the same period of time, Hardy (1974) developed another way to analyze nursing theories. Her analysis method contained some unique criteria when compared to Duffy and Muhlenkamp's and included more criteria related to the process and outcome of theory evaluation. Her evaluation criteria identified the need for the theory to have adequacy, meaning, logic, and pragmatism. She wanted the theory to provide empirical evidence, have the ability to be generalized, contribute to further understanding, and be able to predict outcomes.

These two positions within the same historical time period contain some unique as well as overlapping criteria for the analysis and evaluation of nursing theory.

In the 1980s, Chinn and Jacobs (1983) proposed a combination of the previous two positions and recommended five brief criteria for evaluating nursing theories. They stated that a theory could be evaluated by asking if it had clarity, simplicity, generality, empirical applicability, and consequences. Clarity was further expanded to include semantic clarity, semantic consistency, structural clarity, and structural consistency. Apparently, they felt that semantics and clarity were becoming issues in the nursing community, and they were attempting to address these particular issues.

## THEORY ANALYSIS/CRITIQUE FROM 1990s

In addition to consideration of criteria for evaluation of theories, nursing theorists have proposed steps for the analysis process of nursing theories. Barnum, Meleis, and Fawcett all present several steps for the analysis of a nursing theory.

Recognizing the underlying assumptions of a theoretical work is an analyst's first task in understanding the theory (Barnum, 1998; Meleis, 1997). These assumptions may not be stated but may be inferred by the reader on the basis of other statements made about the given nursing theory in other publications and writings. However, recognizing underlying assumptions may not be possible for some middle range theories, because many of these middle range theories are not constructed by any one particular nursing author but may be the work of multiple authors. It then becomes difficult to understand all of the different assumptions from a variety of publications written by them. In addition, not all middle range theories are named after some nursing author or even have a particular author's name attached to the theory. For example, most of the middle range theories contained in this text do not have a theorist name attached to them, yet they have proved useful in the furtherance of nursing understanding. In addition, there are middle range theories such as Quality of Life, Change Theory, or Reasoned Action that are borrowed from other disciplines unrelated to nursing but are used by nurses to describe and build the understanding of nursing. Nonetheless, there are some middle range theories that do have information available about the underlying assumptions, and for them, it is important to understand and relate these assumptions to the research problem.

Barnum (1990, p. 22) asserts that analysis of a theory demands that the analyst "dig beneath the surface for a deeper insight into a thesis in all its meaning and implications." This "reading between the lines" work may be difficult for some nurses because they may not be comfortable with criticism at this level. Meleis (1997) would like to see reviews of theorists; their education, experience, and professional network; and the sociocultural context of their theories. Because theory development in nursing did not take place in a vacuum, Meleis (1997) feels that it is important to carefully consider the paradigmatic origins of the theory through careful analysis of the references and citations cited by the author. In addition, she wants the analysis to include a thorough review of the assumptions, concepts, propositions, and hypothesis that the author employed, and she wants the theory to be examined for beginnings. Analysis of beginnings looks at where the theory started. Did it begin in the mind of the theorist as an attempt to explain what ought to be, or did it arise out of experience and explain what it is? Fawcett (1995) suggests that analysis needs to include a thorough review of all the author's original works and presentations. However, for some middle range theories, because they are relatively new to the field of nursing, there may not be enough published work produced by a particular author or group of authors for the analyst to read and grasp this level of understanding about the theory's meaning and implications.

Barnum believes that the analyst should determine who or what performs an activity within the theory, as well as to determine who or what is the recipient of the activity. A third area that should be evaluated in each theory is in what context the activity is performed and what the end point of the activity is. Two additional concepts that need to be addressed include the procedures that guide the activity and the energy source of the activity. Other concepts Barnum (1998)considered essential for theory analysis include nursing acts, the patient, and health. Also included for good theory analysis are the relationship of nursing acts to the patient, the relationship of nursing acts to health, and the relationship of the patient to health. These concepts from Barnum are closely associated with the nursing metaparadigm that includes the concepts of nursing, person, health, and environment.

Barnum presents several devices for theory analysis. These devices use common nursing concepts to define nursing theory elements and their interrelationships. They also include determination of the level of theory development, descriptive or explanatory, and the need to discriminate nursing acts from nonnursing acts. Barnum (1990) adds that every nursing theory is based upon one or more dominant principles. These dominant principles contain an idea that is essential for stating or explaining a theory. It is important to identify and consider the nature of each key principle. A principle is a fundamental or basic concept with an explanatory function. It explains the basis upon which the theory rests. The theorist's interpretation

of reality, if it is given, should be analyzed by asking, "What is reality like?" Many of these considerations were geared toward the analysis of grand theories and have to be adapted for use when considering middle range theories. For example, if a middle range theory has been formulated over time by several authors, then it will be difficult, if not impossible, to determine the theorist's interpretation of reality.

Meleis includes internal dimensions as a criterion of her method of theory analysis. Internal dimensions include assumptions and concepts upon which the theory is built. She includes several units of analysis as part of this inquiry. Her units of analysis include content, context, and methods and are similar to the units of analysis contained in Barnum's list. Other items unique to Meleis include the rationale, the system of relations, beginnings, scope, goals, and abstractness. Examining the rationale of a theory's construction provides clarification of how the elements of the theory are united. Meleis wants the analyst to discover the theory's system of relations. This is accomplished by asking the question, "Do relations explain elements or do the elements explain relations?" (Meleis, 1997, p. 258). The scope of a theory determines how broad or narrow is the range of phenomena that the theory covers. Middle range theories keep their scope narrow, helping to make the theory more applicable to research and evidence-based practice projects. The scope of a theory also deals with the breadth of the explanations it attempts to accomplish. The scope is narrower, more specific, and more concrete for middle range theories than it is for grand theories (Fawcett, 1999).

The goals of a theory also need to be examined. Does the theory attempt to describe, explain, predict, or prescribe? Each theory must attempt to accomplish at least one of these goals. Middle range theories can be classified as falling into three distinct categories. These categories are descriptive, explanatory, and predictive (Fawcett, 2000). These three categories are closely aligned with the definition given by Meleis (1997) for a grand theory that includes describing, explaining, and predicting different phenomena.

Abstractness is another point that Meleis says is necessary to examine when analyzing a theory. Analyzing abstractness is an attempt to determine the width of the gaps between the theories, propositions, concepts, and reality. In middle range theories, this gap should be small, or nonexistent, since middle range theories deal with what is and not with what ought to be.

Fawcett (2000) has several recommendations for theory analysis that are similar to Meleis' and

Barnum's. She has two additional components to consider. They are theory context and theory content. Theory context is the environment in which the theory's nursing action takes place. It tells about the nature of the nurses' world and may describe the nature of the client environment. Theory context is also concerned with which nursing metaparadigm concepts are addressed by the theory (Fawcett, 2000). In middle range theories, the focus of the theory may be purposefully limited to just one of the nursing metaparadigm concepts, such as in chronic pain theory.

Theory content identifies the theory elements that are the subject matter of the theory. The content is stated through the concepts and propositions (Fawcett, 2000). Middle range theories should have their content well defined and their concepts clearly stated in the description of the theory.

A theory's process refers to the activities that either the nurse or the client has to perform to implement the theory. This should be the strength of middle range theories as they give clear direction to some process or activity carried out in the application of the theory in research or practice.

## Theory Evaluation

### BARNUM'S THEORY EVALUATION RECOMMENDATIONS

Barnum (1990, p. 20) states that "a thorough criticism (both analysis and evaluation) of a theory requires that attention be given to both aspects of internal and external criticism." Internal criticism refers to the internal construction of how the components of the theory fit together, while external criticism considers the theory and its relationship to people, nursing, and health. Internal criticism requires the reviewer to answer the following questions:

- Given the theorist's underlying assumptions, does the theory logically follow?
- Is the theory consistent with and logical in light of the underlying assumptions?

For external criticism, the reviewer would ask the following questions:

- Do the theory's underlying assumptions ring true?
- Do the assumptions represent the "real world" out there, especially the real world of nursing?

Barnum's criteria for evaluating theories include both internal and external criticism based on specific criteria. Her criteria for judging theories for internal criticism include clarity, consistency, adequacy, logical development, and level of theory development. Her criteria for judging theories using external criticism include reality convergence, utility, significance, discrimination, scope of theory, and complexity (Barnum, 1998).

Internal criticism is first evaluated by deciding the clarity of the theory. Two questions should be answered to determine clarity:

- Does the theory clearly state the main components to be considered?
- Is it easily understood by the reader?

Next on Barnum's list is consistency. Two more questions help to determine if the theory is consistent:

- Does the description of the theory continue to maintain the definitions of the key concepts throughout the explanation of the theory?
- Does it have congruent use of terms, interpretations, principles, and methods?

The next criterion is adequacy. Three questions help to determine if the theory is adequate:

- How completely does the theory speak to the topics it claims to address?
- Are there holes or gaps that need to be filled in by other work or further refinement of the theory?
- Does it account for the subject matter under consideration?

Her fourth criterion is logical development. The quality of this criterion is determined by asking three questions:

- Does the theory logically follow a line of thought of previous work that has been shown to be true or does it launch out into unproven territory with its assumptions and premises?
- Do the conclusions proceed in a logical fashion?
- Are the arguments well supported?

The final criterion for evaluating the internal portion of the theory is the level of theory development, which can be determined by asking the following questions:

- Is it in early development, just at the stage of naming its elements, or has it been around a long time and is able to explain or even predict outcomes?
- How often have different nurse researchers conducted independent research studies applying the theory to different situations and reported the findings in the literature?

Barnum (1998, p. 178) states that "external criticism evaluates a nursing theory as it relates to the real world of man, of nursing, and of health." She recommends that the following criteria should be considered: reality convergence, utility, significance, and capacity for discrimination. In addition, two other criteria may be included: scope and complexity (Barnum, 1998).

Reality convergence deals with how well the theory builds upon the premises from which it is derived and then relates that to reality. Some nursing theorists build on past work and remain within the framework of traditional thinking. Other nurse theorists deconstruct the past and develop a new framework to build upon. These theorists are termed *deconstructionists*. Deconstructionists start with a different set of presuppositions than the historical nursing leaders did, and the resulting nursing theories may not represent the same worldview of nursing as described in the past. At this point, the person doing the evaluation may choose to disagree as to whether a particular theory achieves reality convergence, based primarily on the differences between the beliefs and the values that he or she holds to be true and those proposed by the theory. This part of theory evaluation may have more applicability to grand theories than middle range theories but is an important point to consider, as new and different middle range theories are developed in future.

Utility simply requires that the theory be useful to the nurse researcher employing it. It should suggest subject material that could be investigated and lend itself to methods of inquiry. Middle range theories generally lend themselves to a greater ease of usefulness by nurse researchers than do grand nursing theories. This is because they tend to be very narrow in scope and focused on specific concepts, like health promotion, pain, and quality of life.

The significance of a nursing theory depends upon the extent to which it addresses the phenomena of nursing and lends itself to further research.

Discrimination is the capacity to differentiate nursing from other health-related disciplines through the use of well-defined boundaries. The boundaries need to be clear and precise so that judgments can be made about any given action performed by a nurse.

Barnum includes the scope of a theory as a necessary criterion for external criticism. Important questions to consider here are, does it have a narrow range of scope to help identify it as a middle range theory and does that narrow focus make it easier to use in a research setting?

Complexity is the final criterion in Barnum's list. Complexity is at the opposite pole from the criterion of parsimony. The level of complexity is determined by the number of variables. Middle range nursing theories are less complex than are grand nursing theories because they deal with fewer variables, resulting in a fewer number of relationships between the concepts.

## MELEIS' THEORY EVALUATION RECOMMENDATIONS

Meleis (1997) provides a complex model for theory evaluation. It includes several integral parts: theory description, theory support, theory analysis, and theory critique. She proposes that this complete model represents the necessary elements needed to thoroughly evaluate a theory. Meleis begins the description of her model by listing two criteria that help describe the theory. These two criteria are structural and functional components. Within the criterion of structural components, there are separate units of analysis to consider. The first is assumptions. Assumptions are "givens" in the theory and are based on the theorist's values. They are not subject to testing but lead to the set of propositions that are to be tested. In nursing theories, there are many assumptions made about the concepts included in the nursing metaparadigm and, additionally, to the concepts of human behavior, life, death, and illness. Again, it must be stated that it will not be possible to find the assumptions of all middle range theories.

Another part of Meleis' theory description includes functional components. A functional assessment of a theory carefully considers the anticipated consequences of the theory and its purposes. The units of analysis of the functional components are the theory's focus, that is, the client, nursing, health, nurse–patient interactions, the environment, nursing problems, and nursing therapeutics (p. 251).

Meleis offers several questions to ask when considering the functional components of a nursing theory (p. 254). They include the following:

1. Whom does the theory act upon?
2. What definitions does the theory offer for the elements of the nursing metaparadigm?
3. Does the theory offer a clear idea of what the sources of nursing problems are?
4. Does the theory provide interventions for nurses?
5. Are there guidelines for intervention modalities?
6. Does it provide guidelines for the role of the nurse?
7. Are the consequences of the nurse's actions articulated?

Meleis feels that these criteria are consistent with the ones offered by Barnum.

Another major area of theory evaluation for Meleis is theory support. She includes theory testing in this area. Theory testing consists of four separate tests: tests of utility, tests of nonnursing propositions, tests of concepts, and tests of propositions.

A final area of evaluation in the model is what Meleis calls theory critique. Theory critique is made up of several criteria. Many of her criteria are similar to the ones developed by Barnum, but some are unique to Meleis. The duplicated criteria similar to Barnum's are clarity, consistency, simplicity/complexity, and usefulness. Some unique criteria are tautology/teleology and diagrams.

Tautology considers evaluating the needless repetition of an idea in separate parts of the theory. Overuse of repetition can confuse a reader and make the theory explanation unclear.

Teleology is assessed by considering the extent to which causes and consequences are kept separate in the theory. Meleis (1997) says teleology occurs when the theorist defines concepts by consequences and then introduces totally new concepts, rather than getting to the definitions of the original concepts. As this process continues, there is never a clear definition of the theory's concepts, and the theory remains unclear.

Diagrams are useful to visually see the interrelationship of the concepts to each other before doing research. They can be especially useful for reviewing the strength of statistical correlations between the theory's concepts.

## FAWCETT'S THEORY EVALUATION RECOMMENDATIONS

Fawcett (2000) made the following recommendations to be used for the evaluation of nursing theories. Her criteria include significance, internal consistency, parsimony, testability, empirical adequacy, and pragmatic adequacy. She also recommends that the evaluation of a theory requires judgments to be made about the extent to which a theory satisfies the criteria.

Significance may be determined by asking the following questions: Are the metaparadigm concepts and propositions addressed by the theory explicit? In middle range theories, all aspects of the metaparadigm for nursing are not always covered, and that should not detract from its use by nursing researchers. Are the philosophical claims on which the theory is based explicit? Here again, some middle range theories will be devoid of philosophical claims. Is the conceptual model from which the theory was derived explicit? Are the authors of antecedent knowledge from nursing and adjunctive disciplines acknowledged, and are bibliographical citations given? (Fawcett, 2000, p. 504).

Fawcett's second criterion of internal consistency requires that all the elements of the theory be congruent. These elements may include conceptual model and theory concepts and propositions. In addition, Fawcett suggests that semantic clarity and consistency are required for internal consistency to be maintained. She proposes that the following questions be asked when evaluating the internal consistency of a theory: Are the content and the context of the theory congruent? Do the concepts reflect semantic clarity and consistency? Do the theory propositions reflect structural consistency? (Fawcett, 2000).

Parsimony is concerned with whether the theory is stated clearly and concisely. This criterion is met when the statements clarify rather than obscure the topic of interest. This is as important in middle range theory as it is in grand theory. Even though the scope of the theory may be narrow in a middle range theory, it is still important to be clear and concise in the explanations of the concepts.

The goal of theory development in nursing is the empirical testing of interventions that are specified in the form of middle range theories (Fawcett, 2000). The concepts of a middle range theory should be observable and the propositions measurable. Fawcett (2000, p. 506) suggests that the following questions should be asked when evaluating the testability of a middle range theory: Does the research methodology reflect the middle range theory? Are the middle range theory concepts observable through instruments that are appropriate empirical indicators of those concepts? Do the data analysis techniques permit measurement of the middle range theory propositions?

Empirical adequacy is the fifth step that Fawcett says is necessary in the evaluation of nursing theories. This step requires that assertions made by the theory are congruent with empirical evidence found through studies done using the theory as a basis for research. It usually takes more than one research study to establish empirical adequacy. The end result of using empirical adequacy is to establish the level of confidence in the theory from the best studies yielding empirical results. The question to be considered here is, are the middle range theory's assertions harmonious with the research studies' empirical results?

The final and sixth step in Fawcett's framework for evaluation of nursing theories is the criterion of pragmatic adequacy. This criterion evaluates the extent of how well the middle range theory is utilized in clinical practice. The criterion also requires that nurses fully understand the full content of the theory. In addition, the theory should help move resulting nursing action toward favorable client outcomes. Ask the following questions when evaluating a theory for pragmatic adequacy:

- Do nurses need special education and skill training to apply the theory in clinical practice?
- Is it possible to derive clinical protocols from the theory?
- How often has the theory been used as the basis of nursing research?
- Do favorable outcomes result from using the theory as a basis for nursing actions? (Fawcett, 2000)

Fawcett and Garity (2009) revised and updated Fawcett's (2000) recommendations for evaluating middle range theories in their book *Evaluating Research for Evidence-Based Practice*. In this textbook, they present four key areas to evaluate middle range theories. They outline four areas to consider: significance, internal consistency, parsimony, and testability.

Significance is broken down into two parts to consider: social significance and theoretical significance. Social significance is concerned with the theory's impact on the subject's lifestyle. Theoretical significance is concerned about the theory offering a new insight into people's experience with a certain health condition.

Internal consistency is related to the theory's concepts being operationally and conceptually defined. Semantic consistency is stated as being part of internal consistency and is concerned that all of the concepts used in the middle range theory are used consistently throughout the description and discussion of the theory. The last part of internal consistency is structural consistency. This part is concerned that all of the propositions of the theory are reasonable and that they are organized in such a way that reasonable conclusions can be reached.

Parsimony is concerned with the conciseness with which the theory is explained.

Testability is concerned that each concept used in the theory is observable and thus testable. This area of evaluation asks if the theory has ever been tested with a research study. If so, has the data been analyzed through some reasonable data analysis?

## KOLCABA'S THEORY EVALUATION RECOMMENDATIONS

A recent contribution to this discussion of theory evaluation comes from Kolcaba. According to Kolcaba (2001), there are several criteria that determine a good middle range theory. Her criteria involve evaluation and do not mention steps for theory analysis. They include questions concerning the theory's concepts and propositions and whether or not they are specific to nursing. She also wants to determine if the theory has components that are readily operationalized and can be applied to many situations. She asserts that a middle range theory's propositions can range from causal to associative, depending on their application. The assumptions provided fit the middle range theory. The theory should be relevant for the potential users. The middle range theory should be oriented to outcomes that are important for patients and not merely describe what nurses do. Finally, Kolcaba thinks that middle range theory should describe nursing-sensitive phenomena that are readily associated with the deliberate actions of nurses.

An interesting review process of the Synergy Middle Range Theory (see Chapter on Synergy Model) took place during its development. A committee of experts in the analysis of theoretical and conceptual frameworks was assembled to review this theory in order to identify its strengths and weaknesses and to obtain recommendations regarding the refinement of the model (Sechrist, Berlin, & Biel, 2000). This review committee was made up of the following nurse leaders: Barbara Stevens Barnum, RN, PhD; Marion Broome, RN, PhD; Rose Constantino, RN, PhD; Jacqueline Fawcett, RN, PhD; Edna Menke, RN, PhD; Carolyn Murdaugh, RN, PhD; Patricia Moritz, RN, PhD; Bonnie Rogers, DPH, COHN-S; and Marilyn Frank-Stromborg, EdD, JD, ANP. This esteemed committee developed a review instrument that was organized into six criteria. These criteria included the headings of clarity, consistency, adequacy, utility, significance, and summary. When compared to the recommended criteria listed in this chapter, the expert review committee decided to evaluate the synergy theory on fewer criteria. Their evaluation left out "logical development" and "determining the level of theory development" in the appraisal of internal theory analysis. When determining which criteria to include for the external middle range theory analysis, they chose to reduce the list to just three criteria, leaving out complexity, discrimination, reality convergence, pragmatic, and scope. They did add one new criterion, which may act as a "catchall" for the criteria left out, which they called the summary.

It is evident that there are several distinct differences between the analysis and evaluation process for grand theories and middle range theories. At the same time, there are several similarities. Many of the principles applied to the analysis and evaluation of grand theories can be readily applied to middle range theories and, with some minor modification, can be used to determine the adequacy of a middle range theory. With this in mind, the next section will address the selection of a middle range theory for use in nursing research, evidence-based nursing projects and systematic literature reviews.

## Current Status of Middle Range Theory Evaluation and Review

The evaluation of middle range theories tends to be new in nursing. As described above, nursing scholars have continuously evaluated nursing theories throughout nursing history and made tremendous efforts to develop and refine theory evaluation criteria. However, these efforts rarely considered different types of nursing theories (e.g., grand theories, middle range theories, situation-specific theories, etc.). Despite recent efforts to develop and propose the evaluation criteria by types of theories, very little is still known about the current status of middle range theory evaluation due to a lack of literature on theory evaluation in middle range theories. Indeed, in PUBMED searches, virtually no review articles on theory evaluation in middle range theories could be retrieved. Even when the searches were extended to theory evaluation and theory testing in general, just one review article by Im (2015) was retrieved during the past 10 years.

In 2015, Im (2015) reported her analysis of current status of theory evaluation in nursing in general based on an integrative literature review. This article would be the only one that mentioned about theory evaluation of middle range theories in recent years. In the review, she identified six themes reflecting the current status of theory evaluation process in nursing: (a) rarely using existing theory evaluation criteria; (b) focusing on specifics; (c) using various statistical analysis methods; (d) developing instruments; (e) adopting in practice and education; and (f) evaluating mainly middle range theories and situation-specific theories. In her analysis, she found that only six articles (10.52%) used an existing set of theory evaluation criteria during the past decade. She explained the phenomenon with the fact that nursing scholars in recent years would need to concentrate more on empirical investigations (theory testing) to select the most appropriate and adequate theoretical basis for their research. Also, she found that about 76% of the articles that she reviewed focused on evaluating specific major concepts/subconcepts and/or propositions through their research studies. An interesting finding was that the theory evaluation studies tended to test middle range theories derived from grand theories or specific concepts of grand theories. Furthermore, theory evaluation

studies involved specific populations with/without particular health/illness conditions (62.07%). In her report, she also indicated that various statistical methods (e.g., path analyses, structural equation modeling, and multiple regressions) were used to evaluate nursing theories. Interestingly, in three studies, instruments were developed for theory evaluation, which have rarely been reported in theory evaluation efforts previously. Evidence from practice and education was also used to evaluate specific major concepts and/or propositions in nine studies (15.5%). Finally, she found that theory evaluation during the past decade was mainly conducted to evaluate middle range theories (about 40%) and situation-specific theories (about 35%). In many cases, theory evaluation was simultaneously conducted with theory development by the same authors.

Although little is known about the current status of theory evaluation of middle range theories, one thing clear is that the evaluation of middle range theories is deeply linked to nursing research. As reported in Im's paper, the evaluation of middle range theories involves the development of new instruments that measure the major concepts or subconcepts of middle range theories. Also, the evaluation of middle range theories involves advanced statistical analysis methods to test the relationships among the major concepts and subconcepts of middle range theories. This certainly supports the direct linkage of middle range theories to nursing research that has been claimed by nursing theorists and provides the directions for future evaluation of middle range theories.

## Selecting a Theory for Nursing Research

Before starting to write a proposal, Fawcett (1999) suggests that each investigator become familiar with the research topic and the conceptual model that will guide the study or project. She reiterates that this is done by an immersion into the literature and a thorough study of the topic. In addition, a comprehensive literature search should be done several months before making a proposal of the study. This much time must be given to allow the proper amount of time for reading and thinking about both the content of the proposed study and the conceptual model to provide the basis for the study. It is during this time that the most appropriate middle range theory can be decided upon for use in the research or project.

As nurses shift away from using grand nursing theories and begin to consider using middle range theories, the philosophical underpinnings of the theory itself become of decreased importance. The emphasis shifts from the philosophical basis of the nursing theory to how the middle range theory is applied in research and practice. Thus, time previously spent with the philosophy and background of the theorist can now be devoted to ensuring the proper fit between the research questions to be studied and the middle range theory. Each nurse should ask the following questions about the middle range theory proposed for use in his or her work:

- Does the theory seem to fit the research/ project that you wish to do?
- Is it readily operationalized?
- What has been the primary application for this theory in the past?
- Where has the theory in question been applied and used before?
- How well has the theory performed at describing, predicting, and/or explaining the phenomena that it relates to?
- Does the theory relate to and address the research hypothesis/PICO question in its description and explanation?
- Does the hypothesis/question flow from the research problem/ practice question?
- Does the theory address the primary and secondary questions?
- Are the theory's assumptions congruent with the assumptions that are made for this work?
- Is it oriented to outcomes that are critical to patients and does it not just describe what nurses perform?
- Are validated tools available to test relationships of the theory or do they need to be developed?

The nurse should consider several different middle range theories as possibilities for use. A thorough analysis and evaluation of these theories in question should be done before selecting one. Subsequently, the nurse should become familiar with all aspects of the theory, using the questions provided in the discussion above. It is essential to have a sound understanding and be in agreement with the theory selected before beginning the study. This is accomplished by becoming immersed in the literature about the middle range theory in question and arriving at a thorough and complete understanding of the theory before using it. The nurse researcher should try to understand the middle range theory by identifying all the major concepts. The definitions of these concepts, in turn, should be studied for this particular theory, to make sure that the meanings have not been changed slightly over time as they are described in the literature.

In addition, the major concepts should be examined to determine how they relate to each other. Next, the researcher needs to decide if he or she can accept the premises, rationale, and presuppositions that the nursing theory is based upon before adopting it for use (McKenna, 1997). Finally, it is necessary to determine what means of measurement have been used with previous studies employing this theory. It will be important to know if new measurement tools need to be obtained or if similar tools can be employed for the work to be done.

It is evident that to decide upon and use a middle range theory effectively in nursing, the nurse must do a thorough analysis and evaluation of the middle range nursing theory. The following section will provide the guidance for conducting an evaluation of a middle range theory before selecting it for use in a research study.

## Middle Range Theory Evaluation Process

Before determining if a middle range theory is appropriate for use in a research study or project, apply both internal and external criticism. After careful review of the theory, take into account the following criteria listed here with their definitions. Answer the questions posed for each criterion. Summarize the findings in a concluding paragraph for both internal and external criticism. Finally, make a judgment as to whether the theory could be adapted for use in research.

There are analyses of theory exercises for many of the theories found in this book that are available on "the Point" Web site. After completing the exercise, compare your conclusions about the theory with a nurse who has worked with the theory and completed an analysis.

### INTERNAL CRITICISM

*Adequacy:* How completely does the theory address the topics it claims to address? Are there holes or gaps that need to be filled in by other work or further refinement of the theory? Does it account for the subject matter under consideration?

*Clarity:* Does the theory clearly state the main components to be considered? Is it easily understood by the reader?

*Consistency:* Does the description of the theory address whether it maintains the definitions of the key concepts throughout the explanation? Does it have congruent use of terms, interpretations, principles, and methods?

*Logical development:* Does the theory logically follow a line of thought of previous work that has been shown to be true, or does it launch out into unproven territory with its assumptions and premises? Do the conclusions proceed in a logical fashion? Are the arguments well supported?

*Level of theory development:* Is it consistent with the conceptualization of middle range theory?

## EXTERNAL CRITICISM

*Complexity:* How many concepts are involved as key components in the theory? How complicated is the description of the theory? Can it be understood without lengthy descriptions and explanations? (Considers the number of variables being addressed and exists on a continuum from parsimony—limited number of variables to complex—extensive number of variables)

*Discrimination:* Is this theory able to produce hypotheses that will lead to results that could not be arrived at using some other nursing theory? How unique is this theory to the area of nursing that it addresses? Does it have precise and clear boundaries and definitive parameters of the subject matter?

*Reality convergence:* Do the theory's underlying assumptions ring true? Do these assumptions represent the real world? Do they represent the real world of nursing? Does the theory reflect the real world as understood by the reader?

*Pragmatic:* Can the theory be operationalized in real-life settings?

*Scope:* How broad or narrow is the range of phenomena that this theory covers? Does it stay in a narrow range of scope to keep it a middle range theory? (Narrower implies more applicable to practice; wider implies more global and all-encompassing.)

*Significance:* Will the result of the research that is conducted because of the hypothesis generated by the theory have any impact on the way nurses carry out nursing interventions in the real world, or does it merely describe what nurses do? Does the theory address issues essential, not irrelevant, to the discipline?

*Utility:* Is the theory able to be used to generate hypotheses that are useable by nurses doing research and projects?

## Summary

■ Evaluation of middle range theories involves the development of new instruments to measure the concepts contained within the theory.

■ Evaluation of middle range theories will require the use of advanced statistical analysis to determine the strength of the relationships between the various concepts of the theory

■ In the real world of nursing, theory evaluation is many times done simultaneously with the development of new nursing theories.

■ Middle range theories are directly related to nursing research, and the evaluation of both will be tied together in the future.

---

### CRITICAL THINKING EXERCISES

1. Recently, groups of nurses and nurse theorists alike have migrated to an abbreviated process for middle range theory analysis. What information about the theory is not available from this abbreviated review?

2. Do you think that the shorter method of analysis results in a "good enough" analysis of any one middle range theory? Why or why not?

3. If you were going to use a particular middle range theory for your own work, would you be satisfied with the abbreviated method of analysis before you begin the project?

### REFERENCES

Acton, G. J., Irvin, B. L., & Hopkins, B. A. (1991). Theory-testing research: Building the science. *ANS Advances in Nursing Science, 14*(1), 52–61.

Barnum, B. (1990). *Nursing theory, analysis application, evaluation* (3rd ed.). Glenview, IL: Scott, Foresman, Little Brown.

Barnum, B. J. S. (1994). *Nursing theory: Analysis, application, and evaluation* (4th ed.). Philadelphia, PA: J. B. Lippincott.

Barnum, B. (1998). *Nursing theory: Analysis, application and evaluation* (5th ed.). Philadelphia, PA: Lippincott Williams & Wilkins.

Chinn, P., & Jacobs, M. (1983). *Theory and nursing: A systematic approach.* St. Louis, MO: Mosby.

Chinn, P., & Jacobs, M. K. (1987). *Theory and nursing: A systematic approach.* St. Louis, MO: C. V. Mosby.

Chinn, P. L., & Kramer, M. K. (2010). *Integrated Theory & Knowledge Development in Nursing* (8th ed.). St. Louis, MO: Mosby.

Duffy, M., & Muhlenkamp, A. (1974). A framework for theory analysis. *Nursing Outlook, 22*(9), 570–574.

Ellis, R. (1968). Characteristics of significant theories. *Nursing Research, 17*(3), 217–222.

Fawcett, J. (1995). *Analysis and evaluation of conceptual models of nursing* (3rd ed.). Philadelphia, PA: F.A. Davis.

Fawcett, J. (1999). *The relationship of theory and research* (3rd ed.). Philadelphia, PA: F.A. Davis.

Fawcett, J. (2000). *Analysis and evaluation of contemporary nursing knowledge: Nursing models and theories.* Philadelphia, PA: F.A. Davis.

Fawcett, J. (2005a). Criteria for evaluation of theory. *Nursing Science Quarterly, 18*(2), 131–135. Retrieved from https://doi.org/10.1177/0894318405274823

Fawcett, J. (2005b). Evaluating conceptual-theoretical-empirical structures for science of unitary human beings-based research. Retrieved July 2005, from http://medweb.uwcm.ac.uk/martha/Repository/Fawcett2005.ppt#398,1

Hardy, M. (1974). Theories: Components, development, evaluation. *Nursing Research, 23*(2), 100–107.

Kolcaba, K. (2001). Evolution of the middle range theory of comfort for outcomes research. *Nursing Outlook, 49*(2), 86–92.

McKenna, H. (1997). *Nursing theories and models.* London, UK: Routledge.

Meleis, A. I. (1997). *Theoretical nursing: Development and progress* (3rd ed.). Philadelphia, PA: Lippincott-Raven.

Meleis, A. I. (2010). *Transitions theory: Middle range and situation specific theories in nursing research and practice* (1st ed.). New York, NY: Springer.

Meleis, A. I. (2011). *Theoretical nursing: Development and progress* (5th ed.). Philadelphia, PA: Lippincott Williams & Wilkins.

Moody, L. E., Wilson, M. E., Smyth, K., Schwartz, R., Tittle, M., & Van Cott, M. L. (1988). Analysis of a decade of nursing practice research: 1977-1986. *Nursing Research, 37*(6), 374–379.

Parse, R. (2001). Rosemary Rizzo Parse the human becoming school of thought. In M. Parker (Ed.), *Nursing theories and nursing practice.* Philadelphia, PA: F.A. Davis.

Sechrist K., Berlin, L., & Biel, M. (2000). The synergy model: Overview of theoretical review process. *Critical Care Nurse, 20*(1), 85–86.

# BIBLIOGRAPHY

Alligood, M. R., & Marriner-Tomey, A. M. (2002). *Nursing theory: Utilization and application* (2nd ed.). St. Louis, MO: Mosby.

Barns, B. (1999). *Nursing theories' conceptual and philosophical foundations.* New York, NY: Springer Publishing Company.

Chinn, P., & Kramer, M. (1995). *Theory and nursing: A systematic approach* (4th ed.). St. Louis, MO: Mosby.

Chinn, P., & Kramer, M. (1999). *Theory and nursing: Integrated knowledge development* (5th ed.). St. Louis, MO: Mosby.

Dubin, R. (1978). *Theory building.* New York, NY: The Free Press.

Dudley-Brown, S. (1997). The evaluation of nursing theory: A method for our madness. *International Journal of Nursing Studies, 34*(1), 76–83.

Fawcett, J. (1993). *Analysis and evaluation of nursing theories.* Philadelphia, PA: F.A. Davis.

Fawcett, J. (1994). Analysis and evaluation of nursing theories. In V. Malinski & E. Barrett (Eds.), *Martha E. Rogers: Her life and her work.* Philadelphia, PA: F.A. Davis.

Fawcett, J., & Garity, J. (2009). *Evaluating research for evidence-based nursing.* Philadelphia, PA: F.A. Davis.

George, J. (1995). *Nursing theories: The base for professional nursing practice* (4th ed.). Norwalk, CT: Appleton & Lange.

Gift, A. (1997). *Clarifying concepts in nursing research.* New York, NY: Springer Publishing Company.

Greenwood, J. (Ed.). (2000). *Nursing theory in Australia: Development and application.* Sydney, Australia: Harper Collins.

Huck, S., & Cormier, W. (1996). *Reading statistics & research.* New York, NY: Harper Collins College Publishers.

Im, E. O. (2014). Situation-specific theories from the middle-range transitions theory. *ANS. Advances in Nursing Science, 37*(1), 19–31. Retrieved from https://doi.org/10.1097/ANS.0000000000000014

Im, E. O. (2015). The current status of theory evaluation in nursing. *Journal of Advanced Nursing, 71*(10), 2268–2278. Retrieved from https://doi.org/10.1111/jan.12698

Im, E. O., & Meleis, A. I. (1999). Situation-specific theories: philosophical roots, properties, and approach. *ANS. Advances in Nursing Science, 22*(2), 11–24.

Johnson, D. E. (1974). Development of theory: A requisite for nursing as a primary health profession. *Nursing Research, 23*(5), 372–377.

Kim, H., Kollak, I., & Parker, M. (Eds.). (1990). *Nursing theories in practice.* New York, NY: National League for Nursing, Publ. #15-2350.

McKenna, H. (1997). *Nursing models and theories.* London, UK: Routledge.

McQuiston, C., & Webb, A. (Eds.). (1995). *Foundations of nursing theory.* Thousand Oaks, CA: Sage Publications.

Nicoll, L. H. (1992). *Perspectives on nursing theory.* Philadelphia, PA: J. B. Lippincott.

Nolan, M., & Grant, G. (1992). Middle range theory building and the nursing theory-practice gap: A respite case study. *Journal of Advanced Nursing, 17,* 217–223.

Parker, M. (Ed.). (1990). *Nursing theories in practice.* New York, NY: National League for Nursing.

Parker, M. (Ed.). (1993). *Patterns of nursing theories in practice.* New York, NY: National League for Nursing, Publ. #15-2548.

Parker, M. E. (2000). *Nursing theories and nursing practice.* Philadelphia, PA: F.A. Davis.

Parse, R. R. (1987). *Nursing science: Major paradigms, theories and critiques.* Philadelphia, PA: W B Saunders Co.

Parse, R. R. (2005). Parse's criteria for evaluation of theory with a comparison of Fawcett's and Parse's approaches. *Nursing Science Quarterly, 18*(2), 135–137; discussion 137.

Silva, M. C. (1986). Research testing nursing theory: state of the art. *ANS Advances in Nursing Science, 9*(1), 1–11

Tomey, A. M., & Alligood, M. R. (Eds.). (2002). *Nursing theorists and their work* (5th ed.). St. Louis, MO: Mosby.

Walker, L. O., & Avant, K. C. (1997). *Strategies for theory construction in nursing.* New York, NY: Appleton-Century-Crofts.

Wesley, R. L. (1995). *Nursing theories and models* (2nd ed.). Springhouse, PA: Springhouse.

Whall, A. (1996). The structure of nursing knowledge: Analysis and evaluation of practice, middle range and grand theory. In J. Fitzpatrick & A. Whall (Eds.), *Conceptual models of nursing: Analysis and application* (3rd ed.). Norwalk, CT: Appleton & Lange.

Winstead-Fry, P. (Ed.). (1986). *Case studies in nursing theory.* New York, NY: National League for Nursing.

Young A., Taylor, S. G., & Renpenning, K. (2001). *Connections: Nursing research, theory and practice.* St. Louis, MO: Mosby.

# Application of Middle Range Theories to Project Management

Timothy S. Bredow and Connie Lynn Clark

## Definition of Key Terms

| | |
|---|---|
| **Capstone project** | Often a systematic review of the literature with critical analysis and application of the evidence to address a practice issue or implementation of a change in practice within a professional setting |
| **Decomposition** | The process of breaking down the total work required for a project into smaller levels of work |
| **Deliverables** | Completed documents presented by the project manager to the receiving party of the project |
| **Gantt chart** | A project management tool that provides dates to complete the project tasks in a sequential order and is used by the project manager to keep track of the progress of the project. It is useful to see where tasks are in terms of completion and if more resources are needed to complete the task on time. |
| **Matrix** | A systematic way Garrard (2004) of synthesizing data and findings of published articles that have been selected for a systematic review of the literature. It includes columns with the headings of citation, sample/size, research method, findings/conclusions, and recommendations. |
| **Milestones** | Predetermined dates where significant stages of the project are completely finished |
| **Project manager** | The person in charge of the project to make sure all of the tasks are completed on time and within budget and to the standard agreed upon (project specifications) |
| **Project management** | A prescribed way of working on and through a project to enable the project to be completed on time, within specifications, and within the budget. |
| **Project Overview Statement (POS)** | A written document agreed upon by the project manager and the recipient of the deliverables of the project. Specific deliverables are delineated with agreed-upon specifications for the completed project. |
| **Project scope** | The parameters of the project specifying how large a project will be and helps define what the deliverables will be at completion of the project |
| **Scope creep** | A project management term used to describe how projects can grow in scope over the life of the project resulting in the need for more time, money, and resources. |
| **Scope triangle** | A model of the interrelationship between time, money, and resources |
| **Systematic review of the literature** | A review of the pertinent literature specifically related to key elements of the project. Data collected during this review are oftentimes described by using a single-page matrix that summarizes specific elements of the article reviewed. |
| **Time** | Used in project management to estimate in hours, days, or weeks and how long a task will take to complete. Is part of a Gantt chart used to track progress on the project? |
| **Work-breakdown structure (WBS)** | Similar to a Gantt chart with the addition of the person responsible to complete the task |

Project management has been in use for a long time in the fields of construction, manufacturing, and engineering (Wysocki, 2009). It has only recently been introduced into the health fields and into nursing specifically (Bove, 2009). Skills in project management were necessary for a senior clinical research associate in the medical device division at the 3M Company. There were many projects developing new medical devices. At 3M, each project had a project manager to help keep the project development team on track. Time to market and staying within budget were critical to the team and the project manager. Team size and membership were decided by the scope and complexity of the project. It was unusual to receive extra help to complete the project, so each member had to stay focused on the tasks assigned for the project. With many bright team members who are always thinking of new ways to use something, it was easy to have the project grow in size and complexity as team members would envision new ways of adapting the project to novel applications. This "project creep" (AKA as scope creep) was insidious and sometimes led to delays in meeting set goals and requiring more time and money to investigate. The project manager used several methods to help keep the team on track. One of the most effective strategies employed by the project manager was frequent meetings and communication about the project to compare actual work done as compared to the timeline as portrayed on the Gantt chart. Actually, a modified Gantt chart called a work-breakdown structure (WBS) was used. This chart included not only the task and the time to work on this task but also the people assigned to the task. At the team meetings, each person would report how they were doing at meeting the goals set on the timeline for their assigned task. This was an effective way to keep everybody focused and "on task." When someone had their task up for review at these team meetings, they were said to be "holding the hot potato" as all eyes would be focused on whether or not they met the timeline goal.

This method of working on a project learned on the job at 3M Company can be easily transferred to the university nursing schools and clinical practice settings. This chapter is about using project management to help nurses complete their projects in a quality fashion, on time, and within the budget set for the project.

## Initiation of a Nursing Project

A requirement for degree completion in most masters (MSN) and doctor of nursing practice (DNP) programs is completion of a capstone project.

This may be a systematic review of the literature with critical analysis and application of the evidence to address a practice issue or implementation of a change in practice within a professional setting. The specific requirements of the program and the interests and background of the student will guide the choice of project. The time limits for completion of the project will be dictated by the program. Application of knowledge, skill, and resources is needed to manage, control, and complete a project on time. Strategic planning with use of critical, creative thinking will help ensure successful completion of this goal.

Specifically, this chapter is about applying principles of project management to streamline the process. It is meant to help graduate students and clinical practitioners complete a project on time and according to clinical practice or program requirements. Wysocki (2009) defines project management as: "A sequence of unique, complex, and connected activities that have one goal or purpose and that must be completed by a specific time, within budget, and according to specification" (p. 9). Within this definition is the concept that actions must be completed in a specific order and that there are logical relationships between pairs of activities.

When the project is being solidified in the project manager's mind, it is important to delve into the scientific nursing and related literature to evaluate and discern what is already known about this topic. Every project has at least a few if not several key factors that are interrelated to this main concept. When these key concepts are known to the project manager, it is important to determine if there are any closely related nursing theories that have already been developed that will inform the project at hand. The addition of a theoretical framework at this point in time (not after the project is completed) can help to focus and solidify the project in the project manager's mind. The theory can provide direction as to the trajectory of the project and to help keep the scope of the project in line with the time frame, budget, and resources available to apply and work on the project, and it can also provide an example of how the theory could be used by other practitioners.

## Selection of a Middle Range Theory

Selection of a theory to guide the process of systematic review of the literature and/or implementation of a change in practice is critical to the success of the process. Numerous theories of change have been developed that can be applied in situations of planned change. Resistance to change is human nature; planning for this resistance with identification of facilitators and barriers will assist the graduate student who is leading a change in practice for their capstone project. For example, Lewin's Theory of Planned Change provides a guide for unfreezing current practice, moving to new ways of doing, and sustaining the new reality. See the chapter on change theory for a more in-depth account of this theory. Nursing projects can also be developed to implement a change using a specific middle range theory, for example, self-efficacy, social support, and the other middle range theories presented in this text.

The middle range theory chosen to guide decisions in a systematic review of the literature will be unique to the subject of the review. Part of the evaluation of each literature source is assessing how the proposed recommendations of the project manager align with the theory chosen to guide the systematic review. The chosen theory provides a lens through which to view the issue presented in each literature source. The written summary of the master's capstone includes analysis of the impact of the theory on the issue. Students, who evaluate and view each source through the chosen theory throughout the systematic evaluation process, will find that their analysis of the topic is nearly completed.

## Management of the Project

Bove (2009) defines a project as a temporary endeavor to create a unique product, service, or result. Examples of projects within health care include implementing a new policy or procedure within an acute care setting or initiating a structured outreach program to a vulnerable population within a community setting. For a graduate student, a project may be a completion of the capstone within the specified time. In the clinical settings, the organization may identify the date required for the deliverable. Projects are designed to be completed within a limited time with a defined beginning and end date. This will be very apparent to the graduate student as the educational institution places limits on the time allowed for project completion.

Projects are sometimes done alone by a single person, but many projects will involve several other persons needed to complete the project. Project management works well for a single person but is especially useful when multiple players are involved. So how is a project managed so that the desired results are achieved within the time frame allowed?

The steps of project management are similar to the steps of the nursing process, providing some familiarity to the graduate nursing student. Most nursing projects can be broken down into five phases:

1. Initiation
2. Planning
3. Execution
4. Control
5. Closing

Each step is self-defined. The initiation phase is where the project is selected and defined. Well-defined goals and objectives guide remaining actions in completion of the project. The planning phase can be the most important phase. This phase is where the work plan is developed, including identification of the triple constraints of projects: scope, time, and cost. Planning also includes identification of possible risks and challenges to completion of the project. A contingency plan for handling problems will allow the project to progress on time and within budget. The change process that will be used is also defined in this phase, illustrating direct application of a change theory (see the Change Theory chapter included in this text for specific details). The execution of the project follows the planning. This is where the project is actually carried out in the field. It is where the project gets implemented. Finally, the control phase is where the project manager measures and tracks the project.

Identification of the scope triangle is a key element in project management. The triple constraints in project management are quality, time, and cost.

An increase in any one of these will impact the other two. A foundational and crucial aspect of project management is a statement of the scope of the project. This is a statement that defines the boundaries of the project; in other words, it states what will be done and what will not be done. The need for definition of these boundaries cannot be overstated. Even with this statement, "scope creep" will no doubt occur. Scope creep is any change in the project that was not in the original plan. Creating a scope statement from the outset will allow students and their advisers and clinical practitioner to discern when scope creep begins to occur and address it in a timely manner.

*Quality* refers to the actual quality of the deliverable. At the graduate level, quality is expected to be at a very high level. In most instances, the higher the quality demanded, the higher the cost will become, and there is also an associated increase in the amount of time needed to produce a quality product. When time is at a premium and limited, it is essential to limit the overall scope of the project in order to deliver a high-quality project on time.

As just mentioned, *time* is another element of the scope triangle. The graduate program specifies the amount of time allowed for the project, usually with some limited contingency allowed for needed extensions. The student may set their own time limits within this broader framework due to personal goals. Practitioners will need to especially pay attention to the time factor as many projects are not fully supported with financial reimbursement and the nurse may be working on the project on their own time. It is important to understand that time goes by whether it is used or not and is the prime resource in controlling the project. It needs to be used in the most effective and productive way. One of the most effective ways of managing time is the use of a Gantt chart, described in the next section.

The third side of the scope triangle is *cost*, also known as the budget. Cost may or may not be a concern depending on the project. A critical review of the literature with subsequent analysis and recommendations may be completed with little or no monetary cost. Completion of a change project within a practice setting may cost some money. A wise project manager will be careful to assess the cost of the project up front in the planning/proposal phase so as not to overextend themselves and become unable to finish the project due to a lack of funds. Project managers may need to include planning for the costs of training, resources (human and physical), equipment, and supplies. These estimated costs should be considered and be represented in the Project Overview Statement (POS) at the beginning of the project.

## Tools Used to Plan a Project

### PROJECT OVERVIEW STATEMENT

Many students and clinical practitioners, eager to get going with a project, jump in without the necessary planning that will result in success. It is well known that failure to plan results in planning to fail. There are specific planning tools within project management that help ensure a successful completion of the project. These include the POS, WBS, and the Gantt chart. The POS is a brief statement of the nature of the project. It is the foundation for future planning and execution of the project and the reference document for questions or conflicts related to scope and cost. It contains the following components: the statement of the problem or opportunity, the project goal, the project objectives (which may be viewed as milestones or significant deliverables within the project), success criteria, and the assumptions, risks, and obstacles of the project (conditions that may hinder project success). See Figure 3.1 for the components of a POS and Figure 3.2 for an example.

The POS may need to be accepted by the faculty member or advisor for the capstone and clinical agency management; often, it will include deadlines and deliverables identified by the advisor or manager within a capstone course. Whether its approval is required by the advisor or manager, it is a tool that will define and guide the project to completion if carefully constructed and followed.

| **PROJECT** | **Project Name** |
|---|---|
| **OVERVIEW** | **Project site** |
| **STATEMENT** | **Site contact:** |
| **Goal to solve this problem or opportunity** | |
| **Objectives (specific and measurable)** | |
| **Success Criteria (How will you know the project is successful? What are your main deliverables?)** | |
| **Assumptions, Risks, Obstacles (Think about barriers you may need to overcome)** | |
| **Approved by Advisor** _____ **Date** _____ | |
| **Site Contact Signature** _____ **Date** _____ | |
| **Project Manager** _____ **Date** _____ | |

**Figure 3.1**  Project Overview Statement (POS). (Modified POS adapted from Wysocki, R. (2014))

| *PROJECT* *OVERVIEW* *STATEMENT* | *Project Name* Policy and Procedural Guidelines for Developing a Special Care Plan for Frequent Users of the Emergency Department at XXX. Acute Care Hospitals | *Project Manager* |
|---|---|---|

**Problem/Opportunity (project focus)**

At the present time there are several procedures for developing special care plans for the emergency departments of the acute care hospitals. Having a system wide policy and procedure would ensure consistency of treatment and a better quality of care for those who frequently use the Emergency Department.

**Goal (overall)**

To develop a policy consistent with the mission, vision, and values for use in the emergency departments of H.E. for treatment of individuals who frequently seek treatment in the Emergency Department. To prepare evidenced based procedural guidelines for the emergency department to utilize for frequent users of the emergency department.

**Objectives (specific and measurable)**

- Develop a policy for assessment of patients through collaboration with primary physicians to identify by insert date
- Develop evidence-based procedural guidelines for frequent users of the emergency departments by insert date
- Training of these procedural guidelines will be completed by the Special Care Plans Core team by insert date
- Attendance at the education sessions will meet fifty percent of the employed Point of Entry staff and float personnel

**Success Criteria (How will you know the project is successful?)**

- Procedural guidelines will be approved by the Medical Director and policy committee
- Point of Entry RN Care Managers will work collaboratively with emergency department medical staff to identify patients requiring a special care plan
- Special care plans will be developed utilizing the procedural guidelines consistently throughout the system
- Project guidelines will be written by insert date
- Project education will be completed for Point of Entry RN Care Managers by insert date

**Assumptions, Strengths, Risks, Obstacles**

Assumptions

- The emergency departments will have the information technology to share the care plans throughout the system
- Special Care Plan Core Team will be available to provide education to the staff
- Staff will be accepting of the education

Strengths

- RN Care Managers at the Point of Entry are knowledgeable, friendly, and passionate about encouraging frequent users to develop healthy behaviors
- The RN Care Managers at the point of entry are interested in utilizing a system wide approach to the care plan development for frequent users of the emergency department.

Risks

- The Medical providers will be open to assisting with this process.

Obstacles

- There are varied cultures of clients and personnel in the emergency department
- Collaboration between RN Care Managers and primary medical providers may be difficult due to ownership of this project

| **Prepared by:** Masters Student, RN | **Date:** | Approved By/Date: Project supervisor |
|---|---|---|

**Figure 3.2**   POS example.

## GANTT CHART

The Gantt chart is a tool that can be used by the project manager to visualize the tasks and the time of the project. It is one of the most frequently used tools in project management to depict the project activities and time needed for each. The Gantt chart is a two-dimensional chart with tasks on the vertical axis and time on the horizontal axis. The tasks are listed in order of when they should be completed. The time required for each task is represented by a rectangular bar aligned with each task; the length of the bar corresponds to the duration of the task.

Some of the tasks listed on the Gantt chart will be sequential tasks, meaning they are linear tasks that must be completed in order with one task completed before starting the next. Other tasks may be considered parallel tasks, tasks that can be done at the same time as others. The Gantt chart clearly depicts this with the placement and length of the time bars. Milestones are specific points on the timeline and can be anchor points in the Gantt chart. They specify particular points in time when a deliverable is due or some piece of the project is complete. For students working on a project over a number of semesters, a milestone might include the portion of the project that is due to be turned in at the end of each semester. Figure 3.3 provides an example of a completed Gantt chart.

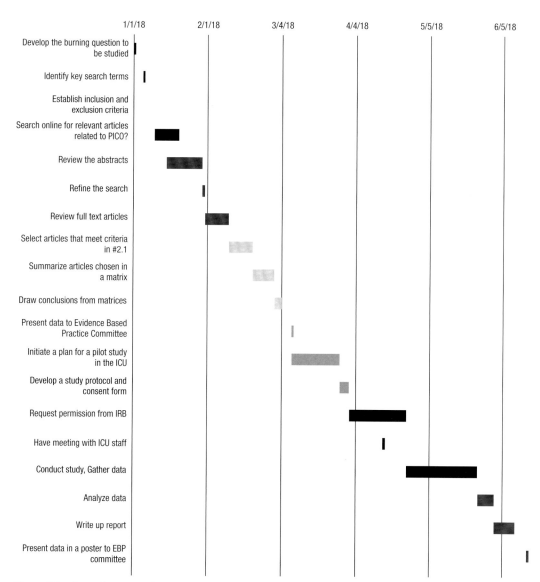

**Figure 3.3**  Gantt chart example.

## WORK BREAKDOWN STRUCTURE

The WBS reduces the most complex project to a set of clearly defined activities. For graduate students, a capstone project, whether a critical review of the literature or a change project, can seem overwhelming unless it is viewed as a series of smaller tasks to complete with set timelines. This is also true for project managers in clinical settings. A WBS describes all of the work that must be done to complete the project (Wysocki, 2009). It is similar to a Gantt chart with the addition of the person assigned to complete the task.

The faculty in the capstone course and/or the faculty advisor will be a resource person for the graduate student in identifying the project requirements and required deliverables. The graduate student handbook may also identify the chapters to be included in the written capstone and be a further resource for the deliverables that are required. For clinical practitioners, their manager may serve as a resource in determining the specific requirements for successful project completion. Once the project is defined and specific deliverables are known, decomposition of the work into discrete tasks can be completed.

Decomposition is the process of breaking down the total work required for a project into smaller levels of work. These smaller levels or portions of work are called activities. Activities are then further divided into tasks, which are even smaller portions of work that make up the activity. Finally, a work package is developed to describe how the tasks will be done, specifically the what, who, when, and how of a task. For the graduate student, the "who" will usually be the student, but may include others such as a university librarian who would assist in obtaining needed evidence from the literature in a critical review of the literature. If the graduate student's project is a change project involving staff in a professional setting, the who could include all who are included in bringing about the change. This group could be formed into a project team, with each team member being assigned specific tasks to perform. For the clinical practitioners, a team of stakeholders often needs to be created.

Decomposition enables the required effort and duration of the project to be estimated and the required resources and schedule of the work to be determined. It is a picture of the work of the project and how all the items of work relate to each other (Wysocki, 2009).

To better construct a complete WBS, post-it notes can be placed on a large surface, like a blank wall. Each task, no matter how small, is written on a post-it note and placed on the wall in the order that it must be accomplished. All project team members need to be present during this exercise to include each and every task that needs to be completed to finish the project. Different team members can post in different colors. When reviewing all of the tasks, as displayed on the wall, movement of tasks into a more efficient order is as easy as moving the post-it note to a different location (Nolan, 2015). As the post-it notes are arranged in the order they need to be completed, it becomes evident that some tasks can be completed at the same time by different people.

When tasks are arranged in the most efficient manner, this is called parallel pathing. Parallel pathing can be accomplished by arraigning tasks within the same time frame as opposed to a linear arrangement of the tasks. This method allows for the timeline to be shortened as individual's complete tasks at the same time rather than waiting for all tasks to be completed one after the other. The post-it note exercise will also identify tasks that must be done before any other work can be done. These tasks are critical to manage as the project will stop until the critical task is finished. The shortest path to completion of the whole project will always pass through the critical tasks and is thus known as the critical path of the project. Passing through a critical task is often referred to as reaching a milestone. The only way to speed up a project is to figure out how to get the critical path done quicker. This can sometimes be accomplished by adding more people to the project. Careful planning can cut timeline length significantly by using the parallel pathing method and concentrating on the critical tasks.

## Setting Priorities

Part of the challenge of the project is setting priorities. By creating the Gantt chart, the sequencing of tasks will become evident in the visual map. Priorities, what must be done before other tasks can be completed, will be shown. University requirements or clinical agency needs will dictate when deliverables are due for the capstone and/or deadlines set by the unit manager.

## Analysis and Evaluation of Outcomes

This is perhaps the most difficult part of project management, as analysis and evaluation can take an extended period of time after the project is implemented to determine if the project actually was a success or not. Complete implementation of a change in practice can take years, and there are many factors outside the project manager's control that can disrupt the best laid plans. Within certain time-constricted situations, success of the project may be determined by whether or not the promised deliverables were met. This is where the use of the POS in the beginning of the planning phase becomes so important. First-time project managers (e.g., graduate student nurses) have a way of proposing grandiose projects that would be impossible to complete in a timely fashion. Success can be achieved when the requirements set out and signed off in the POS were well thought out and reasonable at the start of the project. Sometimes, even reasonable goals and deliverables cannot be met. Were all of the goals and each of the deliverables met or only partially met? Analysis of the reasons why the project turned out the way it did can be an excellent learning tool for the project manager and the project team. Failure as well as success provides excellent learning tools for future projects.

## Summary

■ Understanding the component parts of project management and knowing the specific terms of project management can help nurses work in an ever-changing environment where change is happening at a breakneck speed, but managed on timelines to meet financial and patient satisfaction contingencies.

■ Project management can be a valuable tool to help nurses and nursing students complete their evidence-based practice (EBP), capstone, DNP, dissertation projects, and practice change projects in a quality fashion, on time, and within budget.

■ For projects with only one person doing all the work on the project, the POS and a Gantt chart are recommended. For larger projects needing more managing, nurses should use the POS and the WBS to achieve maximum results.

## CRITICAL THINKING EXERCISES

For this exercise, do one part or all of the parts to experience how project management works:

1. Part One: Think of a project that you might be interested doing at school or at work. Make a list of at least 15 steps (tasks) that would be needed to get the project started and up and going.

2. Part Two: Think of yourself as the project manager and assign different people to complete these tasks. Estimate the amount of time each person will need to work on the task to get it done.

3. Part Three: Figure out how you would shorten the timeline by "parallel pathing" some of the tasks.

4. Part Four: Make a budget for the project. Attach a cost estimate for each task. Some costs can be an hourly rate (or $/h) and some costs can be for materials and expenses to get the task done.

## REFERENCES

Bove, L. A. (2009). Project management for the rest of us. *Caring: Connecting, sharing, and advancing healthcare informatics, 24*(1), 1–2, 4–6.

Garrard, J. (2004[1999]). *Health sciences literature review made easy: The matrix method.* Gaithersburg, MD: Aspen Publishers.

Nolan, T. (2015). Getting started with Agile PM. In: *Agile, DevOps, & More.* Government Finance Officers Association. Retrieved from https://GovLoop.com. Gale Doc Number: Gale|A420323594.

Wysocki, R. (2009). *Effective project management: Traditional, agile, extreme* (5th ed.). Indianapolis, IN: Wiley.

Wysocki, R. (2014). *Effective project management: Traditional, agile, extreme* (7th ed.). Indianapolis, IN: Wiley.

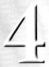

# Pain: A Balance Between Analgesia and Side Effects

Marion Good

## Definition of Key Terms

| | |
|---|---|
| **Analgesia** | Pain relief |
| **Balance between analgesia and side effects** | Patient satisfaction with relief of pain and relief or absence of side effects |
| **Identification of lack of pain or relief of side effect** | Pain intensity greater than the mutual goal; side effects of opioids reported by the patient or observed by the nurse |
| **Intervention, reassessment, and reintervention** | Immediate intervention for pain and side effects; reassessment when peak effect is expected and reintervention if pain and side effects are still unacceptable |
| **Mutual goal setting** | Mutually agreed-upon, safe, realistic goals for relief |
| **Nonpharmacological adjuvant** | Complementary nursing therapies for pain relief (relaxation, music, imagery, massage, and cold) |
| **Pain** | An unpleasant sensory and affective experience associated with tissue damage |
| **Patient teaching** | Patient instruction encouraging attitudes, expectations, and action in reporting pain; obtaining medication, preventing pain during activity, and using complementary therapies |
| **Pharmacological adjuvant** | Analgesic given as a supplement |
| **Potent pain medication** | Opioid analgesic or local anesthetic given systemically or by epidural for acute pain |
| **Regular assessment of pain and side effects** | Report of pain and side effects every 2 hours until under control and then every 4 hours |
| **Side effects** | Unpleasant sensory and affective experiences associated with adverse effects of pain medication |

Pain is the most common reason for people to seek health care. Although pain is known to be a part of life, it is compelling in its unpleasantness and is sometimes overwhelming in its effect. Patients who are in pain endure considerable suffering and are at risk for long-term adverse effects that include slower wound healing, down-regulation of the immune system, chronic pain, and cancer reoccurrence. There are many different types of pain: acute pain of injury, surgery, labor, and sickle cell crisis; chronic pain of musculoskeletal or gastrointestinal disorders; procedural pain of lumbar puncture, venipuncture, and chest tube removal; cancer pain from the enlarging tumor, its metastases, or its treatment; and pain in infants, in the critically ill, and at the end of life. Health care professionals today have a duty and an obligation to identify the source, to treat the cause, and to relieve the pain. Theories have been developed to explain and manage pain, and researchers have an obligation to test interventions for relief.

To study pain, researchers can experimentally induce it in animals and humans using noxious stimuli such as heat, cold, constriction, and sharpness. Or, they can study the pain of humans with painful conditions. In animal research, surgically exposed pain pathways provide information about the transmission of noxious impulses to the thalamus, sensory cortex, and limbic system; however, in animals, the affective component of pain is difficult to discern.

Human patients can report both the sensory and affective components of pain, but experimentally induced pain does not have the whole-person physical and emotional impact over time that clinical pain does. The pain of illness and surgery can limit life functions and arouse existential fears. The emotional impact of these limitations is intense, and it interacts with the sensory pain. Therefore, clinical studies are needed. To measure pain in alert adults who can communicate, clinicians and researchers must ask their patients to indicate a number on a scale. Further, the clinicians must believe the number that their patients tell them. Only the person in pain can tell them what his or her pain is like and describe it in terms of its intensity, quality, duration, and the trajectory over time. Therefore, patient reports of pain are valid.

## Historical Background

### THEORIES OF PAIN MECHANISM

Beginning in the 17th century, scientists proposed various theories of the way pain events are transmitted to the brain and then felt by the person. Early pain theories included direct transmission, proposed by Descartes (Melzack & Wall, 1962), specificity theory by von Frey in 1895 (Moayedi & Davis, 2013), and pattern theories reviewed in Melzack and Wall (1965). Later, evidence of affective pain was demonstrated by Beecher (1959), who showed that pain had a psychological component that could attenuate the transmission of impulses. The gate control theory was a major watershed or paradigm shift in pain theory (Melzack & Wall, 1965). It unified several sensory pain theories and added the affective, motivational, and central control elements, which could modify pain by descending mechanisms from the brain to the dorsal horn.

Discoveries of endogenous opiates in the periaqueductal gray area of the brain and also opioid receptors in the central nervous system produced new scientific theories. In addition, discoveries of catecholamines, serotonin, and neuropeptide receptors produced other new theories. Scientists viewed these newer theories as either supporting or refuting the gate control theory. Some viewed them as components of a more inclusive theory. For example, Melzack (1996) presented his new neuromatrix theory of pain that encompassed existing knowledge about the complexity of pain in humans. Melzack's theory, and the animal and patient research that it stimulated, has transformed our understanding of pain and its mechanisms (Mendell, 2014).

Nurses have created the following middle range descriptive and predictive theories of pain from the perspective of both patients and expert nurses: situation-specific theory (Im, 2006), unpleasant symptoms (Lenz, Pugh, Milligan, Gift, & Suppe, 1997), the paradox of comfort (Morse, Bottorff, & Hutchinson, 1995), a concept of pain (Mahon, 1994), concepts of acute and chronic pain (Simon, Baumann, & Nolan, 1995), nurses' perspective (Slatyer, Williams, & Michael, 2015), the journey to chronic pain (Taverner, Closs, & Briggs, 2014), and effects of chronic pain (Tsai, Tak, Moore, & Palencia, 2003). However, all of these theories describe and explain the *mechanisms and manifestations* of pain. They propose the way pain occurs and is modulated and its associated conditions. Although these theories are very useful, they do not specify effective interventions. Therefore, they are not the *prescriptive theories* needed by nurses for providing and testing interventions (Dickhoff & James, 1968).

### SHIFT TO THEORIES OF PAIN RELIEF

A second watershed in pain theory was a paradigm shift from theories of the mechanisms of pain to theories of relief. In medicine and pharmacology, these included prescriptive and explanatory theories of opioids and of nonopioids such as local anesthetics and nonsteroidal anti-inflammatory drugs (NSAIDs). Opioids, whether taken orally or injected into blood vessels, muscles, or the epidural space, provide potent relief for moderate-to-severe pain. The explanatory theory (mechanism) for this effect was later found to be that opioids attach to mu- and kappa-opioid receptors in the central nervous system. NSAIDs, including aspirin, ibuprofen, acetaminophen, cyclooxygenase-2 (COX-2) inhibitors, and ketorolac, have mechanisms that are different from those of centrally acting opioids. NSAIDs act at the site of the tissue injury to decrease the release of inflammatory substances that sensitize the nerve fibers to respond to the painful stimuli. When they are used as adjuvants, NSAIDs can be opioid sparing but may also interfere with blood clotting.

## DEVELOPMENT OF INTEGRATED PRESCRIPTIVE APPROACHES

A third paradigm shift was the notion that pain alleviation by nurses requires an *integrated* prescriptive approach, proposed in Good and Moore's theory of a balance between analgesia and side effects (Good, 1998; Good & Moore, 1996). Integrated prescriptive pain theories specify the actions that nurses must take to deliver both medical and nursing interventions, for example, pharmacological and nonpharmacological therapies, for relief. This integrative pain alleviation theory for adults (Good & Moore, 1996) was the forerunner of one for children who need assessment of developmental level, coping abilities, and cultural background (Huth & Moore, 1998). Recent evidence-based acute pain management guidelines are consistent with the nursing theory of a balance between analgesia and side effects. Examples are guidelines published by the American Society of Anesthesiologists on Pain Management (2012) and the American Pain Society Quality of Care Task Force (2005). The principles of the Good and Moore theory have stood these tests of time and interdisciplinary agreement and are therefore current for guiding nurses when caring for patients.

# Definition of Theory Concepts

The major concepts of the theory, a balance between analgesia and side effects, are found in Table 4.1, along with theoretical definitions

**Table 4.1    Concepts With Theoretical and Operational Definitions**

| Concepts | Theoretical Definitions | Operational Definitions (Examples) |
|---|---|---|
| **Outcomes** | | |
| Balance between analgesia and side effects | Patient satisfaction with relief of pain and relief or absence of side effects | Patient report of safe and satisfying pain relief with few or no side effects |
| Pain | An unpleasant sensory and affective experience associated with tissue injury following surgery or trauma | Pain intensity on a Visual Analogue Scale |
| Side effects | Unpleasant sensory and affective experiences associated with pain medication | Opioid Side Effects Scale (Good, Seo, Cong, & Huang, 2004) |
| **Proposition 1** | | |
| Potent pain medication | Opioid analgesic or local anesthetic given systemically or by epidural for acute pain | Drug, dose, frequency, route, and method of administration |
| Pharmacological adjuvant | Analgesic given as a supplement | Drug, dose, frequency, route, and method of administration |
| Nonpharmacological adjuvant | Complementary nursing therapies: relaxation, music, imagery, massage, or cold for pain relief | Technique, dose, frequency given, and mastery of use |
| **Proposition 2** | | |
| Regular assessment of pain and side effects | Report of pain and side effects every 2 h until under control and then every 4 h | Pain rating scale<br>Patient report or nurse observation of side effects of opioids |
| Identification of inadequate relief of pain and side effects | Pain/side effect intensity greater than mutual goal | Number and intensity of side effects that are unacceptable to patient/nurse |
| Intervention, reassessment, and reintervention | Immediate intervention for pain and side effects; reassessment when peak effect is expected and reintervention if pain and side effects are still unacceptable | Nurse documentation |
| **Proposition 3** | | |
| Patient teaching | Patient instruction, encouraging attitudes, expectations, and action in reporting pain, obtaining medication, preventing pain during activity, and using complementary therapies | Documentation of nurse instruction or patient use of audio/videotape |
| Mutual goal setting | Mutually agreed-upon, safe, realistic, goals for relief | Nurse discussions with patient daily, including documentation |

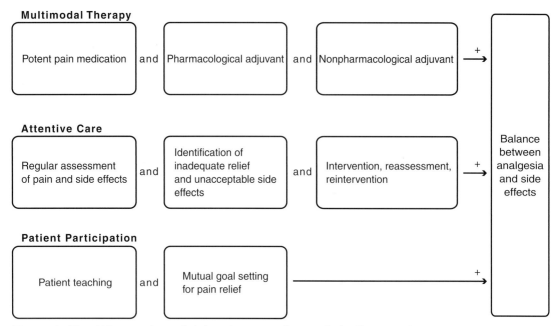

**Figure 4.1**    The middle range theory of a balance between analgesia and side effects prescribes nursing actions to encourage patient participation in using multimodal therapy with attentive care. (Adapted from Good, M. (1998). A middle range theory of acute pain management: Use in research. *Nursing Outlook, 46*(3), 120–124.)

and examples of operational definitions that can be used in research. In addition, Figure 4.1 is a graphic representation of the theory. Acute pain is conceptualized as a multidimensional phenomenon that occurs after surgery or trauma and includes sensory and affective dimensions. Pain in alert adults is what the person reports. The sensory component of pain following damage to body tissues is the localized physical perception of hurt. It is ordinarily termed "sensation of pain." The affective component of pain is the unpleasant emotion associated with the sensation and has been named "distress of pain" (Good et al., 2001), "anxiety" (Good, 1995a), or "unpleasantness" (Price, McGrath, Rafii, & Buckingham, 1983). The sensory and affective components of pain affect each other (Casey & Melzack, 1967; Johnson & Rice, 1974) and can be measured in terms of intensity magnitude.

The concept of *potent pain medication* refers to the major method used for relief. The potent medication may be parenteral opioids, but opioid analgesics have side effects of nausea, vomiting, drowsiness, urinary retention, and respiratory depression. In addition, dependence can also occur. To avoid these side effects, patients often take less analgesic than is needed for adequate relief (Acute Pain Management Guideline Panel, 1992). Epidural analgesia can be achieved with the use of opioids, local anesthetics, or both; these are injected into the epidural space of the spinal

cord. Side effects of epidural analgesia include lower extremity numbness. Other techniques may include regional techniques such as postincisional infiltration with local anesthetics, intra-articular analgesia, and peripheral nerve blocks (American Society of Anesthesiologists Task Force on Acute Pain Management, 2012). These methods often provide insufficient analgesia and uncomfortable side effects. Therefore, physicians often recommend adjuvants.

*Pharmacological adjuvants* may be given because their unrelated mechanism of action increases relief, yet can "spare" the use of strong analgesics and thus reduce their side effects. The American Society of Anesthesiologists Task Force on Acute Pain Management (2012) reports literature that suggests that two routes of administration may be more effective than one and recommends several combinations, such as (a) epidural opioid analgesia combined with oral or systemic analgesics and (b) intravenous opioids combined with oral NSAIDs such as ibuprofen, COX-2 inhibitors (COXIBs) such as celecoxib, or acetaminophen.

*Nonpharmacological adjuvants* to analgesic medication can include relaxation techniques, music, massage, cold, hypnosis, and guided imagery with self-efficacy messages, or pleasant image messages (Box 4.1). Music can be soft, soothing, sedative instrumental music (Good et al., 2000) and can be combined with relaxation or guided imagery.

| BOX 4.1 | **Nonpharmacological Adjuvants** |
| --- | --- |

**Relaxation**
Jaw relaxation (Good et al., 1999)
Autogenic phrases (Green, Green, & Norris, 1979)
Progressive muscle relaxation (Pestka, Bee, & Evans, 2010)
Systematic relaxation (Roykulcharoen & Good, 2004)
Afrocentric relaxation exercise (Campinha-Bacote, Campinha-Bacote, & Allbright, 1992)
Slow rhythmic breathing (Park, Oh, & Kim, 2013)

**Music**
Sedative music (Good et al., 1999, 2010)
Favorite music (Siedlecki & Good, 2006)
Ethnomusic therapy (Campinha-Bacote, 1993; Campinha-Bacote & Allbright, 1992)

**Massage**
Foot massage (Ucuzal & Kanan, 2014)
Massage by patient's companion (Najafi et al., 2014)
Massage in patients with metastatic bone pain (Jane et al., 2011)

**Cold**
Gel pack during coughing after cardiac surgery (Khalkhali, Tanha, Feizi, & Ardabili, 2014)
Cold pack during labor (Shirvani & Ganji, 2014)

**Guided Imagery**
Self-efficacy imagery (Tusek, Church, Strong, Grass, & Fazeo, 1997)
Pleasant imagery (Huth, Broome, & Good, 2004; Lewandowski, 2004; Locsin, 1988)
Hypnosis (Olness, 1981)

Nonpharmacological adjuvants have been studied during emergency treatment, following surgery and trauma, during labor, and during painful procedures.

*Regular pain and side effect assessments* are actions nurses take to identify patient symptoms. The theory then prescribes that nurses treat these symptoms, rather than simply record them. *Identification of inadequate pain relief and side effects* directs the nurse to believe the patient's report of pain and to know what intensity is less than adequate relief. The nurse must consider norms in the postoperative nursing unit and the wide variations in patient responses to pain and analgesics. In hospitals, nurses can request and use rescue orders and dose ranges (e.g., 1 to 2 mg), when the usual dose is insufficient (Gordon et al., 2004). The nurse can also encourage the use of nonpharmacological interventions. All interventions should be followed by *reassessment* when the greatest effect is expected and then *reintervention*, if pain is still not relieved.

*Patient teaching and mutual goal setting* will assist patients in their important role in managing their own pain. It is proposed that nurses teach patients effective attitudes and accurate expectations of pain. Nurses also teach patients to report pain, obtain medication, and use adjuvants. It is proposed that nurses initiate dialogue for mutual goal setting to set realistic relief goals that are acceptable to their patients.

When testing a middle range theory, more specific concepts and testable hypotheses can be deducted from the more general concepts and propositions (Good, 1998). A balance between analgesia and side effects is the general outcome. To deduct more specific concepts, the researcher would think of components of the concept and state their relationships to the general concept. For example, the concept of side effects is a subset of the balance between analgesia and side effects. Subset concepts of sensation and distress of pain can be deducted from the concept of analgesia. In this way, sensation and distress can be studied individually (Good, 1998). Any part of the theory can be examined in research: one concept, new relationships between concepts, part of a proposition, all of a proposition, or the whole theory. In addition, the application to nursing practice or education can be studied.

## Description of the Theory of Pain: A Balance Between Analgesia and Side Effects

The theory of a balance between analgesia and side effects is the first integrative prescriptive middle range pain management theory. Even though it is based on pain management guidelines and is consistent with them, the theory provides a broader and more parsimonious overview. Its general principles of acute pain management are a framework for research and a guide for nursing practice and education. The theorists expect practitioners to use the overall principles, along with the detailed knowledge contained in the professional acute pain guidelines and any current empirical evidence. These overall principles can be used in practice. "Principles" are called "propositions" when referring to the theory or testing them in research. This terminology is a matter of function: principles for practice and theoretical propositions for research. Theory serves as a foundation for research, while research serves as a means to test and generate theory. Both serve the advancement of practice. This theory with its principles/propositions is organized to stimulate additional research and to facilitate

| BOX 4.2 | Assumptions of the Theory of a Balance Between Analgesia and Side Effects |
|---------|---|

1. The nurse and the physician collaborate to effectively manage acute pain.
2. Systemic opioid analgesics or epidural opioids or anesthetic agents are indicated.
3. Medication for side effects is given as needed.
4. Patients are adults with ability to learn, set goals, and communicate symptoms.
5. Nurses have current knowledge of pain management.

the teaching of pain management information to nurses. Furthermore, the theory presents a new perspective that the best pain management practice is an integrated one that combines analgesic medications with nonpharmacological adjuvants, careful nursing care, and patient participation. The goal of the theory is to achieve a more holistic relief outcome than analgesia alone, that is, to balance greater pain relief with fewer side effects of opioids by using the principles.

## SCOPE

The scope for the theory is fairly narrow, encompassing acute postoperative pain or trauma in hospitalized adults. The assumptions of the theory are presented in Box 4.2. They are fairly narrow so that prescriptions can be specific. The theorists meant the theory to be used clinically and tested in adults who have moderate-to-severe acute pain after surgery or trauma. The theory has limits; it does not address the treatment of pain in children, elders, or those with special kinds of acute pain. However, middle range theories have been or can be developed for these phenomena as well.

## PROPOSITIONS

The theory has three prescriptive propositions that can be summarized as follows: In acute pain, (1) multimodal interventions, (2) attentive care, and (3) patient participation are needed for a balance between analgesia and side effects.

The first proposition is about multimodal intervention. It proposes that nurses use potent pain medication plus pharmacological and non-pharmacological adjuvants to achieve a balance between analgesia and side effects. A multimodal effect on pain has been empirically supported. This research support was published by the Acute Pain Management Guideline Panel (1992) and also by Good and colleagues (1999, 2010).

The second proposition is about attentive care. It proposes that nurses assess, intervene, reassess, and reintervene to achieve a balance between analgesia and side effects. The effect on pain is supported by 30 years of research showing that pain is inadequately treated and by findings that regular assessment alone does not produce relief (Good, Auvil-Novak, & Group, 1994). Intervention, followed by reassessment after a strategic interval, and, if necessary, reintervention are needed. Reintervention can involve increasing the dose of analgesic, adding an adjuvant, or both, and reintervention should continue until a satisfactory balance is attained (Good & Moore, 1996).

The third proposition is about patient participation. It proposes that patient teaching and goal setting contribute to a balance between analgesia and side effects (see Fig. 4.1). This proposition is supported by meta-analyses for patient teaching (Devine, 1992; Devine & Cook, 1986; Lovell et al., 2014; Shuldham, 1999). The idea of goal setting for pain management is supported by the expert opinion of the Acute Pain Management Guideline Panel (1992). Patient teaching is a key concept to consider when trying to improve outcomes. It should include ways to obtain medication, report pain, and use a nonpharmacological adjuvant.

## Applications of the Theory

The theory is useful for clinical nursing practice and also for clinical intervention research. Well-designed intervention studies are called randomized controlled trials (RCTs). The theory is useful in alert adult populations in which acute pain following surgery is incompletely controlled by medication alone, and side effects may prevent increasing analgesic medication. The theory has been adopted by postsurgical nursing units as the basis for their postoperative pain management program. It has been used many times to teach graduate nursing students the usefulness and composition of a focused, concrete nursing theory. It can also be used to teach acute pain management to undergraduate students, using the three principles (multimodal interventions, attentive care, and patient participation), along with instruction on current pain management guidelines. Valid and reliable assessment of pain is necessary both for research and more importantly for providing effective pain relief. A number of instruments have been developed to assess different pain experiences and pain in different populations. Table 4.2 is a sample of some of the most commonly used pain assessment instruments.

| Table 4.2 | Instruments to Measure Pain | |
| --- | --- | --- |
| **Category** | **Abbreviation** | **Name of Scale and Citation** |
| Pain | VAS | Visual Analogue Scale[a] |
| Sensory pain | — | VAS Sensation of Pain Scale[a] |
| Sensory pain | — | Numeric Pain Intensity Scale[b] |
| Sensory pain | — | Descriptive Pain Intensity Scale[b] |
| Affective pain | — | VAS Distress of Pain Scale[a] |
| Affective pain | — | Numeric Pain Distress Scale[b] |
| Affective pain | — | Descriptive Pain Distress Scale[b] |
| Affective pain | — | VAS Unpleasantness Scale[c] |
| Affective pain | — | VAS Anxiety of Pain Scale[d] |
| Affective pain | MPQ | McGill Pain Questionnaire[e] |
| Total pain | MPQ-PRI | Pain Rating Index (PRI) |
| Sensory pain | PRI-sensory | Sensory subscale |
| Affective pain | PRI-affective | Affective subscale |
| Pain intensity | MPQ-NWC | Number of Words Chosen |
| Pain intensity | MPQ-PPI | Present Pain Index |
| Pain intensity | MPQ-VAS | Visual Analogue Scale |
| Total, sensory, and affective pain | MPQ-SF | McGill Pain Questionnaire: Short Form[f] |
| Chronic pain | UAB | University of Alabama–Birmingham Pain Behavior Scale[g] |
| Chronic pain | WHYMPI | West Haven–Yale Multidimensional Pain Inventory[h] |
| Cancer pain | BPI | Brief Pain Inventory[i] |
| Cancer pain, relief, mood | MPAC | Memorial Pain Assessment Card[j] |
| 24-h time–intensity | — | Keele's Pain Chart[k] |
| Labor pain | — | Behavioral Index for Assessment of Labor Pain[l] |
| Children's pain | — | Poker Chip Scale[b] |
| Children's pain | — | Word-Graphic Rating Scale[b] |
| Children's pain | — | Oucher Scale[m] |
| Children's pain | — | Wong-Baker FACES Scale[n] |
| Young children's pain | FLACC | Faces, Legs, Activity, Cry, Consolability[o] |

—, No abbreviation.
[a]Good et al. (2001), [b]Acute Pain Management Guideline Panel (1992), [c]Price et al. (1983), [d]McCormack, Horne, and Sheather (1988), [e]Melzack (1975), [f]Melzack (1975), [g]Richards, Nepomuceno, Riles, and Suer (1982), [h]Kerns, Turk, and Rudy (1985), [i]Daut, Cleeland, and Flanery (1983), [j]Fishman et al. (1987), [k]Keele (1948), [l]Bonnel and Boureau (1985), [m]Beyer, Denyes, and Villarruel (1992), [n]Wong and Baker (1988), [o]Merkel, Voepel-Lewis, Shayevitz, and Malviya (1997).

## RESEARCH SUPPORT FOR THE THEORY

The first proposition of the theory has been partially tested. There have been many studies that have found that nonpharmacological adjuvants to analgesics were effective for acute pain. In this section, research support for the following nonpharmacological interventions will be discussed: relaxation, music, massage, and cold therapy. The third proposition has been also been partially tested: patient teaching for pain management. There have been no studies that have tested the second proposition of reassessment and reintervention and no studies that have studied the entire theory.

### Relaxation

Relaxation may be a way to increase patients' participation in their own pain management. An integrated review of relaxation interventions for pain showed they were effective in 8 of the 15 eligible studies. Support was found for (a) progressive muscle relaxation, studied mainly in people with arthritis, (b) jaw relaxation, and (c) systematic relaxation, studied in postoperative pain. The reviewers concluded that more research is needed to confirm the positive findings for these three techniques (Kwekkeboom & Gretarsdottir, 2006). Two RCTs of major abdominal surgical patients showed that jaw relaxation alone (Good et al., 1999) and jaw relaxation combined with soft music resulted in less pain, at both ambulation and rest, during the first 2 postoperative days compared to a control group (Good et al., 2010). Jaw relaxation with music had no effect on salivary cortisol, a measure of stress (Good et al., 1999, 2013). Others studied older patients after abdominal surgery and found that systematic relaxation reduced pain and analgesic use (Rejeh, Heravi-Karimooi, Vaismoradi, & Jasper, 2013). Still others tested jaw relaxation alone in burn patients during dressing changes, but found no effect (Rafii, Mohammadi-Fakhar, & Jamshidi Orak, 2014). Other researchers studied relaxation in patients undergoing upper abdominal surgery to manage the increased pain from the motion of the diaphragm (Topcu & Findik, 2012).

In labor patients, a Cochrane review found that relaxation, yoga, and music may have a role with reducing pain, and increasing satisfaction with pain relief, although the quality of evidence was low (Smith et al., 2018). Future studies should be undertaken to provide a better quality of evidence (Reis, 2012). Benson's relaxation technique reduced pain in women following cesarean section in a pre- and posttest design study (Solehati & Rustina, 2015). Benson's technique was also effective with hemodialysis patients in a randomized 8-week study. The relaxation group had less pain at 8 weeks (Rambod, Sharif, Pourali-Mohammadi, Pasyar, & Raffi, 2014). Relaxation techniques have been shown to give patients more options and more relief than do analgesics alone.

### Music

Music is the most frequently studied nonpharmacological adjuvant for pain management. Many published reviews, meta-analyses, and Cochrane systematic reviews of music for pain were found. Music was effective for postoperative pain (Cepeda, Carr, Lau, & Alvarez, 2006; Hung, Liu, Tsai, & Lin, 2018; Kuhlmann et al., 2018; Song et al., 2018). Music also reduced pain in hospitalized and in critically ill patients (Chlan & Halm, 2013; Cole & LoBiondo-Wood, 2014), and in people with acute, chronic, and cancer pain (Garza-Villarreal, Pando, Vuust, & Parsons, 2017; Huang & Good, 2013; Hung et al., 2018; Lee, 2016; Tsai et al., 2014). Although studies have shown that music is not effective at all times or for all patients, the reviewers conclude that in a variety of medical and surgical conditions, music reduced pain—and the size of the reduction was usually small to medium. The largest individual study was by Good et al. (2010); music combined with relaxation was effective for postoperative pain in three of five testing times in 517 abdominal surgical patients. Reviewers report that the analgesic effect of music appears higher with self-chosen over researcher-chosen music (Garza-Villarreal et al., 2017).

Music is available, safe, inexpensive, and acceptable to many patients, does not add side effects, and in most cases improves patient satisfaction (Gelinas, Arbour, Michaud, Robar, & Côté, 2013). Music should not be used in place of analgesic medication, but adds relief when used along with it. Nevertheless, the many studies supporting the effectiveness of music for pain can only partly inform nurses about whether individual patients should try it (Holden & Holden, 2013). The nurse should always ask patients first whether they would like to try listening to some music for distraction or relaxation along with their pain medication (Chlan & Halm, 2013). Music selections chosen by the patient are often best, because people are more likely to listen to and respond to something they like. On the other hand, some people do not care for music and some do not want to listen to music when they are ill. Some may want to listen to music for other reasons than pain. The reasons offered by people with chronic pain were to gain control over pain; to relieve tension, anxiety, boredom, and loneliness; and to engender thankfulness (Holden & Holden, 2013). For patients who wish to listen to music, nurses should accept that music affects pain and persons differently and that some patients have good relief during the time they are listening to music and some have only a little relief.

### Massage

Studies of the use of massage for pain have provided support for the nonpharmacological part of the first proposition. Following early small studies that suggested that massage therapy could relieve pain, researchers conducted a multisite RCT with patients having advanced cancer. Massage resulted in less pain and better mood in the immediate term (Kutner et al., 2008). A later RCT of patients with metastatic bone pain showed that massage resulted in a significant reduction in pain and that the effects on relaxation were sustained for hours (Jane et al., 2011). In patients who have had coronary artery bypass graft surgery, massage therapy was given by the patient's companion, who was trained by a nurse. In the massage group, pain intensity decreased at all four time points after the intervention, while it did not in the control group (Najafi et al., 2014). In two other studies, massage also had positive results on pain. Foot massage along with analgesic medication provided pain relief immediately after breast surgery, compared to those who received analgesics alone (Ucuzal & Kanan, 2014). In a Veterans Administration hospital, those who received massage as part of their care had pain decreases in the immediate term (Mitchinson, Fletcher, Kim, Montagnini, & Hinshaw, 2014).

Massage therapy is increasingly offered to hospitalized patients for pain and other symptoms. A decade of massage therapy services at a large tertiary medical center was summarized to show the way it developed from early pilot studies to the current program (Rodgers et al., 2014). Two recent meta-analyses found that massage therapy significantly reduced pain after surgery (Kukimoto, Ooe, & Ideguchi, 2017) and in critically ill post–thoracic surgery patients (Boitor, Gelinas, Richard-Lalonde, & Thombs, 2017). However, although patient risk in massage therapies is low, this intervention is not completely without risk (Yin, Gao, Wu, Litscher, & Xu, 2014). There are a variety of types of massage; the clinician is advised to consider the patient's condition and the potential risk and to also be familiar with the technique, preferably in collaboration with a massage therapist.

## Cold

Cold therapy is the oldest analgesic that is still being used clinically. Studies of the use of cold provided initial partial support for the first proposition. Since the advent of easy-to-use cold packs, recent studies have tested the use of cold in innovative ways. One group of researchers found that a cold gel pack reduced the pain associated with coughing and deep breathing following cardiac surgery (Khalkhali et al., 2014). Other researchers found that during chest tube removal, using cold packs around the wound prior to the procedure reduced pain of chest tube removal (Gorji, Nesami, Ayyasi, Ghafari, & Yazdani, 2014; Yarahmadi, Mohammadi, Ardalan, Najafizadeh, & Gholami, 2018). Third, in labor patients, cold packs were applied over the abdomen and back for 10 minutes every half hour during the first phase of labor. Cold packs were also applied over the perineum

for 5 minutes every 15 minutes during the second phase. They found that pain was less in the group that received cold therapy during all parts of active phase and the second stage. In addition, the duration of all phases of labor was shorter in the cold therapy group (Shirvani & Ganji, 2014). A fourth group of researchers found that during tonsillectomy, the intraoperative cooling of the excised area with cold saline reduced postoperative pain during the first 10 days (Shin, Byun, Baek, & Lee, 2014). Principles, techniques, and nursing care involved in cold therapy can be found in McDowell, McFarland, and Nalli (1994). Box 4.3 provides a summary of some of the research that has tested the effectiveness of nonpharmacological adjuvants on pain.

### Extension of the Theory

The portion of the theory regarding the effect of nonpharmacological interventions on pain has been extended to other populations, because of research support. For example, music has reduced chronic pain (Siedlecki & Good, 2006), labor pain (Phumdoung & Good, 2003), arthritis pain (McCaffrey & Freeman, 2003), pain of bone marrow aspiration (Shabanloei, Golchin, Esfahani, Dolatkhah, & Rasoulian, 2010), pain of burn dressing changes (Tan, Yowler, Super, & Fratianne, 2010), and cancer pain (Chiang, 2011; Huang, Good, & Zausniewski, 2010). Also, guided imagery has reduced chronic pain (Lewandowski, 2004), and back massage reduced back pain after abdominal surgery in Asian patients who remain on bed rest after surgery but had no effect on incisional pain (Chin, 1999).

### Patient Teaching

Studies of patient teaching specifically for acute pain management have shown very little support for that part of the third proposition. Patient teaching for pain management after surgery potentially informs and empowers patients by increasing their knowledge and self-efficacy for engaging in postoperative care activities and using their PCA. However, in two studies, brief interventions for PCA use had no effect on pain, whether delivered by pamphlet (Chumbley, Ward, Hall, & Salmon, 2004), anesthetists' teaching and demonstration (Lam, Chan, Chen, & Ngan Kee, 2001), or video (Ihedioha, Vaughan, Mastermann, Singh, & Chaudhri, 2013). A RCT also found that a 5-minute audiotaped teaching intervention for pain management had no effect on pain after abdominal surgery (Good et al., 2010). It taught

| BOX 4.3 | **Examples of Nonpharmacologic Adjuvants Used in Practice** |
|---|---|

Nurses' use of relaxation for postoperative pain, which includes general instructions and specific relaxation techniques, is described in Good (1995b). The empirically tested jaw relaxation technique is included, because it is easy for patients to remember after surgery. When recorded on an audiotape, soft relaxing music could be added. More recently, nurses' use of relaxation for pain management in nursing practice was carefully described by Schaffer and Yucha (2004). They provide a sample of a full-body relaxation script that nurses can read to patients or record on an audiotape for the patient to use independently. They also review the empirical literature that supports the use of relaxation techniques for pain and provide two clinical case studies that illustrate the use of relaxation for neck, back, and headache pain.

Nurses' use of soft music to ease the pain of clinical patients is based on nursing studies in postoperative patients and in patients with the pain of labor, osteoarthritis, cancer, and chronic pain. Based on Nightingale's framework, McCaffrey (2008) discussed nurses' use of music as a healing environment for older adults having surgical, arthritis, and other kinds of pain. She recommends that nurses be given educational sessions to understand the use of music as an intervention in various settings. She encourages assessing preferences, offering a variety of types of music for patients to choose from, using iPods with downloaded music, and bringing music from home, and she lists some composers and CDs that have been used in her studies. Others describe the use of music for labor pain, recommending that women be advised during prenatal childbirth classes of the efficacy of music for pain and relaxation (Zwelling, Johnson, & Allen, 2006). Music should be chosen and obtained in advance, and women should bring their own playing equipment, if it is not available in the hospital. Zwelling et al. (2006) give recommendations for use of complementary therapies in general, including educating the labor and delivery nurses in their use.

The third principle of the theory is that patient teaching and goal setting contribute to balance between analgesia and side effects. Nurses at the bedside can use current guidelines to teach patients to manage pain pharmacologically (McCaffery & Pasero, 1999). An example of a patient and family information sheet for patient-controlled analgesia (PCA) can be found at http://www.greenhosp.org/pe_pdf/pain_PCA.pdf. Setting goals with patients is described in detail by Pasero and McCaffery (2003, 2004). Teaching patients to use a pain rating scale is the first step, and the next step is establishing a comfort–function goal. Examples of comfort–function goals for postoperative patients are given in Pasero and McCaffery (2003). The goal should be documented on the chart, close to the pain scores; if the goal is not met, the pain rating should be addressed with interventions to relieve it. Nurses should consider whether an analgesic can be given or whether to use the range of doses ordered by the physician, call the physician for further orders, and/or add a nonpharmacological therapy. The nurses should then reassess pain and side effects at a time when they are expected to be effective and reintervene if necessary. The health care team's achievement of the comfort–function goals should be monitored in quality improvement plans. Nurses can help patients establish realistic comfort–function goals and should discuss them during shift report and rounds. Pasero and McCaffery (2004) emphasize that pain assessment does not necessarily mean pain relief.

patients to reduce fears of opioid dependency, to use their PCA system, and to tell their nurse about their pain until relief was obtained. Another group of researchers added preemptive analgesia to preoperative teaching for thoracotomy patients, and they did find improvements in pain and analgesia intake. However, it is not clear whether the result was due to the pre-emptive analgesia rather than the patient teaching (Kol, Alpar, & Erdogan, 2014). Each of these investigators used different teaching methods and content. Thus, an effective teaching intervention for patient involvement in their *acute pain* management has not yet been tested. However, a meta-analysis of patient education for cancer pain may provide some direction for teaching patients with acute pain. Optimal strategies included those that were patient-centered and tailored to individual needs, as part of therapeutic relationships (Lovell et al., 2014), in contrast to pamphlets, audiotapes, and videotapes used in acute pain studies.

## SUGGESTIONS FOR ADDITIONAL RESEARCH

The time has come to conduct studies that translate the use of some of these interventions to nursing practice. Studies are particularly needed for postoperative pain, chronic pain, and pain of labor osteoarthritis and cancer. Studies of massage, cold, and patient teaching need further development and testing. In addition, nurses need to study methods of pain management that are relevant in other cultures and countries around the world (Rosa, 2018).

### Relaxation

More studies of jaw relaxation and systematic relaxation are needed following surgery. They need to continue to be tested in various age groups and surgeries and in various countries and cultures, both at ambulation and rest. The whole-body systematic relaxation technique described in Roykulcharoen and Good (2004) should be tested in a replication study and then compared after surgery to jaw relaxation (Good et al., 1999). More research on relaxation is needed in laboring patients to confirm the studies reported here.

Culturally congruent relaxation scripts and voices can be developed and used in practice and research. An excellent example can be obtained from Dr. Josepha Campinha-Bacote, a Cape Verdean transcultural nurse who is an expert on ethnomusic therapy and culturally competent nursing care. She, an African American jazz musician, and her husband developed a tape entitled "Culturally Specific Africentric Relaxation Exercise," which is accompanied by music that is congruent with the African American culture. Nurses could develop such tapes for other cultural and ethnic groups by incorporating principles of ethnomusicology and music therapy.

### Music

Music should continue to be tested and replicated in various painful conditions, such as chronic pain, cancer pain, and procedural pain. Choices of music that are culturally and age appropriate should be offered. Individual studies should be developed in other countries. This work has begun with doctoral graduates who have developed Korean (Good & Ahn, 2008) and Taiwanese music tapes (Chiang, 2011; Huang et al., 2010) to appeal to patients in those countries. Studies are needed to compare slow, sedative music for pain with music with faster tempos. Studies are also needed to compare the effects of different musical instruments or to compare music with lyrics to music without lyrics; these may be influenced by the culture of the participants. Cultural preferences in music for pain need to be studied in the many countries and cultures in the world. Practicing nurses need to become aware of the cultural preferences in their patient populations.

### Massage

There needs to be replication of the initial massage studies for acute pain that were reported earlier in this chapter. In addition, qualitative studies are needed to describe variations in patient reaction to massage. Studies of hand and foot massage for pain in other parts of the body are needed. Various types of massage that are appropriate for a patient condition can be compared for their effectiveness and acceptability to patients. See Harris (2014) for descriptions of types of massage.

### Cold

Replication is needed to support the findings of the studies reported earlier in this chapter. In addition, new ways of using cold can be developed and tested. The new ways would need to be appropriate to the patient condition and should be used in accord with institutional procedures for the use of cold.

### Attentive Care

Attentive care could be studied by using a record review. Researchers could track the actions of nurses who are required to record pain care that includes intervention, reassessment, and reintervention until relief is obtained. Data collection would also include the use of range doses and adjuvant nonpharmacological methods of pain relief and calling the doctor if necessary. This research would describe the extent to which the second proposition is used in practice.

### Patient Teaching and Goal Setting

New methods of patient teaching for use of PCA for postoperative pain need to be developed. The most promising teaching interventions should be tested in research. Setting comfort–function goals could be compared to usual care. Comfort–function goals are discussed by Pasero and McCaffery (2004). Methods to test patient teaching use of adjuvant nonpharmacological methods are also needed. Researchers can use the pain scales listed in Table 4.2. In addition, Box 4.4, Using Middle Range Theory in Research, provides an example of a study designed to further test the theory.

## Use of the Theory in Practice

Nurses have written to the author saying that they use the theory as a basis of practice on their

## USING MIDDLE RANGE THEORY IN RESEARCH    4.4

*Source: Sng, Q. W., Taylor, B., Liam, J. L. W., Klainin-Yobas, P., Wang, W., & He, H. (2013). Postoperative pain management experiences among school-aged children: A qualitative study. Journal of Clinical Nursing, 22, 958–968. doi: 10.1111/jocn.12052*

### PURPOSE/RESEARCH QUESTION

The purpose of the study was to explore the postoperative pain experience of school-aged children.

### RESEARCH DESIGN

Qualitative (phenomenological)

### SAMPLE/PARTICIPANTS

Fifteen children, aged 6 to 12 years old, admitted to pediatric surgical units in a tertiary, public hospital in Singapore. For inclusion, the child's surgery needed to require a minimum of more than 24-hour postoperative hospitalization. They also needed to be considered stable postoperatively.

### DATA COLLECTION

The children were interviewed using a semistructured format, using a guide based on previous research. Each interview took approximately 10 minutes and was audiotaped.

### FINDINGS

Four themes emerged:

1. Children's self-directed actions to relieve pain postoperatively: (a) cognitive behavioral methods, for example, distraction; (b) physical methods, for example, positioning; (c) seeking help from others, for example, informing parents; and (d) pain medication
2. Children's perceptions of parents' actions to relieve their pain: (a) assessing their pain; (b) giving pain medication; (c) using cognitive behavioral methods, for example, distraction; (d) using physical methods, for example, massage; and (e) using emotional support strategies, for example, reassuring words and touch
3. Children's perceptions of nurses' actions to relieve their pain: (a) administering medication; (b) using cognitive behavioral methods, for example, distraction; (c) using emotional support strategies, for example, reassurance; and (d) helping with activities of daily living
4. Suggestions for parents for alleviating postoperative pain: (a) using distraction and (b) being present
5. Suggestions for nurses for alleviating postoperative pain: (a) administering medication, (b) using distraction, and positioning

The researchers concluded that "it is important for health care professionals to value children's roles in their postoperative pain management" (p. 966).

postoperative unit. However, examples of use of the entire theory were not found in the literature. There are articles that describe how nurses use parts of the theory, that is, complementary therapies in addition to analgesics, and patient teaching and goal setting for pain relief. An excellent resource is Complementary & Alternative Therapies in Nursing by Lindquist, Snyder, and Tracy (2014). For an example of use of the theory, see Box 4.5, Using Middle Range Theory in Practice, which provides a detailed description of a specific adjuvant used in practice to promote pain relief.

It would be ideal if an entire postoperative nursing unit would implement the complete theory in caring for their patients. They could first assign readings from this chapter and then hold educational sessions for the nursing staff on pain management, the theory, and the advantages of using evidence-based theories and interventions. In these sessions, nurses could discuss the concepts of the theory and learn what could be offered in terms of analgesics (American Pain Society, 2008) and range orders (Gordon et al., 2004), nonpharmacological adjuvants, patient teaching, and goal setting. They could discuss the day-to-day relief goals and comfort–function goals that they think would be realistic on their unit as patients recover. They could discuss the meaning of attentive care (e.g., intervention, reassessment, and reintervention, until a comfort–function goal is met) (Pasero & McCaffery, 2003, 2004). Since Good et al. (2010) found that an audiotaped patient teaching for pain management intervention was not effective

## USING MIDDLE RANGE THEORY IN PRACTICE | 4.5

*Source: Schaffer, S. D., & Yucha, C. B. (2004). Relaxation and pain management. American Journal of Nursing, 104(8), 75–82.*

### PROBLEM

Analgesics have not consistently provided adequate relief of acute and chronic moderate-to-severe pain nor to related symptoms, such as restlessness, irritability, muscle tension, difficulty concentrating, and sleep problems.

### NURSING INTERVENTION

Relaxation can be taught as an adjuvant to the administration of analgesics. Before teaching a relaxation technique, nurses assess the patient and establish rapport. Teaching is most effective with those patients in mild to moderate pain who have already used nonpharmacological methods and are interested and able to learn a new skill. It should be explained that relaxation is not a substitute for analgesic medications but just a means of enhancing them.

Patients should wear loose, comfortable clothing, be in a comfortable bodily position, and be in a comfortable environment with privacy, dim lighting, and the absence of distractions. The relaxation technique chosen should take into consideration patient preference, provider competency, and relevant contraindications of the method.

Give directions calmly and slowly, using short sentences. Begin by having the patient assume a relaxed body position with body in alignment, properly supported with eyes closed and mouth relaxed and slightly opened. Proceed to teach either breathing techniques or muscle relaxation techniques as a means of promoting relaxation. The techniques can be taught in as little as 15 minutes. For optimal results, the patient should practice the relaxation techniques for 10 minutes twice daily.

---

for pain reduction, nurses on the unit should employ patient-centered strategies that are tailored to individual needs and are part of a therapeutic relationship to teach patients to use their PCA effectively (Lovell et al., 2014; McCaffery & Pasero, 1999).

To use relaxation or music clinically, nurses would need to secure a small amount of funding to provide a modest library on the unit containing relaxation exercises, music, and guided imagery on audiotapes, compact discs, or iPods. It is important to use equipment for playing that could be easily used by the patients. Practice information on using a relaxation intervention can be found in Good (1995b), and information on using a music intervention for pain can be found in Good et al. (2000). Practitioners can use the Numeric Pain Intensity Scale (Table 4.2) to measure pain regularly in adults and any of the children's pain scales that are age appropriate.

Using massage in nursing practice requires knowledge of the patient's condition and avoidance of massaging areas of the body that are likely to be harmed by pressure and motion on the skin. Precautions are discussed in Harris (2014, pp. 263–264). Precautions taken in research with patients following breast surgery can be found in the inclusion and exclusion criteria and the data collection sections in the study by Ucuzal and Kanan (2014, p. 260). These nurse researchers also consulted a massage therapist to train them

in the technique. In nursing practice, consultation with a massage therapist is recommended until nurses on the unit learn the technique and become proficient.

Using cold therapies in nursing practice also requires knowledge of the patient's condition and collaboration with the physician to determine appropriate use. Cold packs are sometimes ordered following some surgeries. For example, following a herniorrhaphy, dental surgery, or a fracture, a cold pack may be ordered for a day or 2 to reduce swelling and pain in the operative site. It is important to use the cold pack in an intermittent manner, so that the tissues do not become too cold. In Table 4.3, there are examples of research evidence to support the use of the theory in the relief of pain.

Using attentive care and intervening until pain is relieved have been incorporated into practice better today than it was 22 years ago when the theory was first published. Today, there is greater attention to pain relief in the United States, due to increased research and improved requirements of the Joint Commission. Nevertheless, nurse educators must continue to teach this principle to students. Nursing educators and administrators in hospitals in which attentive care for pain is not practiced may want to provide some in-service education on pain management and study whether nurses improve in knowledge and in their practice with patients in pain.

**Table 4.3  Examples of Research for Application to Practice**

| Reference | Research Design/Meta-Analysis | Clinical Issue/Research Question | Sample (n)/Participants | Intervention | Outcome |
|---|---|---|---|---|---|
| Gonzales, E. A., Ledesma, R. J. A., Perry, S. M., Dyer, C. A., & Maye, J. P. (2010). Effects of guided imagery on postoperative outcomes in patients undergoing same-day surgical procedures: A randomized, single-blind study. *American Association of Nurse Anesthetists Journal, 78*(3), 181–188 | Randomized, single-blinded, quasi-experimental | To evaluate the effects of guided imagery on postoperative outcomes of patients undergoing same-day surgical procedures | 44 adults (18–71 years old) receiving head or neck surgical procedures. Randomly assigned to one of two groups | Both groups experienced 28 min of privacy with only the treatment group listening to a guided imagery compact disc | The guided imagery group reported significantly less anxiety and pain and left the PACU on average 9 min sooner than did the control group. There were no statistically significant differences in the use of narcotics or satisfaction with the experience |
| Hong, S.-J., & Lee, E. (2012). Effects of structured educational programme of patient-controlled analgesia (PCA) for gynaecological patients in South Korea. *Journal of Clinical Nursing, 21*(23/24), 3546–3555. doi: 10.1111/j.1365-2702.2011.04032.x | A nonequivalent control group, nonsynchronized design | To determine the effects of systematic preoperative education for gynecological patients | 79 patients undergoing gynecological surgery under general anesthesia, 39 in experimental treatment group and 40 in control group | The treatment group received an educational brochure and CD on the use of the PCA, how it is attached to the patient, analgesics and medications used in PCA and their effects, advantages and disadvantages of the PCA, and the lockout period. Education was provided the day before surgery on the unit by the nurse researcher | Pain level and adverse reactions were significantly less for the treatment group. The analgesic dose used and the level of satisfaction with pain control were higher in the treatment group |
| Kwan, M., & Seah, A. S. T. (2013). Music therapy as a non-pharmacological adjunct to pain management: Experiences at an acute hospital in Singapore. *Progress in Palliative Care, 21*(3), 151–157. doi: 10.1179/43291X12Y0000000042 | Descriptive, prospective | To determine the effect of music therapy in the management of pain in patients in an acute care hospital | 44 adult patients (ages 26–92) referred to music therapy for pain management. 37 agreed to participate | Pain assessment was completed as well as patients' needs and strengths, interest, and prior musical experiences before beginning therapy. During therapy, patients were asked to describe their pain through a musical instrument and to work with this pain "sound." Comfort music and relaxation approaches were used based on patients' conditions during the session | Numerical rating of pain intensity decreased following the music therapy session. Responses to open-ended questions following the session revealed a routinely positive experience |
| Rejeh, N., Heravi-Karimmoi, M., Vaismoradi, M., & Jasper, M. (2013). Effects of systematic relaxation techniques on anxiety and pain in older patients undergoing abdominal surgery. *International Journey of Nursing Practice, 19*, 426–470. doi: 10.1111/ijn.12088 | Randomized controlled trial | To investigate the effects of relaxation techniques on pain and anxiety on older patients following elective abdominal surgery | 124 older patients undergoing elective abdominal surgery: 62 in experimental treatment group and 62 in control group | Were provided with information about their surgery and postsurgical protocols. The treatment group was given an audiotape on relaxation exercises, their techniques, importance, and benefits. VAS scales and level of analgesics used were collected on both groups | Experimental/treatment group experienced less pain and anxiety than did the control group. In addition, there was a statistically significant difference in milligrams of morphine used, the treatment group using less |
| Taverner, T., & Prince, J. (2014). Nurse screening for neuropathic pain in postoperative patients. *British Journal of Nursing, 23*(2), 76–80 | Retrospective chart audit | To determine the rate nurses complete patient screening for neuropathic pain signs | 150 charts per unit from three surgical units | Nurses were instructed on the use of the 7-item DN4 for neuropathic pain and how to assess for allodynia (hypersensitivity to touch). Assessments were to be completed every 12 h following surgery | 94% of the audited charts included nurse screening and documentation of neuropathic pain |

# Summary

■ Pain is a universal human experience that has been known since the first human experienced illness, trauma, or labor.

■ Although pain has been studied descriptively for more than a century, it has only recently been studied from a prescriptive nursing perspective.

■ The middle range prescriptive pain management theory of a balance between analgesic and side effects reflects the nursing mission to intervene effectively and holistically to relieve pain and suffering and to prevent their long-term effects.

■ There is increasing empirical support, and nurse researchers can continue to test and to provide support and creative extensions of the theory.

■ Practicing nurses are using the evidence-based principles for effective relief of acute pain in their patients.

## CRITICAL THINKING EXERCISES

1. Compare two scenarios or scripts for nurses and patients engaging in mutual goal setting for pain management after a specific surgical procedure. With peers, analyze each for advantages and disadvantages to the patient and to those who provide care.

2. Analyze the trajectory of patients undergoing a specific surgical procedure and the places they receive nursing care, from the surgeon's office and the decision for surgery, through the pre- and postoperative hospitalization, to recovery at home. Plan the most effective times, amounts of information, and ways nurses can introduce and reinforce the elements of patient teaching for pain management. *The elements are to encourage attitudes, expectations, and actions in reporting pain, obtaining medication, preventing pain during activity, and using complementary therapies.* Describe ways by which this nursing care, delivered in several places, could be streamlined and coordinated with the surgeon's patient teaching.

3. Envision yourself as a leader who is introducing this nursing theory as the basis of postoperative pain management on your unit. Create introductory scripts with arguments for its usefulness to be delivered to the nursing and medical staff. Describe how you would begin to demonstrate its usefulness. Explain your method of presenting its current evidence base. Give the main points of a clinically useable protocol for your unit.

## ACKNOWLEDGMENTS

This chapter was supported in part by the National Institute of Nursing Research (NINR) Grant Number R01 NR3933 (1994–2005), to M. Good, PhD, Principal Investigator, and by the General Clinical Research Center, Case Western Reserve University.

## REFERENCES

Acute Pain Management Guideline Panel. (1992). Acute pain management: Operative or medical procedures and trauma. In: *Clinical practice guideline* (Vol. AHCPR No. 92–0032). Rockville, MD: Agency for Health Care Policy and Research, Public Health Service, U.S. Department of Health and Human Services. Retrieved January 16, 2007 from http://www.ncbi.nlm.nih.gov/books/bv.fcgi?rid=hstat6.chapter.8991

American Pain Society. (2008). *Principles of analgesic use in the treatment of acute pain and cancer pain* (6th ed.). Skokie, IL: Author.

American Pain Society Quality of Care Task Force. (2005). American Pain Society Recommendations for improving the quality of acute and cancer pain management. *Archives of Internal Medicine, 165,* 1574–1580.

American Society of Anesthesiologists Task Force on Acute Pain Management. (2012). Practice guidelines for acute pain management in the perioperative setting: An updated report by the American Society of Anesthesiologists Task Force on Acute Pain Management. *Anesthesiology, 116,* 248–273.

Beecher, H. K. (1959). *Measurement of subjective responses: Quantitative effects of drugs.* New York, NY: Oxford University Press.

Beyer, J. E., Denyes, M. J., & Villarruel, A. M. (1992). The creation, validation, and continuing development of the Oucher: A measure of pain intensity in children. *Journal of Pediatric Nursing, 7*(5), 335–346.

Boitor, M., Gelinas, C., Richard-Lalonde, M., & Thombs, B. D. (2017). The effect of massage on acute postoperative pain in critically and acutely ill adults post-thoracic surgery: Systematic review and meta-analysis of randomized controlled trials. *Heart and Lung, 46*(5), 339–346.

Bonnel, A. M., & Boureau, F. (1985). Labor pain assessment: Validity of a behavioral index. *Pain, 22*(1), 81.

Campinha-Bacote, J. (1993). Soul therapy: Humor and music with African-American clients. *Journal of Christian Nursing, 10*(2), 23–26.

Campinha-Bacote, J., & Allbright, R. J. (1992). Ethnomusic therapy and the dually-diagnosed African American client. *Holistic Nursing Practice, 6*(3), 59–63.

Campinha-Bacote, J., Campinha-Bacote, D., & Allbright, R. J. (1992). *C.A.R.E. I (Culturally-specific Africentric Relaxation Exercise).* A culturally specific relaxation audio cassette. This tape is based on Africentric & Ethnomusic Therapy principles (flute and narrative composition arranged by J. Campinha-Bacote). Contact Dr. Campinha-Bacote at 11108 Huntwicke Place, Cincinnati, OH 45241.

Casey, K. L., & Melzack, R. (1967). Neural mechanisms of pain: A conceptual model. In E. L. Way (Ed.), *New concepts in pain and its clinical management* (pp. 13–31). Philadelphia, PA: F. A. Davis.

Cepeda, M. S., Carr, D. B., Lau, J., & Alvarez, H. (2006). Music for pain relief. *Cochrane Database Systematic Review,* (2), CD004843.

Chiang, L.-C. (2011). Effects of music and nature sounds on pain and anxiety in hospice patients (Unpublished doctoral dissertation). Cleveland, OH: Case Western Reserve University.

Chin, C.-C. (1999). Effects of back massage on surgical stress responses and postoperative pain (Unpublished doctoral dissertation). Cleveland, OH: Case Western Reserve University.

Chlan, L., & Halm, M. A. (2013). Does music ease pain and anxiety in the critically ill? *American Journal of Critical Care, 22*(6), 528–532.

Chumbley, G. M., Ward, L., Hall, G. M., & Salmon, P. (2004). Pre-operative information and patient-controlled analgesia: Much ado about nothing. *Anaesthesia, 59*(4), 354–358.

Cole, L. C., & LoBiondo-Wood, G. (2014). Music as an adjuvant therapy in control of pain and symptoms in hospitalized adults: A systematic review. *Pain Management Nursing, 15*(1), 406–425.

Daut, R. L., Cleeland, C. S., & Flanery, R. C. (1983). Development of the Wisconsin brief pain questionnaire to assess pain in cancer and other diseases. *Pain, 17,* 197–210.

Devine, E. C. (1992). Effects of psychoeducational care for adult surgical patients: A meta-analysis of 191 studies. *Patient Education and Counseling, 19,* 129–142.

Devine, E. C., & Cook, T. D. (1986). Clinical and cost saving effects of psychoeducational interventions with surgical patients: A meta analysis. *Research in Nursing and Health, 9,* 89–105.

Dickhoff, J., & James, P. (1968). A theory of theories: A position paper. *Nursing Research, 17*(3), 197–203.

Fishman, B., Pasternak, S., Wallenstein, S. L., Houde, R. W., Holland, J. C., & Foley, K. M. (1987). The Memorial Pain Assessment Card: A valid instrument for the evaluation of cancer pain. *Cancer, 60*(5), 1151–1158.

Garza-Villarreal, E. A., Pando, V., Vuust, P., & Parsons, C. (2017). Music-induced analgesia in chronic pain conditions: A systematic review and meta-analysis. *Pain Physician, 20*(7): 597–610.

Gelinas, C., Arbour, C., Michaud, C., Robar, L., & Côté, J. (2013). Patients and ICU nurses' perspectives of non-pharmacological interventions for pain management. *Nursing in Critical Care, 18*(6), 307–318.

Gonzales, E. A., Ledesma, R. J. A., Perry, S. M., et al. (2010). Effects of guided imagery on postoperative outcomes in patients undergoing same-day procedures: A randomized, single-blind study. *American Association of Nurse Anesthetists Journal, 78*(3), 181–188.

Good, M. (1995a). A comparison of the effects of jaw relaxation and music on postoperative pain. *Nursing Research, 44*(1), 52–57.

Good, M. (1995b). Relaxation techniques for surgical patients. Complementary modalities/Part 2, Continuing education two hours. *American Journal of Nursing, 95*(5), 39–43.

Good, M. (1998). A middle range theory of acute pain management; use in research. *Nursing Outlook, 46*(3), 120–124.

Good, M., & Ahn, S. (2008). Korean and American music reduces pain in Korean women after gynecologic surgery. *Pain Management Nursing, 9*(3), 96–103.

Good, M., & Moore, S. M. (1996). Clinical practice guidelines as a new source of middle-range theory: Focus on acute pain. *Nursing Outlook, 44*(2), 74–79.

Good M., Albert J. M., Anderson G. C., et al. (2010). Supplementing relaxation and music for pain after surgery. *Nursing Research, 59*(4), 259–269.

Good, M., Albert, J. Arafah, B., et al. (2013). Effects of relaxation/music and patient teaching on salivary cortisol. *Biological Research for Nursing, 15*(3), 317–328. doi: 10.1177/1099800411431301

Good, M., Auvil-Novak, S., & Group, M. (1994). Pain and its management: One year after the guidelines. Paper presented at the AHSR & FSHR Annual Conference, June 12–14. San Diego, CA: Health Services Research.

Good, M., Picot, B., Salem, S., et al. (2000). Cultural responses to music for pain relief. *Journal of Holistic Nursing, 18*(3), 245–260.

Good, M., Seo, Y., Cong, X., & Huang, S.-T. (2004). Development and psychometric properties of the opioid side effects scale for postoperative patients [Abstract]. *The Journal of Pain, 5*(3), 77.

Good, M., Stanton-Hicks, M., Grass, J. M., et al. (1999). Relief of postoperative pain with jaw relaxation, music, and their combination. *Pain, 81*(1–2), 163–172.

Good, M., Stiller, C., Zauszniewski, J., et al. (2001). Sensation and distress of pain scales: Reliability, validity and sensitivity. *Journal of Nursing Measurement, 9*(3), 219–238.

Gordon, D. B., Dahl, J., Phillips, P., et al. (2004). The use of "as-needed" range orders for opioid analgesics in the management of acute pain: A consensus statement of the American Society for Pain Management Nursing and the American Pain Society. *Pain Management Nursing, 5*(2), 53–58.

Gorji, H. M., Nesami, B. M., Ayyasi, M., Ghafari, R., & Yazdani, J. (2014). Comparison of ice packs application and relaxation therapy in pain reduction during chest tube removal following cardiac surgery. *North American Journal of Medical Sciences, 6*(1), 19–24.

Green, E. E., Green, A. M., & Norris, P. A. (1979). Preliminary observation on a new-drug method for control of hypertension. *Journal of the South Carolina Medical Association, 75*(11), 575–582.

Harris, M. (2014). Massage. In R. Lindquist, M. Snyder, & M. F. Tracy (Eds.), *Complementary and alternative therapies in nursing* (7th ed.). New York, NY: Springer.

Holden, R., & Holden, J. (2013). Music: A better alternative than pain? *British Journal of General Practice, 63*(615), 536.

Huang, S. T., & Good, M. (2013). Listening to music as a non-invasive pain intervention. In P. Simon & T. Szabo (Eds.), *Music: Social impacts, health benefits and perspectives* (pp. 105–130). New York, NY: Nova Science Publishers.

Huang, S. T., Good, M., & Zauszniewski, J. A. (2010). The effectiveness of music in relieving pain in cancer patients: A randomized controlled trial. *International Journal of Nursing Studies, 47*(11), 1354–1362.

Hung, T. T., Liu, Y. C., Tsai, P. C., & Lin, M. F. (2018). [The pin-relief efficacy of passive music-based interventions in cancer patients undergoing diagnostic biopsies and surgery: A systematic review and meta-analysis]. *Hu Li Za Zhi 65*(1), 70–82.

Huth, M. M., & Moore, S. M. (1998). Prescriptive theory of acute pain management in infants and children. *Journal of the Society of Pediatric Nurses, 3*(1), 23–32.

Huth, M. M., Broome, M. E., & Good, M. (2004). Imagery reduces children's post-operative pain. *Pain, 110*(1–2), 439–448.

Ihedioha, U., Vaughan, S., Mastermann, J., Singh, B., & Chaudhri, S. (2013). Patient education videos for elective colorectal surgery: Results of a randomized controlled trial. *Colorectal Disease, 15*(11), 1436–1441.

Im, E. O. (2006). A situation-specific theory of Caucasian cancer patients' pain experience. *ANS. Advances in Nursing Science, 29*(3), 232–244.

Jane, S. W., Chen, S. L., Wilkie, D. J., et al. (2011). Effects of massage on pain, mood status, relaxation, and sleep in Taiwanese patients with metastatic bone pain: A randomized clinical trial. *Pain, 152*(10), 2432–2442.

Johnson, J. E., & Rice, V. H. (1974). Sensory and distress components of pain: Implications for the study of clinical pain. *Nursing Research, 23,* 203–209.

Keele, K. D. (1948). The pain chart. *Lancet, 2,* 6–8.

Kerns, R. D., Turk, D. C., & Rudy, T. E. (1985). The West Haven-Yale Multidimensional Pain Inventory (WHYMPI). *Pain, 23*(4), 345.

Khalkhali, H., Tanha, Z. E., Feizi, A., & Ardabili, S. S. (2014). Effect of applying cold gel pack on the pain associated with deep breathing and coughing after open heart surgery. *Iranian Journal of Nursing and Midwifery Research, 19*(6), 545–549.

Kol, E., Alpar, S. E., & Erdogan, A. (2014). Preoperative education and use of analgesic before onset of pain routinely for post-thoracotomy pain control can reduce pain effect and total amount of analgesics administered postoperatively. *Pain Management Nursing, 15*(1), 331–339.

Kuhlmann, A. Y. R., de Rooij, A., et al. (2018). Meta-analysis evaluating music interventions for anxiety and pain in surgery. *British Journal of Surgery, 105*(7), 773–783.

Kukimoto, Y., Ooe, N., & Ideguchi, N. (2017). The effects of massage therapy on pain and anxiety after surgery: A systematic review and meta-analysis. *Pain Management Nursing*, *18*(6), 378–390.

Kutner, J. S., Smith, M. C., Corbin, L., et al. (2008). Massage therapy versus simple touch to improve pain and mood in patients with advanced cancer: A randomized trial. *Annals of Internal Medicine*, *149*(6), 369–379.

Kwan, M., & Seah, A. S. T. (2013). Music therapy as a non-pharmacological adjunct to pain management: Experiences at an acute hospital in Singapore. *Progress in Palliative Care*, *21*(3), 151–157. doi: 10.1179/43291X12Y0000000042

Kwekkeboom, K. L., & Gretarsdottir, E. (2006). Systematic review of relaxation interventions for pain. *Journal of Nursing Scholarship*, *38*(3), 269–277.

Lam, K. K., Chan, M. T., Chen, P. P., & Ngan Kee, W. D. (2001). Structured preoperative patient education for patient-controlled analgesia. *Journal of Clinical Anesthesia*, *13*(6), 465–469.

Lee, J. H. (2016). The effects of music on pain: A meta-analysis. *Journal of Music Therapy*, *53*(4): 430–477. 1365–2168.

Lenz, E. R., Pugh, L. C., Milligan, R. A., Gift, A., & Suppe, F. (1997). The middle-range theory of unpleasant symptoms: An update. *Advances in Nursing Science*, *19*(3), 14–27.

Lewandowski, W. A. (2004). Patterning of pain and power with guided imagery. *Nursing Science Quarterly*, *17*(3), 233–241.

Lindquist, R., Snyder, M., & Tracy, M. F. (2014). *Complementary and alternative therapies in nursing* (7th ed.). New York, NY: Springer.

Locsin, R. (1988). Effects of preferred music and guided imagery music on the pain of selected postoperative patients. *ANPHI Papers*, *23*(1), 2–4.

Lovell, M. R., Luckett, T., Boyle, F. M., et al. (2014). Patient education, coaching, and self-management for cancer pain. *Journal of Clinical Oncology*, *32*(16), 1712–1720.

Mahon, S. M. (1994). Concept analysis of pain: Implications related to nursing diagnoses. *Nursing Diagnosis*, *5*(1), 14–25.

McCaffery, M., & Pasero, C. (1999). *Pain: Clinical manual* (2nd ed.). St. Louis, MO: Mosby.

McCaffrey, R. (2008). Music listening: Its effects in creating a healing environment. *Journal of Psychosocial Nursing and Mental Health Services*, *46*(10), 39–44.

McCaffrey, R., & Freeman, E. (2003). Effect of music on chronic osteoarthritis pain in older people. *Journal of Advanced Nursing*, *44*(5), 517–524.

McCormack, H. M., Horne, D. J., & Sheather, S. (1988). Clinical applications of visual analogue scales: A critical review. *Psychological Medicine*, *18*(4), 1007–1019.

McDowell, J. H., McFarland, E. G., & Nalli, B. J. (1994). Use of cryotherapy for orthopaedic patients. *Orthopedic Nursing*, *13*(5), 21–30.

Melzack, R. (1975). The McGill Pain Questionnaire: Major properties and scoring methods. *Pain*, *1*, 277–299.

Melzack, R. (1996). Gate control theory. *Pain Forum*, *5*(2), 128–138.

Melzack, R., & Wall, P. D. (1962). On the nature of cutaneous sensory mechanisms. *Brain*, *85*, 331.

Melzack, R., & Wall, P. D. (1965). Pain mechanisms: A new theory. *Science*, *150*(3699), 971–979.

Mendell, L. M. (2014). Constructing and deconstructing the gate theory of pain. *Pain*, *155*(2), 210–216.

Merkel, S. I., Voepel-Lewis, T., Shayevitz, J. R., & Malviya, S. (1997). The FLACC: A behavioral scale for scoring postoperative pain in young children. *Pediatric Nursing*, *23*(3), 293–297.

Mitchinson, A., Fletcher, C. E., Kim, H. M., Montagnini, M., & Hinshaw, D. B. (2014). Integrating massage therapy within the palliative care of veterans with advanced illnesses: An outcome study. *American Journal of Hospital & Palliative Care*, *31*(1), 6–12.

Moayedi, M., & Davis, K. D. (2013). Theories of pain: From specificity to gate theory. *Journal of Neurophysiology*, *109*, 5–12.

Morse, J. M., Bottorff, J. L., & Hutchinson, S. (1995). The paradox of comfort. *Nursing Research*, *44*(1), 14–19.

Najafi, S., Rast, S. F., Momennasab, M., et al. (2014). The effect of massage therapy by patients' companions on severity of pain in the patients undergoing post coronary artery bypass graft surgery: A single-blind randomized clinical trial. *International Journal of Community Based Nursing and Midwifery*, *2*(3), 128–135.

Olness, K. (1981). Self-hypnosis as adjunct therapy in childhood cancer: Clinical experience with 25 patients. *American Journal of Pediatric Hematology/Oncology*, *3*, 313–321.

Park, E., Oh, H., & Kim, T. (2013). The effects of relaxation breathing on procedural pain and anxiety during burn care. *Burns*, *39*(6), 1101–1106.

Pasero, C., & McCaffery, M. (2003). Accountability for pain relief: Use of comfort-function goals. *Journal of Perianesthesia Nursing*, *18*(1), 50–52.

Pasero, C., & McCaffery, M. (2004). Comfort-function goals: A way to establish accountability for pain relief. *American Journal of Nursing*, *104*(9), 77–78, 81.

Pestka, E. L., Bee, S. M., & Evans, M. M. (2010). Relaxation therapies. In M. Snyder & R. Lindquist (Eds.), *Complementary and alternative therapies in nursing* (6th ed., pp. 382–396). New York, NY: Springer.

Phumdoung, S., & Good, M. (2003). Music reduces sensation and distress of labor pain. *Pain Management Nursing*, *4*(2), 54–61.

Price, D. D., McGrath, P. A., Rafii, A., & Buckingham, B. (1983). The validation of visual analogue scales as ratio scale measures for chronic and experimental pain. *Pain*, *17*(1), 45–56.

Rafii, F., Mohammadi-Fakhar, F., & Jamshidi Orak, R. (2014). Effectiveness of jaw relaxation for burn dressing pain: Randomized clinical trial. *Pain Management Nursing*, *15*(4), 845–853.

Rambod, M., Sharif, F., Pourali-Mohammadi, N., Pasyar, N., & Raffi, F. (2014). Evaluation of the effect of Benson's relaxation technique on pain and quality of life of haemodialysis patients: A randomized controlled trial. *International Journal of Nursing Studies*, *51*(7), 964–973.

Reis, P. (2012). Cochrane review: Relaxation and yoga may decrease pain during labour and increase satisfaction with pain relief, but better quality evidence is needed. *Evidence Based Nursing*, *15*(4), 105–106.

Rejeh, N., Heravi-Karimooi, M., Vaismoradi, M., & Jasper, M. (2013). Effect of systematic relaxation techniques on anxiety and pain in older patients undergoing abdominal surgery. *International Journal of Nursing Practice*, *19*(5), 462–470.

Richards, J. S., Nepomuceno, C., Riles, M., & Suer, Z. (1982). Assessing pain behavior: The UAB pain behavior scale. *Pain*, *14*(4), 393.

Rodgers, N. J., Cutshall, S. M., Dion, L. J., et al. (2014). A decade of building massage therapy services at an academic medical center as part of a healing enhancement program. *Complementary Therapies in Clinical Practice*, *21*, 52–56. doi: 10.1016/j.ctcp.2014.12.001. pii: S1744-3881(14)00084-X

Rosa, W. E. (2018). Transcultural pain management: Theory, practice, and nurse-client partnerships. *Pain Management Nursing*, *19*(1), 23–33.

Roykulcharoen, V., & Good, M. (2004). Systematic relaxation relieves postoperative pain in Thailand. *Journal of Advanced Nursing*, *48*(2), 1–9.

Schaffer, S. D., & Yucha, C. B. (2004). Relaxation and pain management. *American Journal of Nursing*, *104*(8), 75–82.

Shabanloei, R., Golchin, M., Esfahani, A., Dolatkhah, R., & Rasoulian, M. (2010). Effects of music therapy on pain and anxiety in patients undergoing bone marrow biopsy and aspiration. *AORN Journal*, *91*(6), 746–751.

Shin, J. M., Byun, J. Y., Baek, B. J., & Lee, J. Y. (2014). Effect of cold-water cooling of tonsillar fossa and pharyngeal mucosa on post-tonsillectomy pain. *American Journal of Otolaryngology*, 35(3), 353–356.

Shirvani, M. A., & Ganji, Z. (2014). The influence of cold pack on labour pain relief and birth outcomes: A randomised controlled trial. *Journal of Clinical Nursing*, 23(17–18), 2473–2479.

Shuldham, C. (1999). A review of the impact of pre-operative education on recovery from surgery. *International Journal of Nursing Studies*, 36(2), 171–177.

Siedlecki, S., & Good, M. (2006). Effect of music on power, pain, depression and disability. *Journal of Advanced Nursing*, 54(5), 553–562.

Simon, J. M., Baumann, M. A., & Nolan, L. (1995). Differential diagnostic validation: Acute and chronic pain. *Nursing Diagnosis*, 6(2), 73–79.

Slatyer, S., Williams, A. M., & Michael, R. (2015). Seeking empowerment to comfort patients in severe pain: A grounded theory study of the nurse's perspective. *International Journal of Nursing Studies*, 52(1), 229–239.

Smith, C. A., Levett, K. M., Collins, C. T., et al. (2018). Relaxation techniques for pain management in labour. *Cochrane Database Systematic Review*, (3), CD009514.

Solehati, T., & Rustina, Y. (2015). Benson relaxation technique in reducing pain intensity in women after cesarean section. *Anesthesiology and Pain Medicine*, 5(3): e22236.

Song, M., Li, N. Zhang, X., et al. (2018). Music for reducing the anxiety and pain of patients undergoing a biopsy: A meta-analysis. *Journal of Advanced Nursing*, 74(5): 1016–1029.

Tan, X., Yowler, C. J., Super, D. M., & Fratianne, R. B. (2010). The efficacy of music therapy protocols for decreasing pain, anxiety, and muscle tension levels during burn dressing changes: A prospective randomized crossover trial. *Journal of Burn Care and Research*, 31(4), 590–597.

Taverner, T., Closs, S. J., & Briggs, M. (2014). The journey to chronic pain: A grounded theory of older adults' experiences of pain associated with leg ulceration. *Pain Management Nursing*, 15(1), 186–198.

Topcu, S. Y., & Findik, U. Y. (2012). Effect of relaxation exercises on controlling postoperative pain. *Pain Management Nursing*, 13(1), 11–17.

Tsai, H. F., Chen, Y. R., Chung, M. H., et al. (2014). Effectiveness of music intervention in ameliorating cancer patients' anxiety, depression, pain, and fatigue: A meta-analysis. *Cancer Nursing*, 37(6), E35–E50.

Tsai, P. F., Tak, S., Moore, C., & Palencia, I. (2003). Testing a theory of chronic pain. *Journal of Advanced Nursing*, 43(2), 158–169.

Tusek, D. L., Church, J. M., Strong, S. A., Grass, J. A., & Fazio, V. W. (1997). Guided imagery: A significant advance in the care of patients undergoing elective colorectal surgery. *Diseases of the Colon and Rectum*, 40(2), 172–178.

Ucuzal, M., & Kanan, N. (2014). Foot massage: Effectiveness on postoperative pain in breast surgery patients. *Pain Management Nursing*, 15(2): 458–465.

Wong, D. L., & Baker, C. M. (1988). Pain in children: Comparison of assessment scales. *Pediatric Nursing*, 14(1), 9–17.

Yarahmadi, S., Mohammadi, N., Ardalan, A., Najafizadeh, H., & Gholami, M. (2018). The combined effects of cold therapy and music therapy on pain following chest tube removal among patients with cardiac bypass surgery. *Complementary Therapies in Clinical Practice*, 31, 71–75.

Yin, P., Gao, N., Wu, J., Litscher, G., & Xu, S. (2014). Adverse events of massage therapy in pain-related conditions: A systematic review. *Evidence Based Complementary and Alternative Medicine*, 2014, 480956.

Zwelling, E., Johnson, K., & Allen, J. (2006). How to implement complementary therapies for laboring women. *MCN: The American Journal of Maternal/Child Nursing*, 31(6), 365–370.

# 5 Unpleasant Symptoms

Elizabeth R. Lenz, Linda C. Pugh, and Renee Milligan

## Definition of Key Terms

| | |
|---|---|
| **Performance** | Performance is the multifaceted outcome or result of the symptom experience. It includes functional and cognitive activities. Functional performance includes activities of daily living (ADLs), social interaction, and role performance. Cognitive performance includes knowledge and ability to learn, remember, solve problems, and think abstractly and logically. Quality of life (QoL) can be considered an indicator of performance, because it incorporates both functional and cognitive abilities as perceived by the individual experiencing the symptom(s). |
| **Physiological factors** | Physiological factors are the normal or abnormal functioning of bodily systems. They can influence the experience of symptoms. They may include diseases and dysfunctions, treatments and medications taken in the past or currently, physiological and anatomical abnormalities, comorbidities, diet and nutritional balance, hydration, and amount of exercise. They include the age and gender of the individual. |
| **Psychological factors** | Psychological factors also influence the symptom experience. They include mental state or mood, affective reaction to illness, and the degree of uncertainty and knowledge about the symptoms and their meaning to the individual based on earlier or concurrent experiences. |
| **Situational factors** | Situational factors include aspects of the social and physical environment that surround the person and may influence the experience, interpretation, and reporting of symptoms. They include physical environmental factors, such as heat, humidity, noise, light, safety, and air and water quality. They may include social environmental factors, such as socioeconomic status, marital status, and social support. |
| **Unpleasant symptoms** | Symptoms are the perceived indicators of change in functioning as experienced by patients. They are the subjective indicators of changes in and threats to, or improvement in, health. Generally, they are experienced as unpleasant sensations. |

The theory of unpleasant symptoms (TOUS) is a middle range nursing theory that was developed and intended for application and use by nurses and clinical researchers. The original concept paper appeared in 1995 and was revised in 1997. The theory allows for the presence of multiple symptoms that interact and/or are multiplicative. It implies that experience of one symptom will contribute to the experience of others.

## Historical Background

In 1993, two efforts that emerged from clinical practice and empirical research led to the development of the TOUS. Linda Pugh and Audrey Gift, clinical researchers each studying a single symptom (fatigue and dyspnea, respectively), developed a model that included elements common to both symptoms. Pugh's practice and research specialty were intrapartum fatigue. She teamed with Renee Milligan whose practice and research specialty were postpartum fatigue. Together, they developed a framework for childbearing fatigue that identified common factors related to fatigue across the childbearing period. Both the model and the framework linked antecedent or influencing factors to the symptom of interest and the way in which it is reported by patients. In addition, the symptom was conceptualized as an experience that influences performance outcomes. Noting that the models for the two symptoms were similar, Gift and Pugh realized that similar interventions, such as the use of progressive muscle relaxation, had been proposed and tested for both dyspnea and fatigue. These management techniques were consistent with those proposed for the management of pain.

Both symptom models were usable, but there was a need for a more abstract and inclusive model that could encompass these and other symptoms. Elizabeth Lenz was familiar with the work of all three researchers and had offered critique and support regarding their studies and the theoretical implications. She took the lead to call the collaborators together to further develop the more inclusive model. The team was joined by Frederick Suppe, an eminent philosopher of science with a wealth of experience related to scientific theory and nursing science. The authors began meeting regularly to develop the model, assign writing tasks, and discuss each other's work. The more abstract model that resulted was presented to the nursing scholarly community as an exemplar of a middle range nursing theory (Lenz, Suppe, Gift, Pugh, & Milligan, 1995).

During the next few years, interest in middle range theories increased in the nursing literature. In a later revision and amplification of the TOUS, the authors refined the model to more accurately reflect the complexity and dynamism of clinical situations (Lenz, Pugh, Milligan, Gift, & Suppe, 1997). The likely multiplicity and multiplicative nature of symptoms, the interaction among the influencing factors, and the feedback among the factors, symptoms, and performance were integrated into the theory.

## The Theory of Unpleasant Symptoms

Many models of symptoms focus on one symptom, specifically on its severity or intensity, not on other features such as quality, distress, or duration. The TOUS was one of the earliest to portray multiple symptoms occurring together and relating to each other in an additive or multiplicative manner, potentially catalyzing each other. Thus, this theory, which allows for the presence of multiple symptoms and implies that management of one symptom will contribute to the management of others, is consistent with the large body of current literature that addresses symptom clusters, which are multiple symptoms that occur simultaneously and are related to one another (e.g., Almutary, Douglas, & Bonner, 2017; Ameringer et al., 2015; Blakeman & Stapleton, 2018; Dong et al., 2016; Herr et al., 2015; Huang, Moser, & Hwang, 2018; Lee et al., 2018; Lim, Kim, Kim, & Kim, 2017; Oh, Park, & Seo, 2018; Phigbua et al., 2013; Samantharath, Pongthavornkamol, Olson, Sriyuktasuth, & Sanpakit, 2018; Wang & Fu, 2014).

## Description of the Theory of Unpleasant Symptoms

The TOUS addresses the symptom experience and allows a focus on either multiple symptoms occurring together or a single symptom. It has been used as the theoretical framework to guide many studies of the symptom experience associated with a variety of illnesses, including cancer, chronic obstructive pulmonary disease, heart disease, chronic cough, arthritis, liver cirrhosis, gastric and transplant surgery, multiple sclerosis, and Parkinson's disease. It also has been used as the framework for studies involving the elderly and women experiencing intimate partner violence, pregnancy, and the postpartum (e.g., Blakeman & Stapleton, 2018; French, Crawford, Bova, & Irwin, 2017; Huang et al., 2016, 2018; Lee et al., 2018; Loutzenhizer, McAuslan, & Sharpe, 2015; Oh et al., 2018; So et al., 2013). It has also been used to guide studies of healthy populations under stress, such as parents of hospitalized children (Kim et al., 2017) and family caregivers (Alfheim, Rosseland, Hofso, Smastuen, & Rustoen, 2018; Moriarty, Bunting-Perry, Robinson, & Bradway, 2016). The symptoms are viewed as having either a multiplicative or an additive relationship to one another. Symptoms have antecedent influencing factors that are categorized as physiological, psychological, and situational (environmental). These antecedents are interactive and reciprocal as they relate to one another and to the symptom(s) (Fig. 5.1).

Symptoms have the measurable dimensions of intensity (severity), timing (frequency, duration, trajectory pattern if recurrent, and relationship of onset to precipitating events), distress (the person's interpretation of and reaction to the sensation, which is influenced by the meaning the person assigns to it), and quality (descriptors used to characterize the way the symptom feels and/or its location). The quality dimension may be difficult to measure, depending on the culture and language of the patient and the number of symptoms experienced simultaneously. The dimensions can vary independently but often relate to one another (e.g., Matthie & McMillan, 2014).

The antecedent factors are categorized as physiological, psychological, or situational. Physiological antecedents may include the individual's age, gender, precipitating illness(es) or dysfunction(s), or normal developmental stage (menopause). Additional physiological antecedents can be an event (pregnancy), comorbidities, abnormal blood values, or any other physiological findings that can be attributed to the illness or its treatment (medication, surgery, radiation therapy). Psychological

## Theory of Unpleasant Symptoms

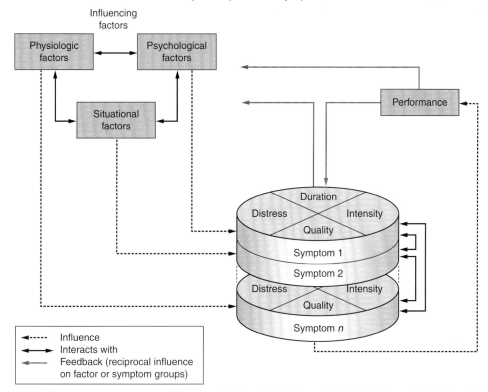

**Figure 5.1**  **Theory of unpleasant symptoms.** (From Lenz, E. R., Pugh, L. C., Milligan, R. A., Gift, A., & Suppe, F. (1997). The middle-range theory of unpleasant symptoms: An update. *Advances in Nursing Science, 19*(3), 14–27. Copyright 1997 by Lippincott, Williams & Wilkins.)

factors affecting the symptom experience may include the person's mood or emotional state, affective reaction to disease, degree of perceived uncertainty about the symptoms or the illness, level of perceived self-efficacy, and the meaning ascribed to the symptoms by the person. Situational factors are contextual. They refer to aspects of the social and physical environment that may affect an individual's symptom experiences and reports of those experiences. Examples include the physical nature of the immediate environment (noise, temperature) and multiple aspects of the social environment (social support, marital status, cultural background, socioeconomic status, occupation, family and work demands, relationships with care providers, and available resources).

In the TOUS, symptoms are hypothesized to affect performance, which includes functional and cognitive domains. Functional performance refers to an individual's ability to perform physical activity, including activities of daily living (ADLs), self-care and self-management, care seeking, and ability to carry out social and personal roles (Park, 2017; Yang & Kang, 2018). Cognitive performance is the ability to concentrate, remember, learn, solve problems, make decisions, reason, and/or think. There is empirical support for relationships between

patterns of cognition and levels of symptoms experienced (e.g., Lee et al., 2018; Yang & Kang, 2018). Some investigators have identified quality of life as a potentially important outcome for research guided by the TOUS (e.g., French et al., 2017; Hsu & Tu, 2014; Oh et al., 2018; Samantharath et al., 2018; Seo, Ryu, & Young, 2018; So et al., 2013).

In the most recent version of the theory (Lenz & Pugh, 2018; Lenz et al., 1997), multiple symptoms are conceptualized as potentially occurring simultaneously and interacting with one another, as are antecedent factors (see Fig. 5.1 for a model of the TOUS). Interactive and reciprocal relationships among the antecedent factors and symptoms are also hypothesized. Symptoms are hypothesized to influence performance. Performance, likewise, reciprocally affects the symptom experience and may change the antecedent factors. Although the TOUS has been criticized for lacking explicit inclusion of interventions (Lee, Vincent, & Finnegan, 2017), its authors and others maintain that it provides a sound basis for designing symptom assessment and management interventions (Lenz & Pugh, 2018; Nguyen, Haas, & Pugh, 2017). See Using Middle Range Theory in Research 5.1, Using Middle Range Theory in Practice 5.2, and Table 5.1 Examples of Research for Application to Practice for examples of the use of the theory.

## USING MIDDLE RANGE THEORY IN RESEARCH   5.1

The TOUS has provided the framework for clinical research projects examining a wide variety of populations and settings. In a recent example, Lee et al. (2018) analyzed baseline data from a longitudinal study of patients with COPD to test a TOUS-based model.

### RESEARCH DESIGN

Cross-sectional baseline data were used for structural equation model testing.

### SAMPLE/PARTICIPANTS

The sample was 282 COPD patients who were participants in a larger study.

### DATA COLLECTION

Data were collected in person and by phone. Influencing factors were dyspnea, anxiety, and depression; the focal symptom was fatigue; the performance outcome was physical performance (measured by physical activity [6-minute walk test; daily steps taken via accelerometer] and strength [grip strength] measures and self-reported physical functioning and role physical scores [SF-36]).

### FINDINGS

Dyspnea was positively related to anxiety, depression, and fatigue; anxiety and depression were positively related to fatigue. Dyspnea was negatively and anxiety was positively related directly to physical performance; however, depression and fatigue were not related to performance in the total sample. Dyspnea had the strongest influence on performance. Fatigue and performance were related in a subsample with moderate illness severity, but not in those with more severe illness.

   Most of the relationships hypothesized in the TOUS were supported. The results underscore the importance of managing multiple symptoms simultaneously to enhance performance outcomes.

## USING MIDDLE RANGE THEORY IN PRACTICE   5.2

### PROBLEM

Several studies have assessed the effectiveness of nursing interventions based on the TOUS. Examples include:
- An interdisciplinary intervention (Collaborative Care to Alleviate Symptoms and Adjust to Illness [CASA]) that integrated physical and psychosocial care by nurses, social workers, and physicians to improve symptoms, depression, and adjustment to illness in persons with chronic heart failure (Bekelman et al., 2014, 2016, 2018)
- An educational intervention for lung cancer patients during radiotherapy that included education about symptom management with focus on reducing stress and coaching about muscle relaxation (Chan, Richardson, & Richardson, 2011)
- A heart failure training program teaching patients to monitor symptoms and respond to changes (Jurgens, Lee, Reitano, & Reigel, 2013)
- An intervention to teach relaxation and sleep hygiene to depressed patients with insomnia (Johnson & Roberson, 2013)

### NURSING INTERVENTION

All interventions involved patient teaching about self-monitoring and strategies to alleviate symptoms; most involved repetition and follow-up.

### FINDINGS

Results were mixed. While most of the interventions achieved desired results, the CASA intervention resulted in improvement in cardiomyopathy, depressive symptoms, and fatigue at 6 months, but no change in pain, shortness of breath, number of hospitalizations, or overall symptom distress; mortality at 12 months did not differ.

**Table 5.1    Examples of Research for Application to Practice**

| References | Research Design/ Meta-Analysis | Clinical Issue/Research Question | Sample (n)/ Population | Intervention | Outcome |
|---|---|---|---|---|---|
| Hinds, P. S., et al. (2019). PROMIS pediatric measures validated in a longitudinal study design in pediatric oncology. *Pediatric Blood & Cancer,* 66(5), e27606. doi: 10.1002/pbc.27606 | Psychometric assessment with longitudinal data collection | Assess responsiveness of PROMIS measures to change over time; assess TOUS-guided association of PROMIS measures, Symptom Distress Scale (SDS), and other demographic and clinical variables | n = 96 pediatric patients in treatment for cancer | PROMIS measures (8), SDS, demographic and clinical variables measured at 3 points in time during a course of chemotherapy | Most PROMIS measures had significant short- and long-term changes and theorized relationships; thus, PROMIS demonstrated concurrent and construct validity, and theorized relationships in the TOUS were supported |
| Huang, H.-C., et al. (2018). Validation of a symptom distress scale in a cirrhotic population using item response theory. *Nursing Research,* 67(6), 359–368 | Psychometric assessment using item response theory–based item analysis | Assess appropriateness of the SDS for assessing distress associated with symptoms experienced by patients with liver cirrhosis | n = 163 outpatients in Taiwan with liver cirrhosis | Interview conducted to administer the SDS and questions about disease duration and severity | Patients reported mild to moderate symptom distress, with highest distress from fatigue, pain, changes in appearance, and itching; persons with more (versus less) severe disease reported more distress from dark urine, drowsiness, and bruising. The SDS is most appropriate for patients with severe symptom distress |
| Park, S. V. (2018). Factors affecting self-care behavior in Koreans with COPD. *Applied Nursing Research,* 38, 29–37 | Cross-sectional description | Describe the level of self-care behavior in Koreans with COPD; determine the effect of symptoms and symptom clusters on self-care behavior | n = 71 persons with exacerbating COPD | Administered MOS SF-36 (for general physical function and general health, COPD Self-Efficacy Scale, Visual Analogue Scale, Modified Medical Research Council Scale, POMS Short Form (for anxiety and depression), MOS Social Support Survey, and Alberto COPD Self-Care Behavior Inventory | Better self-care behavior was predicted by higher education, ED visits in the past year, usual general health perception and education about exacerbation, and lower comorbidities. Persons with high (versus low) cluster scores (dyspnea, anxiety, depression) had better SCB; nurses should monitor self-care behavior and educate patients accordingly |

*(Continued)*

**Table 5.1  Examples of Research for Application to Practice** (Continued)

| References | Research Design/ Meta-Analysis | Clinical Issue/Research Question | Sample (n)/ Population | Intervention | Outcome |
|---|---|---|---|---|---|
| Yang, I.-S., & Kang, Y. (2018). Self-care model based on the theory of unpleasant symptoms in patients with heart failure. *Applied Nursing Research, 43*, 10–17 | Structural equation model testing | Develop and test a hypothetical self-care model, which added self-efficacy to the TOUS-based model | N = 209 patients with heart failure recruited from two Korean medical centers | Interviews were conducted to administer the Hospital Anxiety and Depression Scale; Inventory of Social Supportive Behaviors; physical symptom subscale of the Memorial Symptom Assessment Scale for Heart Failure; self-efficacy, self-care maintenance, and self-care management subscales of the Self-Care of Heart Failure Index; Cardiac Diet and Exercise Self-Efficacy Instrument | Relations of disease severity and anxiety to self-care were mediated by unpleasant symptoms; self-efficacy mediated the effects of depression and social support on self-care. The final model added self-efficacy to the TOUS-based model |
| Oh, H., Park, J., & Seo, W. S. (2018). Identification of symptom clusters and their synergistic effects on quality of life in rheumatoid arthritis patients. *International Journal of Nursing Practice, 25*(2), e12713. doi: 10.1111/ijn.12713 | Hypothetical model testing using path analysis of cross-sectional data | Examine the presence of symptom clusters (pain, fatigue, depression) and their synergistic effects on quality of life (QoL) in rheumatoid arthritis patients; test a hypothetical model of symptom experience based on the TOUS | N = 179 out-patients with rheumatoid arthritis, recruited from a Korean medical center | Administered the following measures: Numeric Rating Scale to measure pain and Fatigue Severity Scale, Hospital Anxiety and Depression Scale, and Short Form of the Health Survey Questionnaire (SF-12) to measure quality of life | Disease activity had direct effects on pain, fatigue, and depression and indirect effects on fatigue and depression, and obesity had a direct effect on fatigue; pain, depression, and fatigue were related; symptom clusters were pain–fatigue, fatigue–depression, and pain–fatigue–depression; pain and fatigue had direct and indirect effects on QoL, whereas pain's effect was indirect through fatigue and depression, with its effect enhanced by its synergism with depression; cluster effects on QoL were synergistic, indicating that clustered symptoms should be treated simultaneously |

# Models That Expand or Modify the Theory of Unpleasant Symptoms

Brant, Beck, and Miaskowski (2010) conducted a systematic review of models related to symptoms or symptom management. The two seminal models they identified were the TOUS and the Theory of Symptom Management (TSM) (Humphreys et al., 2014), an outgrowth of the Symptom Management Model (SMM) (*A Model for Symptom Management, 1994*; Bender, Janson, Franck, & Lee, 2018; The University of California, San Francisco Symptom Management Faculty Group, 1994). Models that have expanded or modified the TOUS include the Symptom Experience Model (SEM) by Armstrong (2003); the Symptoms Experience in Time (SET) model by Henly, Kallas, Klatt, and Swenson (2003); and the Theory of Symptom Self-Management (TSSM) by Hoffman (2013). Yang and Kang's (2018) self-care model added self-efficacy as a predictor of self-care behavior. In addition to the models that have been developed to expand the TOUS, a number of investigators have tested aspects of the theory and, based on their findings, have suggested modifications (Lenz & Pugh, 2018). Brant, Dudley, Beck, and Miaskowski (2016) developed the Dynamic Symptoms Model, which contains some of the same elements as are in the TOUS; however, their model places greater emphasis on interventions. Riegel and colleagues integrated elements of the TOUS, along with other symptom theories, to expand their middle range theory of self-care of chronic illness (Reigel, Jaarsma, Lee, & Strömberg, 2018). It has also been used as a basis for investigator-generated models, which are then tested using path analytic and structural equation modeling techniques (Baydoun, Barton, & Arsinian-Engoren, 2018; Kim et al., 2017; Lee et al., 2018). These techniques have substantiated the importance of including the potential for mediating effects in the TOUS.

## ARMSTRONG'S SYMPTOM EXPERIENCE MODEL

Armstrong (2003) proposed a symptom model that builds on the TOUS but focuses attention on the meaning or perception of the symptom as well as its expression. Multiple co-occurring symptoms can interact and affect the patient's perception of the symptom as a new or recurring event and his or her perception of the ability to deal with the situation. Armstrong further extended the TOUS to include the existential meaning of the symptom(s) to the patient, that is, feelings of vulnerability and

mortality related to the symptom. In Armstrong's modification, antecedents are reorganized as demographic, disease, and individual characteristics. Symptom dimensions are frequency, intensity, and distress (consistent with the TOUS) and the descriptor of symptom meaning. In the TOUS, the individual's interpretation of the symptom's meaning is captured in the level of distress. In the SEM, the consequences of the symptom experience are expanded beyond physical, social, and role performance (and cognitive functioning) to include emotional consequences. Armstrong's model is appropriate to use when the meaning of the symptom is the focus of the investigation or intervention.

## SYMPTOM EXPERIENCE IN TIME MODEL

The SET model was conceptualized by combining the TOUS and the SMM (now the TSM) with a time model for the purpose of examining symptom flow (Henly et al., 2003). In this model, the symptom is initiated by a precipitating event that leads to its onset. The influencing factors of the TOUS are broadened to include nursing metaparadigm concepts of person, health, and environment that may mediate or moderate the symptom. Every symptom has an onset, an experience, a cognitive evaluation, and an emotional response. Symptom dimensions are retained from the TOUS. The cognitive evaluation determines whether the symptom is serious, unpleasant, and/or inexplicable. Each symptom is also evaluated as being chronic or treatable. If treatable, symptom management can take the form of either self-care or help-seeking behavior. The outcomes of these strategies can be changes in the symptom itself, the person, his or her health, and/or the environment.

Time, a factor determining the patterning of a symptom experience, may serve as input to the symptom experience or as output from the symptom management process. It may also be a component of an intervention. Time has different patterns whether considering perceived time, biological/social time, or clock/calendar time. The SET model provides a helpful conceptual amplification of time as an important dimension of the symptom experience.

## THEORY OF SYMPTOM SELF-MANAGEMENT

The TSSM builds upon the TOUS with the aim of improving clinical practice (Hoffman, 2013). The TSSM places considerable importance on perceived self-efficacy for managing one's symptoms and provides a basis for developing strategies for increasing self-efficacy. In addition to being influenced by enhancement strategies, perceived self-efficacy is affected by the symptom experience, patient characteristics (which parallel the influencing factor categories of the TOUS), and functional and cognitive performance outcomes. Perceived self-efficacy is proposed to impact symptom self-management behaviors, which are also influenced by the symptoms and the performance outcomes. The parallels to the TOUS are many; the major differences are explicit emphasis on perceived self-efficacy, which in the TOUS is viewed as a psychological influencing factor, addition of intervention strategies to enhance perceived self-efficacy, and the addition of symptom self-management as a distinct outcome of the symptom experience. With increasing attention to patients' self-managing aspects of their care, the TSSM highlights important considerations.

## Assessment of Symptoms

The TOUS is relevant to practice and can be used as a framework for nursing assessment or care decisions. Symptom experience is subjective; thus, assessment must be tempered by the notion that the severity or distress associated with a symptom reflects the individual's interpretation of that symptom experience. A sensation of the same magnitude might be interpreted quite differently (therefore, rated or described differently) by two individuals. Appropriate symptom assessment and management depend on understanding the symptom involved, the underlying disease or causative factors, the stage of the illness, treatments received previously or concurrently, and the patient's prognosis and overall emotional state and his or her unique life circumstances. Ideally, symptom assessment should paint a total picture for which the TOUS is an excellent guide.

The TOUS can provide a guide for compiling a medical or nursing history, because physiological, psychological, and situational factors provide a framework for identifying symptom antecedents. For instance, physiological factors identified from history taking could include physical sequelae of past illness, injury, or treatment. Psychological factors identified in history taking could include recent or previous depressive incidents or mood changes. Situational factors identified in the history could include family/caregiver issues and living conditions, to include availability of assistance. Symptoms should be assessed using all four dimensions identified in the TOUS in order to provide a full picture of the individual's experience.

## Instruments Used in Empirical Testing

Symptom measures can either focus on one symptom such as pain (Crosta, Ward, Walker, & Peters, 2014; Good, 2017) or address multiple symptoms that are commonly seen in a specific disease entity, the most frequently studied being cancer (Alfheim et al., 2018). Some symptom measures focus only on physical symptoms, while others include both physical and emotional domains. Measures may include only presence, intensity, or frequency, rather than all four dimensions described in the TOUS. Some, such as the Fatigue Symptom Inventory, address both the severity of a symptom and the degree to which it interferes with everyday activities, the latter sometimes used as a proxy measure of distress. In a recent review of instruments used in research about pediatric patients, Von Sadovszky et al. (2018) found several instruments that measured two or more symptom dimensions, but none that addressed all four TOUS dimensions.

Many instruments have been used to measure the other components of the TOUS as well. Among the most commonly used are those that address performance, particularly functional performance measures, which use individuals' reports of their ADLs and roles or others' observations of activity measures (e.g., ability to walk a given distance or range of motion achieved). Many activity measures are limited because they are inappropriate for patients who are in critical condition or at the end stage of life. In addition to the self-report and activity measures, some investigators have used physiological measures, such as spirography or blood values to measure illness severity. Investigators have also used self-report quality-of-life measures to address performance (Hsu & Tu, 2014; Oh et al., 2018). A few examples of the self-report symptom instruments that have been used in applying or testing the TOUS are described briefly in Table 5.2. The article by Von Sadovszky et al. (2018) lists and describes self-report instruments used in pediatric nursing research and practice.

### SELECTION OF INSTRUMENTS

The use of a particular instrument to measure symptom(s), performance, or influencing factors in research or in clinical practice will depend upon what information is needed to answer the research questions being studied and/or the needs and limitations imposed by a particular population or setting. In general, it is preferable to select an existing instrument than to develop a new one, provided it has a good fit to the situation in which it will be used and established reliability and validity (Waltz, Strickland, & Lenz, 2017).

**Table 5.2  Examples of Self-Report Instruments Used to Apply TOUS in Research and Practice**

| Instrument | Concept(s) Measured | TOUS Component Measured | Description |
|---|---|---|---|
| Profile of Mood States (POMS)[a] | Fatigue/inertia (intensity), depressive symptoms | Symptoms (separate sub-scales for specific symptoms); psychological factors; cognitive performance | Long form is comprised of 65 adjectives; for each, respondents indicate the extent to which they are currently experiencing the emotion described. A short form exists |
| Visual Analogue Scale[b] | Most symptoms (e.g., fatigue, pain, dyspnea); has been used primarily to measure symptom intensity, but also other dimensions such as associated distress | Symptoms (single symptom measured at a time) | Subject places mark along a 100-mm line anchored by descriptors (polar opposites) to reflect the intensity of the symptom. Scoring involves measuring the distance from the lowest or left end of the line to the mark |
| Numeric Rating Scale[c] | Most symptoms; most often used to measure intensity; commonly used in clinical practice, especially in pain measurement | Symptoms (single symptom measured at a particular time) | Subject describes the level of the symptom being experienced on a numerical range. The score is the numerical value |
| McGill Pain Questionnaire[d] | Pain | Symptom (single) | Measures sensory, affective, and evaluative dimensions of pain, including the relative intensity of each dimension. Current pain intensity is rated on a 0 distance |
| Brief Fatigue Inventory[e] | Fatigue | Severity and interference associated with symptom | Measures severity of fatigue in the last 24 h and degree of interference with daily functioning. Items (9) are rated on a 10-point scale. Originally developed for cancer-related fatigue, it has been used in persons with other conditions |
| Brief Pain Inventory[f] | Pain | Severity and interference associated with symptom | 11 items measure severity of pain (4) and interference with ADLs (7) in the past week |
| Minnesota Living with Heart Failure Questionnaire[g] | Quality of life; physical and emotional symptoms impacting QoL in HF patients | Disease-specific symptoms (9); performance | A 21-item Likert-type scale measuring quality of life. Patients rate the impact of each of six physical and three emotional symptoms on living during the previous month |
| Medical Outcomes Study Short Form-36 (MOS SF-36)[h] | Symptoms of pain, depressive symptoms, fatigue; performance (functional health), general health status, and quality of life | Symptoms (separate subscales for specific symptoms); physiological and psychological factors; performance | 36 items measure general health; subscales measure mental health, vitality, bodily pain, social functioning, mental health, role limitations, vitality, and perception of general health. Responses are based on how individual reports feeling over the past 4 wk |
| CES-D[i] | Depressive symptoms | Symptoms, psychological factors | Respondents indicate the frequency in the past week with which they experienced each of 20 beliefs and emotions. Designed for use in the general population, it should not be viewed as diagnostic of depression |
| Memorial Symptom Assessment Scale[j] | Physical and psychological symptoms | Severity, frequency, and distress of multiple symptoms | Presence, frequency, intensity, and distress associated with each of 24–32 symptoms. Global, physical, and psychological distress scores and total MSAS score are available. Originally developed for use with cancer patients, it has also been used in patients with other conditions. A 19-symptom short form has been used for patients with COPD and GI illnesses |

*(Continued)*

**Table 5.2    Examples of Self-Report Instruments Used to Apply TOUS in Research and Practice (Continued)**

| Instrument | Concept(s) Measured | TOUS Component Measured | Description |
|---|---|---|---|
| Modified Memorial Symptom Assessment Scale[k] | Physical and psychological symptoms | Symptoms (multiple) | Occurrence, intensity, duration/frequency, and distress associated with each of 8 symptoms. A Thai version[l] added 3 symptoms for a total of 11 |
| MD Anderson Symptom Inventory[m] | Multiple core symptoms most frequently experienced by persons with cancer | Severity of and interference by 13 core symptoms | 19-item scale rating severity (13 items) and interference (6 items) associated with daily functioning in the last 24 h. Translated into multiple languages |
| Fatigue Symptom Inventory[n,o] | Fatigue | Severity and interference with daily activities by fatigue | Two subscales: severity/intensity (3 items) and interference (7 items). Average subscale scores and total scores are calculated |
| Patient Health Questionnaire[p] | Depressive symptoms | Frequency of nine symptoms | 9-item scale in which frequency of nine symptoms that meet criteria for major depression is rated. Total score is calculated |
| Symptom Distress Scale[q] | Distress experienced as a result of physical symptoms | Frequency and intensity of symptoms and degree of distress experienced for each | Each of 21 symptoms is rated in intensity and degree of distress (0–3) experienced |
| Self-Care of Heart Failure Index[r] | Self-care maintenance, management and efficacy in persons with heart failure | Performance of self-care; self-efficacy for self-care | |
| Symptom Screening in Pediatrics Tool[s] | Multiple symptoms in children aged 8–18 | Symptom-specific distress (multiple symptoms) | 15 items administered verbally |
| Pediatric Quality of Life Inventory (PedQL)[t] | Health care quality of life in children and adolescents 2–18 | Health-related quality of life (aspect of performance outcome) | A modular instrument. The generic core scales include 23 items that are usable in healthy or ill pediatric populations. Generic core can be integrated with disease-specific modules. Scales are completed by children or parents (as proxy) |

[a]McNair et al. (1992), [b]Waltz et al. (2010), [c]Kapella et al. (2006), [d]Melzack (1975), [e]Mendoza et al. (1999), [f]Daut et al. (1983), [g]Rector et al. (1987), [h]Ware and Sherbourne (1992), [i]Radloff (1977), [j]Portenoy et al. (1994), [k]Collins et al. (2002), [l]Pongsing (2010), [m]Cleeland et al. (2000), [n]Hann, Denniston, and Baker (2000), [o]Hann et al. (1998), [p]Kroenke, Spitzer, and Williams (2001), [q]Kim, Oh, Lee, Kim, and Han (2006), [r]Riegel, Lee, Dickson, and Carlson (2009), [s]O'Sullivan, Depuis, and Sung (2015), [t]Varni, Burwinkle, Katx, Meeske, and Dickinson (2002); Varni, Seid, and Kurtin (2001).

## Summary

The TOUS has been a comprehensive and useful guide for research and practice in many clinical populations and international settings. The theory is grounded in clinical observations, research, and scientific collaborations. Its basic, interrelated elements are the symptom(s); the physiological, psychological, and situational variables that influence the symptom experience; and its functional and cognitive performance consequences. Symptoms are assumed to vary in intensity, timing, and duration, the distress they generate, and the qualitative ways in which persons experience them. They can occur singly or in clusters.

Having symptoms as the focus of nursing care, rather than simply being an indication of the underlying problem, is relatively new to the nursing literature, but has been prioritized by the National Institute of Nursing Research, in line with the NIH Symptom Science Model (Cashion & Grady, 2015; Moore et al., 2016). Middle range theories like the TOUS help guide clinicians in a comprehensive approach to care (Liehr & Smith, 2017). Nurses can best assess and help manage patients' symptoms within a sound scientific framework. The TOUS has demonstrated high potential for providing the basis for such a framework.

## CRITICAL THINKING EXERCISES

1. Using the theory of unpleasant symptoms as your guide, what would you look for in an assessment tool for patient symptoms?
   a. Do you monitor all symptom dimensions, such as how distressing the symptom is, or do you only ask about symptom severity/intensity?
   b. Do you monitor only one symptom or multiple symptoms?

2. In your patient assessment, how would you include the antecedents to symptoms?

3. How would you use the theory of unpleasant symptoms to plan a comprehensive intervention to alleviate symptoms?
   a. What interventions might you plan that would target the antecedents?
   b. What would you do to intervene regarding symptom distress?

4. What outcome would you use to assess the effectiveness of your interventions?
   a. Would you use an outcome measure that focuses on the physical, role, and/or cognitive performance outcome of symptoms? If so, what measure(s) would that be, specifically?
   b. If you were to have symptom alleviation as your outcome measure, which specific measurement tool would you use?

## REFERENCES

Alfheim, H. B., Rosseland, L. A., Hofso, K., Smastuen, M. C., & Rustoen, T. (2018). Multiple symptoms in family caregivers of intensive care unit patients. *Journal of Pain and Symptom Management, 55*, 387–394.

Almuntary, H., Douglas, C., & Bonner, A. (2017). Towards a symptom cluster model in chronic kidney disease: A structural equation approach. *Journal of Advanced Nursing, 73*, 2450–2461. doi: 10.1111/jan.13303

Ameringer, S. E., Erickson, J. M., Macpherson, C. F., Stegenga, K., & Linder, L. A. (2015). Symptoms and symptom clusters identified by adolescents and young adults with cancer using a symptom heuristics app. *Research in Nursing & Health, 38*, 436–448. doi: 10.1002/NUR.21697

Armstrong, T. S. (2003). Symptoms experience: A concept analysis. *Oncology Nursing Forum, 30*, 601–605.

Baydoun, M., Barton, D. L., & Arsianian-Engoren, C. (2018). A cancer-specific middle-range theory of symptom self-care management: A theory synthesis. *Journal of Advanced Nursing, 74*, 2935–2948. doi: 10.1111/jan.13829

Bekelman, D. S., Allen, L. A., McBryde, C. F., Hattler, B., Fairclough, D. L., Havranek, E. P., … Meek, P. M. (2018). Effect of a collaborative care intervention vs usual care on health status of patients with chronic heart failure: The CASA randomized trial. *JAMA Internal Medicine, 178*(4), 511–519. doi: 10.1001/jamainternmed.2017.8667

Bekelman, D. S., Allen, L. A., Peterson, J., Hattler, B., Havranek, E. P., Fairclough, D. L., … Meek, P. M. (2016). Rationale and study design of a patient-centered intervention to improve health status in chronic heart failure: The Collaborative Care to Alleviate Symptoms and Adjust to Illness (CASA), randomized trial. *Contemporary Clinical Trials, 51*(1), 1–7. doi: 10.1016/j.cct.2016.09.002

Bekelman, D. S., Hooker, S., Nowles, C. T., Main, D. S., Meek, P., McBryde, C, … Heidenreich, P. A. (2014). Feasibility and acceptability of a collaborative care intervention to improve symptoms and quality of life in chronic heart failure: Mixed methods pilot trial. *Journal of Palliative Medicine, 17*, 145–151. doi: 10.1089/jpm.2013.01

Bender, M. J., Janson, S. L., Franck, L. S., & Lee, K. A. (2018). Theory of symptom management. In M. J. Smith & P. R. Liehr (Eds.). *Middle range theory for nursing* (4th ed., pp. 147–178). New York, NY: Springer.

Blakeman, J. R., & Stapleton, S. J. (2018). An integrative review of fatigue experienced by women before and during myocardial infarction. *Journal of Clinical Nursing, 27*, 906–916. doi: 10.1111/jocn.14122

Brant, J. M., Beck, S., & Miaskowski, C. (2010). Building dynamic models and theories to advance the science of symptom management research. *Journal of Advanced Nursing, 66*, 228–240. doi: 10.1111/j.1365-2648.2009.05179

Brant, J. M., Dudley, W. N., Beck, S., & Miaskowski, C. (2016). Evolution of the dynamic symptoms model. *Oncology Nursing Forum, 43*, 651–654. doi: 10.1188/16.onf.651-654

Cashion, A. K., & Grady, P. A. (2015). The National Institutes of Health/National Institutes of Nursing Research Intramural Research Program and the development of the NIH Symptom Science Model. *Nursing Outlook, 63*, 484–487. doi: 10.1016/j.OUTLOOK.2015.03.001

Chan, C. W. H., Richardson, A., & Richardson, J. (2011). Managing symptoms in patients with advanced lung cancer during radiotherapy: Results of a psychoeducational randomized clinical trial. *Journal of Pain and Symptom Management, 41*, 347–357. doi: 10.1016/j.jpainsymman.2010.04.024

Cleeland, C. S., Mendoa, T., Wang, X. S., Chou, C., Harle, M. T., Morrissey, M., & Engstrom, M. C. (2000). Assessing symptom distress in cancer patients. *Cancer, 89*, 1634–1645. doi: 10.10021/1097.1402/20001001<1634::aid-cncr<3.0.CO; 2-v

Collins, J. J., Devine, R. D., Dick, G. S., Johnson, E. A., Kilham, H. A., Pinkerton, C. R., et al. (2002). The measurement of symptoms in young children with cancer: The validation of the memorial symptom assessment scale in children aged 7-12. *Journal of Pain & Symptom Management, 23*, 10–16.

Crosta, Q. R., Ward, T. M., Walker, A. J., & Peters, L. M. (2014). A review of pain measures for hospitalized children with cognitive impairment. *Journal for Specialists in Pediatric Nursing, 12*, 109–118. doi: 10.1111/jspn.12069

Daut, R. L., Cleeland, C. S., & Flaner, R. C. (1983). Development of the Wisconsin brief pain questionnaire to assess pain in cancer and other diseases. *Pain, 17*, 197–210. doi: 10.1016/0304-3959(83)90143-4

Dong, S.T., Costa, D. S. J., Butown, P. H., Lovell, M. R., Agar, M., Belikova, G., … Fayers, P. M. (2016). Symptom clusters in advanced cancer patients: An empirical comparison of statistical methods and the impact on quality of life. *Journal of Pain & Symptom Management, 51*, 88–98. doi: 10.1016/jpainsymman.2015.07.013

French, C. L., Crawford, S. L., Bova, C., & Irwin, R. S. (2017). Change in physiological and situational factors in adults after treatment of chronic cough. *Chest, 152*, 547–562. doi: 10.1016/j.chest.2017.06.024

Good, M. (2017). Pain: A balance between analgesia and side effects. In S. J. Peterson & T. S. Bredow (Eds.), *Middle range theories: Application to nursing research* (4th ed., pp. 49–66). Philadelphia, PA: Wolters Kluwer.

Hann, D. M., Denniston, M. M., & Baker, F. (2000). Measurement of fatigue in cancer patients: Further validation of the fatigue symptom inventory. *Quality of Life Research, 9*, 847 doi: 10.1023/A:1008900413113

Hann, D. M., Jacobsen, P. B., Azzarillo, L. M., Martin, S. C., Curran, S. L., ... Layman, G. (1998). Measurement of fatigue in cancer patients: Development and validation of the fatigue symptom inventory. *Quality of Life Research, 7*, 301. doi: 10.1023/A:1024929829627

Henly, S. J., Kallas, K. D., Klatt, C. M., & Swenson, K. K. (2003). The notion of time in symptom experiences. *Nursing Research, 52*, 410–417.

Herr, J. K., Salyer, J., Flattery, M., Goodloe, L., Lyon, D. E., Kabban, C. S., & Clement, D. G. (2015). Heart failure symptom clusters and functional status—A cross-sectional study. *Journal of Advanced Nursing, 71*, 1274–1287. doi: 10.1111/jan.12596

Hinds, P. S., Wang, J., Cheng, Y. I., Stern, E., Waldron, E., Gross, H., ... Jacobs, S. S. (2019). PROMIS Pediatric measures validated in a longitudinal study design in pediatric oncology. *Pediatric Blood & Cancer, 66*(5), e27606. doi: 10.1002/pbc.27606

Hoffman, A. J. (2013). Enhancing self-efficacy for optimized patient outcomes through the theory of symptom self-management. *Cancer Nursing, 36*, E16–26 doi: 10.1097/NCC.0b013e31824a730a

Hsu, M. C., & Tu, C. H. (2014). Improving quality-of-life outcomes for patients with cancer through mediating effects of depressive symptoms and functional status: A three-path mediation model. *Journal of Clinical Nursing, 23*, 2461. doi: 10.1111/jocn.12399

Huang, H.-C., Chen, M.-Y., Hsieh, L.-W., Chiu, J.-Y., Miao, N. -F., Wu, C.-S., & Lin K.-C. (2018). Validation of a symptoms distress scale in a cirrhotic population using item response theory. *Nursing Research, 67*, 359–368. doi: 10.1097/nnr.0000000000000296

Huang, J., Gu, L. Y., Zhang, L. J., Lu, X. Y., Zhuang, W., & Yang, Y. (2016). Symptom clusters in ovarian cancer patients with chemotherapy after surgery: A longitudinal survey. *Cancer Nursing, 39*(2),106–116. doi: 10.1097/ncc.0000000000000252

Huang, T. Y., Moser, D. K., & Hwang, S. L. (2018). Identification, associated factors, and prognosis of symptom clusters in Taiwanese patients with heart failure. *The Journal of Nursing Research, 26*(1), 60–67.

Humphreys, J., Janson, S., Donesky, K., Dracup, K., Lee, K. A., Puntillo, K., ... The UCSF Symptom Management Faculty Group. (2014). In M. J. Smith & P. Liehr (Eds.), *Middle range theory for nursing* (3rd ed., pp. 141–164). New York, NY: Springer.

Johnson, D., & Roberson, A. (2013). The evaluation of the effectiveness of relaxation training and sleep hygiene education for insomnia of depressed patients. *Clinical Scholars Review, 6*, 39–46. doi: 10.1891/1939-2095

Jurgens, C. Y., Lee, C. S., Reitano, J. M., & Reigel, B. (2013). Heart failure symptom monitoring and response training. *Heart & Lung, 42*, 273–280. doi: 10.1016/j.hrtlng.2013.03.005

Kapella, M. C., Larson, J. L., Patel, M. K., Covey, M. K., & Berry, J. K. (2006). Subjective fatigue, influencing variables, and consequences in chronic obstructive pulmonary disease. *Nursing Research, 55*, 10–17. Accession number: 00006199-300601000-00002. ISSN: 0029-6562

Kim, S. H., Oh, E. G., Lee, W. H., Kim O. S., & Han, K. H. (2006) Symptom experiences in Korean patients with liver cirrhosis. *Journal of Pain and Symptom Management, 31*, 326–334. doi: 10.1016/j.jpainsymman.2005.08.015

Kim, S. J., Kim, H. Y., Park, Y. A., Kim, S. H., Yoo, S. Y., Lee, J. E., & Moon, S. Y. (2017). Factors influencing fatigue among mothers with hospitalized children: A structural equation model. *Journal for Specialists in Pediatric Nursing, 22*, e12171.

Kim, S. K., Kim, H. K., Kang, K. O., & Kim, Y, S. (2019). Determinants of health-related quality of life among outpatients with acute coronary artery disease after percutaneous coronary intervention. *Japan Journal of Nursing Science, 16*, 3–18. doi: 10.1111/JJNS.12209

Kroenke, K., Spitzer, R. L., & Williams, J. B. W. (2001). The PHQ-9: Validity of a brief depression severity measure. *Journal of General Internal Medicine, 16*, 606–613. doi: 10.1046/j.1524-1497.2001.016009606.x

Lee, J., Nguyen, H. Q., Jarrett, M. E., Mitchell, P. H., Pike, K. C., & Fan, V. S. (2018). Effect of symptoms on physical performance in COPD. *Heart & Lung, 47*, 149–156. doi: 10.10106/j.hrtlng.2017.12.007

Lee, S. E., Vincent, C., & Finnegan, L. (2017). An analysis and evaluation of the theory of unpleasant symptoms. *Advances in Nursing Science, 40*(1), E16–E39. doi: 10,1097/ans.0000000000000141

Lenz, E. R., & Pugh, L. C. (2018). The theory of unpleasant symptoms. In M. J. Smith & P. Liehr (Eds.), *Middle range theory for nursing* (4th ed., pp. 179–214). New York, NY: Springer.

Lenz, E. R., Pugh, L. C., Milligan, R. A., Gift, A., & Suppe, F. (1997). The middle range theory of unpleasant symptoms: An update. *Advances in Nursing Science, 19*(3), 14–27.

Lenz, E. R., Suppe, F., Gift, A. G., Pugh, L. C., & Milligan, R. A. (1995). Collaborative development of middle-range nursing theories: Toward a theory of unpleasant symptoms. *Advances in Nursing Science*, 17(3), 1–13.

Liehr, P., & Smith, M. J. (2017). Middle range theory: A perspective on development and use. *Advances in Nursing Science, 40*, 51–63. doi:10.1097/ans.0000000000000162

Lim, K. E., Kim, S. R., Kim, H. K., & Kim, S. R. (2017). Symptom clusters and quality of life in subjects with COPD. *Respiratory Care, 62*, 1203–1211. doi:10.4187/respcare.05374

Loutenhizer, L., McAuslan, P., & Sharpe, D. P. (2015). The trajectory of maternal and paternal fatigue and factors associated with fatigue across the transition to parenthood. *Clinical Psychology, 19,* 15–27. doi: 10.1111/cp.12048

Matthie, N., & McMillan, S. C. (2014). Pain: A descriptive study in patients with cancer. *Clinical Journal of Oncology Nursing, 18*, 205–210. doi: 10.1188/14.cjon.205-210

McNair, D. M., Lorr, M., & Droppelman, M. F. (1992). *The profile of mood states*. San Diego, CA: Educational Testing Service.

Melzack, R. (1975). The McGill pain questionnaire: Major properties and scoring methods. *Pain, 1*, 277–299. http://dx.doi.org/10.1016/0304(75)90044-5

Mendoza, T. R., Wang, X. S., Cleeland, C. S., Morrissey, M., Johnson, B. A., Wendt, J. K., & Huber, S. L. (1999). The rapid assessment of fatigue severity in cancer patients: Use of the brief fatigue inventory. *Cancer, 85*, 1186i–1196. doi: 10.1002/(SICI)1097-0142(19990301)85:5<1186::AID-CNCR24>3.0.CO;2-N

Moore, S. M., Schiffman, R., Waldrop-Valverde, D., Redeker, N. S., McCloskey, D. J., Kim, M. T., ... Grady, P. (2016). Recommendations of common data elements to advance the science of self-management of chronic conditions. *Journal of Nursing Scholarship, 48*(5), 437–447. doi: 10.1111/jnu.12233

Moriarty, H., Bunting-Perry, L., Robinson, J. P., & Bradbury, C. W. (2016). The experience of women who care for spouses with Parkinson's disease and lower urinary tract symptoms. *Journal of Obstetrical, Gynecological, and Neonatal Nursing: JOGNN, 45*, 737–748. doi: 10.1015/j.jogn.2016.04.008

Nguyen, J., Haas, R. E., & Pugh, L. (2017). The application of the theory of unpleasant symptoms to the education and practice of nurse anesthetists. *Nursing & Healthcare International Journal, 1*(4), 000120.

O'Sullivan, C., Depuis, L. L., & Sung, L. (2015). A review of symptom screening tools in pediatric cancer patients. *Current Opinion in Oncology, 27*(4), 285–290. doi: 10.1097/cco,0000000000000197

Oh, H. S., Park, J. S., & Seo, W. S. (2018). Identification of symptom clusters and their synergistic effects on quality of life in rheumatoid arthritis patients. *International Journal of Nursing Practice, 25*(2), e12713. doi: 10.1111/ijn.12713

Park, S. K. (2017). Factors affecting self-care behavior in Koreans with COPD. *Applied Nursing Research, 38*(December), 29–37. doi: 10.1016/j.apnr.2017.09.003

Phigbua, W., Pongthavornkamol, L., Knobf, T. M., Junda, T., Viwatwongkasem, C., & Srimuninnimit, V. (2013). Symptom clusters and quality of life in women with breast cancer receiving adjuvant chemotherapy. *Pacific Rim International Journal of Nursing Research, 17*, 249–267. ISSN:1906-8107

Pongsing, Y. (2010). *Thai Mothers' Reports of Symptoms in Young Children Receiving Chemotherapy* (dissertation). Portland: Oregon Health and Sciences University. Retrieved from http://digitalcommons.ohsu.edu/etd

Portenoy, R. K., Thaler, H. T., Kornblith, A. B., Lepore, J. M., Friedlander-Klar, H., Kiyaau, E. E., … Scher, H. (1994). The Memorial Symptoms Assessment Scale: An instrument for the evaluation of symptom prevalence, characteristics and distress. *European Journal of Cancer, 30A*, 1326–1326. doi: 10.1016/0959-8049(94)90182

Radloff, L. S. (1977). The CES-D scale: A self-report depression scale for research in the general population. *Applied Psychological Measurement, 1*(3), 385–401.

Rector, T. S., Kubo, S. H., & Cohn, J. N. (1987). Patients' self-assessment of their congestive heart failure, part 2: Content, reliability and validity of a new measure of the Minnesota Living with Heart Failure Questionnaire. *Heart Failure, 3*, 198–209.

Reigel, B., Jaarsma, T., Lee, C. S., & Strömberg, A. (2018). Integrating symptoms into the middle-range theory of self-care of chronic illness. *Advances in Nursing Science*, 1–19. doi:10.1097/ans.0000000000000237

Riegel, B., Lee, C. S., Dickson, V. V., & Carlson, B. (2009). An update on the self-care of heart failure index. *Journal of Cardiovascular Nursing, 24*(6), 485–497. doi: 10.1097/jcn.0b013e3181b4baaf

Samantharath, P., Pongthavornkamol, K., Olson, K., Sriyaktasuth, A., & Sanpakit, K. (2018). Multiple symptoms and their influences on health-related quality of life in adolescents with hematologic malignancies undergoing chemotherapy. *Pacific Rim International Journal of Nursing Research, 22*(4), 319–331.

Seo, H. J., Ryu, E. J., & Young, E. M. (2018). Relationships among mood states, social support, symptom experience and quality of life in colorectal cancer patients—Based on the theory of unpleasant symptoms. *Asian Oncology Nursing, 18*(2), 104–113.

So, W. K. W., Leung, D. Y. P., Ho, S. S. M., Lai, E. T. L., Sit, J. W. H., & Chang, C. W. H. (2013). Associations between social support, prevalent symptoms and health related quality of life in Chinese women undergoing treatment for breast cancer: A cross-sectional study using structural equation modeling. *European Journal of Oncology Nursing, 17*, 442–448. doi.10.1016/ejon.2012.11.001

University of California San Francisco School of Nursing Symptom Management Faculty Group: Larson, P., et al. (1994). A model for symptom management. *Image: Journal of Nursing Scholarship, 26*, 272–276. doi: 10.1111/j.1547-5069.1994.tb00333.x

Varni, J. W., Burwinkle, T. M., Katz, E. R., Meeske, K., & Dickinson, P. (2002). The PedQL in pediatric cancer: Reliability and validity of the pediatric quality of life inventory generic core scales, multidimensional fatigue scale, and cancer module. *Cancer, 94*, 2090–2106. Retrieved from https://www.ncbi.nim.gov/pubmed/11932914

Varni, J. W., Seid, M., & Kurtin, P. S. (2001). PedsQ: Reliability and validity of the pediatric quality of life inventory version 4.0 generic core scales in healthy and patient populations. *Medical Care, 39*, 800–812. Retrieved from https://www.ncbi.nim.gov/pubmed/11468499

Von Sadovszky, V., Christensen, E., Jennings, B. M., Miller, S., Hosley, S., Drought, L., & Lenz, E. R. (2018). A systematic review of pediatric self-report symptom measures: Congruence with the theory of unpleasant symptoms. *Journal for Specialists in Pediatric Nursing, 23*(2), e12215. doi: 10.1111/jspn.12215

Waltz, C. F., Strickland, O. L., & Lenz, E. R. (2017). *Measurement in nursing and health research* (5th ed.). New York, NY: Springer.

Wang, D., & Fu, J. (2014). Symptom clusters and quality of life in Chinese patients with lung cancer undergoing chemotherapy. *African Health Sciences, 14*, 49–58. doi: 10.4314/ahs.v14i1.8

Ware, J., & Sherbourne, C. (1992). The MOS 36-item short form health survey (SF-36): Conceptual framework and item selection. *Medical Care, 30*, 473–483.

Yang, I.-S., & Kang, Y. (2018). Self-care model based on the theory of unpleasant symptoms in patients with heart failure. *Applied Nursing Research, 43*, 10–17. doi: 10.1016/j.apnr.2018.06.005

# Self-Efficacy

Barbara Resnick

## Definition of Key Terms

| | |
|---|---|
| **Mastery experience** | The most influential of self-efficacy information is the interpreted result of one's previous performance or mastery experience. Individuals engage in tasks and activities, interpret the results of their actions, use the interpretations to develop beliefs about their capability to engage in subsequent tasks or activities, and act in concert with the beliefs created. |
| **Outcome expectations** | The belief that if a behavior is completed, there will be a certain outcome. Bandura postulates that because the outcomes an individual expects are the result of the judgments of what he or she can accomplish, outcome expectations are unlikely to contribute to predications of behavior. |
| **Self-efficacy** | People's judgments of their capabilities to organize and execute courses of action required to attain designated types of performances. Self-efficacy beliefs provide the foundation for human motivation, well-being, and personal accomplishment. |
| **Social persuasions** | Individuals also create and develop self-efficacy beliefs as a result of the social persuasions they receive from others. These persuasions can involve exposure to verbal judgments of others. |
| **Somatic and emotional states** | Somatic and emotional states, such as anxiety, stress, arousal, and mood, also provide information about efficacy beliefs. People can gauge their degree of confidence by the emotional state they experience as they contemplate an action. |
| **Vicarious experience** | In addition to interpreting the results of their actions, people acquire their self-efficacy beliefs through the vicarious experience of observing others perform tasks. This source of information is weaker than mastery experience in helping to create self-efficacy beliefs, but when people are uncertain about their own abilities or when they have limited prior experience, they are more likely to be influenced by observation reactions. |

Self-efficacy is defined as an individual's judgment of his or her capabilities to organize and execute courses of action. At the core of self-efficacy theory is the assumption that people can exercise influence over what they do. Through reflective thought, generative use of knowledge and skills to perform a specific behavior, and other tools of self-influence, a person will decide how to behave (Bandura, 1977; Bandura, 1986; Bandura, 1995; Bandura, 1997; Bandura, Adams, & Beyer, 1977; Bandura, Reese, & Adams, 1982). To determine self-efficacy, an individual must have the opportunity for self-evaluation or the ability to compare individual output to some sort of evaluative criterion. It is this comparison process that enables an individual to judge performance capability and establish self-efficacy expectation.

## Historical Background

Self-efficacy theory is based on social cognitive theory and conceptualizes person–behavior–environment interaction as triadic reciprocity, the foundation for reciprocal determinism (Bandura, 1977; 1986; 1995; 1997; Bandura et al., 1977; 1982). In the initial study (Bandura et al., 1977) that led to the development of self-efficacy theory, 33 subjects with snake phobias were randomly assigned to three different treatment conditions: (a) enactive attainment, which included actually touching the snakes; (b) role modeling, or seeing others touch the snakes; and (c) the control group. Results suggested that self-efficacy was predictive of subsequent behavior, and enactive attainment resulted in stronger and more generalized (to other snakes) self-efficacy expectations. This early self-efficacy research used an ideal controlled setting in that the individuals with snake phobias were unlikely to seek out opportunities to interact with snakes when away from the laboratory setting. Therefore, there was controlled input of efficacy information. While this ideal situation is not possible in the clinical setting, the theory of self-efficacy has been used to study and predict health behavior change and management in a variety of settings.

## Definition of Theory Concepts

Bandura, a social scientist, differentiated between two components of self-efficacy theory: self-efficacy and outcome expectations. Self-efficacy expectations are judgments about personal ability to accomplish a given task. Outcome expectations are judgments about what will happen if a given task is successfully accomplished. Self-efficacy and outcome expectations were differentiated because individuals can believe that a certain behavior will result in a specific outcome; however, they may not believe that they are capable of performing the behavior required for the outcome to occur.

The types of outcomes people anticipate generally depend on their judgments of how well they will be able to perform the behavior. Those who consider themselves to be highly efficacious in accomplishing a given behavior will expect favorable outcomes for that behavior. Expected outcomes are dependent on self-efficacy judgments. Therefore, Bandura postulated that expected outcomes may not add much on their own to the prediction of behavior. Bandura (Bandura et al., 1977) does state, however, that there are instances when outcome expectations can be dissociated from self-efficacy expectations. This occurs either when no action will result in a specific outcome or when the outcome is loosely linked to the level or quality of the performance. For example, if Mrs. White knows that *even if she* regains functional independence by participating in rehabilitation, she will still be discharged to a skilled nursing facility

rather than back home; her behavior is likely to be influenced by her outcome expectations (discharge to the skilled nursing facility). In this situation, no matter what Mrs. White's performance is, the outcome is the same; thus, outcome expectancy may influence her behavior independent of her self-efficacy beliefs.

Expected outcomes are also partially separable from self-efficacy judgments when extrinsic outcomes are fixed. For example, when a nurse provides care to six patients during an 8-hour shift, the nurse receives a certain salary. When the same nurse cares for 10 patients during the same shift, she receives the same salary. This could negatively impact performance. It is also possible for an individual to believe that he or she is capable of performing a specific behavior but not believe that the outcome of performing that behavior is worthwhile. For example, older adults in rehabilitation may believe that they are capable of performing the exercises and activities involved in the rehabilitation process but may not believe that performing the exercises will result in improved functional ability. Some older adults believe that resting rather than exercising will lead to recovery. In this situation, outcome expectations may have a direct impact on performance.

Outcome expectations are particularly relevant to older adults. These individuals may have high self-efficacy expectations for exercise, but if they do not believe in the outcomes associated with exercise, for example, improved health, strength, or function, then it is unlikely that there will be adherence to a regular exercise program.

### SOURCES OF SELF-EFFICACY JUDGMENT

Bandura (1986) suggested that judgment about one's self-efficacy is based on four informational sources: (a) enactive attainment, which is the actual performance of a behavior, (b) vicarious experience or visualizing other similar people perform a behavior, (c) verbal persuasion or exhortation, and (d) physiological state or physiological feedback during a behavior, such as pain or fatigue. The cognitive appraisal of these factors results in a perception of a level of confidence in the individual's ability to perform a certain behavior. The positive performance of this behavior reinforces self-efficacy expectations (Bandura, 1995).

#### Enactive Attainment

Enactive attainment has been described as the most influential source of self-efficacy information (Bandura, 1977; 1986; 1995; 1997; Bandura et al., 1977). There has been repetition in empirical verification that actually performing an activity strengthens self-efficacy beliefs. Specifically, performance of functional activities (Bisson & Newsam, 2017; Resnick, Gruber-Baldini, et al., 2009), adoption and maintenance of exercise behavior (Ka Wing Ho et al., 2017; Resnick, Galik, Gruber-Baldini, & Zimmerman, 2009; Resnick, Luisi, & Vogel, 2008), and optimal self-management of numerous clinical problems such as HIV (Zhou, Li, Qiao, Zhou, & Shen, 2017), cancer (Soo Hyun, Kisook, & Mayer, 2017), spinal cord and brain injury (Bisson & Newsam, 2017; Soeker, 2017), asthma (Grammatopoulou, Skordilis, Haniotou, John, & Athanasopoulos, 2017), recovery post stroke (Vahlberg, Cederholm, Lindmark, & Hellstrom, 2017), and management of diabetes (Hunt, Grant, & Pritchard, 2012) all strengthened self-efficacy and/or outcome expectations. Enactive attainment generally results in greater strengthening of self-efficacy expectations than do other informational sources.

However, performance alone does not establish self-efficacy beliefs. Other factors, such as preconceptions of ability, the perceived difficulty of the task, the amount of effort expended, the external aid received, the situational circumstance, and past successes and failures all impact the individual's cognitive appraisal of self-efficacy (Bandura, 1995). An older adult who strongly believes that he or she is able to bathe and dress independently because he or she has been doing so for 90 years will not likely alter self-efficacy expectations if he or she wakes up with severe arthritic changes one morning and is consequently unable to put on a shirt. However, repeated failures to perform the activity will impact self-efficacy expectations. The relative stability of strong self-efficacy expectations is important; otherwise, an occasional failure or setback could severely impact both self-efficacy expectations and behavior.

### Vicarious Experience

Self-efficacy expectations are also influenced by vicarious experiences or seeing other similar people successfully performing the same activity. There are some conditions, however, which impact the influence of vicarious experience. If the individual has not been exposed to the behavior of interest, or has had little experience with it, vicarious experience is likely to have a greater impact. In addition, when clear guidelines for performance are not explicated, self-efficacy will be more likely to be impacted by the performance of others. Examples of effective vicarious experience include peer modeling of behaviors as has been done with

spinal cord injury patients (Gassaway et al., 2017) and self-modeling by keeping personal records of behavior (Haylock, 2010).

### Verbal Persuasion

Verbal persuasion involves telling an individual that he or she has the capabilities to master the given behavior and is the most commonly used source of information to strengthen self-efficacy and outcome expectations. Empirical support for the influence of verbal persuasion has been documented since Bandura's early research of phobias (Bandura et al., 1977). Verbal persuasion has proven effective in supporting recovery from chronic illness and in health promotion research. Persuasive health influences lead people with a high sense of self-efficacy to intensify efforts at self-directed change of risky health behavior. For example, verbal persuasion has been used to help strengthen self-efficacy and/or outcome expectations among individuals with regard to smoking cessation (Japuntich et al., 2018; Taniguchi et al., 2017; Tseng et al., 2017), oral health (Wu et al., 2017), breast-feeding and child care (Abbass-Dick et al., 2017; Adams, Morris, Salcedo, & Holmes, 2017; Brockway, Benzies, & Hayden, 2017; Shorey et al., 2017), bone health (Zou, Hamptom, Shade, & Kaku, 2017), pain and fatigue management (Fordham, Chen, Hansen, Lall, & Lamb, 2017; Oliver, Fisher, & Childs, 2017; Van Heest, Mogush, & Mathiowetz, 2017), increasing physical activity (Mirkarimi et al., 2017) and other health promotion activities such as cancer screening (Czajkowska, Hall, Sewitch, Wang, & Komer, 2017; Fowler et al., 2017; Hsiao-Lan et al., 2014), diet interventions (Sharp & Salyer, 2012), and diabetes self-management (Sadler et al., 2017).

### Physiological Feedback

Individuals rely in part on information from their physiological state in order to judge their abilities. Physiological indicators are especially important in relation to coping with stressors, physical accomplishments, and health functioning. Individuals evaluate their physiological state, or arousal, and if aversive, they may avoid performing the behavior. For example, if the older adult has a fear of falling or getting hurt when walking, a high arousal state associated with the fear can limit performance and decrease the individual's confidence in ability to perform the activity. Likewise, if the rehabilitation activities result in fatigue, pain, or shortness of breath, these symptoms may be interpreted as physical inefficacy, and the older adult may not feel capable of performing the activity.

Interventions can be used to alter the interpretation of physiological feedback and help individuals cope with physical sensations, enhancing self-efficacy and resulting in improved performance. Interventions include things such as elimination of pain, fear of falling, or shortness of breath associated with physical activity (Anderson et al., 2017; Coleman, 2011; Vahlberg et al., 2017).

## Relationships Among the Concepts: The Model

The theory of self-efficacy was derived from social cognitive theory and must be considered within the context of reciprocal determinism. The four sources of experience (direct experience, vicarious experience, judgments by others, and derivation of knowledge by inference) that can potentially influence self-efficacy and outcome expectations interact with characteristics of the individual and the environment. Ideally, self-efficacy and outcome expectations are strengthened by these experiences and subsequently moderate behavior. Since self-efficacy and outcome expectations are influenced by performance of a behavior, it is likely that there is a reciprocal relationship between performance and efficacy expectations.

## Application of the Theory in Research

The theory of self-efficacy has been used in nursing research, focusing on clinical aspects of care, education, nursing competency, and professionalism. There have been hundreds of articles in nursing journals using self-efficacy to guide interventions and predict behavior. While the focus of the articles ranges from management of chronic illnesses to education of nurses and parental training, the majority have been related to chronic health problems and participation in health-promoting activities such as exercise, smoking cessation, and weight loss.

The majority of these studies are descriptive in nature, exploring the relationship between self-efficacy expectations and behavior. Although more and more intervention studies are being guided by self-efficacy expectations as noted by the many meta-analyses showing their effectiveness in areas such as smoking cessation (Japuntich et al., 2018; Traavaglini, Li, Brown, & Bennett, 2017), management of osteoarthritis (Brand, Nyland, Henzman,

& Mcginnis, 2013; Zhang et al., 2018), adherence to diet and exercise among cancer survivors (Roberts et al., 2017; Soo Hyun et al., 2017), management of pain (Oliver et al., 2017), increasing physical activity (Higgins, Middleton, Winner, & Janelle, 2017), and management of kidney disease (Li et al., 2011). The interventions described continue to focus mainly on mastery experiences and verbal encouragement usually through education. Although limited, there is some work that is beginning to address the impact of dose effect of the intervention in terms of strengthening self-efficacy (Resnick, Galik, Gruber-Baldini, & Zimmerman, 2011) and testing the impact of different sources of efficacy information such as comparing performance against verbal encouragement (Brock, Cohen, Sourkes, Good, & Halamek, 2017; Resnick et al., 2007). Some research in nursing has shown, for example, that mastery alone was not noted to be more effective than verbal encouragement, physiological feedback, or cueing with self-modeling (Resnick et al., 2007). The most important factor with regard to the use of the theory of self-efficacy in nursing research is that the researcher maintains the behavioral specificity of self-efficacy by developing a fit between the behavior that is being considered and the efficacy and outcome expectations being measured. If the behavior of interest is walking for 20 minutes every day, the self-efficacy measure should focus on the challenges related to this specific behavior (time, fatigue, pain, or fear of falling associated with walking).

### SELF-EFFICACY STUDIES RELATED TO HEALTH BEHAVIORS

Self-efficacy has been used to improve and understand health behaviors with regard to exercise (Maura et al., 2017; Mirkarimi et al., 2017; Resnick, Michael, Griffith, Klinedinst, & Galik, 2014). Specifically, these nursing studies considered the impact of motivational interventions and engaging individuals in exercise activities on self-efficacy expectations and explored relationships between self-efficacy and outcome expectations and exercise behavior. In contrast to Bandura's earlier findings (Bandura, 1997; Bandura et al., 1977), which stressed that self-efficacy expectations were better predictors of behavior than were outcome expectations, in several nursing studies, outcome expectations, rather than self-efficacy expectations, were predictive of exercise behavior (Morrison & Stuifbergen, 2014; Weekes, Haas, & Gosselin, 2014).

Self-efficacy theory has also been used to address health behaviors such as preparing and eating healthy diets (Dinkel et al., 2017; LaChausse, 2017; Oakley, Nelson, & Nickols-Richardson, 2017; Roberts et al., 2017; Sun, Cheng, Bui, Liang, Ng, & Chen, 2017), adherence to immunization recommendations (McCutcheon, Schaar, Herline, & Hayes, 2017), smoking cessation using innovative approaches such as education following screening (Japuntich et al., 2018; Traavaglini et al., 2017), management of bone health (Brand et al., 2013; Nahm et al., 2017; Zhang et al., 2018; Zou et al., 2017), and increasing physical activity (Baruth & Schlaff, 2017; Higgins et al., 2017) among others. In all of these studies, there was consistently a strong association between self-efficacy and the stated health behavior.

## SELF-EFFICACY AND CULTURAL AND NURSING CARE COMPETENCE

Cultural competence in nurses has been considered by using a measure of knowledge of cultural concepts, knowledge of cultural life patterns for specific ethnic groups, and self-efficacy in performing cultural nursing skills (Messler, 2014). Findings indicated that nurses were moderately efficacious in cultural knowledge and abilities. Cultural competence education was also noted to be improved some using an online Facebook intervention for health care professional students (Chang, Guo, & Lin, 2017). Advanced practice nursing students' self-efficacy expectations associated with being able to diagnose depression have also been considered (Delaney & Barrere, 2012). Confidence, or self-efficacy, in being able to identify depression was associated with providing holistic and comprehensive nursing care to adult patients. Self-efficacy expectations associated with improving emergency room nurses' disaster management (Jonson, Paettersson, Rybing, Nilsson, & Prytz, 2017) and improving caregivers' dementia care management are two other areas that have been guided by social cognitive theory (Connor et al., 2009; Lin et al., 2014) as has self-efficacy for providing function-focused care (FFC) across a variety of clinical settings (Resnick, Galik, Petzer-Aboff, Rogers, & Gruber-Baldini, 2008; Resnick et al., 2011). Self-efficacy expectations were associated with the nursing care behaviors of interest (e.g., providing FFC). Lastly, simulation education and lab-related education have been shown to improve self-efficacy for novice nurses across basic nursing techniques (Egenberg, Oian, Eggebo, Arsenovic, & Bru, 2017; Franklin & Lee, 2014; Shahsavari et al., 2017).

## SELF-EFFICACY AND FUNCTIONAL PERFORMANCE

Self-efficacy has been considered with regard to functional performance, particularly with regard to adults undergoing orthopedic interventions (Brady, Straight, & Evans, 2014; Huang, Sung, Wang, & Wang, 2017; Levinger et al., 2017; Resnick et al., 2007; Sullivan, Espe, Kelly, Veilbig, & Kwasny, 2014). Across all these studies, there was an association between self-efficacy expectations and functional performance.

## SELF-EFFICACY AND PATIENT SELF-MANAGEMENT

Nursing research frequently uses self-efficacy theory to address self-care and self-management across a variety of clinical problems. For example, self-efficacy has been used with regard to self-care management of post–acute cardiac events and associated with congestive heart failure self-management (Sharp & Salyer, 2012), diabetes self-care management (Hunt et al., 2012; Sadler et al., 2017; Swoboda, Miller, & Wills, 2017), self-management for asthma (Grammatopoulou et al., 2017), management of HIV (Kekwaletswe, Jordaan, Knkosi, & Morojele, 2017; Tseng et al., 2017; Zhou et al., 2017), managing depression (Mackay, Shochet, & Orr, 2017; Weng et al., 2008), self-management of chronic obstructive pulmonary disease (Donesky et al., 2014; Lee et al., 2013), and management of HIV (Zhou et al., 2017) for prevention and following cancer diagnosis and treatment (Czajkowska et al., 2017; Dockham et al., 2017; Grimmett et al., 2017; Roberts et al., 2017; Soo Hyun et al., 2017), for oral health (Wu et al., 2017), and for pain and fatigue associated with chronic illnesses (Anderson et al., 2017; Fordham et al., 2017; Oliver et al., 2017; Van Heest et al., 2017). Nursing interventions intended to improve adherence to self-care behaviors were guided by self-efficacy theory in these studies, and findings indicated that there were improvements in self-efficacy as well as anticipated behaviors. Using Middle Range Theory in Research 6.1 provides a description of a study that uses self-efficacy for the framework to improve outcomes in individuals with diabetes. The intervention included a group education program followed by 4 weeks of independent use of the Diabetes HealthSense Web site. The intervention resulted in improvements in self-efficacy around diabetes management as well as relevant diabetes management behaviors such as medication adherence and diet and physical activity (Sadler et al., 2017).

**USING MIDDLE RANGE THEORY IN RESEARCH    6.1**

*Source: Sadler, M. D., Saperstein, S. L., Carpenter, C., Devchand, R., Tuncer, D., O'Brian, C., ... Gallivan, J. (2017). Community evaluation of the National Diabetes Education Programs Diabetes Healthsense Website. The Diabetes Educator, 43(5), 476–485.*

**PURPOSE/RESEARCH QUESTION**

The purpose of this study was to test the impact of the Diabetes HealthSense Web site on knowledge, attitudes, and behavior changes that prevent, delay, or facilitate management of diabetes among individuals at risk for diabetes and people with diabetes.

**RESEARCH DESIGN**

A two-group pretest–posttest design was used. Fifteen community sites were randomly assigned to treatment versus control prior to recruitment of participants.

**SUBJECTS/PARTICIPANTS/INTERVENTION**

From the 15 community sites, 311 adults were recruited, 135 in the intervention group and 176 in the control group. The intervention involved a group education session with a diabetes educator followed by 4 weeks of independent use of the Diabetes HealthSense Web site. The comparison or control group received no intervention.

**DATA COLLECTION AND RESULTS**

Outcome measures included self-reported knowledge, self-efficacy, and behaviors that support diabetes prevention or management. Overall linear mixed models showed significant differences between treatment groups for knowledge, stages of change around healthy eating and physical activity, and self-efficacy around healthy eating, physical activity, following provider recommendations, performance of physical activity, and coping behaviors.

**NURSING IMPLICATIONS**

The findings from this study suggest that there may be significant value in the combination of a face-to-face educational program with exposure to a Web site with additional training and resources. This approach is a way to enhance and extend the reach of face-to-face in-person diabetes education. Increasingly nurses, and other members of the health care team, are using Internet-based approaches to provide health education to adults. These approaches provide the verbal encouragement recommended for use by Bandura as a way to strengthen self-efficacy and outcome expectations. The resources and materials online need to be well established and vetted so that they can optimally improve outcomes for those exposed.

## SELF-EFFICACY AND BREAST-FEEDING AND INFANT CARE

Another common use of self-efficacy theory in nursing research is around the area of parenting specifically with regard to breast-feeding and infant care (Adams et al., 2017; Brockway et al., 2017; Costa, Brauchle, & Kennedy-Gehr, 2017; Dinkel et al., 2017; Nikolaus, Graziose, & Nickols-Richardson, 2017; Shorey et al., 2017). Self-efficacy expectations were shown to be associated with breast-feeding and infant care, and interventions to strengthen self-efficacy associated with these behaviors improved adherence to nursing behaviors. Self-efficacy–based interventions around the use of safe car seats and dietary interventions and activities to use with children to prevent obesity were also noted to be effective.

## SELF-EFFICACY AND CANCER CARE

Nurse researchers in the area of oncology identified relationships among self-efficacy, cancer prevention, screening, and adaptation to cancer. Strong self-efficacy expectations predict behaviors such as increased participation in screening programs and adjustment to cancer diagnosis (Dockham et al., 2017; Roberts et al., 2017; Duijts, Bleiker, Paalman, & Beek, 2017; Fowler et al., 2017; Grimmett et al., 2017; Soo Hyun et al., 2017; Tung, Lu, Granner, & Sohn, 2017). Increased self-efficacy is associated with increased adherence to screening activities, treatment, relevant self-care behaviors for management and prevention of cancer such as diet and exercise, and improved psychological symptoms.

## SELF-EFFICACY FOR BONE HEALTH

Self-efficacy interventions have been used to increase adherence to behaviors that are consistent with good bone health such as high-calcium diets and exercise (Nahm et al., 2010, 2017; Qi & Resnick, in press; Zhang et al., 2018). These studies have used education and mastery experiences to strengthen self-efficacy expectations in exercise focused on bone-strengthening exercises, adherence to bone-building medications, and diets high in calcium and vitamin D.

## SELF-EFFICACY FOR CAREGIVERS

Self-efficacy interventions have been used to strengthen caregiving ability across multiple clinical areas. Several studies focused on caregiver confidence to identify clinical problems among older adults with dementia (Piggott, Zimmerman, Reed, & Sloane, 2017) or delirium (Mailhot et al., 2017) and for caregivers for cancer patients (Dockham et al., 2017; Duggleby et al., 2017). Strengthening beliefs in the caregivers' ability to address their care recipients' needs and improve clinical outcomes has emerged as a solution to improve person-centered, individualized care.

## SELF-EFFICACY FOR FALL PREVENTION

Self-efficacy interventions have been used to strengthen self-efficacy expectations related to fear of falling (Vahlberg et al., 2017; Visschedijk, van Balen, Hertogh, & Achterberg, 2013; Ying-Yu, Scherer, Yow-Wu, Lucke, & Montgomery, 2013). Consistently, fear of falling is associated with falls self-efficacy or the confidence that individuals have that they can do routine activities without falling. Strengthening fear of falling is assumed to result in increased performance of the behavior of interest.

## SELF-EFFICACY FOR EXERCISE

Repeatedly, self-efficacy and outcome expectations have been associated with exercise among adults (Galik et al., 2008; Joseph, Ainsworth, Mathis, Hooker, & Keller, 2017; Pekmezi et al., 2017; Resnick et al., 2007; Resnick, Nahm, Shaughnessy, & Michael, 2009; Resnick et al., 2008; Rhodes, Janssen, Bredin, Warburton, & Bauman, 2017). Based on these findings, interventions were developed to strengthen self-efficacy and outcome expectations related to exercise. In addition, the findings from qualitative research identifying the factors that influenced motivation to engage in exercise (Resnick, Pretzer-Aboff, et al., 2008; Resnick & Spellbring, 2000) were used to develop self-efficacy and outcome expectation scales for exercise. Development of self-efficacy expectation measures was based on Bandura's (1977) early work with snake phobias. This approach included a paper and pencil measure that listed activities, from least to most difficult, in a specific behavioral domain. Respondents were given a 100-point scale, divided into 10-unit intervals ranging from 0, which is completely uncertain, to 10, which is completely certain, to identify the extent of confidence the participant had in performing a particular activity (strength of self-efficacy) given the existence of a challenge or benefit. An example of items on a self-efficacy scale for exercise follows:

How confident are you right now that you could exercise three times per week for 20 minutes if:

|  | Not Confident | | Very Confident |
|---|---|---|---|
| 1. The weather was bothering you | 0 | 1 2 3 4 5 6 7 8 9 | 10 |
| 2. You were bored by the program or activity | 0 | 1 2 3 4 5 6 7 8 9 | 10 |

The development of appropriate self-efficacy and outcome expectation measures enables the testing of interventions designed to help participants believe in the benefits and overcome the challenges of performing selected activities. Examples of how this has been done are demonstrated in the WALC (Walk, Address unpleasant symptoms, Learn about exercise, Cueing to exercise) intervention and the Exercise Plus Program (Resnick et al., 2007), the Senior Exercise Self-efficacy Project (Resnick et al., 2008), PRAISEDD, an exercise intervention program for minority older adults living in senior housing (Resnick et al., 2014), and multiple interventions in nursing homes (Galik, Resnick, Hammersla, & Brightwater, 2014; Galik, Resnick, Lerner, Hammersla, & Gruber-Baldini, 2015; Resnick, & Galik, 2013; Resnick, Galik, Vigne, & Carew, 2016; Resnick, Galik, Pretzer-Aboff, et al., 2009; Resnick et al., 2011). All of these interventions incorporated the four sources of information known to influence self-efficacy and outcome expectations. Specifically, they used verbal encouragement, decreasing unpleasant sensations, cueing and role modeling, and the actual performance of the behavior.

Self-efficacy theory has been used as a foundation for FFC interventions, which teach staff how to engage residents in functional and physical activity in a variety of settings. Theoretically based motivational interventions are used with both caregivers and residents. A detailed description of this intervention is provided in Box 6.2.

| BOX 6.2 | Function-Focused Care in Assisted Living (FFC-AL) Intervention |
|---------|----------------------------------------------------------------|

Following pilot testing (Resnick, Galik, Pretzer-Aboff, et al., 2009), FFC-AL was tested using a cluster-randomized controlled trial with a repeated measure design (Resnick et al., 2011). The intervention persisted, and participants were followed over a 12-month period. Four AL communities were matched on ownership, and all were similar in size, staffing, and services. A total of 171 residents and 96 DCWs were recruited from these sites.

The FFC-AL intervention was coordinated and implemented by a research function-focused care nurse (FFCN) with support from an interdisciplinary research team that included advanced practice nurses, social work, and physical therapy. The FFCN worked with the intervention sites 15 hours per week for the first 6 months of the intervention, 8 hours a week for the next 3 months, and 4 hours a week for the final 3 months of the intervention. To assure sustainability of the FFC philosophy, each treatment site identified a staff champion who worked with the FFCN, learned the four components necessary to implement and sustain the FFC philosophy, and helped to institutionalize FFC within the community. Working with the champion, the FFCN implemented the four components of FFC-AL: (a) environment and policy/procedure assessments, (b) education, (c) developing function-focused goals, and (d) mentoring and motivating.

Components were implemented sequentially although overlapped in that once initiated they continued throughout the course of the intervention. Component 1 involved having the FFCN evaluate the environment and community policies and procedures to determine if there were barriers to implementation of an FFC approach. Environments, for example, were evaluated for pleasant walking areas, destination sites, and appropriate bed and chair heights. Findings were discussed during the course of the 12-month study period with AL administrative staff to facilitate appropriate changes. Component 2, the education component, was then implemented, and all staff was invited to attend a 30-minute session on implementing an FFC approach (e.g., benefits of FFC, motivational strategies to engage residents, and recommendations for how to incorporate FFC into routine care activities).

Component 3, individual goal setting, was initiated by the FFCN working closely with the resident, staff champion, and DCWs. Residents' physical capability was evaluated using a Physical Capability Assessment form. This assessment guides the staff to evaluate cognitive status and functional ability (e.g., range of motion and balance) of residents. Goals included things such as walking to the dining room, going to exercise classes, or engaging in personal care activities. The staff was encouraged to

build these goals into the residents' required service plans. Once individual goals were established for all participants, component 4, mentoring and motivating, was initiated. This involved the FFCN and community champion mentoring DCWs and helping them motivate residents to work toward goal achievement. Motivational interventions were used to reward and recognize staff for providing FFC and residents for participating in exercise-related activities. Ongoing informal education and positive role modeling at the bedside related to FFC were provided by the FFCN and staff champion throughout the course of the 12-month intervention.

AL communities randomized to control received FFC-education only. All staff in these communities was invited to attend an educational session on FFC. The education material was identical to that provided to the treatment group, with the exclusion of motivational techniques taught to intervention participants as a way to engage residents in functional and physical activity.

**Study Results**

The majority of the DCWs were female ($n = 95$; 99%) and black ($n = 59$; 62%), with a mean age of 41.7 years (SD = 13.8). The residents were mostly female (80%), white (93%), and widowed (80%) with a mean age of 87.7 years (SD = 5.7). Outcomes for residents included psychosocial domains (mood, resilience, and self-efficacy and outcome expectations for function and physical activity), function, gait and balance, and actigraphy. Outcomes for DCWs included knowledge, performance, and beliefs associated with FFC.

Based on observations, DCWs in treatment sites provided more FFC by 12 months than did those in the control sites. The treatment group increased from providing FFC during 76% of observed care interactions at baseline to 82% at 4 months and 90% at 12 months ($p = 0.001$) compared to the control group, which provided FFC during 75% of care interactions at baseline and 4 months, and then this decreased to 69% of care interactions at 12 months.

Residents in treatment sites demonstrated less decline in function, a greater percentage returned to ambulatory status, and there were positive trends demonstrating more time in moderate-level physical activity at 4 months and more overall counts of activity at 12 months when compared to residents in control sites. Specifically, the control group declined 6.95 points versus 4.33 points for the treatment group, $p = 0.01$, in overall function based on the Barthel Index (scores range from 0 to 100 with higher scores indicative of more independent function). From baseline to 12 months, 13 (17%) residents in the treatment group versus 2

| BOX 6.2 | **Function-Focused Care in Assisted Living (FFC-AL) Intervention** (Continued) |
|---|---|

(4%) residents in the control group resumed walking functional distances versus remaining wheelchair dependent (chi square = 4.94, $p = 0.026$). Although not significantly different, residents in the intervention group showed a greater increase in the amount of time spent in moderate-level physical activity at 4 months ($p = 0.08$). Specifically, the treatment group increased from 0.43 at baseline to 1.00 minute of moderate-level physical activity with 24 hours versus the control group, which had a decline from 0.51 to 0.35 minutes. In addition, the treatment group had an increase in counts of activity from 40,668 at 4 months to 46,960 at 12 months, while the control group declined from 36,834 at 4 months to 32,563 at 12 months ($p = 0.07$). There were no treatment

effects on residents' self-efficacy or outcome expectations, mood, resilience, balance, or gait.

This study supports the use of FFC-AL to change care behaviors among DCWs and suggests that FFC-AL may help prevent some of the persistent functional decline and sedentary behavior commonly noted in these settings.

*Source*: Resnick, B., Galik, E., Gruber-Baldini, A., & Zimmerman, S. (2009). Implementing a restorative care philosophy of care in assisted living: pilot testing of Res-Care-AL. *Journal of the American Academy of Nurse Practitioners, 21*(2), 123–133.; Resnick, B., Galik, E., Gruber-Baldini, A., & Zimmerman, S. (2011). Testing the impact of function focused care in assisted living. *Journal of the American Geriatrics Society, 59*(12), 2233–2240.

## Application of the Theory in Practice

Translation of research findings into practice is not often done in a timely fashion. This is particularly true of research findings that focus on behavior change. There is, however, evidence to demonstrate that the theory of self-efficacy can help direct nursing care. The theory has been particularly helpful with regard to motivating individuals to participate in health-promoting activities such as regular exercise, smoking cessation, weight loss, and going for recommended cancer screenings. Table 6.1 provides examples of studies conducted to test the usefulness of the theory with different populations and desired treatment outcomes.

The ultimate goal of any intervention implemented in a research setting is to maintain the intervention over time and persist in day-to-day clinical practice. FFC interventions were developed so as to be integrated into routine care and continue even at the end of the research activities. It has been demonstrated that FFC interventions persist in clinical settings.

In clinical practice, FFC, like any innovative intervention, requires a champion. The champion can be self-identified or identified by administrative staff to take on the project or focus of care. Champions vary in terms of professional level and administrative position. The champion, however, needs to believe in the benefit of optimizing function and physical activity among older adults and needs to be passionate about helping other caregivers to achieve that type of care. Using Middle Range Theory in Practice 6.3 provides a description of the theory applied to a FFC intervention.

## FUNCTION-FOCUSED CARE INTERVENTION ACTIVITIES

The first step in the implementation of a FFC intervention is to evaluate the current environment and policies within the community. Policy and environmental changes should be established to facilitate implementation of FFC approaches with staff and residents. The communities altered their environments to optimize function in simple ways by doing such things as setting up pleasant and safe walking areas, strategically placing chairs or benches for residents to sit on to rest during a walk, removing clutter from residents' living spaces to encourage ambulation, and developing new, fun activities that incorporate physical activity to replace the commonly provided sedentary activities such as watching a movie. Policy changes to facilitate FFC included new service plan forms, which are required for all AL residents. The new service plan forms develop function and physical activity goals. These goals delineated what the resident was required to do with regard to function and physical activity and how the direct care worker would help the resident achieve his/her goals (e.g., remind the individual to go to exercise class).

Self-efficacy–based mentoring and motivation of staff occurs via ongoing formal and informal education of direct care workers. Following basic education of all staff during a single 30-minute in-service program, all new staff must go through FFC educational session and pass the FFC knowledge test with a score of 80% or greater or repeat the training session. The champion provides monthly oversight to direct care workers in these communities by performing monthly observations

**Table 6.1    Examples of Research for Application to Practice**

| Reference | Research Design/ Meta-Analysis | Clinical Issue/Research Question | Sample (n)/ Participants | Intervention | Outcome |
|---|---|---|---|---|---|
| Roberts et al. (2017) | A systematic review and meta-analysis | Use of digital health behavior change interventions targeting physical activity and diet in cancer survivors | 15 studies included of cancer survivors | Use of digital behavior change interventions | Improved physical activity was noted across seven studies and improvement in body mass index No significant change in fatigue, quality of life, or diet. |
| LaChausse (2017) | A clustered random-ized controlled trial | Fruit and vegetable intake for children | 275 children from 28 schools | Exposure to the Harvest of the Month program, which involved education exposure to fruit and vegetable information | No impact was found on self-efficacy or other behaviors except for fruit and vegetable preferences. There was no effect on eating behaviors |
| Anderson et al. (2017) | A quasi-experimental trial | Improving pain management | 20 health care providers from two large multisite federally qualified health centers in Connecticut and Arizona | Project ECHO Pain videocon-ference case-based learning ses-sions on knowledge and quality of pain care | Those exposed to ECHO were more likely to use formal assessment tools and opioid agreements and refer to behavioral health, and they had better knowledge and self-efficacy associated with pain management and decreased their opioid prescribing |
| Shorey et al. (2017) | A randomized controlled two-group pre- and posttest design | Improving parental out-comes in the immediate postpartum period | 250 participants | Supportive educational pro-grams delivered via a mobile health application for parents during the early postpartum period | Improved parental self-efficacy, social support, and parenting satisfaction at 4 weeks postpartum. There was not dif-ference in postnatal depression scores between groups |
| Sudore et al. (2017) | Comparative effec-tiveness randomized clinical trial | To improve completion of advanced care planning | 414 participants | Exposure to PREPARE a patient-centered advanced care planning Web site with an easy-to-read advance directive to facilitate development of an advanced directive | Improved advanced care planning, improved knowledge, and self-efficacy associated with advanced care planning |

## USING MIDDLE RANGE THEORY IN PRACTICE    6.3

The theory of self-efficacy served as the foundation for the development of an FFC intervention for assisted living (FFC-AL) settings that was used to teach and motivate nursing assistants to provide FFC to residents of AL settings. Once this was established as an effective intervention, a dissemination and implementation project was undertaken to implement FFC-AL into 100 assisted living settings.

*Source: Resnick, B., Galik, E., & Vigne, E. (2014). Translation of function focused care to assisted living facilities. Family and Community Health, 37(2), 101–165.*

### PROBLEM

The majority of older adults who live in AL communities need assistance with bathing, dressing, toileting, and locomotion. They suffer with multiple comorbidities, and many have at least mild comorbidity. They tend to decline in function, engage in limited physical activity, are more likely to become depressed, and experience a lower quality of life. Changes need to be made in the way care is delivered to the residents of AL communities.

### NURSING INTERVENTION

This dissemination and implementation project introduced the FFC philosophy into 99 AL settings in the greater Baltimore area. FFC is a philosophy of care in which nurses acknowledge older adults' physical and cognitive capabilities (e.g., ambulation, hygiene activities) and engage the adults in these activities, integrating them into routine care.

A research nurse facilitator first provided a single full day of education for the in-house champion identified by each setting. That full day reviewed the philosophy of FFC and taught the champion the necessary skills for assessing residents' function and motivation, provided ways to establish goals and alter the service plan to incorporate FFC, and provided the champion with the necessary skills to motivate the staff and the residents to engage in FFC-related activities. The research nurse facilitator worked with a champion monthly in each setting, and together they provided the nursing assistants with an in-service program that introduced them to (a) the philosophy of FFC in this program, contrasting it to more traditional approaches, (b) motivational strategies based on the theory of self-efficacy to motivate residents, (c) integration of FFC activities with personal care activities (bathing, dressing, and feeding), (d) setting resident goals and integration of FFC activities (exercise) during transfers and ambulation, and (e) overcoming challenges in providing FFC. Residents were encouraged, for example, to engage in bed mobility at their highest level, walk to the dining room if having the underlying capability to do so rather than be pushed in a wheelchair, or attend an exercise class. The effectiveness of this approach was evaluated using a number of outcome measures.

### CONCLUSIONS

Evidence of reach was based on our ability to recruit 99 ALs with adoption of the intervention in 78 (78%). There was a significant improvement in policies supporting FFC and in establishing environments that supported FFC. Residents were noted to have fewer transfers to the emergency room or hospital admissions following implementation of FFC approaches in the settings. The changes in settings were maintained for 18 months. Further, we were able to implement all aspects of the intervention although challenges were identified. Future work should incorporate a full stakeholder team within the setting versus just working with the champion on a monthly basis. This will help to keep the stakeholders informed of the process and have them support the direct care workers in providing FFC.

---

of interactions between direct care workers and residents and provides positive feedback to the direct care worker regarding ways in which he/she encouraged and facilitated function and physical activity. Ongoing verbal encouragement was provided to the direct care workers to continue these positive interventions. Examples of effective FFC approaches and role modeling by the research nurse facilitator and champion were also provided to increase functional engagement and physical activity of the resident during routine care activities. Thus, the FFC intervention uses a two-tiered approach with self-efficacy interventions used with direct care workers who then use self-efficacy–based interventions with residents.

Reward systems are established within clinical settings for direct care workers and residents. Direct care workers are recognized for providing exemplary FFC interventions by administrative staff, with gold stars on a bulletin board, or with gift coupons or as a group with a pizza party. Rewards for residents can also be provided via implementation of a "Gifts of the Heart" program in which residents receive tokens or tickets for participating in FFC activities (e.g., a resident who walked to the dining room or attended an exercise class). Residents collect their tokens and then trade them for prizes from a glass display case of gifts.

Taken together, the FFC intervention uses verbal encouragement through education and goal setting, role modeling, ongoing awareness, and changes in the environment and policies to eliminate unpleasant sensations around function and physical activity (e.g., providing places for the residents to rest). In so doing, direct care worker' and residents' self-efficacy and outcome expectations are strengthened, and this innovative philosophy of care persists in the clinical setting.

## Summary

■ The studies done by nurse researchers using the theory of self-efficacy provide support for the importance of self-efficacy and outcome expectations with regard to behavior change.

■ Studies also provide support for the effectiveness of specific interventions that have been tested to strengthen both self-efficacy and outcome expectations and thereby improve behavior. Other variables such as tension/anxiety, barriers to behavior, and other psychosocial experiences impact behavior. Bandura (Bandura, 1986) recognized that expectations alone would not result in behavior change if there was no incentive to perform or if there were inadequate resources or external constraints.

■ Increasingly, it is recognized that use of a comprehensive social–ecological model (SEM) approach, which incorporates intrapersonal, interpersonal (including social networks), environmental, and policy factors, is needed to positively influence preventive health behaviors.

■ Self-efficacy theory is situation specific. It is difficult, therefore, to generalize an individual's self-efficacy from one type of behavior to another.

■ Future nursing research needs to focus on the degree to which specific self-efficacy behaviors can be generalized. To what degree is self-efficacy a dimension of individual humanness, distinct for each person, but consistent across a range of related behaviors for one person?

■ Measurement of self-efficacy and outcome expectations requires the development of valid and reliable, situation-specific scales with a series of activities listed in order of increasing difficulty or by a contextual arrangement in nonpsychomotor skills, such as dietary modification (Marchante et al., 2014; Sterling, Ford, Park, & McAlister, 2014).

■ Scales that are behavior specific can be used as the foundation for assessing an individual's self-care abilities in a particular area. Interventions can then be developed that are relevant for that individual.

■ The Patient-Reported Outcomes Measurement Information System (PROMIS) Program (PROMIS Health Measures, 2017) provides a number of measures of self-efficacy relevant for management of chronic illnesses (Gruber-Baldini, Velozo, Romero, & Shulman, 2017). Specifically, these include the following measures:

| Measure | Description | Full Bank of Items | Short Form |
|---|---|---|---|
| Self-efficacy—general | Confidence in the ability to successfully perform specific tasks or behaviors related to one's health in a variety of situations | 10 | 4 |
| Self-efficacy for managing chronic conditions—manage daily activities | Confidence in performing various activities of daily living (ADLs) without assistance. Items also assess exercise, sexual activities, and managing activities in challenging situations (traveling, bad weather) | 35 | 4, 8 |
| Self-efficacy for managing chronic conditions—manage emotions | Confidence to manage/control symptoms of anxiety, depression, helplessness, discouragement, frustration, disappointment, and anger | 25 | 4, 8 |
| Self-efficacy for managing chronic conditions—manage meds/treatment | Confidence in managing medication schedules of different complexity. Managing medication and other treatments in challenging situations such as when traveling, when running out of medication, and when adverse effects are encountered | 26 | 4, 8 |
| Self-efficacy for managing chronic conditions—manage social interactions | Confidence in participating in social activities and getting help when necessary. Managing communication with others about their medical condition, including communication with health professionals | 23 | 4, 8 |
| Self-efficacy for managing chronic conditions—manage symptoms | Confidence to manage/control their symptoms, to manage their symptoms in different settings, and to keep symptoms from interfering with work, sleep, relationships, or recreational activities | 28 | 4, 8 |

■ A major problem with the use of the theory of self-efficacy in nursing research has been the lack of consideration of outcome expectations. In particular, with regard to exercise in older adults, outcome expectations have been noted to be better predictors of exercise behavior than self-efficacy expectations (Ferrier, Dunlop, & Blanchard, 2010; Resnick et al., 2014).

■ Consideration also needs to be given to the influence of self-efficacy expectations beyond the initiation of behavior to focus more on long-term adherence.

■ Social cognitive theory and the theory of self-efficacy have helped guide nursing research related to behavior change.

■ Ongoing studies are needed to continue to evaluate the impact of both self-efficacy and outcome expectations on behavior change, as well as develop and test interventions that strengthen these expectations.

■ Ongoing studies are needed to establish the value of single approaches (e.g., the use of performance or verbal encouragement) alone versus using multiple sources of efficacy information to optimize outcomes.

## CRITICAL THINKING EXERCISES

1. As a nurse on a medical surgical unit, you are getting ready to discharge a patient home who has just had a hip fracture and an open reduction internal fixation to repair the fracture. She is independent with ambulation using her walker and will have some home physical therapy. Of note, however, she had a bone density scan that indicated severe osteoporosis and has been started on a bisphosphonate and calcium. Your goal at discharge is to increase the likelihood that she will adhere to taking these medications. Address the interventions you would do to ensure this.

2. You have just moved to New Mexico and are very concerned about working with a large percentage of Spanish-speaking older adults. You know little about their culture. Address what interventions you might do for yourself to facilitate this transition in your nursing career.

3. You have just started working on a maternity ward and noted that the mothers admitted who are younger than 20 years of age have a great deal of difficulty with the idea of breast-feeding and how to begin to breast-feed. Develop an intervention that you could implement to optimize your nursing interventions with these individuals.

## REFERENCES

Abbass-Dick, J., Xie, F., Koroluk, J., Alcock Brillinger, S., Huizinga, J., Newport, A., … Dennis, C. L. (2017). The development and piloting of an ehealth breastfeeding resource targeting fathers and partners as co-parents. *Midwifery, 50*, 139–147.

Adams, C. M., Morris, C. E., Salcedo, E. S., & Holmes, J. F. (2017). Dissemination of a child passenger safety program through trauma center community partnerships. *Journal of Trauma Nursing, 24*(5), 300–305.

Anderson, D., Zlateva, I., Davis, B., Bifulco, L., Giannotti, T., Coman, E., & Spegman, D. (2017). Improving pain care with Project ECHO in community health centers. *Pain Medicine, 18*(10), 1882–1889.

Bandura, A. (1977). Self-efficacy: Toward a unifying theory of behavioral change. *Psychological Review, 84*, 191–215.

Bandura, A. (1986). *Social Foundations of Thought and Action*. New Jersey: Prentice Hall.

Bandura, A. (1995). *Self-efficacy in Changing Societies*. New York, NY: Cambridge University Press.

Bandura, A. (1997). *Self-efficacy: The Exercise of Control*. New York, NY: W.H. Freeman and Company.

Bandura, A., Adams, N. E., & Beyer, J. (1977). Cognitive processes mediating behavioral change. *Journal of Personality and Social Psychology, 35*(3), 125–149.

Bandura, A., Reese, L., & Adams, N. (1982). Microanalysis of action and fear arousal as a function of differential levels of perceived self-efficacy. *Journal of Personality and Social Psychology, 43*, 5–21.

Baruth, M., & Schlaff, R. A. (2017). Psychosocial mediators of a group based physical activity intervention in older adults. *Health Science Journal, 11*(4), 1–7.

Bisson, T., & Newsam, C. J. (2017). Short duration high intensity bouts of physical therapy to increase self-efficacy, confidence and function in an individual with incomplete spinal cord injury: A case report. *Physiotherapy Theory and Practice, 33*(11), 888–895.

Brady, A. O., Straight, C. R., & Evans, E. M. (2014). Body composition, muscle capacity, and physical function in older adults: An integrated conceptual model. *Journal of Aging and Physical Activity, 22*(3), 441–452.

Brand, E., Nyland, J., Henzman, C., & Mcginnis, M. (2013). Osteoarthritis: A systematic review and meta analysis comparing arthritis self-management education with or without exercise. *Journal of Orthopaedic & Sports Physical Therapy, 43*(12), 895–910.

Brock, K. E., Cohen, H. J., Sourkes, B. M., Good, J. J., & Halamek, L. P. (2017). Training pediatric fellows in palliative care: A pilot comparison of simulation training and didactic education. *Journal of Palliative Medicine, 20*(10), 1074–1084.

Brockway, M., Benzies, K., & Hayden, K. A. (2017). Interventions to improve breastfeeding self-efficacy and resultant breastfeeding rates: A systematic review and meta analysis. *Journal of Human Lactation, 33*(3), 486–499.

Chang, L-C., Guo, J. L., & Lin, H-L. (2017). Cultural competence education for health professionals from pregraduation to licensure delivered using facebook: Twelve-month follow up on a randomized control trial. *Nurse Education Today, 59*, 94–100.

Coleman, J. F. (2011). Spring forest qigong and chronic pain: Making a difference. *Journal of Holistic Nursing, 29*(2), 118–128.

Connor, K., McNeese-Smith, D., van Servellen, G., Chang, B., Lee, M., Cheng, E., … Vickrey, B. (2009). Insight into dementia care management using social-behavioral theory and mixed methods. *Nursing Research, 58*(5), 348–358.

Costa, U. M., Brauchle, G., & Kennedy-Gehr, A. (2017). Collaborative goal setting with and for children as part of therapeutic intervention. *Disability and Rehabilitation, 39*(16), 1589–1600.

Czajkowska, Z., Hall, N. C., Sewitch, M., Wang, B., & Komer, A. (2017). The role of patient education and physician support in self-efficacy for skin self-examination among patients with melanoma. *Patient Education and Counseling, 100*(8), 1505–1510.

Delaney, C., & Barrere, C. (2012). Advanced practice nursing students' knowledge, self-efficacy, and attitudes related to depression in older adults: Teaching holistic depression care. *Holistic Nursing Practice, 26*(4), 210–220.

Dinkel, D., Tibbits, M., Hanigan, E., Nielsen, K., Jorgensen, L., & Grant, K. (2017). Healthy families: A family based community intervention to address childhood obesity. *Journal of Community Health Nursing, 34*(4), 109–202.

Dockham, B., Titler, M., Shuman, C., Yakusheva, O., Visovatti, M., Ellis, K., … Northouse, L. (2017). Effectiveness of implementing a dyadic psychoeducational intervention for cancer patients and family caregivers. *Supportive Care in Cancer, 25*(11), 3395–3306.

Donesky, D., Nguyen, H. Q., Paul, S. M., & Carrieri-Kohlman, V. (2014). The affective dimension of dyspnea improves in a dyspnea self-management program with exercise training. *Journal of Pain and Symptom Management, 47*(4), 757–771. doi: 10.1016/j.jpainsymman.2013.05.019

Duggleby, W., Ghosh, S., Struthers-Montford, K., Knekolaichukl, C., Cumming, C., Thomas, R., … Swindle, J. (2017). Feasibility study of an online intervention so support male spouses of women with breast cancer. *Oncology Nursing Forum, 44*(6), 765–775.

Duijts, S. F. A., Bleiker, E. M. A., Paalman, C. H., & Beek, A. J. (2017). A behavioural approach in the development of work-related interventions for cancer survivors: An exploratory review. *European Journal of Cancer Care, 26*(5), 961–967.

Egenberg, S., Oian, P., Eggebo, T. M., Arsenovic, M. G., & Bru, L. E. (2017). Changes in self-efficacy, collective efficacy and patient outcome following interprofessional simulation training on postpartum haemorrhage. *Journal of Clinical Nursing, 26*(19/20), 3174–3187.

Ferrier, S., Dunlop, N., & Blanchard, C. (2010). The role of outcome expectations and self-efficacy in explaining physical activity behaviors of individuals with multiple sclerosis. *Behavioral Medicine, 36*(1), 7–11.

Fordham, B., Chen, J., Hansen, Z., Lall, R., & Lamb, S. E. (2017). Explaining how cognitive behavioural approaches work for low back pain: Mediation analysis of the back skills training trial. *Spine, 42*(17), E1031–E1039.

Fowler, S., Klein, W. M. P., Ball, L., McGuire, J., Colditz, G. A., & Waters, E. A. (2017). Using an internet based breast cancer risk assessment tool to improve social cognitive precursors of physical activity. *Medical Decision Making, 37*(6), 657–669.

Franklin, A. E., & Lee, C. S. (2014). Effectiveness of simulation for improvement in self-efficacy among novice nurses: A meta analysis. *Journal of Nursing Education, 53*(11), 607–614.

Galik, E., Resnick, B., Gruber-Baldini, A., Nahm, E., Pearson, K., & Pretzer-Aboff, I. (2008). Pilot testing of the restorative care intervention for the cognitively impaired. *Journal of the American Medical Directors Association, 9*(7), 516–522.

Galik, E., Resnick, B., Hammersla, M., & Brightwater, J. (2014). Optimizing function and physical activity among nursing home residents with dementia: Testing the impact of function-focused care. *Gerontologist, 54*(6), 930–943.

Galik, E., Resnick, B., Lerner, N., Hammersla, M., & Gruber-Baldini, A. L. (2015). Function focused care for assisted living residents with dementia. *Gerontologist, 55*, S26–S30.

Gassaway, J., Johnes, M., Sweatman, W. M., Hong, M., Anziano, P., & DeVault, K. (2017). Effects of peer mentoring on self-efficacy and hospital readmission after inpatient rehabilitation of individuals with spinal cord injury: A randomized controlled trial. *Archives of Physical Medicine and Rehabilitation, 98*(8), 1526–1534.

Grammatopoulou, E., Skordilis, E. K., Haniotou, A., John, Z., & Athanasopoulos, S. (2017). The effect of a holistic self-management plan on asthma control. *Physiotherapy Theory and Practice, 33*(8), 622–633.

Grimmett, C., Haviland, J., Winter, J., Calman, L., Din, A., Richardson, A., … Smith, P. W. F. (2017). Colorectal cancer patient's self-efficacy for managing illness-related problems in the first 2 years after diagnosis, results from the ColoREctal well-being (CREW) study. *Journal of Cancer Survivorship, 11*(5), 634–642.

Gruber-Baldini, A. L., Velozo, C., Romero, S., & Shulman, L. M. (2017). Validation of the PROMIS® measures of self-efficacy for managing chronic conditions. *Quality of Life Research, 26*(7), 1915–1924.

Haylock, P. J. (2010). Advanced cancer: A mind-body-spirit approach to life and living. *Seminars in Oncology Nursing, 26*(3), 183–194.

Higgins, T. J., Middleton, K. R., Winner, L., & Janelle, C. M. (2017). Physical activity interventions differentially affect exercise task and barrier self-efficacy: a meta analysis. *Health Psychology, 38*(8), 89–900.

Hsiao-Lan, W., Christy, S. M., Skinner, C. S., Champion, V. L., Springston, J. K., Perkins, S. M., & Rawl, S. M. (2014). Predictors of stage of adoption for colorectal cancer screening among African American primary care patients. *Cancer Nursing, 37*(4), 241–251.

Huang, T. T., Sung, C. C., Wang, W-S., & Wang, B-H. (2017). The effects of the empowerment education program in older adults with total hip replacement surgery. *Journal of Advanced Nursing, 73*(8), 1848–1861.

Hunt, C. W., Grant, J. S., & Pritchard, D. A. (2012). An empirical study of self-efficacy and social support in diabetes self-management: Implications for home healthcare nurses. *Home Healthcare Nurse, 30*(4), 255–262.

Japuntich, S. J., Sherman, S. E., Joseph, A. M., Clothier, B., Noorbaloochi, S., Danan, E., … Fu, S. S. (2018). Proactive tobacco treatment for individuals with and without a mental health diagnosis: Secondary analysis of a pragmatic randomized controlled trial. *Addictive Behaviors, 76*, 15–19.

Jonson, C-O., Paettersson, J., Rybing, J., Nilsson, H., & Prytz, E. (2017). Short simulation exercise to improve emergency department nurses self-efficacy for initial disaster management: Controlled before and after study. *Nurse Education Today, 55*, 20–25.

Joseph, R. P., Ainsworth, B. E., Mathis, L., Hooker, S. P., & Keller, C. (2017). Utility of social cognitive theory in intervention design for promoting physical activity among African-American women: a qualitative study. *American Journal of Health Behavior, 41*(5), 518–533.

Ka Wing Ho, F., Lobo, H. T. L., Hing Sang Wong, W., Ko Long, C., Tiwari, A. S., Chun Bong, C., … Ip, P. (2017). A sports based youth development program, teen mental health, and physical fitness: An RCT. *Pediatrics, 140*(4), 41–45.

Kekwaletswe, C., Jordaan, E., Knkosi, S., & Morojele, N. (2017). Social support and the mediating roles of alcohol use and adherence self-efficacy on antiretroviral therapy (ART) adherence among ART recipients in Gauteng, South Africa. *Aids and Behavior, 21*(7), 1846–1856.

LaChausse, R. G. (2017). A clustered randomized controlled trial to determine impacts of the Harvest of the Month program. *Health Education Research, 32*(5), 375–383.

Lee, S., Cappella, J. N., Lerman, C., & Strasser, A. A. (2013). Effects of smoking cues and argument strength of antismoking advertisements on former smokers' self-efficacy, attitude, and intention to refrain from smoking. *Nicotine and Tobacco Research, 15*(2), 527–533. doi: 10.1093/ntr/nts171

Levinger, P., Haltam, K., Fraser, D., Pile, R., Ardern, C., Moreira, B., & Talbot, S. (2017). A novel web-support intervention to promote recovery following anterior cruciate ligament reconstruction: A pilot randomised controlled trial. *Physical Therapy in Sport, 27*, 29–37.

Li, T., Wu, H. M., Wang, F., Huang, C. Q., Yang, M., Dong, B. R., & Liu, G. J. (2011). Education programmes for people with diabetic kidney disease. *Cochrane Database of Systematic Reviews,* (6), CD007374.

Lin, S., Hayder-Beichel, D., Rucker, G., Motschall, E., Antes, G., Meyer, G., & Langer, G. (2014). Efficacy and experiences of telephone counselling for informal carers of people with dementia. *Cochrane Database of Systematic Reviews,* (9), CD009126.

Mackay, B., Shochet, I., & Orr, J. (2017). A pilot randomised controlled trial of a school based resilience intervention to prevent depressive symptoms for young adolescents with autism spectrum disorder: A mixed methods analysis. *Journal of Autism and Development Disorders, 47*(11), 3458–3478.

Mailhot, T., Cossette, S., Cote, J., Bourbonnais, A., Cote, M. C., Lamarache, Y., & Denault, A. (2017). A post cardiac surgery intervention to manage delirium involving families: a randomized pilot study. *Nursing in Critical Care, 22*(4), 221–228.

Marchante, A. N., Pulgaron, E. R., Daigre, A., Patiño-Fernandez, A. M., Sanchez, J., Sanders, L. M., & Delamater, A. M. (2014). Measurement of parental self-efficacy for diabetes management in young children. *Children's Health Care, 43*(2), 110–119.

Maura, D., Frits, M., von Heideken, J., Cui, J., Weinblatt, M., & Shadick, N. A. (2017). Physical activity and correlates of physical activity participation over three years in adults with rheumatoid arthritis. *Arthritis Care & Research, 69*(10), 1535–1545.

McCutcheon, T., Schaar, G., Herline, A., & Hayes, R. (2017). HPV awareness and vaccination rates in college aged male athletes. *Nurse Practitioner, 42*(11), 27–34.

Ming-Ling, S., Talley, P. C., Tain-Junn, C., & Kuang-Ming, K. (2017). How can hospitals better protect the privacy of electronic medical records? Perspectives from staff members of health information management. *Health Information Management Journal, 46*(2), 87–95. doi: 10.1177/1833358316671264

Mirkarimi, K., Eri, M., Ghanbari, M. R., Kabir, M. J., Raeisi, M., Ozouni-Davaji, R. B., … Charkazi, A. (2017). Modifying attitude and intention toward regular physical activity using protection motivation theory: A randomized controlled trial. *Eastern Mediterranean Health Journal, 23*(8), 543–550.

Morrison, J. D., & Stuifbergen, A. K. (2014). Outcome expectations and physical activity in persons with longstanding multiple sclerosis. *Journal of Neuroscience Nursing, 46*(3), 171–179.

Nahm, E., Barker, B., Resnick, B., Covington, B., Magaziner, J., & Brennan, P. (2010). Effects of a social cognitive theory-based hip fracture prevention web site for older adults. *Computers, Informatics, Nursing, 28*(6), 371–377.

Nahm, E. S., Resnic, B., Brown, C., Zhu, S, Magaziner, J., Ballantoi, M., … Park, B. K. (2017). The effects of an online theory based bone health program for older adults. *Journal of Applied Gerontology, 36*(9), 1117–1144.

Nikolaus, C. J., Graziose, M. M., & Nickols-Richardson, S. M. (2017). Feasibility of a grocery store tour for parents and their adolescents: a randomized controlled pilot study. *Journal of Nutrition Education and Behavior, 49*(10), 827–837.

Oakley, A. R., Nelson, S. A., & Nickols-Richardson, S. M. (2017). Peer-led culinary skills intervention for adolescents: Pilot study of the impact on knowledge, attitude and self-efficacy. *Journal of Nutrition Education and Behavior, 49*(10), 852–857.

Oliver, S., Fisher, K., & Childs, S. (2017). What psychological and physical changes predict patients' attainment of personally meaningful goals six months following a CBT based pain management intervention? *Disability and Rehabilitation, 39*(22), 2308–2314.

Pekmezi, D., Ainsworth, C., Joseph, R. P., Williams, V., Desmond, R., Menseses, K., … Demark-Wahnefried, W. (2017). Pilot trial of a home-based physical activity program for African American women. *Medicine & Science in Sports & Exercise, 49*(12), 2528–2536.

Piggott, C. A., Zimmerman, S., Reed, D., & Sloane, P. D. (2017). Development and testing of a measure of caregiver confidence in medical sign/symptom management. *American Journal of Alzheimer's Disease & Other Dementias, 32*(7), 373–381.

PROMIS Health Measures. (2017). Retrieved from http://www.healthmeasures.net/explore-measurement-systems/promis/intro-to-promis/list-of-adult-measures

Qi, B., & Resnick, B. (in press). Self-efficacy enhanced education program in preventing osteoporosis among Chinese immigrants. *Nursing Research.*

Resnick, B., & Galik, E. (2013). Using function-focused care to increase physical activity among older adults. *Annual Review of Nursing Research, 31*, 175–208.

Resnick, B., & Spellbring, A. (2000). Understanding what motivates older adults to exercise. *Journal of Gerontological Nursing, 26*(3), 34–42. Retrieved from http://www.ncbi.nlm.nih.gov/entrez/query.fcgi?cmd=Retrieve&db=PubMed&dopt=Citation&list_uids=11111629

Resnick, B., Galik, E., Gruber-Baldini, A., & Zimmerman, S. (2009). Implementing a restorative care philosophy of care in assisted living: pilot testing of Res-Care-AL. *Journal of the American Academy of Nurse Practitioners, 21*(2), 123–133.

Resnick, B., Galik, E., Gruber-Baldini, A., & Zimmerman, S. (2011). Testing the impact of function focused care in assisted living. *Journal of the American Geriatrics Society, 59*(12), 2233–2240.

Resnick, B., Galik, E., Nahm, E., Shaughnessy, M., Michael, K. (2009). Optimizing adherence in older adults with cognitive impairment. In S. A. Shumaker, J. K. Ockene, & K. A. Riekert (Eds.), *The handbook of health behavior change* (3rd ed.). New York, NY: Springer Publishing.

Resnick, B., Galik, E., Petzer-Aboff, I., Rogers, V., & Gruber-Baldini, A. (2008). Testing the reliability and validity of self-efficacy and outcome expectations of restorative care performed by nursing assistants. *Journal of Nursing Care Quality, 23*(2), 162–169.

Resnick, B., Galik, E., Vigne, E., & Carew, A. P. (2016). Dissemination and implementation of function focused care for assisted living. *Health Education & Behavior, 43*(3), 296–304.

Resnick, B., Gruber-Baldini, A., Zimmerman, S., Galik, E., Pretzer-Aboff, I., Russ, K., & Hebel, J. (2009). Nursing home resident outcomes from the Res-Care intervention. *Journal of the American Geriatrics Society, 57*(7), 1156–1165.

Resnick, B., Luisi, D., & Vogel, A. (2008). Testing the senior exercise self-efficacy pilot project (SESEP) for use with urban dwelling minority older adults. *Public Health Nursing, 25*(3), 221–234.

Resnick, B., Michael, K., Griffith, K., Klinedinst, J., & Galik, E. (2014). The impact of PRAISEDD on adherence and initiation of heart health behaviors in senior housing. *Public Health Nursing, 31*(4), 309–316.

Resnick, B., Orwig, D., Yu-Yahiro, J., Hawkes, W., Shardell, M., Hebel, J., … Magaziner, J. (2007). Testing the effectiveness of the exercise plus program in older women post hip fracture. *Annals of Behavioral Medicine, 34*(1), 67–76.

Resnick, B., Pretzer-Aboff, I., Galik, E., Russ, K., Cayo, J., Simpson, M., & Zimmerman, S. (2008). Barriers and benefits to implementing a restorative care intervention in nursing homes. *Journal of the American Medical Directors Association, 9*(2), 102–108.

Rhodes, R. E., Janssen, I., Bredin, S. D., Warburton, D. E. R., & Bauman, A. (2017). Physical activity: Health impact, prevalence, correlates and interventions. *Psychology & Health, 32*(8), 942–975.

Roberts, A., Fisher, A., Smith, L., Heinrich, M., Potts, H., Roberts, A. L., & Potts, H. W. W. (2017). Digital health behaviour change interventions targeting physical activity and diet in cancer survivors: A systematic review and meta-analysis. *Journal of Cancer Survivorship, 11*(6), 704–719.

Sadler, M. D., Saperstein, S. L., Carpenter, C., Devchand, R., Tuncer, D., O'Brian, C., … Gallivan, J. (2017). Community evaluation of the National Diabetes Education Programs Diabetes Healthsense Website. *The Diabetes Educator, 43*(5), 476–485.

Shahsavari, H., Ghiyasvandian, S., Houser, M. L., Zakerimoghadam, M., Kermanshahi, S. S. N., & Torabi, S. (2017). Effect of a clinical skills refresher course on the clinical performance, anxiety and self-efficacy of the final year undergraduate nursing students. *Nurse Education in Practice, 27*, 151–156.

Sharp, P. B., & Salyer, J. (2012). Self-efficacy and barriers to healthy diet in cardiac rehabilitation participants and nonparticipants. *Journal of Cardiovascular Nursing, 27*(3), 253–262.

Shorey, S., Lau, Y. Y., Dennis, C. L., Chan, Y. S., Tam, W. W. S., & Chan, Y. H. (2017). A randomized controlled trial to examine the effectiveness of the home but not along mobile health application educational programme on parental outcomes. *Journal of Advanced Nursing, 73*(9), 2103–2107.

Soeker, S. (2017). The use of model of occupational self-efficacy in improving the cognitive functioning of individuals with brain injury: A pre and post intervention study. *Work, 58*(1), 63–72.

Soo Hyun, K., Kisook, K., & Mayer, D. K. (2017). Self management intervention for adult cancer survivors after treatment: A systematic review and meta analysis. *Oncology Nursing Forum, 44*(6), 719–728.

Sterling, K. L., Ford, K. H., Park, H., & McAlister, A. L. (2014). Scales of smoking-related self-efficacy, beliefs, and intention: Assessing measurement invariance among intermittent and daily high school smokers. *American Journal of Health Promotion, 28*(5), 310–315.

Sudore, R. L., Boscardin, J., Feuz, M. A., McMahan, R. D., Katen, M. T., & Barnes, D. E. (2017). Effect of the PREPARE Website vs an Easy-to-Read Advance Directive on Advance Care Planning Documentation and Engagement Among Veterans: A Randomized Clinical Trial. *JAMA Internal Medicine, 177*(8), 1102–1109. doi: 10.1001/jamainternmed.2017.1607

Sullivan, J. E., Espe, L. E., Kelly, A. M., Veilbig, L. E., & Kwasny, M. J. (2014). Feasibility and outcomes of a community-based, pedometer-monitored walking program in chronic stroke: A pilot study. *Topics in Stroke Rehabilitation, 21*(2), 101–110.

Swoboda, C. M., Miller, C. K., & Wills, C. E. (2017). Impact of goal setting and decision support telephone coaching intervention on diet, psychosocial and decision outcomes among people with type 2 diabetes. *Patient Education and Counseling, 100*(7), 1367–1373.

Taniguchi, C., Tanaka, H., Saka, H., Oze, I., Tachibana, K., Nozaki, Y., …, Sakakibara H. (2017). Cognitive behavioral and psychosocial factors associated with successful and maintained quit smoking status among patients who received smoking cessation intervention with nurses counselling. *Journal of Advanced Nursing, 73*(7), 1681–1695.

Traavaglini, L. E., Li, L., Brown, C. H., & Bennett, M. E. (2017). Predictors of smoking cessation group treatment engagement among veterans with serious mental illness. *Addictive Behaviors, 75*, 103–107.

Tseng, T. Y., Krebs, P., Schoenthaler, A., Wong, S., Sherman, S., Gonzalez, M., … Shelley, D. (2017). Combining text messaging and telephone counseling to increase varenicline adherence and smoking abstinence among cigarette smokers living with HIV: a randomized controlled study. *Aids and Behavior, 21*(7), 1964–1974.

Tung, W. C., Lu, M., Granner, M., & Sohn, H. J. (2017). Assessing perceived benefits/barriers and self-efficacy for cervical cancer screening among Korean American women. *Health Care for Women International, 38*(9), 945–955.

Vahlberg, B., Cederholm, T., Lindmark, B., & Hellstrom, K. (2017). Short-term and long-term effects of a progressive resistance and balance exercise program in individuals with chronic stroke: A randomized controlled trial. *Disability and Rehabilitation, 39*(16), 1615–1622.

Van Heest, K. N. L., Mogush, A. R., & Mathiowetz, V. G. (2017). Effects of a one to one fatigue management course for people with chronic conditions and fatigue. *American Journal of Occupational Therapy, 71*(4), 1–9.

Visschedijk, J., van Balen, R., Hertogh, C., & Achterberg, W. (2013). Fear of falling in patients with hip fractures: Prevalence and related psychological factors. *Journal of the American Medical Directors Association, 14*(3), 218–220.

Weekes, C. V. N., Haas, B. K., & Gosselin, K. P. (2014). Expectations and self-efficacy of African American parents who discuss sexuality with their adolescent sons: An intervention study. *Public Health Nursing, 31*(3), 253–261.

Weng, L., Dai, Y., Wang, Y., Huang H., & Chiang, Y. (2008). Effects of self-efficacy, self-care behaviours on depressive symptom of Taiwanese kidney transplant recipients. *Journal of Clinical Nursing, 17*(13), 1786–1794. doi: 10.1111/j.1365-2702.2007.02035.x

Wu, L., Gao, X., Lo, E. C. M., Ho, S. M. Y., McGrath, C., & Wong, M. C. M. (2017). Motivational interviewing to promote oral health in adolescents. *Journal of Adolescent Health, 61*(3), 378–384.

Ying-Yu, C., Scherer, Y. K., Yow-Wu, W., Lucke, K. T., & Montgomery, C. A. (2013). The feasibility of an intervention combining self-efficacy theory and Wii Fit exergames in assisted living residents: A pilot study. *Geriatric Nursing, 34*(5), 377–382.

Zhang, L., Fu, T., Zhang, Q., Yin, R., Zhu, L., He, Y., … Shen, B. (2018). Effects of psychological interventions for patients with osteoarthritis: A systematic review and meta analysis. *Psychology, Health & Medicine, 23*(1), 1–17.

Zhou, G., Li, X., Qiao, S., Zhou, Y., & Shen, Z. (2017). Psychological and behavior barriers to ART adherence among PLWH in China: Role of self-efficacy. *AIDS Care, 29*(12), 1533–1537.

Zou, J., Hamptom, M. D., Shade, K., & Kaku, L. (2017). Bone health intervention for Chinese immigrants in Santa Clara County. *Orthopaedic Nursing, 36*(4), 293–300.

## WEB RESOURCES

Resources on Albert Bandura's Theory of Self-efficacy. Retrieved from https://positivepsychologyprogram.com/bandura-self-efficacy/

Retrieved from http://study.com/academy/lesson/albert-banduras-theory-of-self-efficacy.html

# Chronic Sorrow

Georgene Gaskill Eakes

## Definition of Key Terms

| | |
|---|---|
| **Chronic sorrow** | Periodic recurrence of permanent, pervasive sadness or other grief-related feelings associated with ongoing disparity resulting from a loss experience |
| **Disparity** | A gap between the current reality and the desired as a result of a loss experience |
| **External management methods** | Interventions provided by professionals to assist individuals to cope with chronic sorrow |
| **Internal management methods** | Positive personal coping strategies used to deal with the periodic episodes of chronic sorrow |
| **Loss experience** | A significant loss, either actual or symbolic, that may be ongoing with no predictable end or a more circumscribed single loss event |
| **Trigger event** | A situation or circumstance or condition that brings the negative disparity resulting from the loss into focus or exacerbates the disparity |

The middle range theory of chronic sorrow, first documented in the literature in 1998 by Eakes, Burke, and Hainsworth, offers a framework for explaining how individuals may respond to both ongoing and single loss events. Moreover, the theoretical model of chronic sorrow provides an alternative way of viewing the experience of grief. The theory of chronic sorrow was inductively derived and subsequently validated from an extensive review of the literature and from the data gathered through 10 qualitative research studies conducted by members of the Nursing Consortium for Research on Chronic Sorrow (NCRCS). Using the Burke/NCRCS Chronic Sorrow Questionnaire, adapted from a guide developed by Burke (1989), as an interview guide, these nurse researchers interviewed 196 individuals who shared their loss experiences as people with chronic conditions, as family caregivers of the chronically ill or disabled, or as bereaved family members.

## Historical Background

The term *chronic sorrow* was introduced into the literature 40 years ago to characterize the recurring episodes of grief experienced by parents of children with disabilities (Olshansky, 1962). This recurring sadness appeared to persist throughout the lives of these parents, although its intensity varied from time to time, from situation to situation, and from one family member to another. Rather than viewing this phenomenon as pathological, Olshansky described chronic sorrow as a normal response to an ongoing loss situation. Professionals were encouraged to recognize the presence of this phenomenon when working with a parent of a disabled child and to support parents' expressions of feelings. Although the term gained wide acceptance in the professional literature, almost two decades passed before there was any documented research on chronic sorrow.

Initial research conducted in the 1980s validated the occurrence of chronic sorrow among parents of disabled young children. Several investigators suggested that the never-ending nature of the loss of the "perfect" child prevented resolution of grief (Burke, 1989; Damrosch & Perry, 1989; Fraley, 1986; Kratochvil & Devereaux, 1988; Wikler, Wasow, & Hatfield, 1981). Moreover, it was this inability to bring closure to the loss experience that was thought to precipitate periodic episodes of re-grief labeled as chronic sorrow. These early studies refined and operationalized the definition of chronic sorrow as a pervasive sadness that was permanent, periodic, and progressive in nature.

# Current Research on Chronic Sorrow

More recent research supports the fact that chronic sorrow is a common experience among family caregivers (Batchelor, 2017; Bettle & Latimer, 2009; Bordonada, 2017; Bowes, Lowes, Warner, & Gregory, 2009; Branch-Smith, 2018; Chang, Huang, Cheng, & Chien, 2018; Clubb, 1991; Copley & Bodensteiner, 1987; Coughlin & Sethares, 2017; Doornbos, 1997; Eakes, 1995; Eakes, Burke, Hainsworth, & Lindgren, 1993; Fraley, 1990; George & Vickers, 2006–2007; Glenn, 2015; Golden, 1994; Gordon, 2009; Hainsworth, 1995; Hainsworth, Busch, Eakes, & Burke, 1995; Hobdell, 2004; Hobdell et al., 2007; Hummel & Eastman, 1991; Johnsonius, 1996; Keamy & Griffin, 2001; Krafft & Krafft, 1998; Liedstrom, Isaksson, & Ahlstrom, 2008; Lindgren, 1996; Lowes & Lyne, 2000; Mallow & Bechtel, 1999; Mayer, 2001; Mercer, 2015; Neilsen, 2013; Nikfarid, Rassouli, Borimnejad, & Alavimajd, 2015; Olwit, Musisi, Leshabari, & Sany, 2015; Patrick-Ott & Ladd, 2010; Phillips, 1991; Rosenberg, 1998; Rossheim & McAdams, 2010; Seideman & Kleine, 1995; Shumaker, 1995; Veltman, 2010; Vitale & Falco, 2014; Whittingham, Wee, Sanders, & Boyd, 2012). The caregivers studied represent a diverse representation of parents of young children with various disabilities, spouses of individuals diagnosed with chronic illnesses, and parents of adult children with debilitating conditions. Moreover, some of the studies cited represent subjects from Taiwan, Iran, Australia and Uganda, adding credence to the international applicability of the theory of chronic sorrow.

The NCRCS, established in 1989 (Eakes, Hainsworth, Lindgren, & Burke, 1991), expanded research on chronic sorrow and explored the relevance of the concept of chronic sorrow among individuals experiencing a variety of loss situations. This group of nurse researchers not only conducted research on chronic sorrow among family caregivers but also investigated individuals affected with chronic conditions and bereaved individuals. Among those diagnosed with a chronic condition, 83% evidenced chronic sorrow (Burke, Hainsworth, Eakes, & Lindgren, 1992; Eakes, 1993; Hainsworth, 1994; Hainsworth, Eakes, & Burke, 1994; Lindgren, 1996). Others have since been validated by the experience of chronic sorrow among those diagnosed with a chronic condition (Isaksson Gunnarsson, & Ahlstorm, 2007; Lichtenstein, Laska, & Clair, 2002; Smith, 2009).

The NCRCS also conducted research studies designed to investigate the occurrence of chronic sorrow among individuals who had experienced a single loss event rather than an ongoing loss. Toward the end, people who had experienced the death of a significant other a minimum of 2 years prior to the study were interviewed. This time lapse was to allow for acute grief to have subsided. Findings revealed that a vast majority (97%) of those interviewed evidenced chronic sorrow (Eakes, Burke, & Hainsworth, 1999). These findings led to further modification of the defining characteristics of chronic sorrow, with recognition that it was ongoing disparity associated with the loss, rather than the ongoing nature of the loss experience as originally thought, that was the antecedent to chronic sorrow. Consequently, chronic sorrow was redefined as permanent, periodic recurrence of pervasive sadness or other grief-related feelings associated with ongoing disparity resulting from significant loss (Eakes, Burke, & Hainsworth, 1998). The necessary antecedent event is involvement in an experience of significant loss. This loss may be ongoing in nature with no predictable end, such as with the birth of a disabled child or diagnosis of a debilitating illness, or it may be more circumscribed as with the death of a loved one. Disparity is created by a loss/situation when an individual's current reality differs markedly from the idealized or when a gap exists between the desired and the actual reality. This lack of closure sets the stage for grief to be periodically reexperienced. That is, the chronic sorrow experience is cyclical and continues as long as the disparity created by the loss remains.

# Middle Range Nursing Theory of Chronic Sorrow

The middle range theory of chronic sorrow (Eakes et al., 1998) was inductively derived and validated through the qualitative studies described above as well as a critical review of existing literature (see Fig. 7.1). Chronic sorrow was reconceptualized based on these findings and is now defined as "the periodic recurrence of permanent, pervasive sadness or other grief-related feelings associated with ongoing disparity resulting from a loss experience" (Eakes et al., 1998, p. 180, 1999). Moreover, chronic sorrow is characterized as pervasive, permanent, periodic, and potentially progressive in nature and continues to be viewed as a normal response to loss. Indeed, the theory of chronic sorrow purports that the periodic return of grief among individuals and caregivers whose anticipated life course has been interrupted continues throughout one's lifetime as

# LIFE SPAN

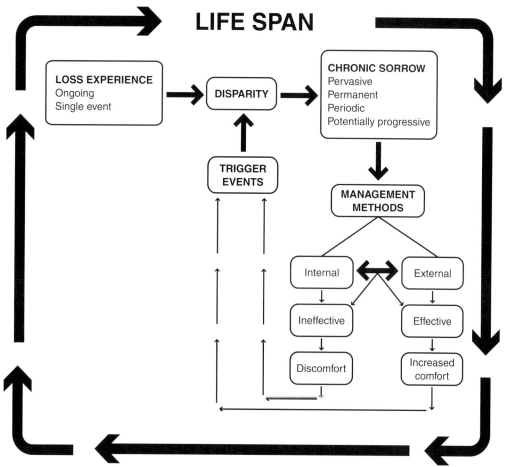

**Figure 7.1**    Theoretical model of chronic sorrow. (From Eakes, G. G., Burke, M. L., & Hainsworth, M. A. (1998). Middle range theory of chronic sorrow. *Image: The Journal of Nursing Scholarship, 30*(2), 179–184.)

long as the disparity created by the loss remains. As stated by Patrick-Ott (2011, p. 110), in reference to manifestation of chronic sorrow in parents of disabled children, "Chronic Sorrow is continual as it moves like waves over a sandy shore such that with each newly understood dimension of the child's significant disability and its meaning for the parent's lifelong care-giving role brings a new tide of chronic sorrow."

The middle range theory of chronic sorrow provides a framework for understanding the reactions of individuals to various loss situations and offers a new way of viewing the experience of bereavement. Although chronic sorrow is viewed as a normal response to the ongoing disparity or void created by significant loss, it is important to note that normalization of the experience in no way diminishes the validity or the intensity of the feelings experienced. At times, feelings can be intense and distressing for the individual experiencing chronic sorrow.

Involvement in an experience of significant loss is the necessary antecedent to the development of chronic sorrow. This may be a loss with no predictable end, such as the birth of a disabled child or diagnosis of a chronic illness, or a more clearly defined loss event such as the death of a loved one. The second antecedent to chronic sorrow is ongoing disparity resulting from the loss. That is, a gap exists between the desired and the actual reality. The lack of closure associated with ongoing disparity sets the stage for chronic sorrow, with the loss experienced in bits and pieces over time. The defining characteristics of chronic sorrow borne out by the research are pervasiveness, permanence, periodicity, and the potential for progressivity. As graphically represented in the theoretical model of chronic sorrow, the experience of chronic sorrow may occur at any point across the life span.

Trigger events, also referenced as milestones, are those situations or circumstances that bring the disparity created by the loss into focus, thereby triggering the grief-related feelings associated with chronic sorrow. Triggers of chronic sorrow have been shown to vary depending on the nature of the loss experience. For affected individuals, chronic sorrow is most commonly triggered when individuals confront disparity with established norms, whether social, development, or personal in nature (Eakes, 1993; Eakes et al., 1993; Hainsworth, 1994; Isaksson & Ahlstrom, 2008; Isaksson et al., 2007), for example, when someone diagnosed with a chronic illness is unable to engage in an activity that they once enjoyed due to exacerbation of their condition.

The most frequent trigger of chronic sorrow among parents of young children with disabilities is disparity associated with developmental milestones (Bowes et al., 2009; Burke, 1989; Clubb, 1991; Coughlin & Sethares, 2017; Damrosch & Perry, 1989; Fraley, 1986, 1990; George & Vickers, 2006–2007; Golden, 1994; Hobdell, 2004; Hobdell et al., 2007; Hummel & Eastman, 1991; Krafft & Krafft, 1998; Mallow & Bechtel, 1999; Olshansky, 1962; Patrick-Ott & Ladd, 2010; Phillips, 1991; Seideman & Kleine, 1995; Shumaker, 1995; Wikler et al., 1981). The chronic sorrow of other family caregivers is often triggered by crises associated with management of the family member's illness and by recognition of the never-ending nature of the caregiving activities (Bettle & Latimer, 2009; Bowes et al., 2009; Branch-Smith, 2018; Coughlin & Sethares, 2017; Eakes, 1995; Eakes et al., 1993; George & Vickers, 2006–2007; Hainsworth, 1995; Hainsworth et al., 1995; Isaksson & Ahlstrom, 2008; Liedstrom et al., 2008; Lindgren, 1996; Nikfarid et al., 2015; Olwit et al., 2015; Patrick-Ott & Ladd, 2010).

The chronic sorrow experience of bereaved individuals is triggered by those situations and circumstances that magnify the "presence of the absence" of the deceased, such as anniversaries and other special occasions (Eakes, Burke, & Hainsworth, 1998, p. 182). In addition, changes in roles and responsibilities necessitated by the death of a loved one may trigger chronic sorrow.

Another key element of the theoretical model of chronic sorrow is management methods. This term is used to refer to both personal coping strategies used by individuals during the chronic sorrow experience (internal) and supportive interventions provided by helping professionals (external). As depicted in the theoretical model, effective internal and external management methods lead to increased comfort and may serve to extend the time between episodes of chronic sorrow.

Effective internal management strategies used by those with chronic sorrow are consistent across the various loss situations. Action-oriented strategies that increase feelings of control are most frequently used to cope with the recurrence grief-related feelings of chronic sorrow (Bordonada, 2017; Burke, 1989; Eakes, 1993, 1995; Hainsworth, 1995; Hainsworth et al., 1994, 1995; Hobdell et al., 2007; Lindgren, 1996). Examples of action-oriented coping include continuing to pursue involvement in interests and activities, gathering information specific to one's loss experience, and seeking out respite opportunities. Other types of coping strategies identified as helpful in dealing with the chronic sorrow experience are labeled as cognitive and interpersonal. Cognitive strategies include adopting a "can-do" attitude and focusing on the positive elements of one's life (Burke, 1989; Eakes, 1993, 1995; Hainsworth, 1995; Hainsworth et al., 1994, 1995; Isaksson & Ahlstrom, 2008). Interpersonal ways of coping include talking with someone close or a trusted professional and interacting with others in a similar situation such as in a support group (Burke, 1989; Eakes, 1993, 1995; Fraley, 1990; Hainsworth, 1995; Hainsworth et al., 1994, 1995; Wikler et al., 1981).

Interventions provided by health care professionals, referred to as external management methods, must be based upon the premise that chronic sorrow is a normal response to a significant loss situation. As long as disparity created by a loss experience remains, one can anticipate that the individual will likely experience chronic sorrow. Indeed, normalization of the periodic re-grief of chronic sorrow is foundational to all other interventions. It is important for professionals to recognize that individuals who have experienced a significant loss may evidence the periodic recurrence of grief-related feelings defined as chronic sorrow. Armed with this awareness, anticipatory guidance may be provided regarding the situations and circumstances likely to trigger episodes of chronic sorrow. Personal coping mechanisms (internal management methods) can be assessed, strengthened, and supported.

In addition, specific interventions provided by heath care professionals, categorized as roles, have been noted as helpful by those experiencing chronic sorrow (Burke, 1989; Copley & Bodensteiner, 1987; Eakes, 1993, 1995; Eakes et al., 1993; Fraley, 1990; Hainsworth, 1995; Hainsworth et al., 1995; Hobdell et al., 2007; Hummel & Eastman, 1991; Isaksson & Ahlstrom, 2008; Wikler et al., 1981). Family caregivers with chronic sorrow derive the most benefit from professional interventions labeled as the role of "teacher/expert." More specifically, these actions include providing situation-specific information in a manner that can be easily understood and giving practical tips for managing caregiving responsibilities (Burke, 1989; Clubb, 1991; Eakes, 1995; Fraley, 1990; Hainsworth, 1995; Hainsworth et al., 1995; Hummel & Eastman, 1991; Warda, 1992; Wikler et al., 1981). Actions associated with the professional role of "empathetic presence" characterized by taking time to listen, offering support, focusing on feelings, and recognizing uniqueness of each individual are also helpful to those who were in a caregiver role (Burke, 1989; Clubb, 1991; Eakes, 1995; Fraley, 1990; George & Vickers, 2006–2007; Gordon, 2009; Hainsworth, 1995; Hummel & Eastman, 1991; Isaksson & Ahlstrom, 2008; Olshansky, 1962; Phillips, 1991; Teel, 1991; Warda, 1992).

For those individuals affected with a chronic or life-threatening condition as well as bereaved persons, the professional role of "empathetic presence" discussed above is perceived as most helpful in dealing with the periodic episodes of chronic sorrow. In addition, the complementary role of "caring professional," evidenced by sensitivity, respectfulness, and nonjudgmental acceptance, and interventions associated with the role of "teacher/expert" are described as beneficial (Burke, 1989; Eakes, 1993; Eakes et al., 1993; Hainsworth et al., 1995, Isaksson & Ahlstrom, 2008).

## Research Applications of Chronic Sorrow

Chronic sorrow has research applications among a variety of populations and across a myriad of loss situations. Identification of the presence of chronic sorrow among affected individuals, family caregivers, and bereaved individuals as well as unique situations such as parental rejection secondary to divorce (McAdams, Dewell, & Holman, 2011) can alert professionals to potential triggers of the recurrent grief and lead to the identification and reinforcement of effective coping mechanisms for those experiencing chronic sorrow.

### EXAMPLE

Bordonada (2017) conducted a study to explore the directional relationship between chronic sorrow among parents with a child diagnosed with autism spectrum disorder (ASD), and family understanding, social support, coping behaviors, and competence were explored. The large study population consisted of 227 females and 162 males aged from 20 to 65 with diverse ethnicity including Caucasians, African Americans, Asians, Hispanics, and Hawaiian/Pacific Islanders. The researcher used the Adapted Burke Questionnaire (Hobdell, 2004) to identify the presence of chronic sorrow as well as the Family Impact of Childhood Disability Scale (Trute & Hiebert-Murphy, 2002), the Multidimensional Scale of Perceived Social Support (Zimet, Dahlem, Zimet, & Farley, 1988), the Coping Health Inventory for Parents (McCubbin et al., 1983), and the Parenting Sense of Competence Scale (Johnston & Mash, 1989) to measure the other variables being studied. It was hypothesized that parents of a child with ASD having higher levels of family understanding, social support, coping behaviors, and competence would have lower levels of chronic sorrow.

Interestingly, the findings revealed a strong positive correlation between family understanding and presence of chronic sorrow and a medium negative relationship between parents' sense of competence and the experience of chronic sorrow. While no significant relationships were found between perceived social support or coping behaviors and incidence of chronic sorrow, the researcher concluded these variables still made a small contribution to the experience of chronic sorrow. Her recommendation was for counselors to address all of these factors in order to enhance their understanding of chronic sorrow among parents of children with ASD.

In reviewing the results of Bordonada's (2017) within the context of the theoretical model of chronic sorrow, one must first recognize that chronic sorrow is a normal and anticipated response to ongoing disparity created by a loss. Chronic sorrow, therefore, is likely to be periodically experienced throughout the existence of the disparate situation/circumstance. It is not surprising that facing the reality of the inherent losses ensconced in having a child with ASD (i.e., family understanding) was found to be positively correlated with evidence of chronic sorrow. Moreover, the association of higher levels of confidence in parenting a child with ASD with reduced evidence of chronic sorrow is consistent with the recognized value of health care professionals arming the individual with knowledge and information (role of "teacher/expert"). It is less clear why the measures of coping and social support were less impactful when examining their relationship with chronic sorrow as interpersonal strategies of talking with someone close, and action-oriented coping strategies such as adopting a "can-do" attitude have previously been shown to be effective strategies. See an additional example of a student work in Using Middle Range Theory in Practice Projects 7.1.

---

**USING MIDDLE RANGE THEORY IN PRACTICE PROJECTS**    **7.1**

*Refer to the following example of a student project using the Middle Range Theory of Chronic Sorrow:*

*Bordonada, T. M. (2017). Examining chronic sorrow among parents of a child with Autism Spectrum Disorder (ASD) (Doctoral Dissertation). Retrieved from http://scholarcommons.sc.edu/etd/4075*

**FIRST ADVISOR**
Jonathan H. Ohrt

**ABSTRACT OF THE STUDY**

The purpose of this quantitative study was to examine the directional relationship between chronic sorrow and each of the following: (a) family understanding, (b) social support, (c) coping behaviors, and (d) competence among parents of a child with autism spectrum disorder (ASD). Specifically, this examination tested the hypothesized directional relationship that parents of a child with ASD scoring higher levels of family understanding, social support, coping behaviors, and competence indicate lower levels of chronic sorrow. A descriptive, correlational research design was employed to examine the research hypothesis. The data was analyzed using structural equation modeling (SEM). The results indicated parents of a child with ASD experience chronic sorrow. Moreover, these findings provide counselors with the knowledge and awareness to support parents of a child with ASD. A discussion of results, implications for counselors, and study limitations is provided.

---

## NCRCS Chronic Sorrow Instrument Development

Historically, research on chronic sorrow has employed qualitative methods with open-ended interview guides used in both face-to-face and telephone interviews with study participants. The Burke/NCRCS Chronic Sorrow Questionnaire (Burke, 1989), with versions adapted for individuals affected with chronic conditions, for family caregivers, and for bereaved individuals, has been used for the majority of studies documented in the literature. This interview guide is composed of 11 open-ended questions that explore feelings experienced at the time of the loss and whether or not they have been reexperienced. Moreover, questions focus on circumstances or situations that trigger recurrence of the grief-related feeling and identification of effective coping mechanisms.

In 2001, two of the original members of the NCRCS undertook the development of a quantitative assessment tool. Questions for the instrument were developed based on the theoretical model and findings from the qualitative studies previously conducted by members of the NCRCS and other researchers. Face and content validity were established by using Lynn's (1986) methodology for establishing validity of an instrument. Once face and content validity of the Burke/Eakes Chronic Sorrow Assessment Tool were established, test–retest reliability studies were conducted. Subjects participating in this aspect of instrument development represented each of the populations previously studied (family caregivers, affected individuals, and bereaved persons). Test–retest correlations for items 4 through 9 (the first three questions assess demographic data) were at acceptable levels, ranging from 0.72 to 0.93. Questions 10 and 11 allow for little variability in responses, and the restricted response range resulted in more marginal test–retest correlations on these items (0.62 and 0.56, respectively) (see Appendix).

## Summary

■ Chronic sorrow has gained increased attention in the past three decades, based in large part on the research endeavors of the Nursing Consortium for Research on Chronic Sorrow (NCRCS). In addition, increased awareness of the changing nature of grief associated with significant losses, whether ongoing in nature or single loss events, has spurred interest in this phenomenon.

■ The theory of chronic sorrow provides a framework for understanding and working with individuals who have experienced significant loss. Specifically, situations and circumstances that trigger chronic sorrow are identified, and management methods deemed helpful to those experiencing chronic sorrow are described.

■ Moreover, the theoretical model of chronic sorrow, along with the Burke/Eakes Chronic Sorrow Assessment Tool, will facilitate further expansion of research on chronic sorrow and provide opportunities for testing of the theory. While studies have identified presence of chronic sorrow among other cultures (Bowes, Lowes, Warner, &

Gregory, 2009; Branch-Smith, 2018; Chang et al., 2018; Isaksson, Gunnarsson, & Ahlstorm, 2007; Langridge, 2002; Nikfarid et al., 2015; Olwit et al., 2015; Rungruangkonkit, 2006), there remains the need for expanded exploration of cultural variations in the experience of chronic sorrow in future research.

■ In addition, relevance of the theory of chronic sorrow to types of loss experiences such as divorce and abuse needs to be further investigated.

■ The middle range theory of chronic sorrow has widespread application for nurses, social workers, counselors, clergy, and others who strive to better understand individuals' responses to loss and to define effective interventions for those experiencing chronic sorrow. Although chronic sorrow is viewed as a normal response to ongoing disparity resulting from a loss, it is important to note that recognition of the periodic re-grief characteristic of chronic sorrow and provision of supportive interventions can provide an increased level of comfort for those experiencing it.

■ At this stage of theory development, attention needs to be directed to the conduct of studies designed to measure outcomes related to provision of documented "helpful" interventions.

## CRITICAL THINKING EXERCISES

1. You are a case manager for a family with a young child diagnosed with cerebral palsy. Explain how the theory of chronic sorrow can be used as a framework for planning care and identifying resources for this family.

2. Expand the application of the theory of chronic sorrow to a population not yet fully studied. Describe the strengths and weaknesses of the theory in relation to the population identified, and discuss if the theoretical premises apply.

3. Draft a research study designed to measure outcomes for the external management strategies described in the theory.

## REFERENCES

Batchelor, L. (2017). *The lived experience of parents with chronic sorrow who are caring for children with a chronic medical condition* (Nursing Theses and Dissertations, Paper 78). Retrieved from http://hdl.handle.net/10950/626

Bettle, A. M. E., & Latimer, M. A. (2009). Maternal coping and adaptation: A case study examination of chronic sorrow in caring for an adolescent with a progressive neurodegenerative disease. *Canadian Journal of Neuroscience Nursing, 31*(4), 15–21.

Bordonada, T. M. (2017). *Examining chronic sorrow among parents of a child with Autism Spectrum Disorder (ASD)* (Doctoral Dissertation). Retrieved from http://scholarcommons.sc.edu/etd/4075

Bowes, S., Lowes, L., Warner, J., & Gregory, J. W. (2009). Chronic sorrow in parents of children with type 1 diabetes. *Journal of Advanced Nursing, 65*(5), 992–1000.

Branch-Smith, C. (2018). *A resiliency perspective of the lived experience of parenting infants and young children with cystic fibrosis in the context of early lung disease surveillance.* Retrieved from http://ro.ecu.edu.au/thesis/1805

Burke, M. L. (1989). *Chronic sorrow in mothers of school-age children with a myelomeningocele disability* (Doctoral dissertation, Boston University, 1989). *Dissertation Abstracts International, 50*, 233B–234B.

Burke, M. L., Hainsworth, M. A., Eakes, G. G., & Lindgren, C. L. (1992). Current knowledge and research on chronic sorrow: A foundation for inquiry. *Death Studies, 16*, 231–245.

Chang, K. J., Huang, X. Y., Cheng, J. F., & Chien, C. H. (2018). The chronic sorrow experience of caregivers of clients with schizophrenia in Taiwan. *Perspectives in Psychiatric Care, 54*, 281–286.

Clubb, R. L. (1991). Chronic sorrow: Adaptation patterns of parents with chronically ill children. *Pediatric Nursing, 17*, 462–466.

Copley, M. F., & Bodensteiner, J. B. (1987). Chronic sorrow in families of disabled children. *Journal of Child Neurology, 2*, 67–70.

Coughlin, M. B., & Sethares, K. A. (2017). Chronic sorrow in parents of children with a chronic illness or disability: An integrative literature review. *Journal of Pediatric Nursing, 37*, 108–116.

Damrosch, S. P., & Perry, L. A. (1989). Self-reported adjustment, chronic sorrow, and coping of parents of children with Down syndrome. *Nursing Research, 38*, 25–30.

Doornbos, M. M. (1997). The problems and coping methods of caregivers of young adults with mental illness. *Journal of Psychosocial Nursing, 35*(9), 22–26.

Eakes, G. G. (1993). Chronic sorrow: A response to living with cancer. *Oncology Nursing Forum, 20*, 1327–1334.

Eakes, G. G. (1995). Chronic sorrow: The lived experience of parents of chronically mentally ill individuals. *Archives of Psychiatric Nursing, IX*, 77–84.

Eakes, G. G., Burke, M. L., & Hainsworth, M. A. (1998). Middle range theory of chronic sorrow. *Image: Journal of Nursing Scholarship, 30*(2), 179–184.

Eakes, G. G., Burke, M. L., & Hainsworth, M. A. (1999). Chronic sorrow: The lived experience of bereaved individuals. *Illness, Crisis, and Loss, 7*(1), 172–182.

Eakes, G. G., Burke, M. L., Hainsworth, M. A., & Lindgren, C. L. (1993). Chronic sorrow: An examination of nursing roles. In S. G. Funk, E. M. Tornquist, M. T. Champagne, & R. A. Wiese (Eds.), *Key aspects of caring for the chronically ill: Hospital and home* (pp. 231–236). New York, NY: Springer.

Eakes, G. G., Hainsworth, M. E., Lindgren, C. L., & Burke, M. L. (1991). Establishing a long-distance research consortium. *Nursingconnections, 4*, 51–57.

Fraley, A. M. (1986). Chronic sorrow in parents of premature children. *Children's Health Care, 15*, 114–118.

Fraley, A. M. (1990). Chronic sorrow: A parental response. *Journal of Pediatric Nursing, 5*, 268–273.

George, A., & Vickers, M. H. (2006–2007). Chronic grief: Experiences of working parents of children with chronic illness. *Contemporary Nurse, 23*, 228–242.

Glenn, A. (2015). Using online health communication to manage chronic sorrow: Mothers of children with rare diseases. George Mason University PhD, 155. UMI Order AA13624279.

Golden, B. (1994). *The presence of chronic sorrow in mothers of children with cerebral palsy* (Unpublished master's thesis). Arizona State University, Tempe.

Gordon, J. (2009). An evidence-based approach for supporting parents experiencing chronic sorrow. *Pediatric Nursing, 35*(2), 115–119.

Hainsworth, M. A. (1994). Living with multiple sclerosis: The experience of chronic sorrow. *Journal of Neuroscience Nursing, 26*, 237–240.

Hainsworth, M. A. (1995). Chronic sorrow in spouse caregivers of individuals with multiple sclerosis: A case study. *Journal of Gerontological Nursing, 21*, 29–33.

Hainsworth, M. A., Busch, P. V., Eakes, G. G., & Burke, M. L. (1995). Chronic sorrow in women with chronically mentally disabled husbands. *Journal of the American Psychiatric Nurses Association, 1*(4), 120–124.

Hainsworth, M. A., Eakes, G. G., & Burke, M. L. (1994). Coping with chronic sorrow. *Issues in Mental Health Nursing, 15*, 59–66.

Hobdell, E. F. (2004). Chronic sorrow and depression in parents of children with neural tube defects. *Journal of Neuroscience Nursing, 36*(2), 82–88, 94.

Hobdell, E. F., Grant, M. L., Valencia, I., Mare, J., Kothare, S. V., Legido, A., & Khurana, D. S. (2007). Chronic sorrow and coping in families of children with epilepsy. *Journal of Neuroscience Nursing, 39*(2), 76–82.

Hummel, P. A., & Eastman, D. L. (1991). Do parents of premature infants suffer chronic sorrow? *Neonatal Network, 10*, 59–65.

Isaksson, A., & Ahlstrom, G. (2008). Managing chronic sorrow: Experiences of patients with multiple sclerosis. *Journal of Neuroscience Nursing, 40*(3), 180–191.

Isaksson, A. K., Gunnarsson, L. G., & Ahlstorm, G. (2007). The presence and meaning of chronic sorrow in patients with multiple sclerosis. *Journal of Clinical Nursing, 16*(11c), 315–324.

Johnsonius, J. (1996). Lived experiences that reflect embodied themes of chronic sorrow: A phenomenological pilot study. *Journal of Nursing Science, 1*(5/6), 165–173.

Johnston, C., & Mash, E. J. (1989). A measure of parenting satisfaction and efficacy. *Journal of Clinical Child Psychology, 18*(2), 167–175.

Keamy, P., & Griffin, T. (2001). Between joy and sorrow: Being a parent of a child with a developmental disability. *Journal of Advanced Nursing, 34*(5), 582–592.

Krafft, S. K., & Krafft, L. J. (1998). Chronic sorrow: Parents' lived experience. *Holistic Nursing Practice, 13*(1), 59–67.

Kratochvil, M. S., & Devereaux, S. A. (1988). Counseling needs of parents of handicapped children. *Social Casework, 68*, 420–426.

Langridge, P. (2002). Reduction of chronic sorrow: A health promotion role for children's community nurses? *Journal of Child Health Care, 6*, 157–170.

Lichtenstein, B., Laska, M. K., & Clair, J. (2002). Chronic sorrow in the HIV-positive patient: Issues of race, gender and social support. *Aids Patient Care and STDs, 16*(1), 27–38.

Liedstrom, E., Isaksson, A., & Ahlstrom, G. (2008). Chronic sorrow in next of kin of patients with multiple sclerosis. *Journal of Neuroscience Nursing, 40*(5), 304–311.

Lindgren, C. L. (1996). Chronic sorrow in persons with Parkinson's and their spouses. *Scholarly Inquiry for Nursing Practice, 10*, 351–367.

Lowes, L. L., & Lyne, P. (2000). Chronic sorrow in parents of children with newly diagnosed diabetes: A review of the literature and discussion of the implications for nursing practice. *Journal of Advanced Nursing, 32*(1), 41–48.

Lynn, M. (1986). Determination and quantification of content validity. *Nursing Research, 35*(6), 382–385.

Mallow, G. E., & Bechtel, G. A. (1999). Chronic sorrow: The experience of parents with children who are developmentally disabled. *Journal of Psychosocial Nursing, 37*(7), 31–35.

Mayer, M. (2001). Chronic sorrow in caregiving spouses of patients with Alzheimer's disease. *Journal of Aging and Identity, 6*(1), 49–60.

McAdams, C. R., III, Dewell, J. A., & Holman, A. R. (2011). Children and chronic sorrow: Reconceptualizing the emotional impact of parental rejection and its treatment. *The Journal of Humanistic Counseling, 50*(1), 27–41.

McCubbin, H. I., McCubbin, M. A., Patterson, J. M., Cauble, A. E., Wilson, L. R., & Warwick, W. (1983). Coping health inventory for parents: An assessment of parental coping patterns in the care of the chronically ill child. *Journal of Marriage and the Family, 45*(2), 359–370.

Mercer, C. (2015). The impact of non-motor manifestations of Parkinson's disease on partners: Understanding and application of chronic sorrow theory. *Journal of Primary Health Care, 7*(3), 221–227.

Neilsen, C. (2013). *Chronic sorrow and illness ambiguity in caregivers of children with sickle cell disease.* Michigan State Thesis. UMI Number: 1549789.

Nikfarid, L., Rassouli, M., Borimnejad, L., & Alavimajd, H. (2015). Chronic sorrow in mothers of children with cancer. *Journal of Pediatric Oncology Nursing, 32*(5), 314–319.

Olshansky, S. (1962). Chronic sorrow: A response to having a mentally defective child. *Social Casework, 43*, 191–193.

Olwit, C., Musisi, S., Leshabari, A., & Sany, I. (2015). Chronic sorrow: Lived experiences of caregivers of patients diagnosed with schizophrenia in Butabika Mental Hospital, Kampala, Uganda. *Archives of Psychiatric Nursing, 29*(1), 43–48.

Patrick-Ott, A. (2011). *The experience of chronic sorrow in parents who have a child diagnosed with a significant disability: Investigating chronic sorrow across parental life* (Doctoral dissertation). Retrieved from ProQuest Dissertation and Theses database (Texas Women's University Library).

Patrick-Ott, A., & Ladd, L. D. (2010). The blending of Boss's concept of ambiguous loss and Olshansky's concept of chronic sorrow: A case study of a family who has significant disabilities. *Journal of Creativity in Mental Health, 5*(1), 74–86.

Phillips, M. (1991). Chronic sorrow in mothers of chronically ill and disabled children. *Issues in Comprehensive Pediatric Nursing, 14*, 111–120.

Rosenberg, C. J. (1998). Faculty-student mentoring. A father's chronic sorrow: A daughter's perspective. *Journal of Holistic Nursing, 16*(3), 399–404.

Rossheim, B., & McAdams, C. (2010). Addressing chronic sorrow of long-term spousal caregivers: A primer for counselors. *Journal of Counseling and Development, 84* (4), 477–482.

Rungruangkonkit, S. (2006). *Understanding the lived experience of depressed Mien refugees who have resided in the United Sates for Ten or more years* (Doctoral dissertation). Available from ProQuest Dissertation and Theses database. UMI #3224283.

Seideman, R. Y., & Kleine, P. F. (1995). A theory of transformed parenting: Parenting a child with developmental delay/mental retardation. *Nursing Research, 44*, 38–44.

Shumaker, D. (1995). *Chronic sorrow in mothers of children with cystic fibrosis* (Unpublished master's thesis). University of Tennessee, Memphis.

Smith, C. S. (2009). Substance abuse, chronic sorrow, and mothering loss: Relapse triggers among female victims of child abuse. *Journal of Pediatric Nursing, 24*(5), 401–412.

Teel, C. S. (1991). Chronic sorrow: Analysis of the concept. *Journal of Advanced Nursing, 16*, 1322–1319.

Trute, B., & Hiebert-Murphy, D. (2002). Family adjustment to childhood developmental disability: A measure of parent appraisal of family impacts. *Journal of Pediatric Psychology, 27*(3), 271–280.

Veltman, M. (2010). Chronic sorrow in children in foster care: An extension of established middle range theory. *Communicating Nursing Research, 43*, 552–552.

Vitale, S., & Falco, C. (2014). Children born prematurely: Risk of parental chronic sorrow. *Journal of Pediatric Nursing, 29*(3), 248–251.

Warda, M. (1992). The family and chronic sorrow: Role theory approach. *Journal of Pediatric Nursing, 7*, 205–210.

Whittingham, K., Wee, D., Sanders, M. R., & Boyd, R. (2012). Predications of psychological adjustment, experienced burden and chronic sorrow symptoms in parents of children with cerebral palsy. *Child: Care, Health and Development, 39*(3), 336–373.

Wikler, L. M., Wasow, M., & Hatfield, E. (1981). Chronic sorrow revisited: Parents vs. professional depiction of the adjustment of parents of mentally retarded children. *American Journal of Orthopsychiatry, 51*, 63–70.

Zimet, G. D., Dahlem, N. W., Zimet, S. G., & Farley, G. K. (1988). The multidimensional scale of perceived social support. *Journal of Personality Assessment, 52*(1), 30–41.

# 8

# Spiritual Care in Nursing Practice (SCiNP)

Lisa Burkhart and Nancy S. Hogan

## Definition of Key Terms

| | |
|---|---|
| **Patient cue** | Verbal, nonverbal, or situational sign that a person is in need of spiritual care |
| **Reflection** | A process of quieting the mind and finding meaning of what happened during a spiritual encounter |
| **Religion** | A social institution where people can express their spirituality as part of an organized belief system |
| **Religiosity** | The human expression of rites and rituals of a faith tradition |
| **Spirit** | Individually defined as that aspect of person that differentiates humans from other living things |
| **Spiritual care** | A purposeful process of helping another find meaning and purpose in life through a mutual connection |
| **Spiritual intervention** | Actualizing spiritual care by promoting patient self-reflection, promoting connectedness between patient and family, and promoting patient connectedness with a Higher Power/God |
| **Spiritual well-being** | A deeper wisdom and peace found through a process of finding meaning and purpose in life |
| **Spirituality** | The expression of meaning and purpose in life |

Spirituality has been a foundational and central dimension of nursing practice, beginning with the Catholic religious orders of the Middle Ages and Florence Nightingale (Nightingale, 1994; O'Brien, 2014; Pesut, 2006; Pesut & Thorne, 2007). Spirituality and spiritual care have recently reemerged over the past several decades as important phenomena within nursing research, standards of practice, and education. Research has demonstrated that spirituality is associated with better physical, psychological, and social dimensions of health, which led to a Joint Commission standard that requires the provision of spiritual care in hospitals, particularly to patients at end of life (Clark, Drain, & Malone, 2003; Joint Commission on Accreditation of Healthcare Organizations, 2003). The American Nurses Association also requires the provision of spiritual care in the Scope and Standards of Nursing Practice (2010a), Social Policy Statement (2010b), and Code of Ethics (2015), and the AACN incorporates spiritual

care in the Essentials of Baccalaureate Education (American Academy of Colleges of Nursing, 2009).

The majority of spirituality and spiritual care theories provide a metaphysical and philosophical accounting of spirituality, along with guidelines in providing spiritual care (Reed, 1991; Watson, 2005). The Spiritual Care in Nursing Practice (SCiNP) theory is a middle range theory focused on spiritual care encounters.

## Historical Background

Spirituality has existed since the beginning of human kind and is grounded in the philosophical question, "What does it mean to be a human being?" Philosophers have different accountings for what is a human being, but the constant thread across philosophers is that humans have a unique dimension of self, called the spirit, and the expression of that spirit, or spirituality, is the exploration of meaning and purpose in life. For example, a human being could be viewed as the way our body or cellular structure is organized (Aristotle, 1976), a unified separate entity within the body (Plato/Socrates, 1997), an evolution of spiritual being (Aquinas, 1949), our individuality with free choice (Kierkegaard, 1989), or a form of evolving energy through space and time that connects us to each other and God (Teilhard de Chardin, 1960a, 1960b). Regardless of how one defines the spirit, the work of "the spirit" is to search for meaning and purpose in life and to transcend who one is today toward who one can become in the future. This process of exploration occurs through self-reflection, relationships with other people, and experiencing literature and the arts. Humans also find meaning and purpose in life through connections with nature and a Higher Power or God.

Spiritual care in Western nursing emerged in the Middle Ages from the Catholic religious orders as a calling from God in Christ's healing ministry (O'Brien, 2014). Nightingale (1994) and Nightingale (1860/1969) recognized spirituality and spiritual care as central to nursing practice and nursing research. Nightingale believed that there was an omnipotent God, which was the source of all Truth: "A Law is nothing else than a 'Thought of God" (Nightingale, 1994, p. 35). It was nurses' role to uncover that Truth through research to learn God's Will and, in practice, to eliminate barriers in the environment so that God could do His Will (Nightingale, 1994). This applied to both specific patient care situations and the development of health care policy (Nightingale/McDonald, 2003).

This conceptualization is consistent with other nursing theories. Watson developed a grand theory of spirituality and focused on the nurse–patient relationship incorporating a metaphysical transpersonal dimension of caring. Her theory also presented 10 carative factors to guide practice (Watson, 1999, 2005). Pamela Reed was one of the first nurse researchers to define spirituality in nursing as the process of finding meaning and purpose in life through connectedness with self, others/environment, and/or a power greater than oneself across time (Reed, 1987, 1991). For example, some individuals experience spirituality internally through self-reflection, transpersonally in close relationships, and/or transcendentally with a Higher Power. This led to her theory of self-transcendence (Reed, 1991).

More recently, spiritual care has been recognized as an essential component of nursing care in the United States and is a requirement in nursing practice and education (AACN, 2009; ANA, 2010a). Providing spiritual care is a health care requirement and is recognized in the international health care database infrastructure, called the Systematized Nomenclature of Medicine (SNOMED CT) (www.nlm.nih.gov/research/umls/snomed/snomed_main.html).

## Empirical Development of the Spiritual Care in Nursing Practice Theory

The reemergence of spiritual care as essential to quality health care demanded the evidence to guide evidence-based spiritual care practice. Early in 2005, the literature converged on a definition of spirituality and the association of spiritual well-being on patient health (Goncalves, Lucchetti, Menezes, & Vallada, 2017), but there was no empirically derived theory of spiritual care in nursing practice.

Burkhart and Hogan (2008) first discovered the SCiNP theory through a grounded theory study using classic Glaserian methods (Glaser, 2001; Glaser & Strauss, 1967). Twenty-five nurse participants who worked across the continuum of care attended one of four focus groups. Theoretical sampling required an additional focus group of nine nurse managers. Findings revealed a purposeful process following seven categorical phases and related subcategories or subprocesses, as shown in Figure 8.1.

The categories are cue from patient, decision to engage or not to engage in spiritual encounter, spiritual care intervention, immediate emotional response, searching for meaning in encounter, formation of spiritual memory, and nurse spiritual well-being. This is a process whereby positive nurse–patient spiritual encounters can lead to positive spiritually growth-filled memories that will increase nurses' spiritual well-being. In contrast, spiritually distressing nurse–patient spiritual encounters can lead to negative, spiritually distress-filled memories that can decrease the nurses' spiritual well-being. However, spiritual distressing encounters can lead to positive, growth-filled memories with reflection. This search for meaning is integral in forming the growth-filled memory. Meaning-filled memories of spiritual encounters lead to greater nurse spiritual well-being. A stronger spiritual well-being supports the nurse's ability to recognize a patient's need for spiritual care in the future (Burkhart & Hogan, 2008).

## Definition of Theory Concepts

Each concept in the theory is defined as follows.

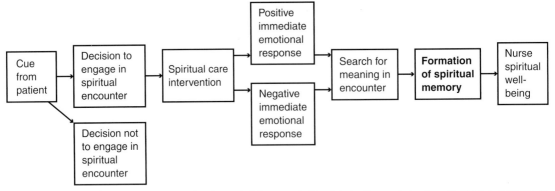

**Figure 8.1**    Spiritual care in nursing practice theoretical framework. (Reprinted with permission from Burkhart, L., & Hogan, N. (2008). An experiential theory of spiritual care in nursing practice. *Qualitative Health Research, 18*(7), 928–938.)

## PATIENT CUE

Spiritual care happens in the moment when the patient expresses a need for spiritual care. Therefore, the first concept in the theory is recognizing the cue, as well as experiencing a patient's openness to engage spiritually. Cues can be verbal (Why is this happening to me? Is God punishing me?), non-verbal (crying, whining, demanding behavior), or situational (receiving a poor prognosis, end of life, learning of life-threatening treatments).

## DECISION TO ENGAGE/NOT ENGAGE

When the nurse recognizes a patient cue, the nurse consciously chooses to engage or not engage in spiritual care. Reasons to not engage include no perceived time, no collegial or institutional support for providing spiritual care, or personal spiritual exhaustion. If the nurse chooses not to engage, spiritual care does not happen.

## SPIRITUAL INTERVENTION

If nurses choose to engage, nurses enter the next phase in the theory of performing spiritual interventions. This third phase is when spiritual care is actualized. Both the patient and nurse spiritually connect, and the nurse engages in one of three types of interventions: promoting patient self-reflection, promoting connectedness between patient and family, and promoting patient connectedness with a Higher Power/God. Promoting patient self-reflection involves discussions that promote the patients' understanding of the meaning in their illness experience. At times, patients are searching for answers to life questions and the meaning of their life experiences. Nurses facilitate that exploration. Promoting connectedness between patient and family involves actions that eliminate barriers and help maintain a spiritual closeness with loved ones. Promoting patient–family connectedness occurs in

many ways and is contingent on patient and family needs. The nurse assesses those needs and individualizes the care to promote meaningful relationships based on that recognized need. Nurses also facilitate patients' connection to a Higher Power, when appropriate. Many patients find meaning by gaining connectedness with God in two ways: by facilitating adherence to religious rites and rituals and through prayer. Facilitating religious rituals requires the nurse to assess religious needs and meet those needs. Nurses also promote spiritual connectedness with God through prayer by praying themselves, by initiating a chaplain referral, or by connecting family or friends to pray with the patient.

## IMMEDIATE EMOTIONAL RESPONSE (POSITIVE/NEGATIVE)

By definition, spiritual encounters are meaningful. Nurses are experiencing mortality, life-changing, and deeply meaningful expressions of love, hope, and, at times, pain. These experiences affect the nurse and lead to either a positive or a negative emotional response. Nurses can leave a spiritual encounter crying, depleted, happy, and/or fulfilled, depending on the nature of the encounter.

## SEARCH FOR MEANING

The emotional release leads to a process of searching for meaning in the encounter. This is a time of finding deeper meaning in those spiritual experiences. Nurses engage in their own spiritual activities, which include reflecting with self, reflecting with others, and faith rituals. Self-reflection is a process of quieting the mind and exploring the meaning of what happened during the spiritual encounter. This can occur when driving home, in the shower, gardening, and/or at bedtime. Nurses also reflect with others, typically with individuals who have had similar spiritual experiences. These individuals include other nurses and chaplains. Many times, family and friends cannot or do not assist in this process because they cannot relate to that nursing spiritual encounter experience. Faith traditions can also provide an opportunity to search for spiritual meaning by attending religious services, reading religious/spiritual materials, and/or praying.

## FORMATION OF A SPIRITUAL MEMORY

This reflective process leads to a memory that stays with the nurse. For many, the memory is so clear; it seems as if it happened recently. These spiritual memories come together to form a cohesive understanding of life experiences. There are three pathways toward the spiritual memory. The degree and type of spiritual reflection that occurs during the "search for meaning phase" lead to different spiritual memories. Positive emotions following a spiritual encounter and meaningful reflection lead to growth-filled spiritual memories and reinforce the joy of nursing practice. A spiritual encounter with a negative emotional response and minimal or negative reflective activities leads to a spiritually distressing memory. However, a spiritual encounter with negative emotions and meaningful reflective activities can lead to a spiritually growth-filled memory. This latter path leads to a deeper wisdom, peace, and feeling privileged in participating in these meaningful experiences. The type of reflective activity affects the memory and cohesive understanding of life experiences.

## SPIRITUAL WELL-BEING

Spiritual well-being is a personal dimension of oneself and is the degree to which one finds meaning and purpose in life. Greater spiritual well-being can lead to spiritual wisdom. This spiritual wisdom can provide strength and insight to support the ability to provide spiritual care to others.

The process of providing spiritual care and finding meaning in spiritual encounters can help the nurse promote his or her own spiritual well-being and can affect whether the nurse decides to engage in spiritual care in the future. Subsequent research was needed to further develop and test the veracity of the theory.

# Instruments Used in Empirical Testing

This phase of theory verification focused on developing an instrument generated from the grounded theory data, representing each of the categories of the theory (Burkhart, Schmidt, &

Hogan, 2011). Initially, 48 items were chosen to represent the seven categories for the instrument development study. To test this initial pool of items, a convenience sample of 298 adult and pediatric acute care, ambulatory, home health, hospice staff, and rehab nurses at two hospitals ($n = 248$) and graduate students at a school of nursing ($n = 50$) completed the instrument. Factor analysis yielded a 17-item tool measuring three of the concepts in the theory: spiritual intervention

| Table 8.1 | Selected Instruments | |
|---|---|---|
| **Author** | **Tool** | **Theory Concept** |
| Daaleman and Frey (2004) | Spiritual Index of Well-Being (SIWB) Subscales: <br> • Life schema <br> • Self-efficacy | Spiritual well-being |
| Paloutzian and Ellison (1991) and Ellison (1983) | Spiritual Well-Being (SWB) Scale Subscales: <br> • Religious well-being <br> • Existential well-being | Spiritual well-being |
| Reed (1987) | Spiritual Perspective Scale (SPS) Subscales: <br> • Values <br> • Interactions | Spiritual intervention Spiritual well-being |
| Taylor, Highfield, and Amenta (1999) | Oncology Nurse Spiritual Care Perspectives Survey (ONSCPS) | Spiritual interventions |
| Peterman, Fitchett, Brady, Hernandez, and Cella (2002) | Functional Assessment of Chronic Illness Therapy, Spiritual Care (FACIT-SP-12) Subscales: <br> • Meaning <br> • Faith | Spiritual well-being |
| Moorhead, Johnson, Maas, and Swanson (2018) | Spiritual Health | Patient cue |
| Burkhart et al. (2011) | Spiritual Care Inventory <br> • Spiritual intervention <br> • Meaning making <br> • Faith rituals | Spiritual intervention Search for meaning Faith rituals |
| Vincensi and Burkhart (2016), | Vincensi Spiritual Assessment Tool | Patient cue |
| Vincensi and Burkhart (2016), and Mamier and Taylor (2015) | The Nurse Spiritual Therapeutics Scale (NSTS)—Vincensi Adaptation | Spiritual interventions |

(4 items), meaning-making reflective practice (10 items), and faith ritual reflective practice (3 items). Recognizing the patient cue and decision to engage in a spiritual encounter was assumed to have occurred prior to the spiritual care intervention. Also, the search for meaning did not factor separately from the spiritual memory, as the survey ultimately measured the memory post–spiritual encounter. Table 8.1 presents this instrument as well as other selected tools that measure spiritual concepts.

## Application of the Theory in Practice

The theory revealed three clinical applications to spiritual care: recognizing the patient cue, providing spiritual interventions, and nurse reflective practices. These three components of spiritual care were integrated into an educational pedagogy as part of a senior capstone clinical practicum. This pedagogy included both face-to-face retreats and

**Table 8.2    Examples of Theory in Practice**

| Citation | Focus |
| --- | --- |
| Caldiera, S., & Hall, J. (2012). Spiritual leadership and spiritual care in neonatology. *Journal of Nursing Management, 20,* 1069–1075. doi: 10.111/jonm.12034 | Each *baby* is an individual and should receive care in a family-centered approach. Spiritual care of this newborn involves provision of privacy, consideration for the environmental conditions, gentleness in care practices, and appropriate touch and encouragement of parental touch. The needs of *parents* in this situation are many: information from staff, assurance of the quality of care their infant is receiving, communication by the staff that they are perceived positively, and a therapeutic relationship with staff. Parents also find that emotional support, a welcoming environment, empowerment and education, and involvement in care were helpful. *Spiritual leadership* promotes workplace spirituality, which is an environment where there is a sense of community, an alignment with organizational values, a sense of making a contribution to society, enjoyment in work, and opportunities for a rich inner life. These can only be achieved when nurses feel they are being cared for by their leader. When this occurs, the nurses are better able to provide spiritual care to their patients. |
| Daaleman, T. P. (2012). A health services framework of spiritual care. *Journal of Nursing Management, 20,* 1021–1029. doi: 10.1111/j.1365-2384.2012.01482.x | Three studies involving dying patients' and their family members' descriptions of (a) providers, types, and outcomes of spiritual care; (b) the process of spiritual care; and (c) outcomes of spiritual care in long-term care facilities. Friends and family were most frequently identified as spiritual care providers, followed by health care workers and clergy. Coping with illness was the most frequently cited spiritual care. The process of providing spiritual care involved presence, opening eyes, and cocreating, a fluid activity between patients, family members, and health care staff. Only 55% of participants were satisfied with their spiritual care experiences. Nurse managers can create a learning environment to help staff integrate spiritual care into their practice. |
| Hodge, D. R. (2015). Administering a two-stage spiritual assessment in healthcare settings: A necessary component of ethical and effective care. *Journal of Nursing Management, 23,* 27–38. doi: 10.111/jonm.12078 | The five rationales for conducting a spiritual assessment as component of nursing care were identified as professional ethics, patient autonomy, the need for an understanding of the knowledge of patients' worldviews, the identification of spiritual assets as a resource for coping, and accrediting and governmental requirements. A two-stage spiritual assessment is recommended with a brief preliminary assessment, followed, if needed, by a more comprehensive assessment or spiritual history. Nurse managers need to help nurses develop an understanding of the strengths and limitations of this approach. |
| Skalla, K. A. (2015). Challenges in assessing spiritual distress in survivors of cancer. *Clinical Journal of Oncology Nursing, 19*(1), 99–104. doi: 10.1188/15.cjon.99-104 | This study concluded that it is feasible to assess spirituality in an outpatient setting using online tools. Participants who were cancer survivors were able to distinguish between personal psychological and spiritual distress. |
| Wynne, L. (2013). Spiritual care at the end of life. *Nursing Standard, 11*(28), 41–45 | The basic tenet is that "spirituality transcends and 'holds together' the physical, psychological and social aspects of terminal illness" (p. 41). Spiritual assessment involves consideration of the relevant rituals and practices of different religions. The HOPE assessment tool can provide a structure for the assessment. H refers to sources of hope, strength, comfort, meaning, peace, love, and connection; O refers to the role of organized religion in the life of the patient; P refers to personal spirituality and practices; and E refers to effects of medical care and end-of-life decisions. Careful assessment and effective communication provide the foundation for the development of a spiritual care plan. Spiritual care should be personal and intimate and delivered with compassion and empathy. |

an online discussion board (Burkhart & Schmidt, 2012). The effectiveness of this program was measured in an RCT pre-/posttest 2 by 2 design with senior nursing students during their capstone clinical immersion course ($n = 59$). Findings revealed a statistically significant increase in students' perceived ability in providing spiritual care, particularly in complex family clinical situations. Findings also indicated a significant increase in the student's use of reflective practices, which students found to help support them during stressful times.

Several international quantitative and qualitative research studies used the SCiNP theory as a conceptual framework (Parsian & Dunning, 2009) or definition of spiritual care (Carr, 2010; Chiang, Lee, Chu, Han, & Hsiao, 2016; Fouka, Plakas, Taket, Boudioni, & Dandoulakis, 2012; Granero-Molina et al., 2014; Koren & Papamiditriou, 2013; Koren et al., 2009; Turan & Karamanoglu, 2012) in the theoretical framework or philosophical underpinnings for their studies.

The SCiNP theory provides the theoretical framework for spiritual care at Loyola University Health System. The electronic health record, using Epic, incorporates a spiritual assessment using a 5-point Likert scale of a patient's initial spiritual need, with "1" as severely compromised and "5" as not compromised. This patient cue recognition is part of the daily documentation flow sheets as a common row for both nursing and chaplain documentation (Burkhart, 2009, 2011; Burkhart & Androwich, 2009). This uses informatics to ease the decision to engage in spiritual care by quickly informing others of this need (minimizing the time constraint and supporting the institutional mission of providing spiritual care) and automatically triggers a chaplain referral to promote an interprofessional response to the patient's spiritual needs.

The chaplain also is available to assist the nurse in reflection post–spiritual encounter if needed (thereby promoting the nurses' meaning-making process). In this model, patients with a "1" or "2" level of spirituality are considered in spiritual distress. This numeric measurement system tabulates the number of patients with spiritual needs in monthly reports based on unit, specialty, or time of day, thereby assisting management in anticipating patient spiritual needs for chaplain staffing. Since Loyola University Health System was one of the early adopters of Epic, this feature is now part of the product and available for other Epic users.

Other examples of spiritual care practices and issues consistent with the theory are found in Table 8.2 with an example of implementing a program to promote spiritual care described in some detail in Using Middle Range Theory in Practice 8.1.

---

## USING MIDDLE RANGE THEORY IN PRACTICE    8.1

*Source: Smith, T., & Gordon, T. (2009). Developing spiritual and religious care competencies in practice: Pilot of a Marie Curie blended learning event. International Journal of Palliative Care, 15(2), 86–92.*

### PROBLEM

Though it is recognized within the profession that holism, which integrates mind, body, and spirituality, is necessary for quality nursing care, "many professionals report barriers to addressing spiritual issues in practice which inhibits the implementation of theory into practice" (p. 86).

### NURSING INTERVENTION

The Marie Curie Cancer Care Spiritual and Religious Care Competencies for Specialist Palliative Care was used to develop a pilot learning event focusing on the development of spiritual care competencies. As part of the planning process, three focus groups were held, attended by registered nurses, hospice volunteers, and health care assistants. The purpose of the groups was identification of the focus and level of the content to be included in the proposed course. Four main themes emerged: self-awareness, communication skills, theoretical knowledge, and professional role.

The course was delivered in a blended learning model with both face-to-face and Internet learning experiences. An online learning development team helped to determine the scope of the content and timing of the learning event. Online learning activities focused on the identified themes, and the online portion of the course was offered over a 5-week period. To complete the course, it required 30 to 60 minutes on a weekly basis. On week 6, a study day was offered, and on week 7, follow-up activities focused on final reflections. Facilitators moderated each activity and encouraged and summarized discussions. Technical problems were addressed by the online learning technologist.

Twelve participants were recruited, and six completed the program. Evaluation of the program from both facilitator and participants revealed that "participants appeared more open to explorations of their own issues and spiritual beliefs, more confident in sharing with each other, and more willing and able to understand their own and others' spiritual needs" (p. 92). The program was considered a success and was placed in a portfolio of learning events that are available on a nationwide basis.

# Application of the Theory in Research

Several recent systemic reviews have explored the relationship between spirituality/spiritual care and health indicators and patient satisfaction (Goncalves et al., 2017; Lewinson, McSherry, & Kevern, 2015; Smith-MacDonald, Norris, Raffin-Bouchal, & Sinclair, 2017), demonstrating inconsistent definitions and measurement of spirituality and spiritual care. Several studies applied the SCiNP theory to guide nursing research in simulation (Desmond, Burkhart, Horsley, Gerc, & Breitschneider, 2018), tool development (Vincensi & Burkhart, 2016), and practice (Coughlin et al., 2017; Vincensi & Solberg, 2017). See Using Middle Range Theory in Research 8.2 and 8.3 as examples.

Desmond et al. (2018) created a spiritual care simulation and performance checklist based on a literature review guided by the SCiNP theory: the simulation script, which included patient cues, and a companion performance checklist, which listed spiritual interventions. Forty RNs participated in the simulation and completed the Spiritual Care Inventory pre–post simulation (Burkhart et al., 2011). The participants, standardized patient, and independent observer completed the performance checklist. Findings supported content, face, construct and predictive validity, as well as interrater reliability. This research provides an evidence-based strategy to teach spiritual care in both education and practice.

Vincensi and Burkhart (2016) developed and evaluated the psychometric properties of two tools to measure spiritual care assessment (or patient cues) and spiritual interventions in nurse practitioner practice. Items were derived from the literature and were evaluated by an expert panel. The subsequent tool was completed by a national sample of nurse practitioners ($n = 133$). Findings demonstrated high internal consistency (>0.70) and convergent and divergent validity. This study described and provides a strategy to measure spiritual care in nurse practitioner practice.

## USING MIDDLE RANGE THEORY IN RESEARCH    8.2

Nursing has as an aim providing holistic care to patients. The domain of spirituality is seen as the most often neglected domain in daily nursing practice.

*Source: Chan, M. F. (2009). Factors affecting nursing staff in practicing spiritual care. Journal of Clinical Nursing, 19, 2128–2136. doi: 10.1111/j.1365-2702.2008.02690.x*

### PURPOSE/RESEARCH QUESTION

This study had two focuses: (a) an examination of nurses' attitudes to practicing spiritual care and (b) the determination of factors associated with nurses' attitudes to practicing spiritual care.

### RESEARCH DESIGN

The design was correlational and retrospective.

### SAMPLE/PARTICIPANTS

The convenience sample was comprised of all nurses working in a Chinese hospital in 2006, with a total of 178 questionnaires distributed. There was a response rate of 61.7%, a total of 110 questionnaires completed and returned.

### DATA COLLECTION

An instrument was developed for this study. It was based on an intensive review of the literature and two previously developed instruments. Ten items were identified and submitted to a panel of experts. The content validity index was 0.92 and confirmation factor analysis established construct validity. Test–retest reliability was also 0.92. Internal consistency of the three subscales, nurses' perceptions, practices, and spiritual care practices, had Cronbach's alpha scores of 0.83, 0.82, and 0.84, respectively. In addition to the instrument, demographic data were collected.

The questionnaires were distributed to nurses by their ward managers with mechanisms for maintaining confidentiality established. Questionnaires were returned via a secure box and were collected 1 week after distribution. "To examine which variables contributed to the practice scores, bivariate analysis including independent t-test and analysis of variance were used to examine difference and Spearman's rho coefficient correlation was used to quantify the relationships between nurses' perceptions and practice level of spiritual care" (p. 2132).

### FINDINGS

The analyses of data revealed that those who were married, previously hospitalized, and employed in the obstetrical and gynecological departments were more likely to have religious beliefs. This group also had higher perception levels of spiritual care and was more likely to be practicing spiritual care.

**USING MIDDLE RANGE THEORY IN RESEARCH   8.3**

Providing spiritual care to patients is a professional nursing responsibility, yet there persists a reluctance to engage in this practice.

*Source: McSherry, W., & Jamieson, S. (2013). The qualitative findings from an online survey investigating nurses' perceptions of spirituality and spiritual care. Journal of Clinical Nursing, 22, 3170–3182. doi: 10.1111/jocn.12411*

### PURPOSE/RESEARCH QUESTION

This study had as its stated purpose providing nurses with an opportunity to express their understandings of spirituality and spiritual care. There were three questions:

1. What do the United Kingdom's Royal College of Nurses (RCN) members understand by the terms spirituality and spiritual care?
2. Do RCN members consider spirituality to be a legitimate area of nursing practice?
3. Do RCN members feel that they receive sufficient support and guidance in these matters?

### RESEARCH DESIGN

The study was descriptive, using a cross-sectional design.

### SAMPLE/PARTICIPANTS

The research was conducted with the population of members of the RCN, nurses, midwives, health care support workers, and students. All 410,000+ members were invited to participate in the study. Only 4,054 members completed the survey, a response rate of slightly less than 1.0%. Though this is an obviously low response rate, it is the largest body of knowledge about nurses' perceptions of spirituality and spiritual care in the United Kingdom.

### DATA COLLECTION

This online survey was adapted from an unpublished questionnaire developed by a graduate student as part of the students Master of Philosophy thesis. It consists of five parts: (a) Spirituality and Spiritual Care Rating Scale, (b) nursing practice, (c) actions, (d) demographics, and (e) response box. The questionnaire was reviewed by a panel of experts to determine content validity. It was piloted with RCN members to establish reliability.

Members received notification of the survey through a bulk e-mail, and in the message, they were directed to the organization's Web site homepage. This site provided a direct link to the survey.

Data were collated using the ProQuest® platform, and a keyword analysis was completed.

### FINDINGS

Five content themes emerged from the data analysis:

1. *Theoretical and conceptual understanding of spirituality.* These included finding meaning and purpose in the midst of life's vicissitudes and living with inner peace and calm. Little mention was made of suffering or evil and its relationship to spirituality.
2. *Fundamental aspects of nursing.* Spirituality was described as essential to the quality of nursing care delivered.
3. *Notion of integration and integrated care.* Spirituality was considered something that is integrated into care—it should not be considered an "add-on."
4. *Education and professional development.* Diversity in opinion was expressed with some supporting formal inclusion of spiritual care instruction into nursing programs and others believing that it would be too restrictive with the possibility of unfound assumptions being made by nurses.
5. *Religious belief and professional practice.* The responses were consistent with the majority of the respondents identifying themselves as Christian. The need for spiritual care practices, with a recognition of the importance for tolerance to diverse beliefs, was expressed. Professional organizations should be helping nurses become more comfortable with providing this type of care.

Coughlin et al. (2017) studied the relationship between provider spiritual beliefs and spiritual care (using the Spiritual Care Inventory) among an interprofessional sample of maternal–child staff in two health systems ($n = 406$). Findings indicated that greater spiritual beliefs were associated with greater intentional spiritual care interventions. This suggests that the spiritual well-being of the provider is associated with the provision of spiritual care.

## Conclusion

Evidence-based theory to guide practice is the gold standard in nursing practice. The SCiNP theory is unique in that its development follows the integration model of the direct linkage between research, theory, and practice. The authors of the SCiNP theory used several kinds of research methods and designs to generate the theory. First, it was empirically derived using a qualitative research method to learn from practicing nurses about their experience of delivering spiritual care and its impact on them and their nursing practice. The theory was then subjected to quantitative research to determine the most parsimonious concepts that define the process of providing spiritual care to patients, and finally the theory was assessed with practice nurses, in a variety of settings, to assess the theory's validity as a research-based practice theory.

## Summary

■ Spiritual care is essential to nursing practice and endorsed by the ANA Scope and Standards of Nursing Practice, Social Policy Statement, and Code of Ethics, and it is incorporated in the AACN Essentials of Baccalaureate Education and is a Joint Commission requirement.

■ The SCiNP theory was empirically derived from grounded theory research and validated psychometrically.

■ An empirically derived instrument to measure practice facilitates research in spiritual care.

■ A theoretically derived educational pedagogy and simulation meet the AACN requirement for spiritual care education.

■ Spiritual care affects both the patient and the nurse. Searching for meaning through reflective practice promotes spiritual well-being.

### CRITICAL THINKING EXERCISES

1. Draw a picture of what spirituality means to you. Compare your picture with the different philosophical perspectives of spirituality and evaluate your own perspective of spirituality.

2. Consider how your view of spirituality is lived out in your nursing practice. How do you identify yourself as a nurse?

3. Think of a time when you provided spiritual care. Consider the phases of the theory and how you were affected by the spiritual encounter. What limits your engagement in spiritual care?

4. In what spiritual practices do you engage? Consider what you do after practicing as a nurse. How do your spiritual practices affect your nursing care?

## REFERENCES

American Academy of Colleges of Nursing. (2009). *Essentials of baccalaureate education for professional nursing practice.* Washington, DC: AACN.

American Nurses Association. (2010a). *Nursing: Scope and standards of practice.* Washington, DC: Author.

American Nurses Association. (2010b). *Nursing's social policy statement* (2nd ed.). Washington, DC: Author.

American Nurses Association. (2015). *Code of ethics for nurses with interpretive statements.* Washington, DC: Author.

Aquinas. (1949). *On spiritual creatures,* Q. 1, Art. 1–2 (M. FitzPatrick, Trans.). Milwaukee, WI: Marquette University Press.

Aristotle. (1976). *De Anima* (R. D. Hicks, Trans.). Cambridge, UK: University Press.

Burkhart, L. (2009). Informatics: Capturing and measuring spiritual care. *Vision, 19*(4), 16–18.

Burkhart, L. (2011). Documenting the story: Communication within a healthcare team. *Vision, 21*(3), 28–33.

Burkhart, L., & Androwich, I. (2009). Measuring spiritual care with informatics. *Advances in Nursing Science, 32*(3), 200–210.

Burkhart, L., & Hogan, N. (2008). An experiential theory of spiritual care in nursing practice. *Qualitative Health Research, 18*(7), 928–938.

Burkhart, L., & Schmidt W. (2012). Measuring effectiveness of a spiritual care pedagogy in nursing education. *Journal of Professional Nursing, 28*(5), 315–321.

Burkhart, L., Schmidt, L., & Hogan, N. (2011). Development and psychometric testing of the spiritual care inventory instrument. *Journal of Advanced Nursing, 67*(11), 2463–2472.

Carr, T. J. (2010). Facing existential realities: Exploring barriers and challenges to spiritual nursing care. *Qualitative Health Research, 20*(10), 1379–1392. doi: 10.1177/1049732310372377

Chiang, Y., Lee, J., Chu, T., Han, C. H., & Hsiao, Y. (2016). The impact of nurses' spiritual health on their attitudes toward spiritual care, professional commitment, and caring. *Nursing Outlook, 64*(3), 215–224.

Clark, P. A., Drain, M., & Malone, M. P. (2003). Addressing patients' emotional and spiritual needs. *Joint Commission Journal on Quality and Safety, 29*(12), 659–670.

Coughlin, K., Mackley, A., Kwadu, R., Shanks, V., Sturtz, W., Munson, D., & Guillen, U. (2017). Characterization of spirituality in maternal–child caregivers. *Journal of Palliative Medicine, 20*(9), 994–997. doi: 10.1089/jpm.2016.0361

Daaleman, T., & Frey, B. (2004). The spirituality index of well-being: A new instrument for health-related quality-of-life research. *Annals of Family Medicine, 2*(5), 499–503.

Desmond, M. B., Burkhart, L., Horsley, T., Gerc, S., & Breitschneider, A. (2018). Development and psychometric evaluation of a spiritual care simulation and companion performance checklist for a veteran using a standardized patient. *Clinical Simulation in Nursing, 4*, 29–44. doi: 10.1016/j.ecns.2017.10.008

Ellison, C. W. (1983). Spiritual well-being: Conceptualization and measurement. *Journal of Psychology and Theology, 11*, 330–340.

Fouka, G., Plakas, S., Taket, A., Boudioni, M., & Dandoulakis, M. (2012). Health-related religious rituals of the Green Orthodox Church: Their uptake and meanings. *Journal of Nursing Management, 20*, 1058–1068. doi: 10.1111/jonm.12024

Glaser, B. G. (2001). *The grounded theory perspective: Conceptualizations contrasted with description.* Mill Valley, CA: Sociology Press.

Glaser, B. G., & Strauss, A. L. (1967). *The discovery of grounded theory: Strategies for qualitative research.* New York, NY: Aldine.

Goncalves, J. P., Lucchetti, G., Menezes, P. R., & Vallada, H. (2017). Complementary religious and spiritual interventions in physical health and quality of life: A systematic review of randomized controlled clinical trials. *PLoS One, 12*(10), e0186539. Retrieved from https://doi.org/10.1371/journal. pone.0186539

Granero-Molina, J., Diaz Cortes, M. M., Marquez Membrive, J., Castro-Sanchez, A. M., Lopen Entrambasaguas, O. M., & Fernandez Sola, C. (2014). Religious faith in coping with terminal cancer: What is the nursing experience? *European Journal of Cancer Care, 23*, 300–309. doi: 10.1111/ecc.12150

Joint Commission on Accreditation of Healthcare Organizations. (2003). *Joint commission resources: 2003 comprehensive accreditation manual for hospitals: The official handbook.* Oakbrook Terrace, IL: Author.

Kierkegaard, S. (1989). In A. Hannay (Ed.), *Sickness unto death.* New York, NY: Penguin.

Koren, M. E., Czurylo, K., Epsom, R., Gattuso, M., Stark, B., Zastrow, P., & Basu, S. (2009). Nurses' work environment and spirituality: A descriptive study. *International Journal of Caring Sciences, 2*(3), 118–125.

Koren, M. E., & Papamiditriou, C. (2013). Spirituality of staff nurses: Application of modeling and role modeling theory. *Holistic Nursing Practice, 27*(1), 37–44.

Lewinson, L. P., McSherry W., & Kevern, P. (2015). Spirituality in re-registration nurse education and practice: A review of the literature. *Nurse Education Today, 35*, 806–814.

Mamier, I. & Taylor, E. J. (2015). Psychometric evaluation of the nurse spiritual care therapeutics scale. *Western Journal of Nursing Research, 37*(5), 679–694.

Moorhead, S., Johnson, M., Maas, M. L., & Swanson, E. (2018). *Nursing outcomes classification (NOC): Measurement of health outcomes* (5th ed.). St. Louis, MO: Elsevier.

Nightingale, F. (1860/1969). *Notes on nursing. What it is and what it is not.* New York, NY: Dover Publications.

Nightingale, F. (1994). In M. D. Calabria, & J. A. Macrae (Eds.). *Suggestions for thought.* Philadelphia, PA: University of Pennsylvania Press.

Nightingale, F. (2003). In L. McDonald (Ed.). *Florence Nightingale on society and politics, philosophy, science, education and literature.* Waterloo, ON: Wilfrid Laurier University Press.

O'Brien, M. E. (2014). *Spirituality in nursing: Standing on holy ground* (5th ed.). Boston, MA: Jones and Bartlett.

Paloutzian, R. F., & Ellison, C. W. (1991). *Manual for spiritual well-being scale.* New York, NY: Life Advance.

Parsian, N., & Dunning, T. (2009). Spirituality and coping in young adults with diabetes: A cross-sectional study. *European Diabetes Nursing, 6*(3), 100–104.

Pesut, B. (2006). Fundamental or foundational obligation? Problematizing the ethical call to spiritual care in nursing. *Advances in Nursing Science, 29*(2), 125–133.

Pesut, B., & Thorne, S. (2007). From private to public: Negotiating professional and personal identities in spiritual care. *Journal of Advanced Nursing, 58*, 396–403.

Peterman, A. H., Fitchett, G., Brady, M., Hernandez, L., & Cella, D. (2002). Measuring spiritual well-being in people with cancer: The functional assessment of chronic illness therapy—Spiritual well-being scale (FACIT-Sp). *Annals of Behavioral Medicine, 24*(1), 49–58.

Plato. (1997). In G. M. A. Grube (Ed.), *Phaedo.* Indianapolis, IN: Hackett.

Reed, P. (1987). Spirituality and well-being in terminally ill hospitalized adults. *Research in Nursing and Health, 10*, 335–344.

Reed, P. G. (1991). Toward a nursing theory of self-transcendence: Deductive reformulation using developmental theories. *Advances in Nursing Science, 13*(4), 64–77.

Smith-MacDonald, L., Norris, J. M., Raffin-Bouchal, S., & Sinclair, S. (2017). Spirituality and mental wellbeing in combat veterans: A systematic review. *Military Medicine, 182*(11/12), e1920–e1940.

Taylor, E., Highfield, M., & Amenta, M. (1999). Predictors of oncology and hospice nurses' spiritual care perspectives and practices. *Applied Nursing Research, 12*(1), 30–37.

Teilhard de Chardin, P. (1960a). *The phenomenon of man.* London, UK: Collins.

Teilhard de Chardin, P. (1960b). *The divine milieu.* London, UK: Collins.

Turan, T., & Karamanoglu, A. Y. (2012). Determining intensive care unit nurses' perceptions and practice level of spiritual care in Turkey. *Nursing in Critical Care, 18*(2), 70–78. doi: 10.1111/j.1478-5153.2012.00538.x

Vincensi, B., & Burkhart, L. (2016). Development and psychometric testing of two tools to assess nurse practitioners' provision of spiritual care. *Journal of Holistic Nursing, 34*(2), 112–122.

Vincensi, B., & Solberg, M. (2017). Assessing the frequency nurse practitioner incorporate spiritual care into patient-centered care. *The Journal for Nurse Practitioners, 13*(5), 368–375.

Watson, J. (1999). *Human science and human care: A theory of nursing.* Boston, MA: Jones and Bartlett.

Watson, J. (2005). *Caring science as sacred science.* Philadelphia, PA: Davis.

# Social Support
Marjorie A. Schaffer

## Definition of Key Terms

| | |
|---|---|
| **Appraisal support** | Affirmation from statements or actions made by another (Kahn & Antonucci, 1980) |
| **Emotional support** | Experience of feeling liked, admired, respected, or loved (Norbeck, Lindsey, & Carrieri, 1981) |
| **Formal support** | Help from professionals, paraprofessionals, or other service providers from structured community organizations (may be paid or unpaid assistance) |
| **Informal support** | Help provided through a person's "lay" social network, such as from family members and friends |
| **Informational support** | Knowledge provided to another during a time of stress that assists in problem solving (House, 1981) |
| **Instrumental support** | Tangible aid, goods, or services (House, 1981) |
| **Negative support** | Interactions that cause stress or are more demanding than helpful (Coyne & DeLongis, 1986) |
| **Perceived support** | Generalized appraisal that individuals are cared for and valued, have others available to them, and are satisfied with relationships (Heller, Swindle, & Dusenbury, 1986) |
| **Social network** | Structure of the interactive process of persons who give and receive help and protection (Langford, Bowsher, Maloney, & Lillis, 1997) |
| **Social support** | (a) "Aid and assistance exchanged through social relationships and interpersonal transactions" (Fleury, Keller, & Perez, 2009, p. 12); (b) "A well-intentioned action that is given willingly to a person with whom there is a personal relationship and that produces an immediate or delayed positive response in the recipient" (Hupcey, 1998b, p. 313) |

Social support is a middle range theory that addresses structure and interaction in relationships. Social support impacts health status, health behavior, and use of health services (Stewart, 1993). As health professionals, nurses often have access to clients' social networks. Through communication with clients and their family members, nurses can intervene to promote or strengthen social support. The literature identifies many positive consequences of social support, including health-promoting behaviors, personal competence, coping, a sense of well-being, self-worth, and decreased anxiety and depression (Langford et al., 1997). Social support is viewed as a protective factor that contributes to reduced mortality, disease, and disability (Waterworth, Rosenberg, Braham, Pescud, & Dimmock, 2014). Research on

social support interventions can provide nurses with knowledge about the most effective strategies for strengthening social support for clients, which contributes to improved health status.

## Historical Background

Cassel (1974), one of the early social support theorists, introduced the term "social support." Based on animal studies, he theorized that strengthening social supports could improve the health of humans. Studies in the early 1970s suggested that social support mediates the negative effects of stress (Roberts, 1984). The "buffer" theory and attachment theory have been the basis for considerable research on the relationship of social support and health (Callaghan & Morrissey, 1993). The buffer theory suggests that social support protects persons from life stressors (Cassel, 1976; Cobb, 1976). The attachment theory holds that the ability to form socially supportive relationships is related to the secure attachments formed in childhood (Bowlby, 1971). In the mid-1970s to the early 1980s, the literature most often described social support in concrete terms, such as an interaction, person, or relationship (Veiel & Baumann, 1992).

In recent years, the term has been used more abstractly, to include perceptions, quality and quantity of support, behaviors, and social systems. Concepts such as social inclusion and social capital have been introduced to expand the importance of community and society as contributors to social support (Jang & Canada, 2014; Wright & Stickely, 2013). The analysis and testing of social support theory have gained multidisciplinary interest and are prominent in nursing and social–psychological literature. Most recently, online social support interventions have been evaluated for effectiveness in strengthening social support. Examples include blogs for family caregivers of persons with dementia, electronic counseling for patients with cancer, online support for parents, an online forum for fathers, social support provided through an Internet weight loss community, online perinatal loss support, and a men's online eating disorder forum (Anderson, Hundt, Dean, Keim-Malpass, & Lopez, 2017; Eriksson & Salzmann-Erikson, 2013; Flynn & Stan, 2012; Holtslander, Kornder, Letourneau, Turner, & Paterson, 2012; Hwang et al., 2010; Merkel & Wright, 2012; Patterson, Brewer, & Stamler, 2013; Pector, 2012; Yli-Uotila, Kaunonen, Pylkkanen, & Suominen, 2016).

## Definition of Theory Concepts

Developers of social support theory have organized definitions of social support by a variety of component labels: aspects, categories, constructs, defining attributes, dimensions, interpersonal transactions, subconcepts, taxonomies, and types as shown in Table 9.1. The variety of definitions of social support provided by theorists illustrates the lack of consensus about the nature of social support. This lack of consensus contributes to complexity in evaluating social support interventions and outcomes, comparing research findings, and developing social support theory.

Although multidimensional definitions predominate, positive interaction or helpful behavior is shared by all social support definitions (Rook & Dooley, 1985). In addition, most social support theories have the assumption that support is given

and received by members of a social network, leading to social integration or a feeling of belonging (Diamond, 1985; Norbeck & Tilden, 1988). Recipients perceive that social support facilitates coping with stressors in their lives (Pierce, Sarason, & Sarason, 1990); high levels of stress may be mediated by social support (Chou, Avant, Kuo, & Fetzer, 2008). Social support is defined as "aid and assistance exchanged through social relationships and interpersonal transactions" (Fleury et al., 2009, p. 12). Social support can be structural, focusing on who provides the support, or functional, emphasizing the act of providing social support activities (Callaghan & Morrissey, 1993; Norwood, 1996). In addition, there are many characteristics that influence the quality and adequacy of social support, such as the stability, direction, and source of support (Stewart, 1989a). Social networks can be described by the number and categories of persons who provide social support: family members, close friends, neighbors, coworkers, and professionals (Tardy, 1985). Hupcey (1998a) suggested that a personal relationship is required for social support to take place, defining social support as "a well-intentioned action that is given willingly to a person with whom there is a personal relationship and that produces an immediate or delayed positive response in the recipient" (Hupcey, 1998b, p. 313).

### EMOTIONAL, INFORMATIONAL, INSTRUMENTAL, AND APPRAISAL SUPPORT

The four theoretical constructs or defining attributes of the theory include emotional, informational, instrumental, and appraisal support (Barrera 1986; Fleury et al., 2009; House, 1981; Tilden & Weinert, 1987). *Emotional support* involves the experience of feeling liked, admired, respected, or loved. *Instrumental support* is the provision of tangible aid, goods, or services. *Informational support* refers to providing information during a time of stress. *Appraisal support* affirms one's actions or statements (House, 1981; Kahn & Antonucci, 1980; Norbeck, 1981).

### NEGATIVE SOCIAL SUPPORT

It is possible for social support to negatively affect one's well-being (Revenson, Schiaffino, Majerovitz, & Gibofsky, 1991). The perception of or the satisfaction with the support one receives (perceived support) is likely to influence the outcome of the support activity (Heller et al., 1986). The support activity could actually be unrecognized or perceived negatively by the recipient. Negative social support is perceived as unhelpful and may

**Table 9.1    Theoretical Multidimensional Definitions of Social Support**

| Label | Support Components |
|---|---|
| Aspects (Cohen, 1992) | Social networks<br>Perceived support<br>Supportive behaviors |
| Categories (Hupcey, 1998a) | Types of support provided<br>Recipients' perceptions<br>Intentions/behaviors of provider of support<br>Reciprocal support<br>Social networks |
| Constructs (Vaux, 1988) | Support network resources<br>Support incidents<br>Support behaviors<br>Support appraisals<br>Support or network orientation |
| Defining attributes (House, 1981) | Emotional support<br>Informational support<br>Instrumental support<br>Appraisal support |
| Dimensions (Cutrona, 1990) | Emotional<br>Esteem (appraisal)<br>Tangible (instrumental)<br>Information<br>Social integration |
| Interpersonal transactions (Kahn, 1979) | Affect—feeling liked or loved<br>Affirmation—of behavior, perceptions, and views<br>Affect—feeling respected or admired<br>Aid—material or symbolic |
| Subconcepts (Barrera, 1981) | Material aid<br>Physical assistance<br>Intimate interaction<br>Guidance<br>Feedback<br>Social participation |
| Taxonomies (Laireiter & Baumann, 1992) | Social integration<br>Network resources<br>Supportive climate and environment<br>Received and enacted support<br>Perception of being supported |
| Types (Wortman, 1984) | Expression of positive affect<br>Expression of agreement<br>Encouragement of open expression of feelings<br>Offer of advice and information<br>Provision of material aid<br>Network of reciprocal help and mutual obligation |

undermine self-esteem. Characteristics of negative social support include stressful or conflicted social networks; misguided or absent support; inappropriate advice; avoidance; disagreement; violations of relationship norms that are interpreted as unpleasant, unwanted, or insensitive; and not receiving expected social support (Brooks & Dunkel-Schetter, 2011; Rook, 2014; Stewart, 1993). In addition, costs to the provider of social support such as overload, overcommitment, and stress-ful emotional involvement may occur (Coyne & DeLongis, 1986; La Gaipa, 1990). The balance of rewards and costs is likely to influence both perceptions and effects of social support. Cost, conflict, reciprocity, and equity are subdimensions that could be measured to capture the negative aspects of social support (Tilden & Galyen, 1987). Assessing the quality of the social support is important. Research shows there's a negative relationship between the quality of social support and caregiver burden (Vrabec, 1997). The amount of conflict in the relationship can result in negative social support that contributes to stress rather than well-being.

## VARIATIONS IN THE THEORY OF SOCIAL SUPPORT

A concept analysis of social support, based on an examination of 200 studies published from 1978 to 1996, revealed that most studies did not include a specific reference to a theoretical definition of social support and that researchers who defined social support often did not use a definition that addressed the interactional nature of social support (Hupcey, 1998b). Although Hupcey suggested that social support exchanges occur in personal relationships, other scholars have discussed examples of social support provided by professionals or outside the context of personal relationships, such as through communication over the Internet.

Professionals can intervene to strengthen existing social support networks for clients or choose to provide social support when it is lacking by helping individuals and families to access resources in the community that strengthen social support. Schaffer and Lia-Hoagberg (1997) concluded that nurses could provide informational support to partners and others important in the social networks of low-income pregnant women that would enhance the emotional, instrumental, informational, and appraisal support available to the women through their existing social networks. Social support was provided by professionals in a program called the New Mothers Network targeted to single, low-income, African American mothers. Program components included an electronic library, a chat group (asynchronous), and e-mail communication. Advanced practice nurses provided informational, appraisal, and emotional support through e-mail discussion and offering encouraging messages in the chat group (Hudson, Campbell-Grossman, Keating-Lefler, & Cline, 2008).

Wright and Bell (2003) explained how social support occurs in computer-mediated support groups. Although communication occurs between participants who do not have close personal relationships, the participants experience emotional support and informational support as they communicate about health-related experiences they have in common. Participants may be more open in expressing emotions since there is greater anonymity and protection from stigmatization in comparison to face-to-face interactions. However, the possibility of negative support exists in the case of hostile messages. Also, there may be greater

difficulty in forming long-term relationships, and a diminished reliance on family and friends may occur. On the positive side, evidence suggests that electronic social support may decrease use of health services (Scharer, 2005).

Overlap of other related concepts with social support is also a concern when defining social support. In a study of nurse-provided telephone social support for low-income pregnant women, Finfgeld-Connett (2005) suggested that the telephone-delivered nursing interventions involved something more than the attributes of social support; she reflected that presence may be a subconcept of social support and that social support may have become the default variable for nursing research studies because of the unavailability of instruments for measuring nursing presence.

## VARIABLES THAT INFLUENCE PERCEPTIONS OF SOCIAL SUPPORT

A number of variables affect the social support that is given and received or experienced. These include perceptions of the need and availability for support, timing, motivation for providing support, duration, direction, life stage, the source of support, and social network.

The provider of the social support first recognizes another's need for social support before determining the response to the need. If there is a mismatch in the provider's and recipient's perceptions of the need for support or the type of support that is provided, the recipient may not consider the support to be helpful (Dunkel-Schetter & Bennett, 1990; Dunkel-Schetter & Skokan, 1990). Providers of support may assume that the recipient who is experiencing stress needs support. If this assumption is inaccurate, the act of support could result in feelings of dependency, inadequacy, and lower self-esteem (Dunkel-Schetter, Blasband, Feinstein, & Herbert, 1992). Research data suggest that the perception of the availability of support is more important for health and well-being than is the actual receiving of the support (Cohen, Gottlieb, & Underwood, 2001).

Timing is also important, because the support needs of the recipient can change relative to the recipient's appraisal of the situation over time (Jacobson, 1986; Norwood, 1996; Tilden, 1986). Social support is a dynamic process influenced by personal characteristics and situations. Changes that affect both the giving and receiving of social support include the nature of relationships from a historical perspective, expectations of support from one's network, and personal coping skills (Lackner, Goldenberg, Arrizza, & Tjosvold, 1994). Cohen, Underwood, and Gottlieb (2000) suggested that individuals may be more receptive to social support interventions when experiencing a crisis.

Motivation for providing social support can affect the quality of the support provided. A sense of obligation on the part of the provider may decrease the recipient's satisfaction with the support (Hupcey, 1998a). Providers of social support are likely to consider the recipient's responsibility and effort relative to the needed support and the costs to the provider that result from the act of support (Jung, 1988). The provider's previous experiences with providing support and previous interactions with the intended recipient will also influence choices of support actions (Hupcey, 1998a).

Duration of the support, referring to length of time or stability of the support, is a consideration for the chronically ill and persons who experience long-term loss (Cohen & Syme, 1985). The long-term effects of stressors on individuals may require ongoing support, as well as support from sources outside the usual social networks. For example, in a longitudinal study of the perceived support and support sources of older women with heart failure, the women identified paid helpers as sources of support at a later time in progression of their illness (Friedman, 1997).

The direction of support may be unidirectional or bidirectional. Bidirectional support is characterized by mutuality and reciprocity (Stewart, 1993). Professional support is usually unidirectional. In family and intimate relationships, the roles of "helper" and "helpee" may alternate (Clark, 1983; Rook & Dooley, 1985). Reciprocity in social support is likely to reduce feelings of burden and strain in providers and inadequacy and lack of control in recipients (Albrecht & Adelman, 1987).

The provision and receiving of social support vary over the life span. Some life stages offer more capability for providing social support, while other life stages require more receiving than giving of social support. Social support needs are greater during times of change and additional stress, such as during the birth of a child or with the loss of strength and function associated with aging.

Individuals often identify family and friends as sources of support in comparison to professionals (Hupcey & Morse, 1997; Schaffer & Lia-Hoagberg, 1997). However, professionals can intervene to enhance the existing social support resources of clients or can act as surrogates to provide support not currently available in the client's social network (Norbeck, 1988). To enhance informal and formal sources of support, professionals can develop and strengthen relationships with personal support networks, mutual aid groups, neighborhood support systems, volunteer programs, and community resources (Chien & Norman, 2009; Froland, Pancoast, Chapman, & Kimboko, 1981). Formal support is more likely to occur in institutional settings. Newsom, Bookwala, and Schulz (1997) found a high degree of formal support for older adults in nursing homes, residential care facilities, and congregate apartments. The instrumental support available in institutional settings was provided primarily by professional and nonprofessional paid staff. These formal support sources may also provide a sizeable amount of emotional support for older adults who have physical and cognitive challenges, because paid staff are more often available for older adults in group residences (Pearlman & Crown, 1992).

The size of the social network is sometimes considered to be an indicator of social support. Key sources of support, including immediate family members and close friends, are distinguished from sources viewed as less important—other relatives, coworkers, church and community members, and professional caregivers (Griffith, 1985). However, a large social network does not necessarily guarantee that a large amount of support is present (Kahn & Antonucci, 1980). The quality of the relationships and availability of persons in the social network, as well as the number of persons in the network, contribute to the enacted social support. A variety of network members can better provide the range of needed social support actions. For example, in one study, persons with a cancer diagnosis perceived spouses or partners as helpful for their physical presence, while friends provided practical help (Dakof & Taylor, 1990). In another study with cancer patients, informational support was perceived as helpful from experts but not from friends or families (Dunkel-Schetter, 1984).

## THE RELATIONSHIP OF SOCIAL SUPPORT AND HEALTH

Heller et al. (1986) posited that two facets of social support, esteem-enhancing appraisal and stress-related, interpersonal transactions, have an effect on health outcomes. They hypothesized that the appraisal or perception of the social interaction is health protective, rather than the social interaction or support activity itself. Esteem-enhancing appraisal results from an assessment of how one is viewed by others. In stress-related interpersonal transactions, network members provide tangible assistance, which facilitates coping. Figure 9.1 illustrates these relationships.

Cohen et al. (2001) described two models that explain how social support influences health. The stress-buffering model holds that social support contributes to health-promoting behaviors in persons who are experiencing stress. Rather than choosing behaviors that may be harmful to health, the support resources strengthen an individual's

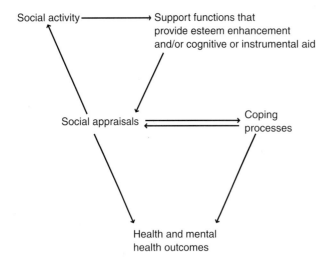

**Figure 9.1** Hypothesized relationships between facets of social support, coping, and health outcomes. (From Heller, K., Swindle, R. W., & Dusenbury, L. (1986). Component social support processes: Comments and integration. *Journal of Consulting and Clinical Psychology, 54*(4), 466–470. Copyright © 1986 by the American Psychological Association. Reprinted with permission.)

perceived ability to cope with a stressful situation (Thoits, 1986). These beliefs lead to a calmer psychological and physiological response to the stressful situation and can decrease negative behavioral responses. In this case, an individual is more likely to have an adaptive response to the stressful situation, thus avoiding a maladaptive response with a greater potential for negative health effects.

The main effect model, the second model described by Cohen et al. (2001), suggests that social support directly impacts psychological and physical health, whether or not an individual is experiencing a stressful situation. Integration into a social network, as contrasted to isolation, can provide social control and peer pressure to engage in health-promoting behaviors and lead to positive psychological states, such as a sense of predictability, stability, purpose, belonging, and security (Cassel, 1976; Hammer, 1981; Thoits, 1983). In addition, social networks can provide multiple sources of information about health care services and may also provide informal health care that prevents progression of illness (Cohen et al., 2001).

Norbeck (1981) proposed a model for using social support as a nursing intervention to improve health outcomes. The social support environment of the client is assessed by determining the need for social support compared to the available social support. An assessment of inadequate social support necessitates developing an intervention plan to increase social support. Possible interventions can focus on strengthening the client's existing social support structure or function or providing direct support during a crisis. According to this nursing process model, adequate social support will result in a positive health outcome; inadequate social support without intervention will result in a negative health outcome.

Research findings have demonstrated the stress-buffering aspects of social support. Social support is a mediator that contributes to improved health outcomes. In a study of women with breast cancer, personal support provided by family and close friends mediated the negative effects of common symptoms contributing to distress during the breast cancer treatment and resulted in improved scores on quality-of-life measures both generally and specific to breast cancer (Manning-Walsh, 2005). Social support during the perinatal period was an important buffer against depression (Li, Long, Cao, & Cao, 2017). In a study of patients discharged from intensive care, instrumental and emotional support had a buffering effect on the physical aspect of quality of life (Tilburgs, Nijkamp, Bakker, & van der Hoeven, 2015). For community-dwelling older adults, social support buffered the negative effects of depression symptoms on life satisfaction (Adams et al., 2016). In a study that used multiple regression analysis to examine the association of race-related stress and hopelessness in African American adults, self-esteem social support (appraisal support) was the strongest predictor of feelings of hopelessness. Self-esteem social support buffered the influence of race-related stress (Odafe, Salami, & Walker, 2017).

Other studies in nursing have resulted in positive relationships between social support and other variables that contribute to improvements in health behavior or positive perceptions about health. In a study of Taiwanese women in early pregnancy, women with higher levels of social support reported less stress; social support along with the additional predictor variables of pregnancy-related nausea and vomiting, perceived stress, and pregnancy planning together explained the variance in maternal psychosocial adaptation (Chou et al., 2008). Keller, Allan, and Tinkle (2006) found that social support from friends increased the time postpartum women spent in physical exercise. In a study of nursing home residents in Norway, Drageset et al. (2009) determined there was a positive relationship between social support and health-related quality of life. In a study of older adults who used senior centers in New York, perceived social support was positively associated with autonomy (Matsui & Capezuti, 2008). Latham and Calvillo (2009) explored predictors of successful diabetes management in a sample of 240 low-income Hispanic people. Social support explained 24% of the satisfaction with quality of life and self on the diabetes quality-of-life measure. Chien and Norman (2009) conducted a literature review to determine the effectiveness of mutual support groups for family caregivers of people with psychotic disorders. Mutual support groups are "informal networks of individuals who share a common experience or issue" (p. 1618). In the review of 25 studies, they found evidence for short-term positive effects on physical and psychosocial health for clients and families. Benefits included more knowledge about the illness and treatment, lower burden and distress, and better coping ability. The researchers suggested that there should be more studies that investigate the long-term effects of mutual support groups.

While social support can contribute positively to health outcomes, negative social exchanges contribute to negative health outcomes. As a stressor, negative social exchanges bring about the release of stress hormones, which, if continued over time, are damaging to the body. The relationship of negative social exchange and negative health outcomes for elders is evident in lower ratings on self-reports on health status, longitudinal studies on links to heart disease, decline of cognitive functioning, and increased disability (Rook, 2014). Bird-Craven and Massey (2013) found that low-income pregnant women who had a distant or no relationship with the baby's father had higher levels of depressive symptoms. Yang, Schorpp, and Harris (2014) investigated how negative social support, measured by social strain, contributed to inflammation, measured by biological markers. Social strain was defined by interpersonal conflict, frequent criticism, and demands from one's social network. While positive social support protected against the risks of inflammation, social strain had a stronger negative influence.

## SOCIAL SUPPORT NURSING ASSESSMENT AND INTERVENTIONS

For nurses, social support can connect family assessment, patient needs, and health outcomes (Hupcey, 1998b). Beeber and Canuso (2005) suggested five critical assessment questions for nurses to help determine effective emotional,

informational, and instrumental social support interventions:

> Who helps you get the day-to-day things you need in your life?
> If you had an emergency, who would you call on for help?
> Who would lend you money to or keep or ask to keep your child(ren) if you needed it?
> Who gives you advice that is useful?
> Who understands your private worries and feelings? (p. 773).

Logsdon and Koniak-Griffin (2005) developed a clinical pathway for social support of postpartum adolescents, which outlines assessment of social support; assessment of related variables such as depression, risk for harm, and high-risk behaviors; and health care provider interventions. They gave examples of specific assessment questions, suggested relevant instruments for the measurement of social support, and identified professional interventions that strengthen existing social support networks. Identified pathway interventions include counseling and teaching about the reality and demands of the postpartum period, common feelings experienced in the postpartum period, options for social support in their network, and the importance of communication as well as providing social skills training and referral for community services. Such interventions can raise the level of perceived appraisal, emotional, informational, and instrumental support.

Vandall-Walker, Jensen, and Oberle (2007) used a grounded theory approach to explore the process of nursing support in a sample of 20 family members from 14 families of critically ill adults hospitalized in intensive care. Family members viewed nursing support as "lightening their load." Initially, nurses engaged family members through the following support activities: acknowledging, welcoming, orienting, relating, trusting, and empathizing. The middle phase focused on sustaining family members through nursing actions of being there, communicating, being accountable, sharing responsibility, negotiating, valuing, promoting family member self-care, and connecting family members to other professionals and services. The final stage of disengaging included providing guidance for decisions, helping to find meaning, and preparing family members to say goodbye, which may involve the client's death or the client leaving the unit. The family members identified nursing support activities that helped them to "get through" the situation, which is different than conceptualizations of support as caring (Vandall-Walker et al., 2007). Many of these nursing actions will likely result in the provision of emotional, informational, instrumental, and appraisal support to families of critically ill adults.

In another intervention example, telephone peer support was provided during the postpartum period to prevent postpartum depression (Dennis, 2010). A peer volunteer initiated telephone conversations for the intervention group. Participants completed the Peer Support Evaluation Inventory (PESI). Mothers reported receiving emotional, informational, and appraisal support through conversations with the peer volunteers. There was a positive relationship between maternal satisfaction and the number and duration of peer contacts. Researchers recommended strengthening appraisal support and matching volunteers to participant characteristics.

## Application of the Theory in Practice

Nurses have the knowledge and expertise to assess the interpersonal and social environments of clients, implement health promotion strategies, and facilitate clients in initiating self-care practices (Tilden, 1985). From a prevention perspective, social support can be viewed as "social inoculation" (Pilisuk, 1982). Through "network therapy," nurses can assess social support adequacy, use existing social support measures, determine the roles of professionals and nonprofessional providers of social support to move clients to increasing independence, and organize and evaluate community support groups (Roberts, 1984). Using Middle Range Theory in Practice 9.1 provides an example of social support interventions nurses can provide to promote wound healing in patients with type 2 diabetes.

An example of preventive support is comprehensive home visitation for vulnerable young mothers provided by public health nurses (Olds et al., 2007). Nurses provided regular home visits to young mothers beginning during their pregnancy and continuing until their children were 2 years of age. The purposes of the visits were to improve pregnancy outcomes, to promote children's healthy development, and to improve the financial self-sufficiency of participating families. Nurses both provided formal support and strengthened informal sources of support. Evaluation of the long-term outcomes through a randomized clinical trial demonstrated positive outcomes for mothers (reduced subsequent birth rate, longer interval between the first and second birth, and more relationship stability) and children (higher academic achievement and lower mortality from preventable causes).

Stewart (1989b) offered a practice application framework consisting of five social support intervention levels: individual, dyadic, groups, community, and social system. Interventions at these levels include strengthening available social support and providing direct social support with the goal of improving health status. At the individual level, a home care nurse could provide informational, appraisal, and emotional support for a pregnant woman placed on bed rest for a high-risk pregnancy. The nurse may also help the woman identify instrumental support for help with household tasks. At the dyadic level of social support, an oncology nurse who is providing care for a woman having a mastectomy would include the woman's partner in social support interventions such as referral to couples' counseling. At the group level, a nurse could refer a patient with multiple sclerosis

---

### USING MIDDLE RANGE THEORY IN PRACTICE  9.1

*Source: Iannino-Renz, R. (2016). The role of social support in persons with type 2 diabetic wounds. MEDSURG Nursing, 25(5), 357–359.*

#### PROBLEM

Diabetic neuropathy, caused by long-term elevation of blood glucose, leads to an inability to sense pain and pressure in lower extremities. Neuropathy is the leading cause of wounds for diabetic patients. One-third of patients with type 2 diabetes experience a diabetic ulcer during their life course. Twenty-five percent of all hospitalizations for diabetes involve a wound related to diabetes.

#### NURSING INTERVENTION

Social support can promote wound healing by improving mood and decreasing stress and anxiety. Nurses can provide informational support through literature and education, daily emotional support while doing wound care, and appraisal support by helping with decisions that facilitate wound healing.

#### CONCLUSIONS

Nurses can offer emotional, instrumental, informational, and appraisal support as they provide wound care to diabetic patients. A review of available research on the topic indicates that social support can promote healing of wounds and improve quality of life for diabetic patients.

and the family members to a support group that would provide informational and emotional support. An example of a community-level support intervention is the Block Nurse Program, which provides informational and instrumental support to isolated elderly in a neighborhood. Finally, a systems example is the establishment of school policy to promote healthy eating. Informational support for parents and school staff, instrumental support through changes in breakfast and lunch offerings to promote healthy eating, and appraisal support through a peer group to encourage positive behavior change all contribute to motivation for healthy eating behaviors. Table 9.2 provides citations and descriptions of specific applications of social support theory in clinical practice.

**Table 9.2    Examples of Theory in Practice**

| Citation | Focus |
| --- | --- |
| Hautsalo, K., Rantanen, A., & Astedt-kurki, P. (2012). Family functioning, health and social support assessed by aged home care clients and their family members. *Journal of Clinical Nursing, 22*, 2953–2962. doi: 10.111/j.1365-2702.2012.04335.x | For older adults living alone, social support is provided by both informal sources, such as families and neighbors, and formal sources, including community services. Emotional support, affirmation, and concrete aid provided through a social network improve quality of life for older people. Home care focuses on providing concrete aid |
| Leahy-Warren, P., McCarthy, G., & Corcoran, P. (2011). First-time mothers: Social support, maternal parental self-efficacy and postnatal depression. *Journal of Clinical Nursing, 21*, 388–397. doi: 10.1111/j.1365-2702.2011.03701.x | Social support for mothers during the postpartum period contributes to successful transition to motherhood. An example is concrete help (instrumental aid) with household tasks from their husbands and mothers during a time that some new mothers may find to be stressful. In addition to instrumental aid, other forms of social support include emotional concern, information, and appraisal from the social network. Appraisal support promotes a sense of competence for new mothers. Social support positively influences their mental health and sense of well-being |
| Petosa, R. L., & Smith, L. H. (2014). Peer mentoring for health behavior change: A systematic review. *American Journal of Health Education, 45*(6), 351–357. doi: 10.1080/193205037.2014.945670 | Peer mentors can promote health behavior change in school settings through providing emotional, information, and appraisal support. Adolescents who generally like to share information informally in their network of friends perceive social support that contributes to a sense of psychological safety and motivation for health behavior change |
| Pinto, S., Schub, T., & Pravikoff, D. (2015). Patient adherence to medical treatment: The effect of social support. Evidence-based Care Sheet. Retrieved from Cinahl Information Systems, a division of EBSCO Information Services | Social support is a resource that contributes to increased adherence to health care treatment. Structural support is provided through social networks (marriage). Functional support refers to actions taken by others. This includes family cohesiveness, emotional support, instruments or practical support, and informational support. Patients who perceive that they have higher levels of social support are more likely to follow the treatment plan. Nursing interventions include assessing social support networks, encouraging supportive communication, providing information in disease management, engaging both the patient and family members in decision making, simplifying the medication regimen, and referring as needed for additional support |
| Sadath, A., Muralidhar, D., Varambally, S., & Gangadhar, B. N. (2017). Does group intervention have benefits on expressed emotion and social support in carers of persons with first episode psychosis? *Social Work in Mental Health, 15*(5), 524–537. doi: 10.1080/15332985.2016.1252826 | A support group intervention for caregivers of persons with first episode psychosis can contribute to improving their perceived social support. When caregivers are encouraged to share their stories and support one another during the group, they may experience informational, emotional, or appraisal support and perceive that support is available to them |
| Sherriff, N., Hall, V., & Panton, C. (2014). Engaging and supporting fathers to promote breast feeding: A concept analysis. *Midwifery, 30*, 667–677. doi: 10.1016/j.midw.2013.07.014 | A concept analysis identified five attributes of father support for breast-feeding: knowledge about breast-feeding, positive attitude to breast-feeding, involvement in the decision-making process, practical support, and emotional support. Health professionals can use these important attributes of father support for breast-feeding to examine current practice, service delivery models, and education |
| Watkins, D. C., & Jefferson, S. O. (2012). Recommendations for the use of online support for African American men. *Psychological Services, 10*(3), 323–322. doi: 10.1037/a0027904 | Although African American men have high levels of psychosocial stress, their distrust of the health care system contributes to a reluctance to use mental health services. Accessibility and anonymity are two characteristics of online support groups that may appeal to African American men. Online communities have the potential to motivate positive health behaviors through emotional, informational, and instrumental support offered by others. Perceived support occurs when the men are satisfied with the support and are able to anticipate support from others |

## Application of the Theory in Research

Cohen et al. (2000) identified three theoretical perspectives for guiding research on social support: (a) The stress and coping perspective holds that social support influences health by protecting people from the negative effects of stress. Supportive actions are viewed as facilitating coping. (b) The social constructivist perspective asserts social support contributes to health through promotion of self-esteem and self-regulation. (c) The relationship perspective addresses how social support within relationships occurs and examines relationship processes, such as intimacy, companionship, and social conflict. The stress and coping perspective predominates in social support research on health outcomes.

Researchers have explored a great variety of nursing practice issues from a social support perspective including topics such as chronic illness, persons who are grieving, the relationship of social support to acute chest complaints, new mothers in stressful situations, and administrative support for nurses. Researchers have also investigated how social support interacts with other variables to predict health outcomes. The majority of studies focus on the individual- or family-level experience of social support. In Middle Range Theory in Research 9.2, there is an example of how social support theory has been used in research. Table 9.3 lists additional examples on social support research in nursing.

### MEASURES OF SOCIAL SUPPORT

Although a great number of social support measures have been developed in several disciplines, many measures do not have adequate reliability and validity testing, and many are situation specific rather than general measures of social support. Available measures address (a) interconnectedness in a social network; (b) received support, based on a person's report of support that was provided; and (c) perceived support, the support a person believes to be personally available to them (Sarason, Sarason, & Pierce, 1990). Researchers have primarily developed situation-specific measures of social support for groups who encounter a common stressor event, such as pregnancy or chronic illness (Stewart, 1993). Of 21 social support instruments reviewed by Stewart (1989a), only 4 were applicable on a general level. Eight measures of social support developed by nurse researchers are described in Table 9.4. The selected instruments represent both general and specific measures of social

---

### USING MIDDLE RANGE THEORY IN RESEARCH    9.2

*Source: Adams, T. R., Rabin, L. A., Da Silva, V. G., Katz, M. J., Fogel, J., & Lipton, R. B. (2016). Social support buffers the impact of depressive symptoms on life satisfaction in old age. Clinical Gerontologist, 39(2), 139–157. doi: 10.1080/07317115.2015.1073823*

#### RESEARCH QUESTION

What is the association of psychosocial and health-related factors with life satisfaction in older community-dwelling adults and the role of social support as a moderator?

#### RESEARCH DESIGN

Nonexperimental

#### SAMPLE/PARTICIPANTS

Participants ($n = 237$) were a subset of older adults participating in a longitudinal, community study on cognitive aging. Eligible participants were 70 or older, lived in the Bronx community in New York, and were English speaking. Participants with dementia, active psychiatric symptoms, nonambulatory status, or sensory disturbances were excluded.

#### DATA COLLECTION

Participants completed a general health survey, a questionnaire on the type and extent of cognitive and physical activity engaged in weekly over the past year, the Geriatric Depression Scale-Short form (GDS-SF), the Adult Manifest Anxiety Scale-Elderly Version (AMAS-E), the Perceived Stress Scale, the Medical Outcomes Study (MOS) Social Support Survey, and Satisfaction With Life Scale (SWLS). For social support, the MOS addresses the availability of affective, informational, emotional, and tangible aspects of social support. The measure has 19 items, which are scored on a Likert-type scale from 1 (none of the time) to 5 (all of the time). The total social support score is a summation of all responses, ranging from 19 to 95. Reliability for this sample was 0.96 (Cronbach's alpha).

#### FINDINGS

In all linear regression analysis models, participants with higher scores on social support and the self-report general health measure had higher scores for life satisfaction ($p < 0.001$). Fewer symptoms of depression, lower perceived stress, higher social support, and higher general health scores were significantly associated with the outcome of higher life satisfaction scores. Researchers determined that social support buffered the negative impact of depressive symptoms on life satisfaction.

**Table 9.3    Examples of Research for Application to Practice**

| Reference | Research Design/Meta-Analysis | Clinical Issue/Research Question | Sample (n)/Population | Intervention | Outcome |
|---|---|---|---|---|---|
| Fallatah, F., & Edge, D. S. (2014). Social support needs of families: The context of rheumatoid arthritis. *Applied Nursing Research, 28*, 180–185. doi: 10.1016/j.apnr.2014.10.004 | Qualitative; semistructured interview guide; organized data into tables to analyze social support needs of family members and relatives with rheumatoid arthritis (RA) | Exploration of family member experience of providing social support to their relative with RA and forms of support they required | Seven family members who had a relative living with rheumatoid arthritis in Canada; diverse in age, gender, and ethnic identity | NA | All participants provided emotional and instrumental support to their relative; social support for participants included mutual social support in the relationship with their relative and emotional and instrumental support (e.g., transportation, meals) from extended family members |
| Graven, L. J., & Grant, J. (2013). The impact of social support on depressive symptoms in individuals with heart failure. *Journal of Cardiovascular Nursing, 28*(5), 429–443. doi: 10.1097/JCN.0b013e3182578b9d | Systematic review of quantitative and qualitative studies; 15 articles met inclusion criteria | Examination of literature on the impact of social support on symptoms of depression in heart failure patients | Outpatient and hospitalized patients with heart failure | NA | 11 of 15 articles reported significant findings; social support had a positive impact on reduction and prevention of depression or symptoms in heart failure patients |
| Letourneau, N., Stewart, M., Masuda, J. R., Anderson, S., Cicutto, L., McGhan, S., & Watt, S. (2012). Impact of online support for youth with asthma and allergies: A pilot study. *Pediatric Nursing, 27*, 65–73. doi: 10.1016/j.pedn.2010.07.007 | Mixed method; standardized measures for all variables; open-ended questions; postintervention and exit interviews. Social support was measured by Multidimensional Scale of Perceived Social Support (MSPSS) | Investigation of (a) support-seeking coping, (b) support satisfaction and support needs, (c) social network size, (d) loneliness and social isolation, and (e) self-efficacy | 28 youth between 11 and 16 with physician-diagnosed asthma and/or allergies | Online peer training mentorship program for youth—3 mo of support moderated by trained peer mentors and health professionals | Trends in data show likelihood of benefits to providing support online. Social isolation and loneliness were reduced. "Youth reported gaining confidence and a sense of normality from talking to other youth" (p. 71) |
| Maycock, B., Binns, C. W., Dhaliwal, S., Tohotoa, J., Hauck, Y., Burns, S., & Howat, P. (2013). Education and support for fathers improves breastfeeding rates: a randomized controlled trial. *Journal of Human Lactation, 29*(4), 484–490. doi: 10.1177/0890334413484387 | Randomized controlled trial | Investigation of effects of antenatal education and postnatal support targeted to fathers to increase initiation and duration of breast-feeding | 695 couples in eight public hospitals in Australia | Antenatal education session; 6-wk postnatal social support package of printed information (informational support), birth congratulatory note to fathers, beer can holder bearing the study logo, and resources to assist in reducing fathers' anxiety (emotional support) and increase problem-solving abilities | For intervention group, breast-feeding rate was significantly greater at 6 wk, 81.6%, compared to 75.2% in control group, odds ratio 1.46 (95% CI, 1.01–2.13) |

*(Continued)*

**Table 9.3  Examples of Research for Application to Practice** (Continued)

| Reference | Research Design/ Meta-Analysis | Clinical Issue/ Research Question | Sample (*n*)/ Population | Intervention | Outcome |
|---|---|---|---|---|---|
| Sammarco, A., & Konecny, L. M. (2010). Quality of life, social support, and uncertainty among Latina and Caucasian breast cancer survivors: A comparative study. *Oncology Nursing Forum, 37*(1), 93–99 | Descriptive, comparative study; instruments included Social Support Questionnaire (Northouse, 1988) | What is the difference between Latina and Caucasian breast cancer survivors in perceived social support, uncertainty, and quality of life? | 182 Caucasian and 98 Latina breast cancer survivors | NA | Caucasians reported higher levels of perceived social support in comparison with Latinas. "To address the value of familialism, efforts should be made to remove barriers that may impede family involvement in the care of Latina breast cancer survivors" (p. 98) |
| Tilburgs, B., Nijkamp, M. D., Bakker, E. C., & van der Hoeven, H. (2015). The influence of social support on patients' quality of life after an intensive care unit discharge: A cross-sectional survey. *Intensive and Critical Care Nursing, 31*, 336–342. doi: 10.1016/j.iccn.2015.07.002 | Cross-sectional survey | Determination of influence of instrumental, emotional, and informative support on the quality of life of former intensive care unit (ICU) patients | 88 former intensive care patients in The Netherlands | NA | With more instrumental or emotional support, patients had fewer role limitations due to physical problems; patients preferred receiving social support from family members rather than from friends, professional caregivers, or fellow former ICU patients |
| Stewart, M., Simich, L., Shizha, E., Makumbe, K., & Makwarimba, E. (2012). Supporting African refugees in Canada: Insights from a support intervention. *Health and Social Care in the Community, 20*(5), 516–527. doi: 10.1111/j.1365-2524.2012.01069.x | Qualitative analysis of interviews | What types of social support were provided in the intervention? Additionally, intervention processes, participants' perceptions, issues discussed in the face-to-face support groups and telephone dyads, facilitator perceptions, benefits and challenges, and recommended changes were evaluated | Somali (*n* = 39) and Sudanese (*n* = 29) refugees from Canada | Eight support groups in urban centers, consisting of 5–12 participants, facilitated by a peer and a professional. Met biweekly for face-to-face sessions over 6 mo. Peer facilitators delivered supplementary one-to-one telephone support between group sessions | Types of support provided included emotional, informational, and affirmational support. "Refugees felt encouraged because they could bring their problems to the group and seek support. This social support intervention resulted in increased social integration, decreased loneliness, and expanded repertoire of coping strategies" (p. 525) |

**Table 9.4    Selected Social Support Instruments Developed by Nurse Researchers**

| Instrument | Social Support Components | Description | Sample Item |
|---|---|---|---|
| Interpersonal Relationships Inventory (IPRI) Tilden et al. (1990) | Social support Reciprocity Conflict | • 39 items (13 for each subscale)<br>• 5-point agree/disagree scale<br>• Subscales used separately<br>• Internal consistency and test–retest reliability<br>• Construct validity for social support and conflict subscales | Someone believes in me (support) I let others know I care (reciprocity) Wish people were more sensitive (conflict) |
| Norbeck Social Support Questionnaire (NSSQ) Norbeck et al. (1981, 1983) | Affect Affirmation Aid Loss Duration of relationship Frequency of contact | • Identify persons in network<br>• 5-point scale on extent of support provided for nine questions<br>• Internal consistency and test–retest reliability<br>• Construct validity | How much does this person make you feel liked or loved? |
| Social Support Questionnaire (SSQ) Northouse (1988) Perceived Resource Questionnaire (PRQ-85) Weinert (1987, 1988) | Sources of social support Amount of social support Intimacy Social integration Nurturance Worth Assistance | • 40 items<br>• Sources—spouse, family member, friends, nurse, physician<br>• 5-point Likert type agree/disagree scale<br>• Internal consistency reliability and concurrent validity<br>• Part 1—identifies resources and satisfaction with help<br>• Part 2—25 items on perceived social support; seven-point agree/disagree scale<br>• Internal consistency reliability—part 2<br>• Construct validity—part 2 | If I need advice, there is someone who would assist me to work out a plan for dealing with the situation |
| Support Behaviors Inventory (SBI) Brown (1986) | Perceived degree of experiential support during pregnancy—satisfaction with partner support and satisfaction with other support | • 11 items on shortened version<br>• 6-point satisfied/dissatisfied scale<br>• Internal consistency reliability for total support score on shortened version | Tolerates my ups and downs and unusual behaviors |
| Social Support in Chronic Illness Survey (SSCII) Hilbert (1990) | Intimate interaction Guidance Feedback Maternal aid Behavioral assistance Positive social interaction | • 38 items<br>• 6-point satisfied/dissatisfied scale<br>• Internal consistency reliability<br>• Content validity | Commented favorably when he or she noticed me doing something that the health team recommended |
| Postpartum Support Questionnaire Logsdon, Usui, Birkimer, and McBride (1996) | Material support Emotional support Informational support Comparison support | • 34 items—self-report or interview<br>• Eight options—not important to very important<br>• Two scales for importance and support<br>• Internal consistency reliability | Takes worries seriously |
| Supportive Needs of Adolescents Breastfeeding Scale (SNAB) Grassley, Spencer, and Bryson (2013) | Instrumental support Emotional support Appraisal support Informational support | • 20 items<br>• Rate supportive nurse behaviors on the helpfulness of the behavior from 0 to 5<br>• Internal consistency reliability | Provided for privacy that I wanted when I was with BF |

Note: *Additional Measures of Social Support Used by Nurse Researchers*
- Family Functioning, Health, and Social Support (FAFHES)—Social support portion has 37 items for aid, affirmation, and affect subscales (Astedt-Kurki, Tarkaa, Rikala, Lehti, & Paavilainen, 2009).
- Family Support for Exercise Scale (Sallis, Grossman, Pinski, Patterson, & Nader, 1987).
- Friend Support for Exercise Scale (Sallis et al., 1987).
- Interpersonal Support Evaluation List (ISEL)—15 items include appraisal, belonging, and tangible support (Cohen, Mermelstein, Kmarack, & Hoberman, 1985; Owen, 2003).
- Medical Outcome Study Social Support Survey (Holden, Lee, Hockey, Ware, & Dobson, 2014; Sherbourne & Stewart, 1991).
- Multidimensional Scale of Perceived Social Support (MSPSS)—12 items include significant other, family, and friend subscales (Zimet, Dahlem, Zimet, & Farley, 1988).
- Postpartum Social Support Questionnaire (PSSQ) (Hopkins & Campbell, 2008).
- Social Support for Physical Activity Scale—4 items measure support from kin, nonkin, and health care workers (Cousins, 1996).

support and have been psychometrically analyzed. None of the instruments are applicable to young children. Additional measures of social support that have been used by but not developed by nurse researchers are listed at the bottom of the table.

Cohen et al. (2000) propose the following questions for researchers to consider when selecting a social support measure of perceived or received support:

What supportive functions are relevant for this population? (i.e., appraisal support, emotional support, informational support, instrumental support).

Should I measure received support as well as perceived support?

How long a measure do I need?

Should I use a composite score or separate scale scores?

Should I include measures of unsupportive interactions as well as support?

How should I assess support from specific network members?

Should I measure both availability and satisfaction with support?

Will I need to adapt the measure for a specific population?

Will I need to adapt the measure for a particular stressor?

Will I need to adapt the measure for an intervention study?

For example, researchers adapted the Norbeck Social Support Questionnaire (NSSQ) for a study on social support in low-income pregnant women (Schaffer & Lia-Hoagberg, 1997). Two items were added to the NSSQ to measure informational support specific to pregnancy that was provided by others in order to determine the relationship of social support to prenatal health behaviors.

Most measures of social support are self-reports. Al-Dwaikat and Hall (2017) completed a systematic review to evaluate measures of social support used in studies of persons with diabetes type 2. Of 48 studies, most were general measures of perceived social support and only 17% of the studies measured both positive and negative support. They found that 25% of the studies used the Medical Outcomes Study-Social Support Survey (MOS-SSS).

Newsom et al. (1997) discussed the challenge of measuring social support for the cognitively impaired. They suggested that proxy and observational measures of social support may be an alternative strategy for determining the adequacy of social support for persons who cannot provide an accurate self-report. Proxies, such as nursing home staff and primary caregivers, can provide information about social network contacts and interactions. Observational methods include recording interaction behaviors and videotaping. A coding system can be used to label the source of the support, the type of support, the recipient response, and other characteristics of the support interaction.

An example of a measure of social support with a very specific focus is the Child and Adolescent Social Support Scale for Healthy Behaviors (CASSS-HB), which can be used by nurses working with children and adolescents in a clinical or school setting to measure social support for healthy behaviors (Cullum & Mayo, 2015). Initial psychometric testing demonstrated adequate reliability and validity. Sixty self-report items represent twelve themes that are repeated five times; social support subscales include the social support sources of parent, teacher, classmates, close friends, and people in my school. Items focus on health behaviors such as physical activity and healthy eating.

Some researchers have used qualitative approaches for investigating social support, although quantitative measures appear to be predominant. In Finland, nurse researchers asked one open-ended question to explore perceptions of social support after the death of a spouse: "What helped you cope with your grief?" (Kaunonen, Tarkka, Paunonen, & Laippala, 1999). The researchers used content analysis to classify the data by the structure of social relationships and the social support functions of aid, affirmation, and affect in relationships (Kahn, 1979). Lugton (1997) used a strategy called social contact analysis, in addition to interview data, to explore the social support experienced by women treated for breast cancer. Participants drew their social networks, with self at center, using shorter lines for closer relationships and arrows to indicate whether the relationship involved support, strain, or both. The researcher then asked participants to describe how professional and informal persons in the social network had responded to the illness of the participant in supportive and nonsupportive ways. Types of support that facilitated adjustment were emotional support, companionship, practical help, opportunities for confiding, experiential support (from others who had experienced breast cancer), and sexual identity support.

Evans, Donelle, and Hume-Loveland (2012) conducted a content analysis of messages posted in an online postpartum depression support group over 6 months. The analysis revealed that the online discussion provided emotional, informational, and instrumental support for women who were experiencing postpartum depression. Participants were able to express their feelings, perceived they were understood, and could share their emotional distress.

## Challenges to Social Support Theory Development and Research

Future efforts in social support theory development and research need to move from a description of the relationship of social support and health outcomes to the investigation of interactional characteristics, negative aspects, gender and cultural contexts, causal relationships in social support, and effective social support interventions. In particular, multilevel interventions that address both interpersonal support and community-level environmental support could contribute to knowledge about cost-effective social support strategies for improving the health status of populations.

Because researchers have used a variety of definitions of social support and have measured different aspects of social support, it is difficult to compare study results (Heitzmann & Kaplan, 1988; Roberts, 1984). Hupcey (1998b) commented that many other concepts, such as marital status and frequency of contact, have often been included in definitions of social support. To determine effectiveness of social support, an understanding of the perceptions of the providers of social support as well as those of the recipient merits further exploration (Hupcey, 1998b). The reciprocity of social support is an interactional variable that can contribute to understanding effective social support interventions.

Middle range social support theory development could be enhanced by greater exploration of the negative effects of informal social support. Many social support measures do not include negative aspects of relationships (Al-Dwaikat & Hall, 2017; Krishnasamy, 1996; Stewart, 1993). In a review of 50 studies on social support and caregiver burden, Vrabec (1997) recommended further examination of the amount of conflict in the social support network as a predictor of caregiver burden. The Interpersonal Relationships Inventory (IPRI) is one of the few measures that attempts to encompass the full context of relationships through inclusion of reciprocity and conflict subscales (Tilden, Nelson, & May, 1990).

Al-Dwaikat and Hall (2017) made the following recommendations for guiding selection of social support measures in nursing research, education, and practice: (a) identify aspects of social support for measurement, (b) use the specific aims of the study to determine conceptualization of relationships between social support and outcomes, and (c) complete a critical review of the psychometric properties of each measure specific to the population.

Social support measures also need to be sensitive to the cultural context (Ducharme, Stevens, & Rowat, 1994). Higgins and Dicharry (1991) evaluated the Personal Resources Inventory Part 2 (PRQ) for its applicability to Navajo women. They found that 10 of the 25 items were not applicable to Navajo culture. The 10 items were considered too personal because in the Navajo culture, family problems and feelings are not discussed with others. Different cultural groups may vary in perceptions of the number of persons they consider to be a part of their social network, as well as the relative importance of the different components of social support. Expectations for independence and help may differ. Some types of assistance could be expected and appreciated by one culture and be interpreted as shameful by another culture.

In a study on types of social support in African Americans with cancer, Hamilton and Sandelowski (2004) found that although the broad categories of social support were applicable to the African American sample, strategies for perceived helpful social support differed from Caucasian populations. African Americans perceived presence and distracting activities as emotional support in contrast to verbal expressions of problems. Instrumental support included offers of prayer and other kinds of assistance that were less often identified in other studies of social support.

Martinez-Schallmoser, MacMullen, and Telleen (2005) suggested specific assessment questions that are adapted to the social support needs of the Mexican American pregnant women population. The meaning of social support across cultures needs further exploration. In addition, males are a neglected population in social support research (Langford et al., 1997). Qualitative research approaches could be useful for discovering meanings of social support across cultures.

Causality in social support research needs further exploration. Researchers have conducted many descriptive and correlational studies that link social support to positive health outcomes, but fewer studies substantiate causal links (Callaghan & Morrissey, 1993). The impact of health status on how people seek and receive support has been explored less often than the effects of social support on health status (Stewart, 1993). Changes in health status are likely to influence the amount of and components of social support that are needed. With increased stress resulting from threats to health, social support actions can facilitate positive or problem-focused coping. Moreover, the balance of reciprocity in relationships and the amount of conflict present may change in response to health status changes. One question suggested by Cohen et al. (2001) for future study is whether persons with chronic illness decrease their provision of support, resulting in an imbalance in the social network (reciprocity). The explosion of social media and networking is another important focus for research on social support interventions. A comparison of interventions delivered through different modes of communication (face-to-face, telephone, Internet) on specific types of support would add to understanding how to deliver effective social support interventions.

There are a limited number of controlled intervention studies that evaluate the contribution of social support to health outcomes. Therefore, an important priority is evaluating the effectiveness of social support interventions used in nursing practice. Cohen et al. (2000) summarized lessons gained from a summary of controlled intervention studies on social support outcomes. Social support interventions that were longer in duration appeared to have greater effectiveness in comparison with brief interventions. The authors determined that teaching individuals about using support resources was a worthwhile intervention. In social support research design, it is important to address the interpersonal barriers individuals may experience in maintaining successful relationships and the attitudinal barriers that social support recipients may possess. Authors noted that interventions, which promote support from individuals' natural networks, may not be useful for all populations, such as abusive mothers or individuals facing overwhelming life stress.

## MIDDLE RANGE THEORY APPLICATION: STUDENT PROJECT  9.3

### SUMMARY OF PROJECT

Public health nurses (PHNs) provided school and home visits to teens enrolled in a Pregnant and Parenting Teen Program. A graduate student collaborated with PHNs to explore teen and PHN perspectives on the mentor–mentee relationship. As mentors, PHNs use interactions in their relationships with teens to provide information, support, and affirmation of healthy choices and actions (Schaffer & Mbibi, 2014). The student interviewed 11 teen mothers who participated the program about their experience of being mentored by a PHN. The student collaborated with the nursing program advisor who interviewed seven PHNs that provided home and school visits to the teen mothers.

### USE OF MIDDLE RANGE THEORY

Mentors provide information and affirmation support to the teen mothers. This support promotes a greater level of independence and contributes to success in life roles. Teen mothers must balance the responsibilities of pregnancy and parenting with the tasks of their adolescent developmental stage. The social support provided by PHNs in mentoring relationships with teen mothers facilitates their coping and management of stressors in their lives (Schaffer & Mbibi, 2014).

### PROJECT OUTCOME

The student participated in interview data analysis and presented results of the interviews to PHN staff and their supervisor at a staff meeting. Three of six themes resulting from interviews with teen parents reflected the social support experienced by the teen in the mentoring relationship with the PHN: (a) The PHN is part of their support network, (b) the PHN helps with important decisions, and (c) the PHN helps to build the teen's independence. The teens also talked about the support provided by family members and other helping professionals, such as social workers and teachers. Out of eight themes resulting from the analysis of the PHN interviews, four themes reflected social support: (a) sticking with the teen (emotional support), (b) honoring persons (appraisal support), (c) giving information (informational support), and (d) facilitating decisions (instrumental support).

### RECOMMENDATIONS/CONCLUSIONS

To effectively provide social support in mentoring teen mothers, PHNs need continuing education about mentorship, including an emphasis on cultural influences. Supervision is important because the opportunity for monitoring and debriefing will promote best practices for mentoring teen mothers. PHNs also must manage professional boundaries as they provide mentoring over time to teen mothers. Ethical principles for guiding mentoring relationships (Dancer, 2003) can be used by PHNs to reflect on the quality and safety of the social support they provide in mentoring relationships: (a) Am I keeping my promises? (b) Am I giving choices that are valued by the teen? (c) Am I promoting good for the teen and her child? (d) Am I preventing potential harm? (e) Am I being fair in distributing resources and my time to the teens in my caseload?

To further develop understanding of the linkages of social support to health outcomes, theoretically based social support interventions need to be tested in controlled intervention trials across varied settings and age groups (Ducharme et al., 1994). Cohen et al. (2001) suggested that more intervention research should be conducted on promising interventions, such as support groups and support provided in dyads (partner or peer support). In addition, research on interventions that focus on strengthening the social support environments at a community or systems level can develop knowledge about how to use social support to improve the health status of populations. Multilevel interventions may be the most effective. Rook and Dooley (1985) described two categorical approaches to social support interventions—individual and environmental. Individual interventions are used to change how a person perceives or seeks support, while an environmental approach targets the community to improve the social support climate. Social support is likely to be maximized with the implementation of both approaches. Research methods used to test the effectiveness of social support interventions need to be tailored to the intervention level. Measures for any level should include the potential negative aspects of social support in the person's interactions and environment, which, if not considered, can confound the interpretation of study findings. Evaluation of social support interventions at the individual, dyadic, and group levels is likely to focus on the perceptions of social support actions and available support. Evaluation of social support interventions at the community and systems levels emphasizes analysis of social support available in networks and the environment (Middle Range Theory Application: Student Project 9.3).

## Summary

■ There is a lack of consensus on the definition of social support.

■ There are numerous measures of social support; many are for specific situations.

■ Future theory development should include negative aspects of social support and provision of support at the community and societal levels.

■ Future research on social support should address the effectiveness of social support interventions, including support from social media and networking.

■ Social support theory is important to nurses because it can explain and suggest nursing interventions to improve health outcomes.

## CRITICAL THINKING EXERCISES

1. Compare two options for providing a social support intervention for parents of children diagnosed with a chronic mental illness: (a) a nurse-led monthly face-to-face meeting of parents (with child care provided) and (b) an asynchronous Internet discussion for the parents.

2. Look at the list of definitions of key terms. Use the key terms to analyze the nature of the social support experience that could be expected from each of the two interventions.

3. Analyze how each of the interventions is consistent or inconsistent with Hupcey's definition of social support.

4. Design evaluation studies, using both quantitative and qualitative approaches, to measure the experience of social support and effectiveness of the intervention for each of the two options. Consider the reliability and validity of suggested measurement strategies.

5. Analyze how the following variables may affect the experience of social support in each of the two options: perceptions of the need for and availability of support, timing, motivation for providing support, duration, direction, life stage, sources of social support, and social network.

6. Analyze the potential effectiveness (improved health outcomes and coping) resulting from professional or nurse-provided social support versus enhancement of social support provided by personal relationships and social networks for parents of children with a chronic mental illness.

## REFERENCES

Adams, T. R., Rabin, L. A., Da Silva, V. G., Katz, M. J., Fogel, J., & Lipton, R. B. (2016). Social support buffers the impact of depressive symptoms on life satisfaction in old age. *Clinical Gerontologist*, 39(2), 139–157. doi: 10.1080/07317115.2015.1073823

Albrecht, T., & Adelman, M. (1987). Communication networks as structures of social support. In T. Albrecht & M. Adelman (Eds.), *Communicating social support* (pp. 40–61). Newbury Park, CA: Sage.

Al-Dwaikat, T. N., & Hall, L. A. (2017). Systematic review and critical analysis of measures of social support used in studies of persons with Type 2 Diabetes. *Journal of Nursing Measurement*, 25(2), E74–E107. doi: 10.1891/1061-3749.25.2.E74

Anderson, J. G., Hundt, E., Dean, M., Keim-Malpass, J., & Lopez, R. P. (2017). "The church of online support": Examining the use of blogs among family caregivers of persons with dementia. *Journal of Family Nursing*, 23(1), 34–54. doi: 10.1177/1074840716681289

Astedt-Kurki, P., Tarkka, M., Rikala, M., Lehti, E., & Paavilainen, E. (2009). Further testing of a family nursing instrument (FAFES). *International Journal of Nursing Studies, 46*, 350–359.

Barrera, M. (1981). Social support in the adjustment of pregnant adolescents: Assessment issues. In B. Gottlieb (Ed.), *Social networks and social support* (pp. 69–96). Beverly Hills, CA: Sage.

Barrera, M. Jr. (1986). Distinctions between social support concepts, measures, and models. *American Journal of Community Psychology, 14*(4), 413–445.

Beeber, L. S., & Canuso, R. (2005). Strengthening social support for the low-income mother: Five critical questions and guide for intervention. *Journal of Obstetric, Gynecologic & Neonatal Nursing, 34*(6), 769–776.

Bird-Craven, J., & Massey, A. R. (2013). Lean on me: Effects of social support on low socioeconomic-status pregnant women. *Nursing and Health Sciences, 15*, 374–378.

Bowlby, J. (1971). *Attachment*. London, UK: Pelican.

Brooks, K. P., & Dunkel-Schetter, C. 2011. Social negativity and health: Conceptual and measurement issues. *Social and Personality Psychology Compass, 5*(11), 904–918.

Brown, M. A. (1986). Social support during pregnancy: A unidimensional or multidimensional concept? *Nursing Research, 35*(1), 4–9.

Callaghan, P., & Morrissey, J. (1993). Social support and health: A review. *Journal of Advanced Nursing, 18*, 203–210.

Cassel, J. (1974). Psychosocial process and "stress": Theoretical perspectives. *International Journal of Health Services, 4*(3), 471–482.

Cassel, J. (1976). The contribution of the social environment to host resistance. *American Journal of Epidemiology, 104*(2), 107–123.

Chien, W., & Norman, I. (2009). The effectiveness and active ingredients of mutual support groups for family caregivers of people with psychotic disorders: A literature review. *International Journal of Nursing Studies, 46*, 1604–1623.

Chou, F., Avant, K. C., Kuo, S., & Fetzer, S. J. (2008). Relationships between nausea and vomiting, perceived stress, social support, pregnancy planning, and psychosocial adaptation in a sample of mothers: A questionnaire survey. *International Journal of Nursing Studies, 45*, 1185–1191.

Clark, J. S. (1983). Reactions to aid in communal and exchange relationships. In J. D. Fisher, D. Nadler, & B. M. DePaulo (Eds.), *New directions in helping: Vol 1. Recipient reactions to aid* (pp. 281–305). New York, NY: Academic Press.

Cobb, S. (1976). Social support as a moderator of life stress. *Psychosomatic Medicine, 38*, 300–314.

Cohen, S. (1992). Stress, social support, and disorder. In H. O. Veiel & U. Baumann (Eds.), *The meaning and measurement of social support* (pp. 109–204). New York, NY: Hemisphere Publishing Corporation.

Cohen, S., Gottlieb, B. H., & Underwood, L. G. (2001). Social relationships and health: Challenges for measurement and intervention. *Advances in Mind–Body Medicine, 17*, 129–141.

Cohen, S., Mermelstein, R., Kmarack, T., & Hoberman, H. M. (1985). Measuring the functional components of social support. In I. G. Sarason & B. R. Sarason (Eds.), *Social support: Theory, research and applications*. Boston, MA: Martinus Nijhoff Publishers.

Cohen, S., & Syme, S. L. (1985). Issues in the study and application of social support (pp. 73–94). In S. Cohen & S. L. Syme (Eds.), *Social support and health* (pp. 3–32). New York, NY: Academic Press.

Cohen, S., Underwood, L. G., & Gottlieb, B. H. (Eds.). (2000). *Social support measurement and intervention a guide for health and social scientists*. New York, NY: Oxford University Press.

Cousins, S. O. (1996). Exercise cognition among elderly women. *Journal of Applied Sport Psychology, 8*, 131–145.

Coyne, J. C., & DeLongis, A. (1986). Going beyond social support: The role of social relationships in adaptation. *Journal of Consulting and Clinical Psychology, 54*, 454–460.

Cullum, K. G. H., & Mayo, A. M. (2015). A review of the child and adolescent social support scale for healthy behaviors. *Clinical Nurse Specialist, 29*(4), 198–202. doi: 10.1097/NUR.0000000000000142

Cutrona, C. E. (1990). Stress and social support: In search of optimal matching. *Journal of Social and Clinical Psychology, 9*(1), 3–14.

Dakof, G., & Taylor, S. (1990). Victim's perception of social support: What is helpful from whom? *Journal of Personality and Social Psychology, 58*(1), 80–89.

Dancer, J. M. (2003). Mentoring in healthcare: Theory in search of practice? *Clinician in Management, 12*, 21–31.

Dennis, C. (2010). Postpartum depression peer support: Maternal perceptions from a randomized controlled trial. *International Journal of Nursing Studies, 47*, 560–568. doi: 10.1016/j.ijnurstu.2009.10.015

Diamond, M. (1985). A review and critique of the concepts of social support. In R. A. O'Brien (Ed.), *Social support and health: New directions for theory and research* (pp. 1–32). Rochester, NY: University of Rochester Press.

Drageset, J., Eide, G. E., Nygard, H. A., Bondevik, M., Nortvedt, M. W., & Natvig, G. K. (2009). The impact of social support and sense of coherence on health-related quality of life among nursing home residents—A questionnaire survey in Bergen, Norway. *International Journal of Nursing Studies, 46*, 66–76.

Ducharme, F., Stevens, B., & Rowat, K. (1994). Social support: Conceptual and methodological issues for research in mental health nursing. *Issues in Mental Health Nursing, 15*, 373–392.

Dunkel-Schetter, C. (1984). Social support and cancer: Findings based on patient interviews and their implications. *Journal of Social Issues, 40*(4), 77–98.

Dunkel-Schetter, C., & Bennett, T. L. (1990). Differentiating the cognitive and behavioral aspects of social support. In B. R. Sarason, I. G. Sarason, & G. R. Pierce (Eds.), *Social support: An interactional view* (pp. 267–296). New York, NY: Wiley.

Dunkel-Schetter, C., Blasband, D., Feinstein, L., & Herbert, T. (1992). Elements of supportive interactions. When are attempts to help effective? In S. Spacapan & S. Oskamp (Eds.), *Helping and being helped* (pp. 83–114). New York, NY: Academic Press.

Dunkel-Schetter, C., & Skokan, L. A. (1990). Determinants of social support provision in personal relationships. *Journal of Social and Personal Relationships, 7*(4), 437–450.

Eriksson, H., & Salzmann-Erikson, M. (2013). Supporting a caring fatherhood in cyberspace—An analysis of communication about caring within an online forum for fathers. *Scandinavian Journal of Caring Sciences, 27*, 63–69. doi: 10.1111/j.1471- 6712.2012.01001.x

Evans, M., Donelle, L., & Hume-Loveland, L. (2012). Social support and online postpartum depression discussion groups: A content analysis. *Patient Education and Counseling, 87*, 405–410.

Finfgeld-Connett, D. (2005). Telephone social support or nursing presence? Analysis of a nursing intervention. *Qualitative Health Research, 15*(1), 19–29.

Fleury, J., Keller, C., & Perez, A. (2009). Social support theoretical perspective. *Geriatric Nursing, 30*(2S), 11–14.

Flynn, M., & Stan, A. (2012). Social support in a men's online eating disorder forum. *International Journal of Men's Health, 11*(2), 150–169. doi: 10.3149/jmh.1102.150

Friedman, M. M. (1997). Social support sources among older women with heart failure: Continuity versus loss over time. *Research in Nursing and Health, 20*, 319–327.

Froland, C., Pancoast, D., Chapman, D., & Kimboko, P. (1981). *Helping networks and human services*. Beverly Hills, CA: Sage.

La Gaipa, J. J. (1990). The negative effects of informal support systems. In S. Duck (Ed.), *Personal relationships and social support* (pp. 122–139). London, UK: Sage.

Grassley, S., Spencer, B. S., & Bryson, D. (2013). The development and psychometric testing of the Support Needs of Adolescents Breastfeeding Scale. *Journal of Advanced Nursing, 69*(3), 708–716. doi: 10.1111/j.1365-2648.2012.06119.x

Graven, L. J., & Grant, J. (2013). The impact of social support on depressive symptoms in individuals with heart failure. *Journal of Cardiovascular Nursing, 28*(5), 429–443. doi: 10.1097/JCN.0b013e3182578b9d

Griffith, J. (1985). Social support providers: Who are they? Where are they met? And the relationships of network characteristics to psychological distress. *Basic and Applied Social Psychology, 6*(1), 41–60.

Hamilton, J. B., & Sandelowski, M. (2004). Types of social support in African Americans with cancer. *Oncology Nursing Forum, 31*(4), 792–800.

Hammer, M. (1981). "Core" and "extended" social networks in relation to health and illness. *Social Science and Medicine, 17*, 405–411.

Heitzmann, C. A., & Kaplan, R. M. (1988). Assessment of methods for measuring social support. *Health Psychology, 7*(1), 75–109.

Heller, K., Swindle, R. W., & Dusenbury, L. (1986). Component social support processes: Comments and integration. *Journal of Consulting and Clinical Psychology, 54*(4), 466–470.

Higgins, P. G., & Dicharry, E. K. (1991). Measurement issues addressing social support with Navajo women. *Western Journal of Nursing Research, 13*(2), 242–255.

Hilbert, G. A. (1990). Measuring social support in chronic illness. In O. L. Strickland & C. F. Waltz (Eds.), *Measurement of nursing outcomes* (Vol. 4, pp. 79–95). New York, NY: Springer Publishing Company.

Holden, L., Lee, C., Hockey, R., Ware, R. S., & Dobson, A. J. (2014). Validation of the MOS Social Support Survey—6 item (MOS-SSS-6) measure with two large population-based samples of Australian women. *Quality of Life Research, 23*, 2849–28530. doi: 10.1007/s11136-014-07541-5

Holtslander, L., Kornder, N., Letourneau, N., Turner, H., & Paterson, B. (2012). Finding straight answers: Identifying the needs of parents and service providers of adolescents with type 1 diabetes to aid in the creation of an online support intervention. *Journal of Clinical Nursing, 21*, 2419–2428. doi: 10.1111/j.1365-2702.2012.04182.x

Hopkins, J., & Campbell, S. B. (2008). Development and validation of a scale to assess social support in the postpartum period. *Archives of Women's Mental Health, 11*, 57–65. doi: 10.1007/s00737-008-0212-5

House, J. S. (1981). *Work stress and social support*. Englewood Cliffs, NJ: Prentice Hall.

Hudson, D. B., Campbell-Grossman, C., Keating-Lefler, R., & Cline, P. (2008). New mothers network: The development of internet-based social support intervention for African American mothers. *Issues in Comprehensive Pediatric Nursing, 31*, 23–25.

Hupcey, J. E. (1998a). Clarifying the social support theory–research linkage. *Journal of Advanced Nursing, 27*(6), 1231–1241.

Hupcey, J. E. (1998b). Social support: Assessing conceptual coherence. *Qualitative Health Research, 8*(3), 304–318.

Hupcey, J. E., & Morse, J. M. (1997). Can a professional relationship be considered social support? *Nursing Outlook, 45*, 270–276.

Hwang, K. O., Ottenbacher, A. J., Green, A. P., et al. (2010). Social support in an Internet weight loss community. *International Journal of Medical Informatics, 79*, 5–13. doi: 10.1016/j.ijmedinf.2009.10.003

Iannino-Renz, R. (2016). The role of social support in persons with type 2 diabetic wounds. *MEDSURG Nursing, 25*(5), 357–359.

Jacobson, D. E. (1986). Types and timing of social support. *Journal of Health and Social Behavior, 27*, 250–264.

Jang, E., & Canada, K. E. (2014). New directions for the study of incarcerated older adults: Using social capital theory. *Journal of Gerontological Social Work, 57*, 858–871. doi: 10.1080/01634372.2014.900841

Jung, J. (1988). Social support providers: Why do they help? *Basic and Applied Social Psychology, 9*, 231–240.

Kahn, R. L. (1979). Aging and social support. In M. W. Riley (Ed.), *Aging from birth to death: Interdisciplinary perspectives* (pp. 77–91). Boulder, CO: Westview Press.

Kahn, R. L., & Antonucci, T. C. (1980). Convoys over the life course: Attachment, roles, and social support. In P. B. Baltes & G. Brim (Eds.), *Life span development and behavior* (Vol. 3, pp. 253–283). New York, NY: Academic Press.

Kaunonen, M., Tarkka, M., Paunonen, M., & Laippala, P. (1999). Grief and social support after the death of a spouse. *Journal of Advanced Nursing, 30*(6), 1304–1311.

Keller, C., Allan, J., & Tinkle, M. B. (2006). Stages of change, processes of change, and social support for exercise and weight gain in postpartum women. *Journal of Obstetric, Gynecologic & Neonatal Nursing, 35*(2), 232–240.

Krishnasamy, M. (1996). Social support and the patient with cancer: A consideration of the literature. *Journal of Advanced Nursing, 23*(4), 757–762.

Lackner, S., Goldenberg, S., Arrizza, G., & Tjosvold, I. (1994). The contingency of social support. *Qualitative Health Research, 4*(2), 224–243.

Laireiter, A., & Baumann, U. (1992). Network structures and support functions theoretical and empirical analyses. In H. O. Veiel & U. Baumann (Eds.), *The meaning and measurement of social support* (pp. 33–55). London, UK: Hemisphere Publishing Corporation.

Langford, C. P. H., Bowsher, J., Maloney, J. P., & Lillis, P. (1997). Social support: A conceptual analysis. *Journal of Advanced Nursing, 25*(1), 95–100.

Latham, C. L., & Calvillo, E. (2009). Predictors of successful diabetes management in low-income Hispanic people. *Western Journal of Nursing Research, 313*, 364–387.

Li, Y., Long, Z., Cao, D., & Cao, F. (2017). Social support and depression across the perinatal period: A longitudinal study. *Journal of Clinical Nursing, 26*, 2776–2783. doi: 10.1111/jocn.13817

Logsdon, M. C., & Koniak-Griffin, D. (2005). Social support in postpartum adolescents: Guidelines for nursing assessments and interventions. *Journal of Obstetric, Gynecologic, and Neonatal Nursing, 34*(6), 761–768.

Logsdon, M. C., Usui, W., Birkimer, J. C., & McBride, A. B. (1996). The postpartum support questionnaire: Reliability and validity. *Journal of Nursing Measurement, 4*(2), 129–142.

Lugton, J. (1997). The nature of social support as experienced by women treated for breast cancer. *Journal of Advanced Nursing, 25*(6), 1184–1191.

Manning-Walsh, J. (2005). Social support as a mediator between symptom distress and quality of life in women with breast cancer. *Journal of Obstetric, Gynecologic, and Neonatal Nursing, 34*(4), 482–493.

Martinez-Schallmoser, L., MacMullen, N. J., & Telleen, S. (2005). Social support in Mexican American childbearing women. *Journal of Obstetric, Gynecologic, and Neonatal Nursing, 34*(6), 755–760.

Matsui, M., & Capezuti, E. (2008). Perceived autonomy and self-care resources among senior center users. *Geriatric Nursing, 29*(2), 141–147.

Merkel, R. M., & Wright, T. (2012). Parental self-efficacy and online support among parents of children diagnosed with type 1 diabetes mellitus. *Pediatric Nursing, 38*(6), 303–308.

Newsom, J. T., Bookwala, J., & Schulz, R. (1997). Social support measurement in group residences for older adults. *Journal of Mental Health and Aging, 3*(1), 47–66.

Norbeck, J. S. (1981). Social support: A model for clinical research and application. *Advances in Nursing Science, 3*(4), 43–59.

Norbeck, J. S. (1988). Social support. *Annual Review of Nursing Research, 6,* 85–109.

Norbeck, J. S., & Tilden, V. P. (1988). International research in social support: Theoretical and methodological issues. *Journal of Advanced Nursing, 13,* 173–178.

Norbeck, J. S., Lindsey, A. M., & Carrieri, V. L. (1981). The development of an instrument to measure social support. *Nursing Research, 30*(5), 264–269.

Norbeck, J. S., Lindsey, A. M., & Carrieri, V. L. (1983). Further development of the Norbeck social support questionnaire: Normative data and validity testing. *Nursing Research, 32*(1), 4–9.

Northouse, L. (1988). Social support in patients' and husbands' adjustment to breast cancer. *Nursing Research, 37,* 91–95.

Norwood, S. L. (1996). The social support Apgar: Instrument development and testing. *Research in Nursing and Health, 19,* 143–152.

Odafe, M. O., Salami, T. K., & Walker, R. L. (2017). Race-related stress and hopelessness in community-based African American adults: Moderating role of social support. *Cultural Diversity and Ethnic Minority Psychology, 23*(4), 561–569. doi: 10.1037/cdp0000167

Olds, D. L., Kitzman, H., Hanks, C., Cole, R., Anson, E., Sidora-Arccoleo, K., .... Bondy, J. (2007). Effects of nurse home visiting on maternal and child functioning: Age-9 follow-up of a randomized trial. *Pediatrics, 120*(4), 832–845.

Owen, A. E. (2003). *Evaluation of differences in depression, defensiveness, social support, and coping between acute and chronic CHD patients hospitalized for myocardial infarction and unstable angina* (Unpublished doctoral dissertation). Department of Philosophy College of Arts and Sciences University, South Florida.

Patterson, B., Brewer, J., & Stamler, L. L. (2013). Engagement of parents in on-line social support interventions. *Journal of Pediatric Nursing, 28,* 114–124. doi: 10.1016/j.pedn.2012.05.001

Pearlman, D. N., & Crown, W. H. (1992). Alternative sources of social support and their impacts on institutional risk. *Gerontologist, 32,* 527–535.

Pector, E. A. (2012). Sharing losses online: Do internet support groups benefit the bereaved? *International Journal of Childbirth Education, 27*(2), 19–25.

Pierce, G. R., Sarason, B. R., & Sarason, I. G. (1990). Integrating social support perspectives: Working models, personal relationships, and situational factors. In S. Duck (Ed.), *Personal relationships and social support* (pp. 173–189). London, UK: Sage.

Pilisuk, M. (1982). Delivery of social support: The social inoculation. *American Journal of Orthopsychiatry, 52,* 20–31.

Revenson, T., Schiaffino, K., Majerovitz, S., & Gibofsky, A. (1991). Social support as a double-edged sword: The relation of positive and problematic support to depression among rheumatoid arthritis patients. *Social Science and Medicine, 33*(7), 807–813.

Roberts, S. J. (1984). Social support—Meaning, measurement, and relevance to community health nursing practice. *Public Health Nursing, 1*(3), 158–167.

Rook, K. S. (2014). The health effects of negative social exchanges in later life. *Generations: Journal of the American Society on Aging, 38*(1), 15–23.

Rook, K. S., & Dooley, D. (1985). Applying social support research: Theoretical problems and future directions. *Journal of Social Issues, 41*(1), 5–28.

Sallis, J. F., Grossman, R. M., Pinski, R. B., Patterson, T. L., & Nader, P. R. (1987). The development of scales to measure social support for diet and exercise behaviors. *Preventive Medicine, 16,* 825–836.

Sarason, B. R., Sarason, I. G., & Pierce, G. R. (1990). *Social support: An interactional view.* New York, NY: John Wiley.

Schaffer, M. A., & Lia-Hoagberg, B. (1997). Effects of social support on prenatal care and health behaviors of low-income women. *Journal of Obstetric, Gynecologic, and Neonatal Nursing, 26*(4), 433–440.

Schaffer, M. A., & Mbibi, N. (2014). Public health nurse mentorship of pregnant and parenting adolescents. *Public Health Nursing, 31*(5), 428–437. doi: 10.1111/phn.12109

Scharer, K. (2005). Internet social support for parents: The state of the science. *Journal of Child and Adolescent Psychiatric Nursing, 18*(1), 26–35.

Sherbourne, C. S., & Stewart, A. L. (1991). The MOS Social Support Survey. *Social Science and Medicine, 31*(6), 705–714.

Stewart, M. J. (1989a). Social support instruments created by nurse investigators. *Nursing Research, 38*(5), 268–275.

Stewart, M. J. (1989b). Social support intervention studies: A review and prospectus of nursing contributions. *International Journal of Nursing Studies, 26*(2), 93–114.

Stewart, M. J. (1993). *Integrating social support in nursing.* Newbury Park, CA: Sage.

Tardy, C. H. (1985). Social support measurement. *American Journal of Community Psychology, 13*(2), 187–202.

Thoits, P. A. (1983). Multiple identities and psychosocial well-being: A reformation and test of the social isolation hypothesis. *American Sociological Review, 48,* 174–187.

Thoits, P. A. (1986). Social support as coping assistance. *Journal of Consulting and Clinical Psychology, 54*(4), 416–423.

Tilburgs, B., Nijkamp, M. D., Bakker, E. & van der Hoeven, H. (2015). The influence of social support on patients' quality of life after an intensive care unit discharge: A cross-sectional survey. *Intensive and Critical Care Nursing, 37*(1), 336–342. doi: 10.1016/j.iccn.2015.07.002

Tilden, V. P. (1985). Issues of conceptualization and measurement of social support in construction of nursing theory. *Research in Nursing and Health, 81,* 199–206.

Tilden, V. P. (1986). New perspectives on social support. *The Nurse Practitioner, 11,* 60–61.

Tilden, V. P., & Galyen, R. D. (1987). Cost and conflict: The darker side of social support. *Western Journal of Nursing Research, 9*(1), 9–18.

Tilden, V. P., Nelson, C. A., & May, B. A. (1990). The IPR inventory: Development and psychometric characteristics. *Nursing Research, 39*(6), 337–343.

Tilden, V. P., & Weinert, S. C. (1987). Social support and the chronically ill individual. *Nursing Clinics of North America, 22*(3), 613–620.

Vandall-Walker, V., Jensen, L., & Oberle, K. (2007). Nursing support for family members of critically ill adults. *Qualitative Health Research, 17,* 1207–1218.

Vaux, A. (1988). *Social support—Theory, research, and intervention.* New York, NY: Praeger.

Veiel, H. O., & Baumann, U. (1992). The many meanings of social support. In H. O. Veiel & U. Baumann (Eds.), *The meaning and measurement of social support* (pp. 1–9). New York, NY: Hemisphere.

Vrabec, N. J. (1997). Literature review of social support and caregiver burden, 1980 to 1985. *Image: The Journal of Nursing Scholarship, 29*(4), 383–388.

Waterworth, P., Rosenberg, M., Braham, R., Pescud, M., & Dimmock, J. (2014). The effect of social support on the health of Indigenous Australians in a metropolitan community. *Social Science & Medicine, 119*, 139–146. doi: 10.1016/j.socscimed.2014.08.0350277-9536

Weinert, C. (1987). A social support measure: PRQ85. *Nursing Research, 36*(5), 273–277.

Weinert, C. (1988). Measuring social support: Revision and further development of the personal resource questionnaire. In O. L. Strickland & C. F. Waltz (Eds.), *Measurement of nursing outcomes* (Vol. 1, pp. 309–327). New York, NY: Springer Publishing Company.

Wortman, C. B. (1984). Social support and the cancer patient: Conceptual and methodologic issues. *Cancer, 53*(10), 2339–2362.

Wright, K. B., & Bell, S. B. (2003). Health-related support groups on the Internet: Linking empirical findings to social support and computer-mediated communication theory. *Journal of Health Psychology, 8*(1), 39–54.

Wright, N., & Stickely, T. (2013). Concepts of social inclusion, exclusion, and mental health: A review of the international literature. *Journal of Psychiatric and Mental Health Nursing, 20*, 71–81. doi: 10.111/j.1365-2850.2012.01889.x

Yang, Y. C., Schorpp, K., & Harris, K. M. (2014). Social support, social strain and inflammation: Evidence from a national longitudinal study of U.S. adults. *Social Science & Medicine, 107*, 124–135.

Yli-Uotila, T., Kaunonen, M., Pylkkanen, L., & Suominen, T. (2016). Facilitators and barriers for electronic social support. *Scandinavian Journal of Caring Sciences, 30*, 547–556. doi: 10.1111/scs.12277

Zimet, G. D., Dahlem, N. W., Zimet, S. G., & Farley, G. K. (1988). The multidimensional scale of perceived social support. *Journal of Personality Assessment, 52*, 30–41.

# 10 Caring

Danuta M. Wojnar

## Definition of Key Terms

| | |
|---|---|
| **Being with** | Being emotionally present to the other by conveying ongoing availability, sharing feelings, and monitoring that the one providing care does not burden the one cared for. (p. 163) |
| **Caring** | A nurturing way of relating to a valued other toward whom one feels a personal sense of commitment and responsibility. (Swanson, 1991, p. 165) |
| **Doing for** | Doing for the other what he or she would do for the self if it were at all possible. Doing for the other means providing care that is comforting, protective, and anticipatory, as well as performing duties skillfully and competently while preserving the person's dignity. (p. 164) |
| **Enabling** | Facilitating the other's passage through life transitions and unfamiliar events by informing, explaining, supporting, focusing on relevant concerns, thinking through issues, and generating alternatives. Enabling promotes the client's personal healing, growth, and self-care. (p. 164) |
| **Knowing** | Striving to understand an event as it has meaning in the life of the other. Knowing involves avoiding assumptions about the meaning of an event to the one cared for, centering on the other's needs, conducting in-depth assessment, seeking verbal and nonverbal cues, and engaging the self of both. (p. 163) |
| **Maintaining belief** | Sustaining faith in the other's capacity to get through an event or transition and face a future with meaning. The goal is to enable the other so that within the constraints of his or her life they are able to find meaning and maintain a hope-filled attitude. (p. 165) |

Nursing, like other health professions, is based on the ideal of service to humanity. At the core of nursing values lies the ideal of altruistic caring that is guided by theory, research, and a code of ethics. Nursing is focused on creating caring–healing environments that assist individuals, families, and communities to attain or maintain a state of optimal wellness in their life experiences from birth, through adulthood, until the end of life (Swanson & Wojnar, 2004). Most individuals choose nursing as a profession because of their desire to care for others. With advances in nursing science, there has been an escalating interest in the concept of caring in nursing. Over the past few decades, philosophical debates, research, and theory development have ensued to define the concept of caring, articulate caring behaviors, and identify outcomes of caring for patients, families, nurses, organizations, and society. Also of deep concern is detecting and eliminating barriers to caring in clinical practice. Among several prominent frameworks, Swanson's

middle range theory of caring has achieved popularity among practitioners because of its simplicity, elegance, relevance, and ease of application in education, research, and clinical practice.

## Historical Background

Nursing has a long legacy as a caring–healing profession. In the 19th century, Florence Nightingale, the matriarch of modern-day nursing, expressed a belief that caring for the sick is based on the understanding of persons and environment. She saw the uniqueness of nursing in creating optimal environments for restoring the health of individuals, a vision that has now been in operation for over 100 years (Chinn & Kramer, 2004). Nurse theorists, such as Benner (1984), Benner and Wrubel (1989), Boykin (1994), Leininger (1981, 1988), Swanson (1991, 1993, 1998, 1999a,b,c), Swanson-Kauffman (1985, 1986, 1988a,b), Swanson-Kauffman and

Roberts (1990), and Watson (1979, 1988, 1999), have reaffirmed the importance of caring for the profession through philosophical debates, theory development, and groundbreaking research. These scholars have led the profession in reminding nurses that caring is essential for delivery of sound nursing care.

## Theory Development

Swanson's interest in the caring science has been a rapid process. As a novice nurse, she was drawn to working in clinical sites that had a clearly articulated vision for professional nursing practice and actively supported primary care nursing (Swanson, 2001). During the theorist's doctoral studies at the University of Colorado, the concept of caring went to the forefront of her professional and scholarly activities, and from that point on, caring and miscarriage have become the foci of her scholarship. For her doctoral dissertation, Swanson set out to conduct descriptive phenomenological investigation of 20 women who had recently miscarried and to identify what types of caring behaviors they considered most helpful (Swanson, 1991). Inductive data analysis led Swanson to the development of a Caring Model with five distinct caring processes: *knowing, being with, doing for, enabling,* and *maintaining belief* (Swanson, 1991, 1993; Swanson-Kauffman, 1985, 1986, 1988a). These caring processes provided foundation for the development of Swanson's middle range theory of caring.

In a subsequent investigation, Swanson focused on exploring caring from the perspective of 19 professional caregivers and seven parents of infants hospitalized in the Neonatal Intensive Care Unit (NICU) (Swanson, 1990). She discovered that the caring processes she had identified through her dissertation research were also applicable to parents and professionals who were responsible for taking care of babies in the NICU. Swanson was not only able to retain and refine the definitions describing the acts of caring but was also able to propose that clinical care in a complex environment requires balance of caring for self and others, attaching to others as well as one's role, managing responsibilities, and avoiding bad outcomes for self, others, and society (Swanson, 1990). The next phase in development of Swanson's caring theory was the "Caring and the Clinical Nursing Models Project" in which Swanson explored how a group of young mothers who received a long-term public health nursing intervention recalled and described nurse caring (NC) (Swanson-Kauffman, 1988b). Based on the findings of this study, Swanson defined caring as a concept and refined the definitions of caring processes (Swanson, 1993).

Subsequently, Swanson's scholarship has shifted to conducting a meta-analysis of data-based publications about caring (Swanson, 1999a) and instrument development. Swanson established psychometric properties of several instruments to measure caring, including Caring Other Scale (Table 10.1) and Caring Professional Scale (Table 10.2). Among other measures, she used

| Table 10.1 | Caring Mate/Caring Other Scale | | | | | |
|---|---|---|---|---|---|---|
| | **As of Late, to What Extent Does Your Mate:** | **Not at All** | **Occasionally** | **About Half the Time** | **Often** | **All of the Time** |
| 1. | Strive to understand what miscarriage means to you? | 1 | 2 | 3 | 4 | 5 |
| 2. | Share in your feelings about miscarriage? | 1 | 2 | 3 | 4 | 5 |
| 3. | Do extra things to help you out? | 1 | 2 | 3 | 4 | 5 |
| 4. | Just be with you? | 1 | 2 | 3 | 4 | 5 |
| 5. | Provide you with opportunities to discuss the miscarriage if you want to or need to? | 1 | 2 | 3 | 4 | 5 |
| 6. | Keep you informed about how she is feeling about the miscarriage? | 1 | 2 | 3 | 4 | 5 |
| 7. | Support you emotionally? | 1 | 2 | 3 | 4 | 5 |
| 8. | Believe in you and your ability to get through tough times? | 1 | 2 | 3 | 4 | 5 |
| 9. | Maintain hope that your plans to have children will all work out as you desire? | 1 | 2 | 3 | 4 | 5 |
| 10. | Do little things to show she cares? | 1 | 2 | 3 | 4 | 5 |

Swanson, K. M. (1999a). Research-based practice with women who have had miscarriages. *Image: The Journal of Nursing Scholarship, 31*(4), 339–345; Swanson, K. M. (2000). Predicting depressive symptoms after miscarriage: A path analysis based on Lazarus' paradigm. *Journal of Women's Health & Gender-based Medicine, 9*(2), 191–206.

**Table 10.2    Caring Professional Scale**

| Was the Nurse, Provider, etc., You Just Met With: | Yes Definitely | Mostly | About Half and Half | Occasionally | No, Not at All | Not Applicable |
|---|---|---|---|---|---|---|
| Comforting? | 1 | 2 | 3 | 4 | 5 | N/A |
| Positive? | 1 | 2 | 3 | 4 | 5 | N/A |
| Informative? | 1 | 2 | 3 | 4 | 5 | N/A |
| Clinically competent? | 1 | 2 | 3 | 4 | 5 | N/A |
| Understanding? | 1 | 2 | 3 | 4 | 5 | N/A |
| Personal? | 1 | 2 | 3 | 4 | 5 | N/A |
| Caring? | 1 | 2 | 3 | 4 | 5 | N/A |
| Supportive? | 1 | 2 | 3 | 4 | 5 | N/A |
| An attentive listener? | 1 | 2 | 3 | 4 | 5 | N/A |
| Centered on you? | 1 | 2 | 3 | 4 | 5 | N/A |
| Technically skilled? | 1 | 2 | 3 | 4 | 5 | N/A |
| Aware of your feelings? | 1 | 2 | 3 | 4 | 5 | N/A |
| Visibly touched by your experience? | 1 | 2 | 3 | 4 | 5 | N/A |
| Able to offer you hope? | 1 | 2 | 3 | 4 | 5 | N/A |
| Respectful of you? | 1 | 2 | 3 | 4 | 5 | N/A |

I. About the nurse, physician, provider, etc.

**Directions:** It is very important that you give us honest feedback on your experience. When you are done, your evaluation will be placed in a sealed envelope and will not be seen by your nurse, provider, etc.

Please answer the questions about the nurse, provider, etc. you just met with.

the above instruments to determine the impact of support after miscarriage on women (Swanson, 1999b,c, 2000; Swanson, Connor, Jolley, Pentinato, & Wang, 2007; Swanson, Karmali, Powell, & Pulvermakher, 2003) and couples (Huffman, Schwartz, & Swanson, 2015; Swanson, Chen, Graham, Wojnar, & Petras, 2009). Most recently, Jansson and colleagues (2017) provided validation of the revised Impact of Miscarriage Scale for Swedish conditions and compared the experiences of Swedish and American couples after miscarriage, while Wojnar, Swanson, and Adolfsson (2011) developed a conceptual model of miscarriage based on international datasets from heterosexual and lesbian couples who miscarried.

## Definitions of Theory Concepts

In 1993, Swanson refined her theory by making explicit her beliefs about the four phenomena of concern to the discipline of nursing: nursing, person/client, health, and environment. The concept of caring, central to the theory, as well as caring processes (knowing, being with, doing for, enabling, and maintaining belief) are clearly defined and arranged in a logical sequence (see the structure

of caring, Figure 10.1, which depicts how caring is delivered). Swanson also made explicit her beliefs about what it means for nurses to practice in a caring manner to promote health and healing of others. Chinn and Kramer (2004) and Meleis (1997) maintain that the simplicity and clarity of a theory refer to a theory with a minimal number of concepts. Simplicity and clarity of language used to define the concepts allow practitioners to understand and apply Swanson's theory in practice.

### NURSING

Swanson (1991, 1993) defines nursing as informed caring for the well-being of others. She posits that the discipline is informed by scientific knowledge from nursing and related fields and by knowledge derived from the humanities, clinical practice, and cultural values and beliefs (Swanson, 1993).

### PERSON

Persons are defined as "unique beings who are in the midst of becoming and whose wholeness is made manifest in thoughts, feelings, and behaviors" (Swanson, 1993, p. 352). Swanson asserts that life experiences of each individual are influenced

**The Structure of Caring**

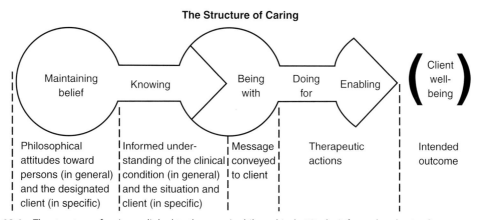

Figure 10.1    The structure of caring as linked to the nurse's philosophical attitude, informed understandings, message conveyed, therapeutic actions, and intended outcome. (Reprinted with permission from Swanson, K. M. (1993). Nursing as informed caring for the well-being of others. *Image: The Journal of Nursing Scholarship, 25*(4), 352–357.)

by a complex interplay of genetics, spiritual endowment, and the person's capacity to exercise free will. Therefore, persons both shape and are shaped by the environment in which they live.

Persons are viewed as dynamic, growing, self-reflecting, yearning to be connected with others, and spiritual beings. Swanson posits that spiritual endowment connects each human being to an eternal and universal source of goodness, mystery, life, creativity, and serenity. The spiritual endowment may be a soul, higher power/Holy Spirit, positive energy, or, simply, grace; free will equates with choice and the capacity to decide how to act when confronted with a range of possibilities (p. 352). Yet, she also maintains that limitations set by race, class, gender, sociopolitical system, or access to care might prevent individuals from exercising free will. Hence, acknowledging free will mandates nursing discipline to honor individuality and consideration of a whole range of possibilities that might be acceptable or desirable to the patients, families, and communities for whom nurses care.

According to Swanson, the "other," whose personhood nursing discipline serves, refers to individuals, families, groups, and societies. With this understanding of personhood, nurses are mandated to take on leadership roles in advocating for human rights, equal access to health care, and other humanitarian causes. Lastly, when nurses think about the "other" to whom they direct their caring, they also need to think of self, other, nurses, and the practice of nursing as the designated "other/recipient" of their caring.

## HEALTH

According to Swanson (1993), to experience health and well-being is to have a subjective, meaning-filled

experience of wholeness that involves a sense of integration and becoming wherein all levels of being are free to be expressed including human spirituality, thoughts, feelings, intelligence, creativity, relatedness, femininity, masculinity, and sexuality, to name just a few. Therefore, reestablishing wholeness involves a complex process of curing and healing at the physical, mental, psychosocial, and spiritual levels.

## ENVIRONMENT

Swanson (1993) defines environment as situational rather than physical and views environment as any situation that influences or is influenced by the designated client. Environment is ever changing at the cultural, social, biophysical, political, and economic realms, and by any context that influences or is influenced by the designated client. She believes that in nursing, the terms "environment" and "person/client" can be viewed interchangeably, since the environment may be specified to the intraindividual level of a specified client. The "client" may be at the cellular level and the "environment" may be the tissues or body of which the cell is a component. The client may be an entire community and its environment, including cultural, social, and political aspects (p. 353). Therefore, when Swanson's theory is used in research or clinical practice, one must remember that what is considered an environment in one situation may be considered a client in another.

## CARING

Swanson believes that Nurse Caring (NC) is grounded in a belief in people and their capacities. Therefore, caring is defined as a nurturing way of relating to a valued other toward whom one feels a personal sense of commitment and responsibility. Swanson maintains that caring involves five processes: (a) knowing, (b) being with, (c) doing for, (d) enabling, and (e) maintaining belief. For detailed definition of the caring processes, refer to the beginning of the chapter, Definitions of Key Concepts section.

## Description of the Theory of Caring

### PHILOSOPHICAL FOUNDATION

Swanson has drawn on various philosophical and theoretical sources while developing her theory of caring. In the chapter "The Program of Research on Caring," Swanson (2001) recalled that early on in her career, knowledge obtained from formal nursing education and clinical practice made her acutely aware of the centrality of caring to preserving human dignity and promoting healing. Swanson also acknowledged several nurse scholars for influencing her beliefs about nursing and caring. She credits Dr. Jacqueline Fawcett for helping her understand the unique role of nursing in caring for others and importance of altruistic caring for the persons' well-being. Swanson also acknowledges Dr. Jean Watson for encouraging her to inductively study caring. While Drs. Swanson and Watson sustain a deep friendship and respect for each other's scholarship, they both view their scholarship as complementary. Yet, both scholars see their theories of caring and their programs of research on caring as unique and the congruency of their findings as adding credibility to their individual work (Swanson, 2001). Lastly, Swanson credits Dr. Kathryn M. Barnard for encouraging her to test and apply her theory of caring through randomized clinical trials.

Swanson's theory was developed empirically, using inductive methodology. According to Chinn and Kramer (2004), inductive reasoning involves inducing of hypotheses and relationships by observing or living through phenomena before reaching definite conclusions. Swanson's theory of caring was inductively developed through descriptive phenomenological inquiry with women who had miscarried (Swanson-Kauffman, 1985, 1986, 1988a,b), caregivers of vulnerable infants in the Neonatal Intensive Care Unit (NICU) (Swanson, 1990), and socially at-risk mothers who had received long-term care from master's prepared public health nurses (Swanson, 1991).

### THEORETICAL ASSUMPTIONS

Swanson purports that caring, which she defines as "a nurturing way of relating to a valued other toward whom a nurse feels a sense of commitment and responsibility" (1991, p. 162), is not unique to the domain of perinatal nursing. Instead, she posits, caring is an essential component of nurse–client relationship in any setting. Swanson also purports that caring occurs in every nurse–client relationship that involves skillful application of caring processes (knowing, being with, doing for, enabling, and maintaining belief). She also posits that regardless of the amount of nursing experience, caring is influenced by the nurse's attitude (maintaining belief), understanding of client's experience (knowing), verbal and nonverbal interaction with the client (being with), enabling (believing in the client's capacity to live through difficult transitions), and outcomes of caring (intended outcomes of nursing process). Swanson purports that caring processes coexist and overlap and cannot be delivered in a linear way or in separation from one another. Lastly, Swanson claims that if she had truly identified and defined the universal aspects of caring, then her caring processes should ring true in any situation where caring is a part of an interpersonal relationship. Swanson (1993) depicted the caring processes and the relationships between them in the structure of caring (see Fig. 10.1).

## Examples of the Theory Application in Research

Reynolds (1971) suggests that a functional theory is one that can be applied in clinical practice and research. Swanson has persevered in the development of her theory from the point of defining the concept of caring and caring processes in her Caring Model to the development of middle range theory of caring, descriptive research to determine human responses to miscarriage over time, and theory testing using randomized controlled trial design.

Specifically, in her dissertation research, the theorist analyzed data obtained from in-depth interviews with 20 women who have recently miscarried. Two theoretical models were proposed as a result of this phenomenological investigation: (a) the Human Experience of Miscarriage Model and (b) the Caring Model. In the Caring Model that Swanson proposed, the processes of knowing, being with, doing for, enabling, and maintaining belief, gives meaning to nursing acts labeled as caring (Swanson-Kauffman, 1985, 1986, 1988a,b).

Findings of this investigation provided the foundation for the development of middle range theory of caring at a later time.

As part of her postdoctoral studies, Swanson conducted another phenomenological investigation, in which she explored "what it was it like to be a provider of care to vulnerable infants in the NICU." As a result of this study, Swanson (1990) found that the caring processes she identified with women who miscarried were also applicable to parents, physicians, and nursing staff responsible for taking care of infants in the Neonatal Intensive Care Unit (NICU). Therefore, Swanson decided to retain the wording describing the acts of caring and propose that holistic care in a complex environment like NICU embraces balance of *caring* (for self and the one cared for), *attaching* (to others and roles), *managing responsibilities* (assigned by self, others, and society), and *avoiding bad outcomes* (Swanson, 1990).

In a later investigation, Swanson (1991) explored what it had been like for socially at-risk mothers to receive supportive, long-term nursing interventions. As a result of this study, she was finally able to define caring and further refine the definitions of caring processes. Collectively, findings of Swanson's research with women who have miscarried, caregivers in the NICU, and socially at-risk mothers provided the foundation for expanding the Caring Model into the middle range theory of caring (Swanson, 1991, 1993).

Swanson tested her theory of caring with women who miscarried in several investigations funded by the National Institutes of Health, National Institutes of Nursing Research, and other funding sources. Swanson's (1999a, b) intervention study with 242 women who miscarried focused on examining the effects of caring-based counseling sessions on the women's processing of loss and their emotional wellness in the first year after loss. Additional aims of the study were to examine the effects of the passage of time on healing and to design strategies to monitor caring interventions. The main findings of this investigation were that caring was effective in decreasing the participants' overall disturbed mood, depression, and anger. Moreover, all study participants (treated or not) who assigned less personal significance to miscarrying had higher levels of self-esteem and less anxiety, anger, and confusion. In other words, the findings of the study demonstrated that while passing of time had positive effects on women's healing after miscarriage, caring interventions had a positive impact on decreasing the overall disturbed mood, anger, and level of depression. The second aim of this investigation was to monitor the caring variable and identify whether caring was delivered as intended. In this

investigation, caring was monitored in three different ways: (a) approximately 10% of counseling sessions were transcribed and data were analyzed using inductive and deductive content analysis; (b) before each caring session, the counselor completed McNair, Lorr, and Droppelman's (1981) Profile of Mood States to monitor whether her own mood was associated with women's ratings of caring after each session, using the investigator-developed Caring Professional Scale. After each session, the counselor completed an investigator-developed Counselor Rating Scale and took narrative notes about the counseling session. The most noteworthy finding of monitoring caring was that the majority of participants were highly satisfied with caring received during counseling sessions, suggesting that caring was delivered as intended.

In 2009, Swanson and her research team published results from the National Institutes of Health (NIH)-funded intervention research "Couples Miscarriage Healing Project" (see Using Middle Range Theory in Research 10.1) conducted with ($N = 341$) heterosexual couples over a period of 1 year after loss (Swanson et al., 2009). The study was conducted to determine the effects of miscarriage on couples in committed heterosexual relationships and to identify effective ways of helping couples heal both as individuals and as couples subsequent to miscarriage. Study participants (couples) were randomly assigned to one of three treatment groups: (a) NC (three counseling sessions with a nurse), (b) self-caring (three videos and workbook modules), (c) combined caring (one NC session and three videos and workbook modules), or (d) a control group (no intervention). Interventions, based on Swanson's caring theory and Meaning of Miscarriage Model, were offered 1, 5, and 11 weeks after enrollment. Differences in rates of recovery were estimated via multilevel modeling conducted in a Bayesian framework. Swanson et al. (2009) found that caring-based interventions delivered by a registered nurse had the overall broadest positive impact on couples' resolution of grief and depression. In addition, grief resolution was accelerated by self-caring intervention for women and combined nurse and self-caring intervention for men, suggesting that Swanson's caring theory is an effective framework to facilitate healing of individuals and couples in clinical practice.

Reynolds (1971) asserts that a useful theory provides a sense of understanding and applicability in research, education, and practice. The caring theory has been the theoretical foundation for numerous research studies, masters and doctoral dissertations, and scholarly projects of undergraduate and graduate nursing students. Literature

## USING MIDDLE RANGE THEORY IN RESEARCH    10.1

Source: Swanson, K. M., Chen, H., Graham, J. C., Wojnar, D. M., & Petras, A. (2009). Resolution of depression and grief during the first year after miscarriage: A randomized controlled trial of couples-focused interventions. Journal of Women's Health, 18(8), 1245–1257.

### PURPOSE/RESEARCH QUESTION

The purpose of this study was to examine the effects of three couple-focused interventions and a control condition on women and their partners' resolution of depression and grief during the 1st year after miscarriage.

### RESEARCH DESIGN

A randomized controlled clinical trial (RCT) was used in this study.

### SAMPLE/PARTICIPANTS

Three hundred and forty-one couples participated in the study. They were enrolled within the first 12 weeks after pregnancy loss.

### DATA COLLECTION

Subsequently, couples who met the inclusion criteria were randomly assigned to nurse caring (NC) intervention that entailed three counseling sessions: self-caring (SC) that consisted of three videos and workbook modules, combined caring (CC) that included one counseling session plus three SC modules, or controlled condition in which no treatment was offered. Interventions were based on Swanson's caring theory and Meaning of Miscarriage Model. They were offered 1, 5, and 11 weeks after enrollment. Outcomes included depression (CES-D) and grief, pure grief (PG), and grief-related emotions (GRE). Couples' perceptions of Caring Professional and Caring Mate and Caring Other Scales in the aftermath of loss were also administered to all participants. Differences in rates of recovery were estimated via multilevel modeling conducted in a Bayesian framework.

### FINDINGS

Swanson et al. (2009) found that Bayesian odds (BO) ranging from 3.0 to 7.9 favored NC over all other conditions for accelerating women's resolution of depression. BO of 3.2 to 6.6 favored NC and no treatment over SC and CC for resolving men's depression. BO of 3.1 to 7.0 favored all three interventions over no treatment for accelerating women's PG resolution, and BO of 18.7 to 22.6 favored NC and CC over SC or no treatment for resolving men's PG. BO ranging from 2.4 to 6.1 favored NC and SC over CC or no treatment for hastening women's resolution of GRE. BO from 3.5 to 17.9 favored NC, CC, and control over SC for resolving men's GRE. Swanson et al. (2009) concluded that NC had the overall broadest positive impact on couples' resolution of grief and depression. In addition, grief resolution (PG and GRE) was accelerated by SC for women and CC for men.

review of computerized databases (MEDLINE, CINAHL, and Digital Dissertations) indicates that Swanson's theory and research have been cited or otherwise utilized in over 160 data-based publications, while the article "Nursing as informed caring for the well-being of others" (Swanson, 1993) alone has been cited over 50 times. Applications of Swanson's caring theory in research include the following publications: Kish and Holder's (1996) exploration of clinical scholarship in practice; Yorkston, Klasner, and Swanson's (2001) guidelines for practitioners working with patients who have multiple sclerosis; Quinn, Smith, Ritenbaugh, and Swanson's (2003) guidelines for assessing impact of healing relationships in nursing; Sikma's (2006) study of caring with elderly population; Kavanaugh, Moro, Savage, and Mehendale's (2006) research with vulnerable populations; Sandblom's (2006) analysis of grief and depression after miscarriage

among couples with history of infertility; Wojnar's (2007) research with lesbian couples who miscarry; and Wojnar's et al. (2011) comparisons of lesbian and heterosexual couples' experiences of miscarriage using international datasets. Most recently, researchers applied Swanson's theory in working with pediatric patients including supporting parent–child interactions during painful procedures (Bai, Swanson, Harper, Santacroce, & Penner, 2018; Bai, Swanson, & Santacroce, 2018) and supporting children hospitalized for heart surgery and their parents (Wei et al., 2016; Wei, Roscigno, & Swanson, 2017).

### APPLICATIONS OF THE THEORY IN EDUCATION AND CLINICAL PRACTICE

In recent decade, Swanson's theory has also been successfully adapted as a framework for

| BOX 10.2 | Examples of the Theory Application in Education and Practice |
|----------|-------------------------------------------------------------|

**Application of the Theory in Education**
- Dalhousie University in Halifax, Nova Scotia, Canada, has embraced Swanson's theory of caring as a framework to guide teaching and professional formation of student nurses.

**Application of the Theory in Clinical Practice**
- Nurses at IWK Health Centre, a tertiary level hospital in Halifax, Nova, Scotia, Canada, have selected Swanson's theory of caring as representative of the caring–healing legacy of nursing profession and relevant to the clinical practice.

## CRITICAL THINKING EXERCISES

1. Think about a time when you felt that you or someone close to you experienced caring in the health care environment. What was it like to experience caring? What did the practitioner say or do? How consistent were his or her actions with caring processes identified by Swanson? Alternatively, think about a situation when caring was not delivered. What was missing in your interaction with that practitioner?

2. Think about a situation in your clinical practice when your interaction with the client did not go smoothly. Consider key definitions identified in Swanson's theory and reflect on what caring processes were missing from that interaction. In what ways could that interaction be improved?

3. Consider Swanson's theory of caring as a theoretical framework for a research study relevant to your clinical practice. In what ways would it be applicable?

professional nursing practice by various universities and practice settings across the United States, Canada, and Sweden (see Box 10.2). According to Chinn and Kramer (2004), the situations in which the theories may be applied should not be limited. Clearly, it has been demonstrated that Swanson's theory of caring may be used effectively to establish therapeutic relationships with diverse populations, far beyond the perinatal context, to promote the individuals' wellness across lifespan (Swanson, 1999c), making it generalizable to any nurse–client relationship and any clinical setting. Hence, it offers a framework for enhancing contemporary nursing practice while bringing the discipline to its traditional caring–healing roots.

## Summary

■ The usefulness of Swanson's theory of caring has been demonstrated in research, education, and clinical practice.

■ The belief that caring has a pivotal role in the practice of professional nursing had its beginning in the theorist's clinical practice, in the influence of her mentors, and in the findings from her phenomenological investigations.

■ Her later works, including meta-analysis of research on caring (Swanson, 1999a,b,c), have demonstrated generalizability and applicability of the theory of caring in education, clinical nursing practice, and research beyond perinatal context.

■ NC, as demonstrated by Swanson in research with women who miscarried, caregivers in the Neonatal Intensive Care Unit, and socially at-risk mothers, recognizes the importance of attending to the wholeness of human experiences and needs.

## REFERENCES

Bai, J., Swanson, K. M., Harper, F. W. K., Santacroce, S. J., & Penner, L. A. (2018). Longitudinal analysis of parent communication behaviors and child distress during cancer port start procedures. *Pain Management Nursing, 19*(5), 487–496. doi: 10.1016/j.pmn.2018.01.002

Bai, J., Swanson, K. M., & Santacroce, S. J. (2018). Observational coding systems of parent-child interactions during painful procedures: A systematic review. *Pain Practice, 18*(1), 130–145. doi: 10.1111/papr.12588

Benner, P. (1984). *From novice to expert.* Menlo Park, CA: Addison-Wesley.

Benner, P., & Wrubel, J. (1989). *The primacy of caring.* Menlo Park, CA: Addison-Wesley.

Boykin, A. (1994). *Living a caring-based curriculum.* New York, NY: National League for Nursing.

Chinn, P. L., & Kramer, M. K. (2004). *Integrated knowledge development in nursing* (6th ed.). St. Louis, MO: Mosby.

Huffman, C. S., Schwartz, T. A., & Swanson, K. M. (2015). Couples and miscarriage: The influence of gender and reproductive factors on the impact of miscarriage. *Women's Health Issues, 25*(5), 570–578. doi: 10.1016/j.whi.2015.04.005

Jansson, C., Volgsten, H., Huffman, C., Skoog Svanberg, A., Swanson, K. M., & Stavreus-Evers, A. (2017). Validation of the revised Impact of Miscarriage Scale for Swedish conditions and comparison between Swedish and American Couples' experiences after miscarriage. *European Journal of Contraception and Reproductive Healthcare, 22*(6), 412–417. doi: 10.1080/13625187.2017.1409346

Kavanaugh, K., Moro, T. T., Savage, T., & Mehendale, R. (2006). Enacting a theory of caring to recruit and retain vulnerable participants for sensitive research. *Research in Nursing and Health, 29*(3), 244–252.

Kish, C. P., & Holder, L. M. (1996). Helping to say goodbye: Merging clinical scholarship with community service. *Holistic Nursing Practice, 10*(3), 74–82.

Leininger, M. M. (1981). The phenomenon of caring: Importance of research and theoretical considerations. In M. M. Leininger (Ed.), *Caring: An essential human need.* Thorofare, NJ: Slak.

Leininger, M. M. (1988). Leininger's theory of nursing: Cultural care diversity and universality. *Nursing Science Quarterly, 1*(4), 152–160.

McNair, D. M., Lorr, M., & Droppleman, L. F. (1971). *Profile of mood states: Manual.* San Diego, CA: Educational and Industrial Testing Service.

Meleis, A. I. (1997). *Theoretical nursing: Development and progress.* Philadelphia, PA: Lippincott-Raven.

Quinn, J., Smith, M., Ritenbaugh, C., & Swanson, K. M. (2003). Research guidelines for assessing the impact of the healing relationship in clinical nursing. *Alternative Therapies in Health and Medicine, 9*(31), 69–79.

Reynolds, P. D. (1971). *A primer of theory construction.* Indianapolis, IN: Bobs-Merrill.

Sandblom, S. (2006). Does a history of infertility affect the grief and depression response in couples experiencing a spontaneous miscarriage? (Unpublished master thesis), Seattle, WA: University of Washington School of Nursing.

Sikma, S. (2006). Staff perceptions of caring: The importance of a supportive environment. *Journal of Gerontological Nursing, 32*(6), 22–29.

Swanson, K. M. (1990). Providing care in the NICU: Sometimes an act of love. *Advances in Nursing Science, 13*(1), 60–73.

Swanson, K. M. (1991). Empirical development of a middle range theory of caring. *Nursing Research, 40*(3), 161–166.

Swanson, K. M. (1993). Nursing as informed caring for the well-being of others. *Image: The Journal of Nursing Scholarship, 25*(4), 352–357.

Swanson, K. M. (1998). Caring made visible. *Creative Nursing, 4*(4), 8–11, 16.

Swanson, K. M. (1999a). Research-based practice with women who have had miscarriages. *Image: The Journal of Nursing Scholarship, 31*(4), 339–345.

Swanson, K. M. (1999b). The effects of caring, measurement, and time on miscarriage impact and women's well-being in the first year subsequent to loss. *Nursing Research, 48*(6), 288–298.

Swanson, K. M. (1999c). What's known about caring in nursing: A literary meta-analysis. In A. S. Hinshaw, J. Shaver, & S. Feetham (Eds.), *Handbook of clinical nursing research* (pp. 31–60). Thousand Oaks, CA: Sage.

Swanson, K. M. (2000). Predicting depressive symptoms after miscarriage: A path analysis based on Lazarus' paradigm. *Journal of Women's Health & Gender-based Medicine, 9*(2), 191–206.

Swanson, K. M. (2001). A program of research on caring. In M. E. Parker (Ed.), *Nursing theories and nursing practice* (pp. 411–420). Philadelphia, PA: Davis.

Swanson, K. M. (2002). Caring professional scale. In J. Watson (Ed.), *Assessing and measuring caring in nursing and health science.* Seattle, WA: Springer Publishing Company.

Swanson, K. M. Chen, H., Graham, J. C., Wojnar, D. M., & Petras, A. (2009). Resolution of depression and grief during the first year after miscarriage: A randomized controlled trial of couples-focused interventions. *Journal of Women's Health, 18*(8), 1245–1257.

Swanson, K. M., Connor, S., Jolley, S. N., Pettinato, M., & Wang, T. (2007). The context and evolution of women's responses to miscarriage over the first year after loss. *Research in Nursing & Health, 30*(1), 2–16.

Swanson, K. M., Karmali, Z., Powell, S., & Pulvermahker, F. (2003). Miscarriage effects on interpersonal and sexual relationships during the first year after loss: Women's perceptions. *Psychosomatic Medicine, 65*(5), 902–910.

Swanson, K. M., Kieckhefer, G., Powers, P., & Carr, K. (1990). Meaning of miscarriage scale: Establishment of psychometric properties (Abstract). *Communicating Nursing Research, 25*, 365.

Swanson, K. M., & Wojnar, D. (2004). Optimal healing environments in nursing. *Alternative Therapies in Health and Medicine, 10*(1), 43–51.

Swanson-Kauffman, K. M. (1985). Miscarriage: A new understanding of the mother's experience. *Proceedings of the 50th anniversary celebration of the University of Pennsylvania School of Nursing,* Philadelphia, PA, 63–78.

Swanson-Kauffman, K. M. (1986). Caring in the instance of unexpected early pregnancy loss. *Topics in Clinical Nursing, 8*(2), 37–46.

Swanson-Kauffman, K. M. (1988a). The caring needs of women who miscarry. In M. M. Leininger (Ed.), *Care, discovery and uses in clinical and community nursing* (pp. 55–71). Detroit, MI: Wayne State University Press.

Swanson-Kauffman, K. M. (1988b). There should have been two: Nursing care of parents experiencing the perinatal death of a twin. *Journal of Perinatal and Neonatal Nursing, 2*(2), 78–86.

Swanson-Kauffman, K. M., & Roberts, J. (1990). Caring in parent and child nursing. *Knowledge about care and caring: State of the art and future development.* Washington, DC: American Academy of Nursing.

Watson, J. (1979). *Nursing: The philosophy and science of caring.* Boston, MA: Little & Brown.

Watson, J. (1988). New dimensions of human caring theory. *Nursing Science Quarterly, 1*, 175–181.

Watson, J. (1999). *Nursing: Human science and human care: A theory of nursing.* Sudbury, MA: Jones & Barlett.

Wei, H., Roscigno, C. I., & Swanson, K. M. (2017). Healthcare providers' caring: Nothing is too small for parents and children hospitalized for heart surgery. *Heart and Lung, 46*(3), 166–171. doi: 10.1016/j.hrtlng.2017.01.007

Wei, H., Roscigno, C. I., Swanson, K. M., Black, B. P., Hudson-Barr, D., & Hanson, C. C. (2016). Parents' experiences of having a child undergoing congenital heart surgery: An emotional rollercoaster from shocking to blessing. *Heart & Lung: The Journal of Critical Care, 45*(92), 154–160. doi: 10.1016/j.hrtlng.2015.12.007

Wojnar, D. (2007). Miscarriage experiences of lesbian birth and social mothers: Couples' perspective. *Journal of Midwifery and Women's Health, 52*(5), 479–485.

Wojnar, D. M., Swanson, K. M., & Adolfsson, A. S. (2011). Confronting the inevitable: A conceptual model of miscarriage for use in clinical practice and research. *Death Studies, 35*(6), 536–558.

Yorkston, K. M., Klasner, E. R., & Swanson, K. M. (2001). Communication in multiple sclerosis: Understanding the insider's perspective. *American Journal of Speech Language Pathology, 10*, 126–137.

# 11

# Interpersonal Relations

Sandra J. Peterson

## Definition of Key Terms

| | |
|---|---|
| **Communication** | A skill necessary to understand the nurse–patient relationship; composed of "spoken language, rational and nonrational expressions of wishes, needs, and desires, and the body gesture" (Peplau, 1991, p. 289) |
| **Interpersonal relations** | Any process that occurs between two people. The interpersonal processes between nurse and patient are identified as the core of nursing (Forchuk, 1993) |
| **Nursing situation** | What occurs between the nurse and the patient; thus, the interaction of the individual thoughts, feelings, and actions of both |
| **Observation** | A skill necessary to understand the nurse–patient relationship. Its aim, "as an interpersonal process, is the identification, clarification, and verification of impressions about the interactive drama, of the pushes and pulls in the relationship between nurse and patient as they occur" (Peplau, 1991, p. 263) |
| **Personality** | "… Pattern that is relatively stable and that characterizes persisting situations in the life of an individual … total assets and liabilities that determine an individual action" (Peplau, 1991, pp. 164, 165). Nurses attempt to provide experiences for patients that promote personality development |
| **Phases of nurse–patient relationship** | Four overlapping but generally sequential aspects of the relationship identified as orientation, identification, exploitation, and resolution |
| **Psychobiological experiences** | Factors that influence the functioning of personalities, providing energy that is converted into constructive or destructive behavior. The primary source of this energy is anxiety |
| **Psychological tasks** | "Tasks encountered in the process of learning to live with people as an aspect of formation and development of personality and as an aspect of the tasks demanded of nurses in their relations with patients" (Peplau, 1991, p. 159), for example, counting on others, delaying satisfaction, identifying self, and participating with others |
| **Recording** | Methods used to create documents of nurse–patient interactions, primarily for the purpose of student learning |
| **Roles in nursing** | Set of functions that nurses use in the context of nurse–patient situations as a means of helping the patient, identified as stranger, resource person, teacher, leader, surrogate, and counselor |

"When the history of nursing theory comes to be written few names will be seen to have been more influential than that of Hildegard Peplau" (Welch, 1995, p. 53). Peplau, who developed the theory of interpersonal relations, is identified as the first contemporary nurse theorist (McKenna, 1997). Sills (1978) credits Peplau with clarifying the relationships between nursing theory, practice, and research. "Theory was used to guide nursing practice. Theory was tested in the real world of practice" (Sills, 1978, p. 122).

Although Peplau entitled her work a conceptual frame of reference, she also referred to it as a theory (Peplau, 1992, p. 13). Peplau produced a testable theory, identifying her work as a "source of hypotheses that may be examined with profit in all nursing situations" (Peplau, 1991, p. ix). The theory of interpersonal relations is currently labeled as a middle range theory (Armstrong & Kelly, 1995; Fawcett, 2000; O'Toole & Welt, 1989). Peplau, herself, defined the scope of her theory as in the middle range. She referred to it as "a partial theory for the practice of nursing as an interpersonal process" (Peplau, 1991, p. 261).

Initially developed with a focus on phenomena of most concern to psychiatric nurses, the theory of interpersonal relations is applicable to all nurses (Peplau, 1964, 1992). Peplau (1997) claimed that "the nurse–patient relationship is the primary human contact that is central in a fundamental way to providing nursing care" (p. 163). The stated purpose of her theory is the improvement of nurses' relations with patients. This is achieved through the nurse's understanding of his or her own behavior, helping others identify personally experienced difficulties, and applying principles of human relations to the problems that arise in the context of relationships (Peplau, 1991, p. xi). This process results in a nursing situation in which both the patient and the nurse learn and grow. A growth-producing relationship with others is a goal that transcends any particular nursing specialty, and in her description of the theory, Peplau (1952, 1991) used examples of patients with a variety of health issues, for example, a woman diagnosed with lymphosarcoma, a child having surgery on his hand to correct a congenital problem, a woman in labor, and a man with a coronary occlusion.

## Historical Background

What makes Peplau's theory of interpersonal relations so remarkable is that it was conceived during a period in nursing's history when nurses had little or no independent role and little or no investment in the development of nursing theory. Peplau was educated and began her nursing practice, as described in her own words, at a time when "we were absolutely not allowed to talk to a patient, because if we did we might say the wrong thing" (Welch, 1995, p. 54). It was not until the late 1930s while working as a staff nurse at Mount Sinai Hospital, New York, that she discovered "there was more to nursing than just this doing activity, because there we were allowed to talk to the patients" (Welch, 1995, p. 54). In the 1940s, Peplau found psychiatric nursing still focused on activities, for example, helping patients with tasks of daily living, which included cleaning patients' rooms and doing patients' laundry (Peplau, 1985, p. 31). It was out of her desire to be more useful to patients that the idea of interpersonal relations theory was developed.

Peplau used both deductive and inductive methods in her theory development work (Reed, 1995).

Deductively, she integrated ideas from a number of theories into her theory of interpersonal relations. She was influenced by the work of Sigmund Freud, particularly his interest in unconscious motivation. Harry S. Sullivan's theory of interpersonal relations also contributed to her thinking about interpersonal processes in nursing. For example, she refers to his concepts of anxiety, self-system, and modes of experiencing. Also incorporated into her theory are elements from developmental psychology and learning theory (Armstrong & Kelly, 1995; Lego, 1980) and the ideas of the humanistic psychologists, Abraham Maslow, Rollo May, and Carl Rogers (Gastmans, 1998).

Peplau defined her inductive approach in both general and specific terms. The inductive approach for concept naming that she described included several steps:

1. Observing behaviors for which no explanatory concepts are available
2. Seeking to repeat those observations in others, under similar conditions
3. Noting regularities concerning the nature of the data being observed
4. Naming the phenomena (Peplau, 1989, p. 28)

These steps would be followed by further observation, resulting in the phenomenon becoming more clearly defined, which then allowed for testing with additional patients. "Eventually, useful interventions would be derived from the explanation of the phenomenon and the effects of these interventions upon it also tested" (Peplau, 1969, p. 28).

Peplau's specific inductive process of theory development involved using data from student–patient interactions. "I just happened to hit upon the notion of sitting students down with one patient for a long time and then study what they did with patients" (Peplau, 1985, p. 31). It was from these observations that psychotherapy by nurses in the context of the interpersonal relationship emerged.

Her theory of interpersonal relations, first appearing in 1952 in the book *Interpersonal Relations in Nursing*, has been published unchanged several times. During the 1950s and 1960s, her theory was used and tested in the challenging environment of state psychiatric hospitals. Some of this work is reported in *Basic Principles of Patient Counseling* published in 1964 by Smith, Kline, and French (Sills, 1978, p. 124). In four decades since its inception, interpersonal theory has been expanded by Peplau and other nurse scientists (Peplau, 1991, p. vi). For example, work on therapeutic milieu, crisis, and family therapy has been based on Peplau's theory. Sills (1978) conducted a review of three major nursing journals from 1972 to 1977 (one published for the first time in 1963). She identified 93 citations of Peplau's work and concluded that "it [is] remarkable that twenty-five years after the publication of *Interpersonal Relations in Nursing* that it, with no revisions, is still found useful. And … that utilization increases" (Sills, 1978, p. 125).

## Definitions of Theory Concepts

Although not specified at the time of the development of the theory in 1952, each domain of the traditional metaparadigm of nursing is addressed by Peplau. Her definitions of these major domain concepts are useful in understanding the rather complex theory of interpersonal relations.

### NURSING

The foundation of her theory is her definition of nursing. Perhaps, what is unique, but not unexpectedly so, is the primacy of the nurse–patient relationship in her definition. She defines nursing as an interpersonal process, intended to be therapeutic. It "is a human relationship between an individual who is sick or in need of health services" (Peplau, 1991, pp. 5, 6) and a nurse who has appropriate preparation to respond to the need. The use of technical procedures in nursing is acknowledged but relegated to a secondary role.

### PERSONS

In her theory, Peplau includes two persons as components: the nurse and the client or, more often, the patient (O'Toole & Welt, 1989; Peplau, 1992). Peplau (1952) initially defined man as:

> An organism that lives in an unstable equilibrium (i.e., physiological, psychological, and social fluidity) and life is the process of striving in the direction of stable equilibrium, that is, a fixed pattern that is never reached except in death (p. 82).

Forchuk (1991) revised that definition, omitting the terms "organism" and "equilibrium" because they represent a more "mechanical, closed-system perspective" (p. 55) that is inconsistent with Peplau's view of humans as growth seeking. A person is a relational being experiencing "interacting expectations, conceptions, wishes, and desires, as well as feelings when … in situations with other persons" (O'Toole & Welt, 1989, p. 5). This perspective on persons as relational beings is fundamental to the theory.

### Nurse

The nurse is identified as a professional with definable expertise (Peplau, 1992). This expertise should include the ability to "identify human problems that confront patients, the degrees of skill used to meet situations, and be able to develop with patients the kind of relationships that will be conducive to improvement in skill" (Peplau, 1991, p. xiii). The nurse also possesses "a unique blend of ideals, values, integrity, and commitment to the well-being of others" (Peplau, 1988, p. 10).

### Patient

The patient is defined first as a person, deserving of "all the humane considerations: respect, dignity, privacy, confidentiality, and ethical care" (Peplau, 1992, p. 14), but a person who has problems that now require the services of a nurse. Ideally, the patient participates actively in the nurse–patient relationship (O'Toole & Welt, 1989, p. 57).

### HEALTH

Peplau (1952) described health as "a word symbol that implies forward movement of personality and other human processes in the direction of creative, constructive, productive, personal, and community living" (p. 12). In addition, she identified two processes that are necessary for health: (a) biological, for example, absorption and elimination, and (b) social, which promotes physical, emotional, and social well-being (pp. 12–13).

### ENVIRONMENT

Peplau focused on the issue of environment as milieu, using the term to describe a therapeutic environment (O'Toole & Welt, 1989, p. 78). The milieu is composed of structured (e.g., ward government) and unstructured components. The unstructured components consist of the complex relationships between patients, staff, visitors, and other patients, which are often neglected and yet have a significant impact on patient outcomes. Milieu ideally involves the creation of an atmosphere conducive to recovery.

## Description of Theory of Interpersonal Relations

Peplau implied a philosophical foundation to her theory of interpersonal relations and provided two basic assumptions, which have been expanded by others, using the initial publication of the theory as the primary source. Peplau did not label the propositional statements in her theory as such; instead, they are integrated into her discussion of the components of the theory.

## PHILOSOPHICAL FOUNDATIONS

There are some different perspectives on the nature of the philosophical underpinnings of Peplau's theory of interpersonal relations in nursing. Sellers (1991) labels the theory:

> … a mechanistic, deterministic, persistence onto-logical view; an epistemology that is consistent with the totality paradigm, with its emphasis on a received view of knowledge and logical posi-tivism; and an axiology that values stability, tra-ditionalism, and nursing's close alignment with medicine. (p. 158)

Sellers did not support these conclusions with examples from the theory. Since the complexity of Peplau's theory makes it difficult to categorize, it is not surprising that others have considered it from a different philosophical perspective.

More recently, existential phenomenology has been identified as the philosophical foundation of Peplau's theory (Gastmans, 1998). Consistent with phenomenology, observation of patients as a fun-damental task of nursing is seen as contextual and value laden. It requires openness to and involve-ment with patients' existential situations. "Nursing has a human interpretive character" (Gastmans, 1998, Phenomenology and Nursing Science, para. 5) with the nurse–patient relationship at its core. Interpretations are meaning-seeking activities that arise as the nurse participates with the patient. This participation with the patient is described as respectful, communicating positive interest, and nonjudgmental regard (Peplau, 1991). Peplau uses the term "professional closeness" (Peplau, 1969) to summarize these characteristics that allow the nurse to communicate care when participating with patients.

Although most of Peplau's philosophy is imbed-ded in her writings, she does delineate six "beliefs about patients" (Peplau, 1964). She identifies these as her "philosophy about patients and their care" (p. 30), attributed primarily to psychiatric nurses but applicable to all patients:

1. All behavior is purposeful, has meaning, and can be understood.
2. The nurse must observe what is going on; she must interpret what is observed, and then she must decide action on the basis of her interpretations.
3. The nurse meets the needs of the patient.
4. The nurse–patient interaction—the verbal and nonverbal exchanges in the nursing sit-uation—can influence recovery.
5. The personality of the patient is somehow involved in his illness.
6. There are some ideas about nursing care that relate to the word *anxiety* (pp. 30–35).

## ASSUMPTIONS

In the initial publication of her theory, Peplau (1952) listed two guiding assumptions, emphasiz-ing the importance of the nurse's own growth and development in establishing helpful interpersonal relationships with patients. Others have expanded that list through personal correspondence with Peplau and review of her writings. Table 11.1 pro-vides a list of the assumptions of the theory of interpersonal relations.

These 13 assumptions serve to illustrate the com-plexity of Peplau's theory of interpersonal relations.

## THEORY DESCRIPTION WITH PROPOSITIONAL STATEMENTS

The core of the theory, the relationship between nurse and patient, is composed of phases, ful-filled through roles, influenced by psychobiologi-cal experiences, and requires attending to certain psychological tasks. Peplau also identified methods that can assist the nurse to develop understanding of the nurse–patient relationship. The description of the theory is presented using the same sequence as Peplau (1952, 1991) did in her seminal work, *Interpersonal Relations in Nursing*.

### Composed of Phases

Peplau (1991) initially defined four phases of the nurse–patient relationship: orientation, identifica-tion, exploitation, and resolution. Forchuk (1991) later reconceptualized these phases into three, with the working phase replacing the identification and exploitation phases. These phases are considered overlapping and interlocking, with each phase possessing characteristic functions. They are expe-rienced in every nursing situation.

**Phase of Orientation.** There are four functions that nurses use during orientation: (a) *provide the resources* of specific, needed information to help the patient understand the problem and the health care situation, (b) *serve as a counselor* to encourage the patient to express thoughts and feelings related to the problem situation, (c) *act as surrogate* fam-ily members so that the patient can reenact and examine relevant issues from prior relationships, and (d) *use technical expertise* to attend to con-cerns or issues that require the use of professional devices. These nursing functions assist the patient to address the needs experienced during the phase of orientation.

The patient needs to recognize and understand the extent of the difficulty and the help that is needed to address it. Orienting the patient to the nature of the problem requires that the nurse acts

| Table 11.1 | Assumptions of the Theory of Interpersonal Relations |
|---|---|
| **Source** | **Assumptions** |
| Identified by Peplau (1952) | 1. "The kind of person each nurse becomes makes a substantial difference in what each patient will learn as he is nursed throughout his experience with illness" (p. xii).<br>2. "Fostering personality development in the direction of maturity is a function of nursing and nursing education; it requires the use of principles and methods that permit and guide the process of grappling with everyday interpersonal problems or difficulties" (p. xii). |
| Based on correspondence with Peplau (Forchuk, 1993) | 3. Nursing can claim as its uniqueness the responses of clients to the circumstances of their illnesses or health problems (1989, p. 28).<br>4. Because illness provides an opportunity for learning and growth, nurses can assist clients to further develop their intellectual and interpersonal competencies, during the illness experience, by gearing nursing practices to evolving such competencies through nurse–client interactions (1989, p. 28). Peplau references Gregg and Mereness in the development of this fourth assumption (Forchuk, 1993, p. 6). |
| Inferred from Peplau's writings (Forchuk, 1993) | 5. Psychodynamic nursing crosses all specialty areas of nursing. It is not synonymous with psychiatric nursing because every nurse–client relationship is an interpersonal situation in which recurring difficulties of everyday life arise (summarized from Peplau (1952), introduction).<br>6. Difficulties in interpersonal relations recur in varying intensities throughout the life of everyone (Peplau, 1952, p. xiv).<br>7. The need to harness energy that derives from tension and anxiety connected to felt needs to positive means for defining, understanding, and meeting productively the problem at hand is a universal need (Peplau, 1952, p. 26).<br>8. All human behavior is purposeful and goal seeking in terms of feelings of satisfaction and/or security (Peplau, 1952, p. 26).<br>9. The interaction of nurse and client is fruitful when a method of communication that identifies and uses common meanings is at work in the situation (Peplau, 1952, p. 284).<br>10. The meaning of behavior to the client is the only relevant basis on which nurses can determine needs to be met (Peplau, 1952, p. 226).<br>11. Each client will behave, during crisis, in a way that has worked in relation to crises faced in the past (Peplau, 1952, p. 255). |
| Inferred from Peplau's writings (Sellers, 1991) | 12. The function of personality is to grow and to develop. Nursing is a process that seeks to facilitate development of personality by aiding individuals to use those compelling forces and experiences that influence personality in ways that ensure maximum productivity (p. 73).<br>13. Because illness is an event that is experienced along with feelings that derive from older experiences but are re-enacted in the relationship of nurse to patient, the nurse–patient relationship is an opportunity for nurses to help patients to complete the unfinished psychological tasks of childhood to some degree (p. 59). |

as both a resource person and a counselor. As a resource person, the nurse provides specific information about the problem confronting the patient and helps the patient see the personal relevance of the information. As a counselor, the nurse encourages the patient to be actively involved in identifying and assessing the problem.

The patient also needs to recognize and use the professional services offered. The nurse serves as a resource person to help the patient identify the range and limitations of services provided. It is important for the patient to know what can be expected from the nurse. In order for the patient to move successfully to the next phase in the nurse–patient relationship, he or she must harness the energy from the tension and anxiety created by felt needs in a constructive fashion to define, understand, and resolve the problem.

The counseling role of the nurse is vital in dealing with the patient's anxiety. The nurse must understand the meaning of the situation to the patient and be alert to evidence of anxiety manifested by apathy, dependency, or overaggressiveness or terror and panic if the patient fails to deal with it. As a resource person, the nurse helps the patient understand the meaning of the anxiety-promoting events he or she is experiencing in the health care environment. In the counseling role, the nurse encourages the expression of expectations and feelings by responding unconditionally to the patient. This is accomplished through nondirective listening, encouraging the patient to focus on the problem and express related feelings, without offering advice, reassurance, suggestions, or persuasions. This establishes the foundation for the work of the next phase of the relationship.

**Phase of Identification.** During this phase, the patient can selectively begin to identify with some of the individuals who are offering help in one of the three ways: with interdependence/participation, independence/isolation, or dependence/helplessness. This identification is based on the degree to which the patient believes the nurse will be helpful and on the nature of his or her past relationships.

The patient who responds interdependently feels less powerless and identifies with and expresses the attitudes of cheerfulness, optimism, and problem solving that he or she perceives in the nurse. Under these conditions, the patient may express feelings that are not normally considered acceptable (e.g., helplessness or self-centeredness). These expressions are seen as potentially growth producing if the nurse accepts the feelings and continues to meet the needs of the patient.

Not all patients can identify with the nurse offering help because of the influence of earlier negative relationships with others. This experience often leads to a response that is independent or isolative. At this time, the nurse in the surrogate family member role may provide the patient with the opportunity to have new and more positive relational experiences.

Other patients may identify with the nurse too quickly, which can result in an overly dependent response to the nurse. These patients want all their needs to be met by others with no expectations placed on them. This not uncommon response limits the possibility of growth through the experience.

It is important for the nurse to consider the phenomenon of leadership during the identification phase. The nurse attempts to provide opportunities for the patient to assume responsibility in the situation that promotes more constructive rather than imitative learning. The patient is encouraged to develop the skills to perceive, focus, and interpret cues in the situation, and then respond appropriately, independent of the nurse.

**Phase of Exploitation.** During this phase, the patient feels comfortable enough to take full advantage of the services being offered and experience full value from the relationship with the nurse. Varying degrees of dependence and self-directedness are manifested with vacillation between the states. Ideally, the patient begins to identify and orient self to new goals besides solving the immediate problem, for example, in the case of a hospitalized patient, the goal of functioning at home.

**Phase of Resolution.** As old needs are met, they are replaced by new goals that began to be formulated while the patient engaged in (i.e., exploited) the use of the services provided by the nurse. It is hoped that the patient will experience a sense of security and release that occurs because he or she received help in the time of need. This security is accompanied by less reliance on and decreasing identification with helping persons and increasing reliance on self to deal with the problem. This is the result of a nurse–patient relationship that is characterized during all phases by (a) an unconditional, patient-focused, and ongoing relationship that provides for the patient's needs, (b) a recognition of and appropriate response to cues that indicate the patient's desire and readiness to grow, and (c) a shift of power from nurse to patient as patient assumes responsibility for achieving new goals (Peplau, 1991, pp. 40, 41).

### Fulfilled Through Roles

The roles of nursing are defined by nurses, endorsed by patients, influenced by society, and promoted by the professional literature. Peplau identified the roles that she considered most relevant to nurse–patient situations and delineated principles for the successful fulfilling of those roles. The roles she identified were as follows:

1. *Stranger*: The nurse approaches the patient with respect and positive interest.
2. *Resource person*: The nurse answers questions using level of functioning, psychological readiness, psychological atmosphere, and relevance of the questions to formulate the response.
3. *Teacher*: The nurse considers what patients already know and level of interest to develop learning situations that enable patients to learn through experience.
4. *Leader*: The nurse engages patients as active participants in planning their care.
5. *Surrogate*: The nurse recognizes that patients often respond to him or her as they would to a person from their past and uses that recognition to help patients deal constructively with their feelings and learn new ways or relating to others.
6. *Counselor*: The nurse observes and listens to patients in a way that helps patients develop fully understanding of themselves, their feelings, and actions.

### Influenced by Psychobiological Experiences

The psychobiological experiences of needs, frustration, conflict, and anxiety influence the functioning of personalities. These experiences are also sources of energy that can result in both constructive and destructive actions. It is through understanding these experiences that individuals can learn to become more productive human beings (Peplau, 1991).

**Needs.** Although Peplau identifies needs as both physiological and psychological, her emphasis is on those that are psychological in nature. Security, new experiences, affection, recognition, and mastery are identified as psychological needs. If needs are unmet, they lead to increasing tension or anxiety. When needs are met, new and more health-producing ones may emerge.

**Frustration.** Frustration occurs when fulfillment of a need or pursuit of a goal is blocked. The primary goal identified by Peplau (1991) is the need for a "feeling of satisfaction and/or security" (p. 86). Frustration can be manifested as aggression and/or anxiety. The individual defends self from anxiety by (a) modifying the goal to one for which success is more likely, (b) giving up on the goal with the possibility of dissociation of feelings occurring, and/or (c) adopting fixed responses (e.g., stereotyping and delusions). It is important for the nurse and patient to communicate in order to clarify goals and arrive at mutually acceptable ones.

**Conflict.** Another issue that the nurse and patient deal with in their interpersonal relationship is conflicting goals. Conflicting goals are often unrecognized and are expressed in the behavioral responses of hesitation, tension, vacillation, or complete blocking.

Blocking occurs when approaching a goal is completely incompatible with avoiding another one (approach–avoidance conflict). The most common example is the desire to go home (approaching goal) that coexists with the desire to not leave the perceived safety of the hospital (avoiding goal). Fear results and can express itself as withdrawal or avoidance. If that which is feared can be identified, the nurse can act as a resource person by providing information and experiences that can reduce the strength of avoidance. Individuals often are required to make choices between two desirable goals (approach–approach conflict). The nurse is most helpful by fulfilling the counselor role in this situation. Listening in a way that encourages the expression of feelings allows the individual to recognize the factors that influence the choice to be made.

**Unexplained Discomfort/Anxiety.** As previously noted, anxiety or unexplained discomfort, as Peplau sometimes referred to it, can occur when there are unmet needs, obstacles to goals, or conflicting goals. Anxiety is often associated with guilt, doubt, fears, and obsessions. Both patients and nurses experience this feeling state that influences behavior productively or destructively through the energy it produces. The nurse helps reduce the anxiety to a more manageable and useful level by his or her presence as someone who will listen and provide for the patient's physical needs.

### Requires Attending to Certain Psychological Tasks

Psychological tasks are those related to learning to live with others. Peplau addresses the tasks of (a) learning to count on others, (b) learning to delay satisfaction, (c) identifying oneself, and (d) developing skills in participation. These tasks occur not only as an aspect of the development of personality but also as features of nurse–patient relationships. During this relationship, the nurse has the opportunity to help patients develop in areas of task deficit. In order to provide this assistance, the nurse uses the previously discussed roles and understanding of the previously examined psychobiological experiences. In addition, in order to understand his or her own personality and the patient's, the nurse needs to appreciate the psychological tasks of infants and children as identified by Sigmund Freud and Richard Havighurst (Peplau, 1991, p. 166) and the acculturation processes that enable those tasks to be successfully completed.

**Counting on Others.** The first psychological task of the infant is the development of healthy dependence. The nurse encounters varying degrees of both healthy dependency and dependency longings in nursing situations. In response to those situations, nurses help patients learn that they are trustworthy so that patients can become more aware of their needs and to express those needs more effectively (Peplau, 1991, p. 181). There are a number of positive consequences of having needs met. The patient experiences a feeling of self-worth and as a result begins to collaborate with the nurse in his or her growth. In addition, as needs are met, new, more mature ones can emerge.

**Delaying Satisfaction.** The socialization of a child includes the lesson of deferring to the wishes of others and delaying gratification of one's own wishes, a lesson that is dependent on having already learned that those being deferred to are also those that can be counted upon. According to Peplau (1991), this lesson takes place primarily during the process of toilet training.

Peplau (1991) identified principles that are consistent with healthy toilet training and general socialization activities that help the nurse establish rapport with patients and assist them in developing the ability to delay gratification of needs:

1. Show unconditional interest and acceptance.
2. Encourage expression of needs and feelings.
3. Provide times in which demands are met and times when they are not met.
4. Promote participation in decision-making so that patients can become more self-directing.
5. Allow for some "hoarding," which reinforces feelings of security.
6. Encourage sharing, which can only occur when there is freedom from coercion.

The goal is for patients to learn that delaying gratification can be experienced without an overwhelming sense of anxiety.

**Identifying Oneself.** Self-identity or concept of self enhances or distorts relationships with others, a fact that is true for both the patient and the nurse. This sense of self develops initially through a child's interactions with adults as he or she learns to rely on others and delay gratification in relation to needs. The way the child is appraised during these interactions results in three possible views of self: (a) a sense of competency to identify wants and needs, (b) a sense of helplessness and dependence on others, or (c) a sense of distrust in others. A nurse can assist a patient struggling with self-concept by:

1. Being value neutral
2. Communicating hope and acceptance
3. Avoiding the problematic responses of praise, blame, and indifference

The nurse who exhibits these characteristics can enhance the patient's concept of self and ability to experience interdependent relationships with others.

**Participating With Others.** When individuals participate in making decisions that affect them, they are more likely to understand the decisions, be involved in implementing them, and appreciate the contributions of others to the ultimate decision. This task of participating with others is composed of the abilities to compromise, compete, and cooperate. This participatory approach serves to improve the patient's skills in meeting problems. Peplau (1991) describes a three-step process:

1. Assist the patient to identify the problem.
2. Collaborate to "achieve a decision on what is possible, what can be done, and then move into other items that have been mentioned and other *possible courses of action* that can be taken in behalf of and with the co-operation of the patient" (Peplau, 1991, p. 248).
3. Encourage the patient to try out what has been proposed.

### Nursing Methods Used to Understand Interpersonal Processes

Observation, communication, and recording are three basic skills that are "valuable to the use of nursing as an interpersonal process that is therapeutic and educative for patients" (Peplau, 1991, p. 309). Peplau considered these three operations as integral to the nursing process.

**Observation.** "The aim of observation in nursing, when it is viewed as an interpersonal process, is the identification, clarification, and verification of impressions about the interactive drama, of the pushes and pulls in the relationship between nurse and patient, as they occur" (Peplau, 1991, p. 263). Observation as described by Peplau is composed of four components: (a) intuitive impressions or hunches, (b) hypothesis statements, (c) organized observations based on the hypothesis, and (d) judgment formations.

Peplau (1991) provides a classification of types of observer–observed relationships that the nurse can use to gather evidence: (a) spectator; (b) interviewer; (c) collector, that is, using reports and records to help form partial impressions; and (d) participant, that is, involvement in activities with the patient that allow for observation.

**Communication.** One of the basic tools of nursing is communication, which requires "awareness of means of communication; spoken language, rational and nonrational expressions of wishes, needs, and desires, and the body gesture" (Peplau, 1991, p. 289). Use of words or verbal communication can convey facts, focus on everyday events, and provide interpretations. Spoken language can reveal personal realities or express hidden meanings, but it can also avoid conveying anything meaningful.

There are two main principles for effective verbal communication: clarity and continuity. Clarity occurs when there is a common frame of reference or when specific efforts are made to arrive at mutual understanding. Continuity occurs when the connections between ideas and the related feelings, events, or themes expressed through the ideas are made evident. Following up on what patients say communicates that what they said is important and that as individuals they are worthwhile.

The nurse's self-awareness is one of the primary conditions for achieving understanding. For a nurse, this awareness enables her to express congruence in the use of words, their relevance, and related actions. Awareness provides the primary distinction between rational and nonrational communications. Rational expressions more likely occur when individuals see themselves rather than others as a source of personal security and when they are oriented toward the future rather than oriented to the past. Nonrational expressions communicate in more ambiguous and indirect ways than rational expressions. It is the nurse's responsibility to interpret the meaning of the communication by considering the symbols being used to express the underlying emotions.

In addition to the spoken word, gestures can be considered either rational or nonrational expressions. "The body as a whole, as well as parts of it, act as expressional instruments that communicate to others the feelings, wishes, and aspirations of an individual" (Peplau, 1991, p. 304). Underactivity and overactivity are examples of whole-body gestures. Hand gestures (e.g., clenched fist) and facial grimaces (e.g., biting a lip) are examples of more specific gestures. The nurse's responsibility is to observe gestures and attempt to understand both what he or she and the patient are communicating to each other. Arriving at understanding or meaning is a complicated and ongoing process of observation and communication.

**Recording.** Peplau focuses primarily on recording for the purpose of student learning. In addition to charting in medical records, students need additional forms that provide a means of examining the relationship. The purpose is to achieve insight into the student nurse's own behavior and the ways the patients responded. The ultimate goal of recordings, as well as observation and communication, is nurse–patient relationships that result in improved health outcomes for the patient.

## Applications of the Theory: Research

Peplau's theory of interpersonal relations remains relevant as a foundation for scientific inquiry and nursing practice. A review of the literature, 2007–2017, revealed over 100 publications in which Peplau's work was cited. Theory of interpersonal relations is of interest internationally, with publications by nurse scientists from Australia, Brazil, Canada, China, Denmark, Great Britain, India, Iran, Ireland, the Netherlands, New Zealand, Nigeria, Portugal, Slovenia, Sweden, and Turkey.

Among the citations to Peplau's work are a biography (Winship, Bray, Repper, & Hinshelwood, 2009), book chapters on her theory (Butts & Rich, 2015; George, 2011; Parker & Smith, 2010), editorials and tributes (Wills, 2010; Zauszniewski, 2009), doctoral dissertations (Brown-O'Hara, 2013; Moss, 2015), and numerous articles using her theory as a framework for research or a basis for nursing

care practices. In addition, there are articles that describe her theory (McCarthy & Aquino-Russell, 2009) and present her contributions from historical perspectives (Caldwell, Sclafani, Piren, & Torre, 2012; D'Antonio, Beeber, Sills, & Naegle, 2014; Silverstein, 2008; Winship, Bray, Repper, & Hinshelwood, 2009).

The theory has served as a framework for studying a variety of research questions, using both qualitative and quantitative methods. Although originally a theory designed to describe therapeutic relationships between nurses and psychiatric patients (Forchuk & Reynolds, 2001; Forchuk et al., 2000; Tofthagen, 2004), it is currently used to examine the nature of relationships with other populations.

For instance, in qualitative research published in English focusing on nursing practice, the theory has provided the framework to study women: (a) living in rural American during pregnancy (Evans & Bullock, 2017; Evans, Deutsch, Drake, & Bullock, 2017), (b) experiencing antepartum depression (2014), and (c) parenting as a single mother with minimal financial resources (Porr, Drummond, & Olson, 2012).

Peplau's theory has also been used to study individuals during times of crisis or stress. For example, qualitative studies have focused on (a) experiences of adolescent victims of dating violence (Draucker, Cook, Martsolf, & Stephenson, 2012), (b) development of palliative care guidelines for cancer patients and their families (Thelly & Priyalatha, 2013), (c) role of psychosocial nurses in caring for patients with cancer (Arving, 2011), and (d) helping roles in working with survivors of sexual violence (Courey, Martsolf, Draucker, & Strickland, 2008).

Peplau's theory has also served as the conceptual framework for qualitative research that focused on nursing education, for example, Boulton and O'Connell's (2017) study of students' perceptions of faculty support in relation to experience of stress and substance misuse, Reid et al.'s (2014) study of simulation to teach interpersonal skills for working with children, and Bernsston and Hildingh's (2013) study of the perspectives of nursing students specializing in prehospital emergency care.

The quantitative studies focus on both nursing practice and nursing education. New to the body of research are several randomized control studies. Table 11.2 provides examples of nursing research using quantitative methods published in English from 2007 to 2017.

As noted in the table, nurse scientists have begun to explore the usefulness of Peplau's theory in cross-cultural contexts. Using Middle Range Theory in Research 11.1 describes one such study.

**Table 11.2    Examples of Research Using Theory of Interpersonal Relations**

| Citation | Focus |
|---|---|
| Boulton, M., & O'Connell, K. A. (2017). Nursing students' perceived faculty support, stress, and substance misuse. *Journal of Nursing Education, 56*(7), 404–411. doi: 10.3928/01484834-20170619-04 | Relationship of nursing students' perception of faculty support with their level of stress and substance use |
| Hagerty, T. A., Samuels, W., Norcina-Pala, A., & Gigliotti, W. (2017). Peplau's theory of interpersonal relations: An alternate factor structure for patient experience data? *Nursing Science Quarterly, 30*(2), 160–167. doi: 1077/0894318417693286 | Use of Peplau's theory to demonstrate nurses' impact on the experience of hospitalized patients |
| Scheidenhelm, S., & Reitz, E. (2017). Hardwiring bedside shift report. *The Journal of Nursing Administration, 47*(3), 147–153. doi: 10.1097/NNA.0000000000000457 | Use of standardized bedside report to establish trusting relationship with patients and improve their level of satisfaction |
| Ward, J. (2016). The empathy enigma: Does it still exist? Comparison of empathy using students and standardized actors. *Nurse Educator, 41*(3), 134–138. doi: 10.1097/NNE.0000000000000236 | Use of simulation in both pediatric and adult situations to increase students' level of self-reported empathy |
| Radtke, K. (2013). Improving patient satisfaction with nursing communication using bedside shift report. *Clinical Nurse Specialist, 27*(1), 19–25. | Effect of bedside shift report using Peplau's theory to improve patient satisfaction with nurse communication |
| Kourosh, Z., Maqhsoudi, S., Dashtebozorgi, B., Hghighzadeh, M. S., & Javadi, M. (2014). The impact of Peplau's therapeutic model on anxiety and depression in patients candidate for coronary artery bypass. *Clinical Practice & Epidemiology in Mental Health, 10*, 159–165. doi: 10.2174/1745017901410010159 | Use of therapeutic communication to reduce anxiety and depression of patients who were scheduled for coronary artery bypass surgery |
| Shen, J. J., Xu, Y., Staplers, S., & Bolstad, A. L. (2014). Using the interpersonal skills tool to assess interpersonal skills of internationally educated nurses. *Japan Journal of Nursing Science, 1*(3), 171–179. doi: 10.1111/jjns.12018 | Determination of the interpersonal skill level of internationally educated nurses |
| Washington, G. T. (2013). The theory of interpersonal relations applied to the preceptor—New graduate relationship. *Journal for Nurses in Professional Development, 29*(1), 24–29. doi: 10.1097/DCC.ObO13e3182619b4c | Impact of residency program on the performance anxiety for new nursing graduates |
| Washington, G. T. (2012), Performance anxiety in new graduate nurses. *Dimensions of Critical Care Nursing, 31*(5), 295–300. doi: 10.1097/DCC.0b013e3182619b4c | Impact of professional relationship factors on performance anxiety in graduate nurses |
| Aghamohammadi-Kalkhoran, M., Karimollahi, M., & Abdi, R. (2011). Iranian staff nurses' attitudes toward nursing students. *Nurse Education Today, 31*(5), 477–481 | Attitudes of Iranian staff nurses toward nursing students during their clinical rotations |
| Anderson, K. H., Ford, S., Robson, D., Cassis, J., Rodriques, C., & Gray, R. (2010). An exploratory, randomized controlled trial of adherence therapy for people with schizophrenia. *International Journal of Mental Health Nursing, 19*, 340–349. Retrieved from www.wiley.com/bw/journal.asp?ref=1445-8330 | Use of adherence therapy to improve compliance with antipsychotic medication regime in people with psychosis |
| Beeber, L. S., Holditch-Davis, D., Perreria, K., Schwartz, T. A., Lewis, V., Blanchard, H., …, Goldman, B. D. (2010). Short-term in-home intervention reduces depressive symptoms in early Head Start Latina mothers of infants and toddlers. *Research in Nursing and Health, 33*(1), 60–76. doi: 10.1002/nur.20363 | Use of in-home culturally appropriate psychotherapy intervention to reduce symptoms of depression in Latina mothers of toddlers and infants |
| Gallgher-Lepack, S., Sheibel, P., & Gibson, C. C. (2009). Integrating telehealth in nursing curricula: Can you hear me now? *Online Journal of Nursing Informatics (OJNI), 13*(2), 1089–9758. Retrieved from http://ojni.org/ | Impact of a faculty development program on informatics and computer competencies and the subsequent ability of students to establish relationships with patients using telehealth techniques |
| Erci, B., Sezgin, S., & Kacmaz, Z. (2008). The impact of therapeutic relationship on preoperative and postoperative patient anxiety. *Australian Journal of Advanced Nursing, 26*, 59–66. Retrieved from www.ajan.com.au | Effect of the Interpersonal Relations Model based on phases of therapeutic relationship on perioperative anxiety |

**Table 11.2    Examples of Research Using Theory of Interpersonal Relations** (Continued)

| Citation | Focus |
|---|---|
| Oflaz, F., Hatipoglu, S., & Aydin, H. (2008). Effectiveness of psycho-education intervention on post-traumatic stress disorder and coping styles of earthquake survivors. *Journal of Clinical Nursing*, *17*, 677–687. doi: 10.1111/j.1365-2702.2007.02047.x | Comparison of psychoeducation (based on phases of therapeutic relationship) alone, medication alone, with combined approach to reduce anxiety and improve coping of survivors of earthquake in Turkey |
| Mariani, B. S. (2007). *The effect of mentoring on career satisfaction of registered nurses and intent to stay in the nursing profession* (Unpublished doctoral dissertation). Widener University School of Nursing, Chester, PA. | Effect of mentoring as a representation of an interpersonal relationship on career satisfaction of nurses and their intent to stay in the profession |

## USING MIDDLE RANGE THEORY IN RESEARCH    11.1

*Source: Beeber, L. S., Holditch-Davis, D., Perreria, K., Schwartz, T. A., Lewis, V., Blanchard, H., …, Goldman, B. D. (2010). Short-term in-home intervention reduces depressive symptoms in early Head Start Latina mothers of infants and toddlers. Research in Nursing and Health, 33(1), 60–76. doi: 10.1002/nur.20363*

### PURPOSE/RESEARCH QUESTION

The purpose of the study was to test the effect of an intervention based on Peplau's theory of interpersonal relations on depressive symptoms of Latina mothers of infants and toddlers. Hypothesis 1 stated: "mothers who received the intervention would demonstrate significantly less depressive symptom severity, report less child behavioral aggression and fewer concerns about child social-emotional functioning, and demonstrate greater maternal responsiveness midway through the intervention (T2: 14 weeks), at the conclusion of the intervention (T3: 22 weeks), and 1 month following completion of the intervention (T4: 26 weeks) compared to mothers who received usual care" (p. 62).

### RESEARCH DESIGN

Experimental (pretest/posttest).

### SAMPLE/PARTICIPANTS

The sample comprised 80 newly immigrated, Latina mothers with depressive symptoms who had infants or toddlers. They were recruited for Early Head Start programs located in southeastern United States. The mothers spoke only Spanish or had limited English proficiency.

### DATA COLLECTION

Peplau's theory provided the structure for the intervention that consisted of 16 in-home contacts made by teams of English-speaking master's prepared psychiatric nurses and trained Spanish language interpreters. The focuses of the intervention were (a) reduction of depressive symptoms and their interpersonal sources, (b) choice and use of social support, (c) management of stressful life issues and interpersonal disputes, and (d) development of strategies to increase responsiveness to the child. The CES-D, Spanish version, was used to determine depressive symptoms; child aggression was measured by the Child Behavior Checklist (CBCL), Spanish version, and the Ages and Stages Questionnaire-Social–Emotional (ASQ-SE); and responsiveness to child was assessed using the Maternal–Child Observation (MCO) and the Home Observation for Measurement of the Environment (HOME).

### FINDINGS

The findings were supportive of Peplau's theory:

1. There was a statistically significant greater decrease in depressive symptoms for the mothers receiving the intervention than those who received usual care, T2, $p = 0.02$; T3, $p = 0.01$; and T4, $p = 0.02$.
2. Reports of aggression decreased in the intervention group from T1 to T4 ($p = 0.03$), whereas they increased in the usual care group during the same time frame.
3. There were no statistically significant differences between the two groups related to maternal interactions and responsiveness.

Instrument development to study the nature of nurse–patient relationships began in the 1960s, with the most recent instrument published in 2011 (Dearing & Steadman, 2011). The relatively few numbers of instruments may be explained in part by the phenomenological nature of the theory (Haber, 2000) and in part by its complexity. Table 11.3 provides an overview of some of those instruments.

Peplau has contributed to both the processes used to develop nursing's body of knowledge and the content of that knowledge base. "Optimistically,

legitimatization of practice-derived theory in the 1990s will make theory-testing and hypothesis-generating qualitative research related to Peplau's model a priority for nurse researchers in the new millennium" (Haber, 2000, pp. 59, 60). Peplau and others have suggested research needs or questions for this new millennium. Peplau (1964) identified the following questions for nurses in general hospital settings:

1. How do nurses distinguish between a demand and a need of a patient?

| Table 11.3 | Instruments Used to Test Theory of Interpersonal Relations | |
|---|---|---|
| **Instrument** | **Reference** | **Description** |
| Social Interaction Inventory | Methven, D., & Schlotfeldt, R. (1962). The social interaction inventory. *Nursing Research*, 11(2), 83–88. | Inventory composed of 30 common nurse–patient situations in which the stress faced by the patient and his or her family is identified. For each situation, responses representing five different types are given (i.e., expression of concern that encourages verbalization; expression of sympathy and giving reassurance; inquiry into tangential aspects of the situation; explanations, justifications, or defense of nurse's point of view; rejection or denunciation of patient's need). Validity is described. |
| Therapeutic Behavior Scale | Spring, R., & Turk, H. (1962). A therapeutic behavior scale. *Nursing Research*, 11(4), 214–218. | Tool to rate nurses' responses to patients as therapeutic or nontherapeutic in relation to approach, level, topic, focus, and consistency. Validity and reliability data are included. |
| Facilitative Level of a Therapeutic Relationship | Aiken, L., & Aiken, J. (1973). A systematic approach to the evaluation of interpersonal relationships. *American Journal of Nursing*, 73, 863–867. | Tool to evaluate the implementation of the five core dimensions (empathic understanding, positive regard, genuineness, concreteness, and self-exploration) using a five-point scale of descriptors of nurse's or patient's behaviors. No data on validity or reliability are included. |
| Working Alliance Inventory (WAI) | Horvath, A. O., & Greenberg, L. (1986). The development of the Working Alliance Inventory. In L. Greenberg, & W. Pinsof (Eds.), *Psychotherapeutic process: A research handbook* (pp. 529–556). New York, NY: Guilford Press. | 36-item instrument, with parallel forms for client and therapist to self-report sense of bonding and tasks and goals of the developing therapeutic relationship. Validity and reliability data are included. |
| Relationship Form | Forchuk, C., & Brown, B. (1989). Establishing a nurse–client relationship. *Journal of Psychosocial Nursing and Mental Health Services*, 27(2), 30–34. | 7-point analog scale of the stages of the nurse–patient relationship, using brief descriptions of both the nurse's and the client's roles at each stage. Validity and reliability data are provided. |
| Engagement with Health Care Provider | Bakken, S., Holzemer, W. L., Brown, M. A., Powell-Cope, G. M., Turner, J. G., Inouye, J., … Corless, I. B. (2000). Relationships between perception of engagement with health care provider and demographic characteristics, health status, and adherence to therapeutic regimen in persons with HIV/AIDS. *AIDS Patient Care and STDs*, 14, 189–197. | 13-item scale on which clients rate the nature of their interactions with health care provider using a four-point scale with 1 = always true and 4 = never true. Focuses on issues such as listening, caring, mutuality in decision-making, and respect. Reliability data are provided. |
| Self-Assessment of the Interpersonal Relationship Scale (SAIRS) | Dearing, K. S., & Steadman, S. (2011). The psychometric properties of the self-assessment of the Interpersonal Relationship Scale. *Perspectives in Psychiatric Care*, 47(4), 176–182. doi: 10.1111/j.1744-6163.2010.00287.x | 31-item scale to be rated by health care professional. All items were stated in terms consistent with a therapeutic relationship and rated on a five-point scale: strongly agree, agree, not sure, disagree, and strongly disagree. Three traits are measured: receptive, core, and complimentary. |

2. What is the language behavior during the nurse–patient exchange in the general hospital?

3. How do patients develop sufficient flexibility to incorporate body image changes into views of self after major surgery or major life experiences? What nursing interventions are most helpful to patients during this process?

4. How does the one-to-one relationship fit into the present and the future health care delivery system? (pp. 81, 82).

Perhaps, the most fundamental and pervasive question that researchers of the nurse–patient relationship can ask and attempt to answer is, What aspects of the nurse–patient relationship contribute to the welfare and well-being of patients? (Caris-Verhallen, Kerkstra, & Bensing, 1997). The promotion of the welfare of patients is core to all nursing theories, but for Peplau, the means of achieving that goal focuses on the attributes and behaviors of both the nurse and the patient and in the dynamic interaction that occurs between them.

## Applications of the Theory: Practice

Peplau's theory of interpersonal relations has remained popular with nurses, in earlier years particularly those practicing psychiatric–mental health nursing. Surveys of psychiatric nurses in Canada and the United States found over half of them claiming to use Peplau's theory in their practices (Forchuk, 1993, p. 28). Most recently in the field of mental health, the theory has been used to (a) provide a foundation for care in community-based centers for psychosocial care (Fernandes & de Miranda, 2016), (b) conceptualize the role of mental health consultant liaison (Merritt & Procter, 2010), (c) prepare nurse therapists (Vandermark, 2006), (d) promote therapeutic relationships (Stockman, 2005), (e) care for depressed and potentially suicidal elderly (Campbell, 2001), and (f) prioritize care in community mental health settings (Bonner, 2001).

The theory has also been used to consider practice issues of general concern to nurses, for instance, (a) presence (Zblock, 2010), (b) shared decision-making (Wills, 2010), (c) quality of life (McCarthy & Aquino-Russell, 2009), (d) altered body image (Wiest, 2006), patient autonomy (Moser, Houtepen, & Widdershoven, 2007), (e) power struggles (Kozub & Kozub, 2004), (f) process of aging (Wadensten & Carlsson, 2003), (g) intentionality (Ugarriza, 2002), (h) stress reduction using reminiscence (Puentes, 2002), and (i) explanation of symptoms (Mahoney & Engebretson, 2000).

Examples of application to practice in the last 10 years demonstrate how useful the theory is in a broad range of nursing situations. The theory has been used to (a) care for patients in end-stage kidney disease (Graham, 2006), (b) promote computer-mediated communication (Hrabe, 2005), (c) serve as a foundation for assessing needs in a patient with heart failure (Davidson, Cockburn, Daly, & Fisher, 2004), (d) work with younger residents in long-term care setting (Schafer & Middleton, 2001), (e) improve palliative care (Wallace, 2001), and (f) support parents of children with severe meningococcal disease (Haines, 2000). Peplau's theory has also served as a foundation to educate (a) faculty and students on telehealth through distance learning methods (Gallgher-Lepack, Sheibel, & Gibson, 2009), (b) patients undergoing urinary diversion to promote their recovery (Marchese, 2006), (c) antepartal patients on prevention of prematurity (Tiedje, 2004), and (d) emigrants on cross-cultural health promotion practices (Kater, 2000). Using Middle Range Theory in Practice 11.2 provides an example of the theory applied to a specific practice issue, and Table 11.4, Examples of Theory in Practice, includes descriptions of several applications, demonstrating the usefulness with different populations and different settings.

## Applications of the Theory: Theory and Model Development

Peplau's theory of interpersonal relations is being integrated into new conceptualizations of nursing as a discipline. Using her theory as well as others, Plummer and Molzahn (2009) suggest as a major concept in the metaparadigm quality of life rather than health. Peplau's theory of interpersonal relations has also served as a foundation for the development of other middle range theories and models applicable to practice. Examples include (a) the Model of Simple Reminiscence (Puentes, 2002), (b) Cultural Competence (Warren, 2002), (c) Client–Nurse Interaction Phase of Symptom Management Model (Haworth & Dluhy, 2001), and (d) Interface of Anthropology and Nursing Model (Mahoney & Engebretson, 2000). But Peplau's contributions to nursing are not limited to the content of her theory. She is credited with promoting the "scholarship of nursing practice" (Reed, 1996), integrating nursing practice with a process for ongoing development of nursing's knowledge base.

## USING MIDDLE RANGE THEORY IN PRACTICE　11.2

*Source: Doyle, C., & Buckley, S. (2012). An account of nursing a child with complex needs in the home. Nursing Children and Young People, 24(5), 19–22.*

The seven roles of the nurse as identified by Peplau are applied to working with children with long-term health care needs in their homes. This article provides specific examples of how the roles were realized in these situations. "The main challenges [are] related to feeding, breathing and neurological problems" (p. 19).

### PROBLEM

There are an increasing number of seriously ill children who are likely to be technology-dependent and require medical and nursing care throughout their lifetime. Home is the best environment for these children but that means that appropriate resources must be available for the child and the family care givers.

### NURSING INTERVENTION

Peplau identified seven roles: stranger, resource, teacher, counselor, surrogate, leader, and technical expert. Each is needed by the nurse in working with the child with complex needs and his or her family.

Stranger—is applicable during the first encounter with the family. Respect and positive interest are shown, usually in an informal setting. Ordinary courtesies are often exchanged.

Resource—is used as a source of expertise on a variety of clinical and technical issues. Specific questions often related to a larger issue are answered.

Teacher—is often a mutual role. Family members share their ability to perform specific nursing skills, and the nurse teaches a variety of nursing techniques (e.g., positioning and unblocking feeding tubes).

Counselor—is needed as family members share their concerns. This requires good communication skills, especially the ability to engage as an active listener. Some of the primary issues are dealing with the reality of their child's "life-limiting condition" (p. 21) and how to cope with the ongoing needs of the child.

Surrogate—requires the nurse care for the child with love and compassion, that is, mothering care.

Leader—provides democratic leadership and advocate. Serving as advocate can be needed when working with the multidisciplinary team. But acting as a democratic leader and advocate is often required on a daily basis.

Technical expert—is needed when dealing with the technical equipment needed to care for the seriously ill child. The nurse assists and teaches parents how to use new equipment safely and effectively and finds ways to keep the equipment as unobtrusive as possible.

### Table 11.4　Examples of Theory in Practice

| Citations | Focus |
|---|---|
| Hochberger, J. M. & Lingham, B. (2017). Utilizing Peplau's interpersonal approach to facilitate medication self-management for psychiatric patients. *Archives of Psychiatric Nursing, 31*(1), 122–124. doi: 10.1015/japnu.2016.08.006 | Peplau's theory, emphasizing education and interpersonal skills, is used to assist patients to realize their highest level of functioning. Nurses assume the roles of teaching, supporting, and partnering to promote shared decision-making. The goal is to prepare psychiatric patients to manage their own medications. |
| Davis, J. H. (2016). Faculty roles and processes for NCLEX-RN outcomes: A theoretical perspective. *Teaching and Learning in Nursing, 11*, 171–174. doi: 10.1016/j.teln.2016.07.001 | The phases of the nurse–patient relationship were used by faculty members in their work with students to prepare them for success as a student, particularly preparing them for taking the licensure exam. Specific examples of actions for each phase are identified. |
| Fernandes, R. L., & de Miranda, F. A. N. (2016). Analysis of the theory of interpersonal relationships: Nursing care in psychosocial care centers. *Journal of Nursing UFPE/Revista de Enfermagen UFPE, 10*(2), 880–886. doi: 10.5202/reuol.6884-59404-2-SM-1.100sup201624 | The principles of the therapeutic relationship with the goal of nurses and patients sharing in the identification of problems and solutions are used with patients in Psychosocial Care Centers in Brazil. The phases of the relationship are specifically described for this population. |
| Deane, W. H., & Fain, J. A. (2015). Incorporating Peplau's Theory of Interpersonal Relations to promote holistic communication between older adults and nursing. *Journal of Holistic Nursing, 34*(1), 35–41. doi: 10.1177/08980101155 | The phases of the nurse–patient relationship are described, focusing on the nature of verbal and nonverbal communication for each phase. The goal is that students learn to communicate holistically, able to use both active listening and focusing. It is suggested that the theory be used as a framework for structuring classroom, clinical past-conferences, and skill laboratory activities. |

**Table 11.4   Examples of Theory in Practice** (Continued)

| Citations | Focus |
|---|---|
| Gugel, F., Keitte, P., Tourinho, S. V., Monteiro, F., & Iwata, A. (2014). Collective consultation of growth and development of the child the light of the theory of Peplau. *Anna Nery School Journal of Nursing/Escola Ann Nery Revista de Enfermagem*, *18*(3), 539–543. doi: 10. 5935/1414-8145.20140077 | Each phase of the interpersonal relationship between nurse and patients (in this instance the family caregivers) is described with specific issues related to promoting healthy growth in development in the child. The nature of this relationship should be on empowering the caregiver resulting in mutuality. |
| Searl, K. R., McAllister, M., Dwyer T., Krebs, K. L., Anderson, C., Quinney, L., & McClellan, S. (2014). Little people, big lessons: An innovative strategy to develop interpersonal skills in undergraduate nursing students. *Nurse Education Today*, *34*(9), 1201–1206. doi: 10.1016/j.nedt.2014.04.004 | The phases of interpersonal relationships are applied to the nurse–child relationship with simulation used to provide opportunities for students to apply the theory of and practice the skills using puppets. |
| Berntsson, T., & Hildingh, C. (2013). The nurse–patient relationship in pre-hospital care—From the perspective of Swedish specialist ambulance nursing students. *International Emergency Nursing, 21*, 257–263. doi: 10.1016/j.ienj.2012.10.003 | The actions of the ambulance team during the prehospital experience are identified using Peplau's stages of the nurse–patient relationship. In practice, the identification and resolution phases occurred more than once. |
| Radtke, K. (2013). Improving patient satisfaction with nursing communication using bedside shift report. *Clinical Nurse Specialist, 27*(1), 19–25. doi: 10.10797NUR.0b013e3182777011 | Peplau and Lewin's theories were integrated to improve communication between nurses, patients, and their families by instituting a practice of conducting change-of-shift reports at the patients' bedside. The goal was to improve patient-focused care and thus patient satisfaction. The project did result in an increase in patient satisfaction with communication with nurses. |
| Senn, J. F. (2013). Peplau's theory of interpersonal relations: Application in emergency and rural nursing. *Nursing Science Quarterly, 26*(1), 31–35. doi: 10.1177/089431842466744 | In emergency department settings, the nurse uses the phases of the nurse–patient relationship over a limited time, usually 4 h or less. Because anxiety is a major feature of most patient visits to the emergency department, Peplau's approach to helping patients experiencing anxiety is most applicable. In rural settings, the nurse–patient relationship is necessary for achieving quality patient outcomes. Empathy and active listening are most important. |
| Nwinee, J. P. (2011). Nwinee socio-behavioral self-care management nursing model. *West African Journal of Nursing, 22*(1), 91–98. | Rosenstack' Health Belief Model, King's Theory of Goal Attainment, and Peplau's Theory of Interpersonal Relationships were combined to create a model that is used to help diabetic clients maintain compliance with self-care management. |
| Parent, E., & Scott, L. (2011). Pediatric posterior fossa syndrome (PFS): Nursing strategies in the post-operative period. Improving patient satisfaction with nursing communication using bedside shift report. *Canadian Journal of Neuroscience Nursing, 33*(2), 24–31. | Peplau's theory of interpersonal relationships was applied to working with families of hospitalized children. The children had surgery to treat posterior fossa syndrome. Specific nursing roles, for example, stranger, teacher, and counselor, were considered as they related to phases of the relationship. |
| Penckofer, S., Byrn, M., Mumby, P., & Ferrans, C. E. (2011). Improving subject recruitment, retention, and participation in research through Peplau's theory of interpersonal relations. *Nursing Science Quarterly, 24*(2), 146–151. doi: 10.1177/0894318411399454 | Peplau's theory was found to be successful for recruitment and retention of subjects to a clinical trial of a psychoeducational program to address depression in women with type 2 diabetes. The issues of trust and anxiety as they related to the study were considered as the theory was applied to the orientation, working, and termination phases of the nurse–patient relationship. |
| Merritt, M. K., & Procter, N. (2010). Conceptualising the functional role of mental health consultation-liaison nurse in multi-morbidity, using Peplau's nursing theory. *Contemporary Nurse, 34*(2), 158–166. doi: 10.5172/conu.2010.34.2.158 | The transition from inpatient treatment to the community is challenging for patients with mental health diagnoses. MHCLN plays a significant role during this experience. The actions of the MHCLN are identified for each phase of the relationship, and six roles as identified by Peplau are defined with the specific needs of these patients as a focus. |

# Summary

■ Peplau is acknowledged as the first theorist of the modern era of nursing.

■ Her theory of interpersonal relations in nursing focuses on the stages experienced, the nursing roles used, and the issues addressed in the context of the nurse–patient relationship.

■ In the nursing profession, the primacy of the nurse–patient relationship is still recognized, and Peplau's phenomenological approach to theory development is still valued.

■ "Peplau's work has been influential, particularly (though not exclusively) in mental health nursing and 'her ideas have provided an architectural design for the practice of a discipline'" (Pearson, 2008, p. 80). Her theory has been used in a variety of practice settings and with many different populations.

■ Peplau was able to pull together "loose, ambiguous data and put them into systematic terms that could be tested, applied, and integrated into the practice of psychiatric nursing" (Lego, 1980, p. 68).

■ Because of its complexity, research on the theory of interpersonal relations is not a simple undertaking; further testing of Peplau's theory could make significant contributions to nursing's body of knowledge.

## CRITICAL THINKING EXERCISES

1. In what ways might Peplau's theory of interpersonal relations need to be revised to be most useful to nurses in a health care environment in which contact time between nurse and client is limited?

2. The surrogate role is not one that is frequently mentioned in recent nursing practice literature. Is that role as defined by Peplau relevant to nursing practice as currently experienced? If so, in what way? If not, why?

3. Peplau's theory focuses on the one-to-one therapeutic relationship between a nurse and a patient. Are the phases of relationships, roles of the nurse, psychobiological experiences encountered in the relationship, and psychological tasks described by Peplau relevant in other nursing contexts, for example, in relationships between nurses? If so, what are some examples of these contexts? If not, why?

## REFERENCES

Armstrong, M. E., & Kelly, A. E. (1995). More than the sum of their parts: Martha Rogers and Hildegard Peplau. *Archives of Psychiatric Nursing, 9*(1), 40–44.

Arving, C. (2011). Creating a new profession in cancer nursing? Experiences of working as a psychosocial nurse in cancer care. *Journal of Clinical Nursing, 20*(19/20), 2939–2947.

Bakken, S., Holzemer, W. L., Brown, M. A., Powell-Cope, G. M., Turner, J. G., Inouye, J., … Corless, I. B. (2000). Relationships between perception of engagement with health care provider and demographic characteristics, health status, and adherence to therapeutic regimen in persons with HIV/AIDS. *AIDS Patient Care and STDs, 14*, 189–197.

Bernsston, T., & Hildingh, C. (2013). The nurse-patient relationship in pre-hospital emergency care—From the perspective of Swedish specialist ambulance nursing students. *International Emergency Nursing, 21*, 257–263. doi: 10.1016/j.ienj.2012.10.003

Bonner, G. P. (2001). *Touched by violence and caring for the violator: The lived experiences of nurses who were assaulted by their patients in psychiatric settings* (Doctoral dissertation). Retrieved from CINAHL database (UMI No. AAI3519436).

Boulton, M., & O'Connell, K. A. (2017). Nursing students' perceived faculty support, stress, and substance misuse. *Journal of Nursing Education, 56*(7), 404–411. doi: 10.3928/01484834-20170619-04

Brown-O'Hara, P. (2013). *Influence of academic coaching on: Baccalaureate nursing students' academic success, perceptions of the academic coaching relationship, perceived NCLE-RN exam readiness and success on NCLEX-RN exam* (Doctoral dissertation). Retrieved from CINAHL database (UMI No. AAI3570585).

Butts, J. B., & Rich, K. L. (2015). *Philosophies and theories for advanced nursing practice* (2nd ed.). Boston, MA: Jones & Bartlett.

Caldwell, B. A., Sclafani, M., Piren, K., & Torre, C. (2012). The evolution of advanced practice role in psychiatric nursing in New Jersey: 1960–2010. *Issues in Mental Health Nursing, 33*(4), 217–222. doi: 10.3109/01612840.2011.647253

Caris-Verhallen, W., Kerkstra, A., & Bensing, J. (1997). The role of communication in nursing care for elderly people: A review of the literature. *Journal of Advanced Nursing, 25*, 915–933.

Courey, T. J., Martsolf, D. S., Draucker, C. B., & Strickland, K. B. (2008). Hildegard Peplau's theory and the health care encounters of survivors of sexual violence. *Journal of the American Psychiatric Nurses Association, 14*, 136–143. doi: 10.1177/1078390308315613

D'Antonio, P., Beeber, L., Sills, G., & Naegle, M. (2014). The future in the past: Hildegard Peplau and interpersonal relations in nursing. *Nursing Inquiry, 21*(4), 311–317. doi: 10.1111/nin.12056

Davidson, P., Cockburn, J., Daly, J., & Fisher, R. S. (2004). Patient-centered needs assessment: Rationale for a psychometric measure for assessing needs in heart failure. *Journal of Cardiovascular Nursing, 19*(3), 164–171.

Dearing, K. S., & Steadman, S. (2011). The psychometric properties of the self-assessment of the Interpersonal Relationship Scale. *Perspectives in Psychiatric Care, 47*(4), 176–182. doi: 10.1111/j.1744-6163.2010.00287.x

Draucker, C. B., Cook, C. B., Martsolf, D. S., & Stephenson, P. S. (2012). Adolescent dating violence and Peplau's dimension of the self. *Journal of the American Psychiatric Association, 18*(3), 175–188. doi: 10.1177/1078390312442743

Evans, E. C., & Bullock, L. F. C. (2017). Supporting rural woman during pregnancy: Baby BEEP nurses. *MCN: The American Journal of Maternal Child Nursing, 42*(1), 50–55. doi: 10.1097. NMC.0000000000000305

Evans, E. C., Deutsch, N. L., Drake, E., & Bullock, L. (2017). Nurse-patient interaction as a treatment for antepartum depression: A mixed method analysis. *Journal of the American Psychiatric Nurses Association*, 23(5), 347–359. doi: 10.1177/1078390317705449

Fawcett, J. (2000). *Analysis and evaluation of contemporary nursing knowledge: Nursing models and theories*. Philadelphia, PA: F.A. Davis.

Fernandes, R. L., & de Miranda, F. A. N. (2016). Analysis of the theory of interpersonal relationships: Nursing care in psychosocial care centers. *Journal of Nursing UFPE On Line*, 10(Suppl 2), 880–886. doi: 10.5205/reuol.6884-59404-2-1002sup201624

Forchuk, C. (1991). Peplau's theory: Concepts and their relations. *Nursing Science Quarterly*, 4(2), 54–60.

Forchuk, C. (1993). *Hildegard E. Peplau: Interpersonal nursing theory*. Newbury Park, CA: Sage.

Forchuk, C., & Reynolds, W. (2001). Clients' reflections on relationships with nurses: Comparisons form Canada and Scotland. *Journal of Psychiatric and Mental Health Nursing*, 8, 45–51. Retrieved from onlinelibrary.wiley.com

Forchuk, C., Westwell, J., Martin, M., Bamber-Azzapardi, W., Kosterewa-Tolman, D., & Hux, M. (2000). The developing nurse–client relationship: Nurses' perspectives. *Journal of the American Psychiatric Nurses Association*, 6, 3–10. doi: 10.1177/107839030000600102

Gallgher-Lepack, S., Sheibel, P., & Gibson, C. C. (2009). Integrating telehealth in nursing curricula: Can you hear me now? *Online Journal of Nursing Informatics (OJNI)*, 13(2), 1089–9758. Retrieved from http://ojni.org/

Gastmans, C. (1998). Interpersonal relations in nursing: A philosophical-ethical analysis of the work of Hildegard E. Peplau. *Journal of Advanced Nursing*, 28, 1312–1319. Retrieved from http://gateway1.ovid.com/ovidweb.cgi

George, J. B. (2011). *Nursing theories: The base for professional practice* (6th ed.). Boston, MA: Pearson.

Graham, J. (2006). Nursing theory and clinical practice: How three nursing models can be incorporated into the care of patients with end stage kidney disease. *CANNT Journal*, 16(4), 28–31.

Haber, J. (2000). Hildegard E. Peplau: The psychiatric nursing legacy of a legend. *Journal of the American Psychiatric Nurses Association*, 6(2), 56–62.

Haines, C. (2000). Use of a theoretical framework in pediatric intensive care to provide support for parents of children with severe meningococcal disease. *Nursing in Critical Care*, 5, 87–97. Retrieved from http://www.wiley.com/bw/journal.asp?ref=1362-1017

Haworth, S. K., & Dluhy, N. M. (2001). Holistic symptom management: Modeling the interaction phase. *Journal of Advanced Nursing*, 36, 302–310. Retrieved from www.journalofadvancednursing.com

Hrabe, D. P. (2005). Peplau in cyberspace: An analysis of Peplau's interpersonal relations theory and computer-mediated communication. *Issues in Mental Health Nursing*, 26(4), 397–414.

Kater, V. (2000). A tale of teaching in two cities. *International Nursing Review*, 47, 121–125. Retrieved from http://onlinelibrary.wiley.com/journal/10.1111/(ISSN)1466-7657

Kozub, M. L., & Kozub, F. M. (2004). Dealing with power struggles in clinical and educational settings. *Journal of Psychosocial Nursing and Mental Health Services*, 42(2), 22–31.

Lego, S. (1980). The one-to-one nurse–patient relationship. *Perspectives in Psychiatric Care*, 18(2), 67–89.

Mahoney, J. S., & Engebretson, J. (2000). The interface of anthropology and nursing guiding culturally competent care in psychiatric nursing. *Archives of Psychiatric Nursing*, 14, 183–190. doi: 10.1053/apnu.2000.8657

Marchese, K. (2006). Using Peplau's theory of interpersonal relations to guide the education of patients undergoing urinary diversion. *Urologic Nursing*, 26(5), 363–371. Retrieved from http://www.suna.org/cgi-bin/WebObjects/SUNAMain.woa/wa/viewSection?s_id=1073743840&ss_id=536872962

McCarthy, C. T., & Aquino-Russell, C. (2009). A comparison of two nursing theories in practice: Peplau and Parse. *Nursing Science Quarterly*, 22, 34–40. doi: 10.1177/0894318408329339

McKenna, H. (1997). *Nursing theories and models*. London, UK: Routledge.

Merritt, M. K., & Procter, N. (2010). Conceptualizing the functional role of mental health consultation-liaison nurse in multi-morbidity using Peplau's nursing theory. *Contemporary Nurse*, 34, 158–166. Retrieved from http://www.contemporarynurse.com/

Moser, A., Houtepen, R., & Widdershoven, G. (2007). Patient autonomy in nurse-led shared care: A review of theoretical and empirical literature. *Journal of Advanced Nursing*, 57(4), 357–365.

Moss, R. L. (2015). *Communication skill of novice psychiatric nurses with aggressive psychiatric patients* (Doctoral dissertation). Retrieved from CINAHL database (UMI No. AAI3685393).

O'Toole, A. W., & Welt, S. R. (1989). *Interpersonal theory in nursing practice: Selected works of Hildegard E. Peplau*. New York, NY: Springer.

Parker, M. E., & Smith, M. C. (2010). *Nursing theories and nursing practice* (3rd ed.). Philadelphia, PA: F.A. Davis

Pearson, A. (2008). Dead poets, nursing and contemporary nursing practice (4). *International Journal of Nursing Practice*, 14, 79–80. doi: 10.1111/j.1440-172X.2008.00682.x

Peplau, H. E. (1952). *Interpersonal relations in nursing*. New York, NY: G.P. Putnam's Sons.

Peplau, H. E. (1964). Psychiatric nursing skills and the general hospital patient. *Nursing Forum*, 3(2), 28–37.

Peplau, H. E. (1969). Professional closeness—As a special kind of involvement with a patient, client or family group. *Nursing Forum*, 8, 343–360.

Peplau, H. E. (1985). Help the public maintain mental health. *Nursing Success Today*, 2(5), 30–34.

Peplau, H. E. (1988). The art and science of nursing: Similarities, differences and relations. *Nursing Science Quarterly*, 1, 8–15.

Peplau, H. E. (1989). Theory: The professional dimension. In A. W. O'Toole, & S. R. Welt (Eds.), *Interpersonal theory in nursing practice: Selected works of Hildegard E. Peplau* (pp. 21–30). New York, NY: Springer.

Peplau, H. E. (1991). *Interpersonal relations in nursing: A conceptual frame of reference for psychodynamic nursing*. New York, NY: Springer.

Peplau, H. E. (1992). Interpersonal relations: A theoretical framework for application in nursing practice. *Nursing Science Quarterly*, 5(1), 13–18.

Peplau, H. E. (1997). Peplau's theory of interpersonal relations. *Nursing Science Quarterly*, 10(4), 162–167.

Plummer, M., & Molzahn, A. E. (2009). Quality of life in contemporary nursing theory: A concept analysis. *Nursing Science Quarterly*, 22(2), 134–140. doi: 10.1177/0894318409332807

Porr, C., Drummond, J., & Olson, K. (2012). Establishing therapeutic relationships with vulnerable and potentially stigmatize clients. *Qualitative Health Research*, 22(3), 384–396. doi: 10.1177/1049732311421182

Puentes, W. J. (2002). Simple reminiscence: A stress-adaptation model of the phenomenon. *Issues in Mental Health Nursing*, 23(5), 497–511.

Reed, P. G. (1995). A treatise on nursing knowledge development for the 21st century: Beyond postmodernism [Electronic version]. *Advances in Nursing Science*, 17(3), 70–84.

Reed, P. G. (1996). Transforming practice knowledge into nursing knowledge—A revisionist analysis of Peplau. *Image: The Journal of Nursing Scholarship*, 28, 29–33. Retrieved from http://gateway1.ovid.com/ovidweb.cgi

Reid, K. S., McAllister, M., Dwyer, T., Krebs, K. L., Anderson, C. L., & McLellan, S. (2014). Little people, big lessons: An innovative strategy to develop interpersonal skills in undergraduate nursing students. *Nurse Education Today*, 34(9), 1201–1206. doi: 10.1016/j.nedt.2014.04.004

Schafer, P., & Middleton, J. (2001). Examining Peplau's pattern integrations in long-term care. *Rehabilitation Nursing*, *26*, 192–197. Retrieved from http://www.researchgate.net/journal/0278-4807_Rehabilitation_nursing_the_official_journal_of_the_Association_of_Rehabilitation_Nurses

Sellers, S. C. (1991). *A philosophical analysis of conceptual models of nursing* (Unpublished doctoral dissertation). Iowa State University, Ames, IA.

Sills, G. M. (1978). Hildegard E. Peplau: Leader, practitioner, academician, scholar, and theorist. *Perspectives in Psychiatric Care*, *16*(3), 122–128.

Silverstein, C. M. (2008). From the front lines to the home front: A history of the development of psychiatric nursing in the U.S. during the World War II era. *Issues in Mental Health Nursing*, *29*, 719–737. doi: 10.1080/01612840802129087

Stockman, C. (2005). A literature review of the progress of the psychiatric nurse–patient relationship as described by Peplau. *Issues in Mental Health Nursing*, *26*, 911–919. doi: 10.1080/01612840500248197

Thelly, A. S., & Priyalatha (2013). A qualitative study to study the lived experience of cancer patients and their family members in a view to develop a palliative care guideline for the nursing personnel at selected hospitals in Bangalore. *International Journal of Nursing Education*, *5*(2), 7–11. doi: 10.5958/j.0974-9357.5.2.055

Tiedje, L. B. (2004). Teaching is more than telling: Education about prematurity in a prenatal clinic waiting room. *MCN: The American Journal of Maternal/Child Nursing*, *29*(6), 373–379.

Tofthagen, R. (2004). An encounter between two realities: What experiences do psychiatric nurses gain from their efforts to create a helping relationship with psychotic patients? *Nordic Journal of Nursing Research and Clinical Studies*, *24*(2), 4–9.

Ugarriza, D. N. (2002). Intentionality: Applications within selected theories of nursing. *Holistic Nursing Practice*, *16*(4), 41–50. Retrieved from http://journals.lww.com/hnpjournal/pages/default.aspx

Vandermark, L. M. (2006). Awareness of self and expanding consciousness: Using nursing theories to prepare nurse-therapists. *Issues in Mental Health Nursing*, 363–371. doi: 10.1080/01612840600642885

Wadensten, B., & Carlsson, M. (2003). Nursing theory views on how to support the process of ageing. *Journal of Advanced Nursing*, *42*, 118–124. Retrieved from http://www.journalofadvancednursing.com/

Wallace, P. R. (2001). Improving palliative care through effective communication. *International Journal of Palliative Nursing*, *7*, 86–90. Retrieved from http://www.ijpn.co.uk/

Warren, B. J. (2002). The interlocking paradigm of cultural competence: A best practice approach. *Journal of the American Psychiatric Nurses Association*, *8*(6), 209–213.

Welch, M. (1995). Hildegard Peplau in a conversation with Mark Welch. Part I. *Nursing Inquiry*, *2*(1), 53–56.

Wiest, D. A. (2006). Impact of conceptual nursing models in a professional environment. *Topics in Emergency Medicine*, *28*(2), 161–166.

Wills, D. E. (2010). Sharing decisions with patients: Moving beyond patient-centered-care. *Journal of Psychosocial Nursing and Mental Health Services*, *48*(3), 1–5.

Winship, G., Bray, J., Repper, J., & Hinshelwood, R. D. (2009). Collective biography and the legacy of Hildegard Peplau, Annie Altschul and Eileen Skellern: The origins of mental health nursing and its relevance to the current crisis in psychiatry. *Journal of Research in Nursing*, *14*(6), 505–517. doi: 10.1177/1744987109347039

Zauszniewski, J. A. (2009). Mentoring our next generation: Time to dance. *Journal of Child and Adolescent Psychiatric Nursing*, *22*(3), 113–114.

## SELECTED WORKS BY PEPLAU

Peplau, H. E. (1984). Help the public maintain mental health. *Nursing Success Today*, *2*(5), 30–34.

Peplau, H. E. (1986). The nurse as counselor. *Journal of American College Health*, *35*(11), 11–14.

Peplau, H. E. (1987). Interpersonal constructs for nursing practice. *Nurse Education Today*, *7*(5), 201–208.

Peplau, H. E. (1989). Future directions in psychiatric nursing from the perspective of history. *Journal of Psychosocial Nursing*, *27*(2), 18–21, 25–28, 39, 40.

Peplau, H. E. (1994). Quality of life: An interpersonal perspective. *Nursing Science Quarterly*, *7*(1), 10–15.

Peplau, H. E. (1995). Some unresolved issues in era of biopsychosocial nursing. *Journal of the American Psychiatric Nurses Association*, *1*(3), 92–96.

Peplau, H. E. (1996). Fundamental and special—The dilemma of psychiatric mental nursing—Commentary. *Archives of Psychiatric Nursing*, *10*(4), 162–167.

## SELECTED WORKS ON PEPLAU'S THEORY

Beeber, L. S. (1998). Treating depression through the therapeutic nurse–patient relationship. *The Nursing Clinics of North America*, *33*(1), 153–157.

Beeber, L., Anderson, C. A., & Sills, G. M. (1990). Peplau's theory in practice. *Nursing Science*, *3*(1), 6–8.

Bonner, G. (2001). Mental health. The concept of priority as it relates to a community mental health team. *British Journal of Community Nursing*, *6*, 86–93. Retrieved from www.bjcn.co.uk/

Campbell, D. M. (2001). Learning to care. *Assignment*, *7*, 25–38.

Comley, A. L. (1994). A comparative analysis of Orem's self-care model and Peplau's interpersonal theory. *Journal of Advanced Nursing*, *20*(4), 755–760.

Feely, M. (1997). Using Peplau's theory in nurse-client relations. *International Nursing Review*, *44*(4), 115–120.

Forchuk, C. (1991). A comparison of the works of Peplau and Orlando. *Archives of Psychiatric Nursing*, *5*(1), 38–45.

Forchuk, C. (1991). Conceptualizing the environment of the individual with chronic mental illness. *Issues in Mental Health Nursing*, *12*, 159–170.

Forchuk, C. (1994). Preconceptions in the nurse–client relationship. *Journal of Psychiatric and Mental Health Nursing*, *1*(3), 145–149.

Fowler, J. (1994). A welcome focus on a key relationship: Using Peplau's model in palliative care. *Professional Nurse*, *10*(3), 194–197.

Fowler, J. (1995). Taking theory into practice: Using Peplau's model in the care of a patient. *Professional Nurse*, *10*(4), 226–230.

Greg, D. E. (1978). Hildegard E. Peplau: Her contributions. *Perspectives in Psychiatric Care*, *16*(3), 118–121.

Martin, M. L., Forchuk, C., Santopinto, M., & Butcher, H. K. (1992). Alternatives approaches to nursing practice: Application of Peplau, Rogers, and Parse. *Nursing Science Quarterly*, *5*(2), 80–85.

Samhammer, J., & Myers, H. B. (1964). Learning in the nurse–patient relationship. *Perspectives in Psychiatric Care*, *2*(3), 20–29.

Schroder, P. J. (1979). Nursing intervention with patients with thought disorders. *Perspectives in Psychiatric Care*, *17*(1), 32–39.

Zauszniewski, J. A. (2010). Mentoring our next generation: Time to dance. *Journal of Child and Adolescent Psychiatric Nursing*, *22*, 113–114. doi: 10.1111/j1744-6171.2009.00191x

Zblock, D. M. (2010). Nursing presence in contemporary nursing practice. *Nursing Forum*, *45*, 120–124. Retrieved from http://onlinelibrary.wiley.com/journal/10.1111/(ISSN)1744-6198

# 12 Attachment

Trine Klette and Sandra J. Peterson

## Definition of Key Terms

| | |
|---|---|
| **Affective empathy** | An individual's congenital tendency to identify with the emotions of others |
| **Attachment** | An innate psychobiological urge to form lasting bonds with a primary caregiver |
| **Care** | Watchful and gentle ways of attending to the needs of others |
| **Cognitive empathy** | A developmentally conditioned ability to understand and take the perspective of others |
| **Comfort** | Activities based on an individual's capacity for sensitivity and empathy whose goal is to relieve distress |
| **Early interaction** | Dyadic activities performed by a child and its caregiver |
| **Health** | Composite process and phenomenon including experience of physical well-being, sense of logical coherence, meaningful social functioning, and feeling of security |
| **Internal working model** | Basic assumptions about oneself, others, and the interaction with others |
| **Nursing care** | Theoretical and training-based knowledge and skills in ways of attending to the basic needs of individuals or groups of individuals, independent of age, sex, ethnic background, or beliefs, with regard to context and the given environments |
| **Patterns of attachment** | The distinct ways an individual tends to behave when feeling distressed |
| **Sensitivity** | The ability to perceive and understand signals from others |

## Historical Background

Attachment theory was first presented by John Bowlby in 1957 in the form of three lectures for the British psychoanalytic society. In the first lecture, "The nature of the child's tie to its mother," Bowlby claimed that the human child is ready to enter into interaction and relations from the moment he or she is born. By proposing this, Bowlby opposed two of the dominant theories on child development at that time: the theory of secondary drive and the theory of object relations (Klette, 2007). Building on Freud's work on the subconscious and transference but opposing his theories of psychosexual phases and aggression as basic developmental forces, Bowlby proposed that it is the real-life interactions and experiences that are most important for an individual's psychological health. The actual satisfaction or denial of basic needs during the upbringing years (not fantasies or phases) is the basis for an individual's capacity to enter into and maintain social relations. This is seen as fundamental to psychological health. By making this claim, Bowlby moved attention on human development and functioning from intrapersonal conflicts to interpersonal relations.

## Description of Attachment Theory

Integrating knowledge from medicine, ethology, learning theories, developmental biology, and psychology, John Bowlby presented the theory on human attachment. Observations of animal behaviors had been of great importance when he stated that all primates are conditioned to seek proximity to a caregiver for the purpose of protection and survival (Harlow, 1958). Having an inborn, specific repertoire of communicative expressions and functions, human infants are normally able to exhibit specific behaviors to establish and maintain proximity to caregivers (Simpson & Belsky,

2008). These are smiling and vocalizing (signaling behaviors), crying and screaming (aversive behaviors), and sucking and clinging (active behaviors). During childhood and adolescence, these behaviors mature and integrate and will vary in strength until they are *referred to the backseat* as Bowlby put it (Bowlby, 1958). But all the attachment-related behaviors are maintained at different levels of activity and will be used in new combinations throughout life. When danger or threats occur, they may be demonstrated just as strongly as in childhood, especially crying and clinging.

Initially, it was the observations of children's responses to separations from their primary caregivers that had caught Bowlby's attention. These observations led among others to the description of three phases of reactions to such separations: protest, grief, and denial. The longer the separations had lasted and the younger the child had been when the separation had occurred, the more serious the psychological disturbances were observed to be (Bowlby, 1960). Attachment theory describes how and why an infant organizes and integrates behavior focused on a specific mother figure during the first year of life. Because the first attachment relationship is of vital importance to the child, separation from the primary caregiver is experienced as utterly threatening. According to the theory, attachment relationships are the products of a behavior response system, which "supervise" the physical presence and the psychological availability of the mother figure and activate/regulate attachment behavior directed at her (Ainsworth & Bowlby, 1989; George & Solomon, 1996). From a biologic point of view, such behavior enhances the infant's probability of survival and later reproduction. As long as the infant feels safe, the attachment figure functions as a secure base for exploration, play, and other social activities. But when the child feels distressed, the goals of exploration are normally overruled by the need for protection from the caregiver. Between 8 and 18 months, separations from the primary caregiver cause particularly intense distress in a child. Even though the attachment system never locks down, it becomes increasingly invisible over the years (Bowlby, 1958).

## Definition of Key Concepts

### ATTACHMENT

Bowlby described the core of attachment to be a child's preferred wish for contact with its primary caregiver when feelings of threats occur (Bowlby, 1958). The establishment of attachment

relationships develops through phases. The first three take place between birth and the age of 3. From 7 months to 3 years of age, the three primary functions of attachment are most noticeable:

1. *Proximity maintenance*: staying close to and resisting separations from the attachment figure
2. *Safe haven behavior*: turning to the attachment figure for support and comfort
3. *Secure base behavior*: using the attachment figure as a base for exploration and other nonattachment activities

The fourth phase, which begins about 3 years of age, normally implies a child's increased ability to take the caregiver's perspective and develop a "goal-corrected partnership" with the caregiver (Posada et al., 1995; Simpson & Belsky, 2008).

### INTERNAL WORKING MODELS

On the basis of the child's needs and demands and the caregiver's responses, basic beliefs, expectations, and attitudes about relationships develop. Such mental representations were termed *internal working models* by Bowlby (1988). The development and integration of the internal working model include and affect the psychological, physiological, social development, and functioning of the child (Hofer, 1994; Luecken, 2000; Roisman et al., 2009; Schore, 1994). The core in a child's working model of the world is the comprehension of who the attachment figure is, where it can be found, and how it can be expected to respond when called upon. The perception of how acceptable the child is in the eyes of the caregiver is seen as the core in the child's inner working model of the self. A child growing up with available, predictable, and supportive parents tends to construct an internal working model of itself as capable and worthy of help and support. Children experiencing little or unpredictable response and support or have caregivers who threaten, harm, or abandon them tend to develop internal working models of themselves as unworthy, unloved, or ineffective. Some of these children might, however, develop positive internal working models of their caregivers to be able to live in and tolerate the relationship. Regardless of the upbringing, as an internal working model matures and integrates, it becomes gradually subconscious and automatic.

### PATTERNS OF ATTACHMENT

Bowlby's collaboration with psychologist Mary Ainsworth represented a breakthrough with regard to further research and application of attachment theory. Based on a study of attachment-related behavior among families with small children in Baltimore, Ainsworth was able to describe certain distinct patterns of attachment behavior (Ainsworth, Blehar, Waters, & Wall, 1978). These patterns were, respectively, termed *secure, anxious avoidant*, and *anxious ambivalent*. Ainsworth also constructed the classic observational method for studying attachment behavior in children between 8 and 18 months: "The Strange Situation Procedure" (Ainsworth & Bell, 1970). The procedure, lasting for about 20 minutes, consists of seven episodes including two short separations between the child and the caregiver. In the first separation episode, the child is left with a stranger, and in the second, it is left alone. Since the attachment system is open and visible at this age, trained coders will be able to ascribe the children to either of the following categories:

*Secure attachment*: A securely attached child is generally described as emotionally open and straightforward, claiming comfort and protection from the caregiver when distressed and able to settle down and eventually exhibit creative playfulness when they feel secure. The secure pattern is associated with available, predictable, and sensitive caregiving.

*Anxious avoidance*: A child who has developed an anxious–avoidant pattern of attachment generally tries to suppress or hide open manifestations of negative emotions and reactions when distressed, avoiding eye contact with the caregiver and often using toys as a distraction. This pattern is associated with relatively consistent distant, reserved, rejecting, or punitive caregiving. Maltreated children with this pattern are most likely to have been victims of physical and emotional abuse (Weinfeld, Sroufe, Egeland, & Carlson, 2008).

*Anxious ambivalence*: Children who develop an anxious ambivalent pattern of attachment show mixed emotions toward their caregiver when distressed. Conspicuous helplessness and passivity alternate with outbursts of aggression or fear. A child with an anxious ambivalent pattern of attachment tends not to explore the surroundings very much but concentrates its attention on the caregiver's whereabouts. The pattern of anxious ambivalence is associated with unpredictable caregiving, where the caregiver tends to follow his/her own impulses rather than consistently responding to the signals and needs of the child. Maltreated children displaying this pattern of attachment are most likely to have been victims of neglect (Weinfeld et al., 2008). Ainsworth described two subpatterns of anxious ambivalence.

By describing the pattern of attachment and developing a procedure for observing attachment behavior in small children, attachment research developed rapidly (Cassidy & Shaver, 2008). It soon became clear, however, that some children could not be ascribed to any of the original patterns described by Ainsworth. These children, who exhibited a confusing mixture of behavioral responses, often combined with tics and other bodily oddities, were eventually described as disorganized with regard to attachment (Main & Hesse, 1990; Main & Solomon, 1990).

*Disorganized attachment*: Disorganized attachment is particularly associated with fearful and/or frightening parenting that makes it impossible for the child to develop a coherent attachment pattern. Prolonged isolation, neurological problems, and pharmacologic interventions have later been added to the precursors for disorganized attachment. It has been speculated that the seemingly meaningless body movements seen in many children with disorganized attachment correspond to what is described as conflict behavior in animals. That is, the movements are expressions of the impossible in the child's situation, caught as it is between the drive and the need to seek closeness to and protection from the caregiver and the impulse to fight or flee from the very same person.

*Earned secure*: Adults have been observed who, despite strong evidence of unloving parents and a harsh upbringing, appear coherent and balanced with regard to attachment in the Adult Attachment Interview.\* These individuals were described as "earned secure" (Hesse, 2008; Pearson, Cohn, Cowan, & Cowan, 1994). Studies indicate that attachment-related behavior is as stable and robust with earned security as with natural security. Alternative secure attachment and psychological treatment seem to account for such positive changes of an attachment strategy.

## Attachment as a Basic Need

By describing the basic human needs, Abraham Maslow (1999) made a great contribution to the works of a variety of disciplines, including nursing. Although the need for attachment is not explicitly addressed in Maslow's pyramid, it is touched upon through (the needs for) shelter, protection, security, family, relationships, and so on. It is, however, strongly indicated by research that the need for attachment not only is a need in its own right but also in fact is a central one. With great respect to Maslow's invaluable work, a pyramid that is

---

\* The Adult Attachment Interview is a semistructured interview about attachment-related episodes from the childhood to the present (George, Kaplan, & Main, 1985).

modified to integrate attachment needs is suggested in Figure 12.1.

## Attachment and Care

Attachment theory gives strong evidence to the importance of meeting a child's need for contact and closeness with understanding, respect, and warmth. It also gives evidence on the importance of care in general and in cases of disease, illness, and loss in particular. Individual care factors known to promote attachment security are availability, predictability, and sensitivity. Socially contributing factors are extended networks, education, stable incomes, preventive health care, and a general social stability (Cassidy & Shaver, 2008; Killén, Klette, & Arenevik, 2006; Solomon & George, 1996).

Individuals who have received adequate care during childhood tend to be open and trusting toward others and also exhibit empathy and caring behavior toward the needs of others. Individuals who have experienced rejection, abuse, and little comfort and protection during childhood tend to withdraw, trivialize, or dismiss care needs. Individuals who have been exposed to unpredictable and neglectful care seem to alternate between passivity and intrusive behavior (Klette, 2007).

Attachment relationships will be formed throughout life, and when first formed, such relationships tend to be strong and important, for better or worse. Attachment theory offers an opportunity to understand, observe, and change some apparently fixed premises for human behavior. Instead of assigning behaviors merely to genetic conditions and individual dispositions, attachment theory and research have shown that crucial social behavior is *learned* through interaction and care (see Fig. 12.2).

## Attachment and Health

Health is understood as a process and phenomenon that includes experience of physical well-being, sense of logical coherence, meaningful social functioning, and the feeling of security. Seen in this light, secure attachment accounts for many positive health-related conditions and functions. Among other things, a marked lack of securely attached individuals is found in various clinical psychiatric samples (van Ijzendoorn, Goldberg, Koonenberg, & Frenkel, 1992). As mentioned earlier, basic beliefs/expectations/attitudes and patterns of self-protective behavior tend to reemerge in times of threats, illness, or loss (Bretherton & Munholland, 2008). Bowlby described the early behaviors (crying, clinging, etc.) as *old soldiers* who are put to rest, but who will rise again when needed. How and to which extent the old soldiers will fight will vary according to the attachment strategy of the individual. Signs of secure attachment are, among other things, trust and ability to ask for and make use of help and care. Securely attached individuals also tend to be more balanced and flexible than individuals with other attachment experiences, and they are better able to regulate and adjust their feelings and reactions to a stressful situation. Evidence of connections between child abuse and

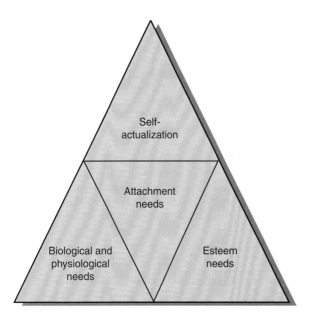

**Figure 12.1** Maslow's pyramid modified to integrate attachment needs.

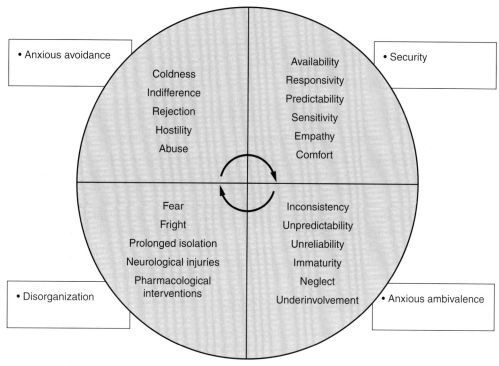

**Figure 12.2** Factors underlying the patterns of attachment.

neglect, various diseases, and anxious and disorganized attachment is significant (Klette, 2008). A pioneering study by McWilliams and Bailey (2010) shows strong association between adult attachment ratings and a number of health conditions. The study findings support that insecure (i.e., anxious) attachment is a risk factor for disease and chronic illness, particularly conditions involving the cardiovascular system. See also Donovan and Leavitt (1985), Reite and Field (1985), Spangler, Schieche, Ilg, Maier, and Ackerman (1994), and Hofer (2003) for studies of associations between attachment and psychobiology.

Epigenetics is a new research area that offers significant insights into the interaction between genes and environment. Among others, studies show that the quality of care received in early age influences the development of the brain and behaviors by altering processes that control the expression of the DNA. Enzymes that block, repair, and switch functions of the genes on and off are described. The findings indicate that psychiatric diseases are related to stress in relation to primary caregivers or significant others in childhood (Donovan & Leavitt, 1985; Fosse, 2009; Heim, Newport, Bonsall, Miller, & Nemeroff, 2003; Luecken, 2000; Szyf, McGowan, & Meaney, 2008).

## Development and Change

If the upbringing conditions of a child remain unaltered, the basic attitudes, expectations, and behavioral strategies also tend to remain unchanged. If the conditions change for the better, the internal working model and the pattern of attachment may change in a more secure direction. If the conditions change for the worse, they may change in an anxious or even disorganized direction. Earned security indicates that attachment status can be altered throughout life, but it appears to become increasingly resistant to change. The problem with changing status of attachment is probably not least due to the subconscious and automatic character of the internal working model. But also the common tendency to believe that an attachment pattern is the product of individual dispositions probably accounts for this. The first years and the puberty period seem to be most susceptible to attachment-related influence and change, but the attachment system also tends to open up for adaptation during pregnancy and in the postpartum period as well as in cases of loss, illness, or disease. According to Bowlby, the ability to change is reduced with age, but changes occur throughout life, which means that an individual is always open to positive influence.

## Applications of Attachment Theory: Research

Attachment theory research highlights the importance of preventive health care directed at families with small children. Guidance, practical help, and emotional support with regard to behaviors that facilitate secure attachments appear to be among the best ways to promote health and prevent disease. Obtaining knowledge about attachment may help many parents to improve their interactive behaviors. Others will need much supervision and close follow-up to be able to change destructive patterns. Some parents, independent of the investments made, will still not be able to change, and therefore, alternative care should be found. Virginia Henderson's concepts of strength, will, and knowledge may prove very useful in assessing and addressing attachment-related health behaviors. They can be seen as corresponding to the phenomena of the internal working model: expectations, attitudes, and assumptions.

Although it is known to be of great importance for health care behaviors, the phenomenon of will is still quite elusive and unclear. Henderson equaled will to "love of life," and psychologist Rollo May (1969) describes will not as an independent ability or special personality trait, but as a product of care. Will and wish cannot be the basis of care, but rather the opposite, they are found in and manifest themselves as liberated and activated care. By describing the internal working model and the patterns of attachment, Bowlby and Ainsworth provided new insights into the phenomenon of will. Some patients apparently do not, despite huge investments, want to change their self-destructive behaviors or engage in health-preventive activities. Taking the patient's attachment experiences into account may prove valuable when planning interventions. A definition of will as *the ability to be or do something, rooted in attachment experiences*, is suggested.

Much of the current research is published either in nonnursing journals or by international nurses. Published research demonstrates the applicability of attachment theory across cultures and to populations throughout the life span. Intergenerational transmission of attachment has been a focus of a number of research studies. Şen and Kavlak (2012) considered the adult attachment patterns of mothers and grandmothers in Turkey; Cassibba, Coppola, Sette, Curci, and Costantini (2017)

examined attachment security across three generations; Bar-On and Scharf (2016) examined the similarities and differences in attachment relationships between fathers and sons; Cassibba, Granqvist, and Costantini (2013) considered mother's attachment security as a predictor of children's sense of closeness to God; Özcan, Boyacioğlu, and Tomruk (2016) studied the relationship between the attachment patterns of mothers who experienced childhood trauma and suffer with a psychiatric disorder and the trauma and attachment styles of their children; and Behrens, Haltigan, and Bahm (2016) considered the intergenerational transmission gap, particularly as it relates to security.

Research has been conducted to consider the attachment issues of premature infants (Tilokskulchai, Phatthanasiriwethin, Vichitsukon, & Serisathien, 2002), infants with low birth weights (Gathwala, Singh, & Balhara, 2008; Wolke, Eryigit-Madzwamuse, & Gutbrod, 2014), infants with orofacial clefts (Habersaat et al., 2013), infants from low-income Korean families (Lee, McCreary, Breitmayer, Kim, & Yang, 2013), irritable infants (Sherman, Stupica, Dykas, Ramos-Marcuse, & Cassidy, 2013), and paternal involvement in breast-feeding (Viana Rêgo, Alves e. Souza, Assis da Rocha, & Santos Alves, 2016).

There has also been an interest in research of attachment among the elderly. For instance, (a) Cicirelli (2010) concluded that attachment networks were important for maximum adaptation in old age; (b) Verdecias, Jean-Louis, Zizi, Casimir, and Browne (2009) found in the elderly possible associations between secure attachment styles and positive but subjective measures of sleep; (c) Gillath, Johnson, Selcuk, and Teel (2011) demonstrated a relationship between securely attached older adults and the maintenance of social ties with subsequent low levels of depression; (d) Falk, Wijk, Persson, and Falk (2013) identified accepting frailty, looking on the bright side of life, reconciling to one's biography, and feeling valued as the four dimensions that enabled individuals to construct attachment in a residential care facility; and (e) Loetz et al. (2013) found that in palliative care situations, there is a dialectical balance between security and separation, phenomena common in both attachment and spirituality.

Attachment theory has also been the focus of research on nurses and nursing students. Examples of research on attachment of these individuals include the study of (a) attachment styles of staff caring for dementia patients (Kokkonen, Cheston, Dallos, & Smart, 2014), (b) the impact of nursing education on the attachment styles of students in Turkey (Kaya, 2010), and (c) the effect of parental and peer attachments on Egyptian and Saudi nursing students' academic success (Gemeay, Ahmed, Ahmad, & Al Mahmoud, 2015).

The Gemeay et al. study was cross-cultural in nature. A cross-cultural study of attachment was also conducted by Gojman et al. (2012). They compared the experiences of intergenerational attachment between Spanish-speaking adults of middle to high socioeconomic status in urban setting and Indian adults in rural setting in Mexico. Interestingly, they found attachment theory to be cross-culturally robust.

## MEASURES OF ATTACHMENT THEORY

A number of measurements have been developed since Ainsworth's strange situation, and great advances have been made in measuring attachment throughout the life span. Table 12.1 summarizes other measures of maternal–child attachment and attachment experiences of children from infancy through adolescence. In addition to the measures identified in the table, Q-set methods have been used to assess attachment in preschool-aged children (Waters & Deane, 1985). The research described in Using Middle Range Theory in Research 12.1 provides an example of an instrument used in the study of attachment.

A number of instruments have been developed to assess attachment in adults. The Attachment Script Assessment (ASA) is a narrative measure using a set of prompt words to create a story about an attachment issue (Waters & Rodrigues-Doolabh,

2004). The more common approaches include the Adult Attachment Interview (AAI) that assesses general and specific memories of childhood (Hesse, 2008) and the Adult Attachment Projective Picture System (AAP), which involves telling stories based on picture stimuli (George & West, 2012). Self-reporting questionnaires have also been used to assess attachment in adults. Bartholomew and Horowitz (1991) developed a four-category model of attachment and the Relationship Questionnaire (RQ) to measure the styles. To assess secure attachment styles in adults with intellectual challenges, the Manchester Attachment Scale-Third party observational measure (MAST) was developed. This measure uses a Likert scale competed by professional informants to determine attachment behaviors (Penketh, Hare, Flood, & Walker, 2014).

# Applications of Theory: Practice

As with applications of attachment theory to research, the theory can be used in practice throughout the life span. This use begins with the newborn population and proves useful until the later years of life. For instance, to promote parental attachment with newborns, nurses can foster nurturing touch by allowing parents as much access to their new child during the first hour of his/her life and throughout their time in the hospital. Breast-feeding provides prolonged times of contact between mother and child. The U.S. Baby-Friendly

**Table 12.1    Measures of Attachment in Children**

| Instrument | Focus | Citation |
|---|---|---|
| Maternal Attachment Inventory (MAI) | Maternal affectionate attachment (questionnaire) | Muller, M. E. (1994). A questionnaire to measure mother to infant attachment. *Journal of Nursing Measurement, 2*(2), 129–141 |
| Preschool Assessment of Attachment (PAA) | Patterns of attachment in 18-month to 5-year-old children (observation) | Crittenden, P. M. (1992). Quality of attachment in the preschool years. *Development and Psychopathology, 4,* 209–241 |
| Attachment Story Completion (ASCT) | Attachment style in response to a stress-inducing stories (recorded interview) | Bretherton, I., Ridgeway, D., & Cassidy, J. (1990). Assessment internal working models of the attachment relationship. In M. T. Greenberg, D. Cicchetti, & E. M. Cummings (Eds.), *Assessment in the preschool years: Theory research and interventions.* Chicago, IL: Chicago University Press |
| Child Attachment Interview (CAI) | Relationships with parents and attachment-related events in 3- to 8-year-olds (semistructured interview | Target, M., Fonagy, P., & Schmueli-Goetz, Y. (2003). Attachment representations in school-aged children: The development of the Child Attachment Interview (CAI). *Journal of Child Psychotherapy, 29*(2), 171–186 |
| Attachment Interview for Childhood and Adolescence | Organization of transition from late childhood to early adolescence (interview) | Ammaniti, M., Van Ijzendoorn, M. H., Speranza, A. M., & Tambelli, R. (2000). Internal working models of attachment during late childhood and early adolescence: An exploration of stability and change. *Attachment & Human Development, 2*(3), 328–346. doi: 10.1080/14616730010001587 |

**USING MIDDLE RANGE THEORY IN RESEARCH    12.1**

*Source:* Killén, K., Klette, T., & Arenevik, E. (2006). Tidlig mor-barn samspill i norske familier (early mother–child interaction in Norwegian families). *Tidskift for Norsk Psykologforening, 43,* 694–701.

## PURPOSE/RESEARCH QUESTION

The aim of the study was to investigate relations between early mother–child interaction and the development of attachment.

## RESEARCH DESIGN

Prospective longitudinal design.

## PARTICIPANTS

There were 293 mother–child dyads, observed from 3 months until 4½ years old. The participants were from different socioeconomic districts in Norway and also included dyads from mother–child institutions.

## DATA COLLECTION

The procedures used in the study were the Care Index (see below), Ainsworth's strange situation, and a short questionnaire concerning education, income, social network support, drug abuse, and medical diagnoses.

### Care Index

The Care Index is a scoring system for observing parent–child interaction under nonthreatening conditions on the basis of short videotapes (Crittenden, 2000). Sensitivity to the child's signals is the central concept that the Care Index coding system is built around. Crittenden defines adult sensitivity as a behavior pattern that pleases the child most, increases its well-being, and reduces its distress, and it is seen as a dyadic concept. According to the definition, it also incorporates the child's temperament and mother's empathy. The mothers' behavior is scored by a two-point scoring system on the three dimensions: sensitive, passive, or controlling (open or hidden). The child's behavior is scored on four dimensions: cooperative, difficult, passive, or compulsive compliant. The behaviors scored include seven elements: (a) facial expression, (b) vocal expression, (c) position and body contact, (d) expression of affection, (e) turn-taking contingent, (f) control, and (g) choice of activity. The first four of these aspects are assessment of affect within the dyad. The final three refer to temporal contingencies. The two points could both be placed on one dimension (for instance, sensitive), or they might be split (for instance, between sensitive and controlling). The sum of the score should always be 14 points. Obtaining between 11 and 14 points on the sensitive and cooperative scales can, according to Crittenden, be considered sufficient for the "sensitive" and "cooperative" categories. Scores between 7 and 10 points are classified as "adequate (for adults) and mixed cooperative (for infants)." Less than six sensitive or cooperative items should yield classifications of "inept" (5 to 6) and "at risk" (0 to 4), which can be "controlling" and/or "unresponsive" (for adults) and "difficult" and/or "passive" (for infants). The Care Index is considered useful in applied settings to screen for risk, guide intervention, and assess some outcomes of treatment. When used diagnostically, it is emphasized that the data provided by the Care Index would constitute only one part of information, which could be useful in conjunction with other information.

| Crittenden's Sensitivity Scale (Crittenden, 2000) | | Proposed Sensitivity Scale | |
| --- | --- | --- | --- |
| 13–14 points | Mutual delight, joy in one another; a dance | 8–14 points | "Good enough" mother–child interaction |
| 11–12 points | Smooth, pleasing interaction; playful shared positive affect | | |
| 9–10 points | Quite satisfactory play; no problems, but no dance | | |
| 7–8 points | Adequate play, but noticeable periods of dyssynchrony (either controlling or unresponsive) | | |
| 5–6 points | Clear, unresolved problems; limited playfulness, but no evidence of hostility or lack of empathy (unresponsiveness) | 5–7 points | Mother–child interaction at "risk" |

**USING MIDDLE RANGE THEORY IN RESEARCH   12.1 (Continued)**

| Crittenden's Sensitivity Scale (Crittenden, 2000) | | Proposed Sensitivity Scale | |
|---|---|---|---|
| 3–4 points | Clear lack of empathy; nevertheless, some feeble (insufficient or unsuccessful) attempts are made to respond to infant; lack of playful quality | 0–4 points | "Maltreatment" interaction between mother and child |
| 0–2 points | Total failure to perceive or attempt to sooth infant's distressed state; no play | | |

**RESULTS**

From the Care Index, strong correlations were found between education, social network, social stress factors, and the mothers' sensitivity at the first two observations. At 6 to 7 months, but not at 3 to 4 months, there were observed significant differences in sensitivity between mothers exposed to, respectively, low and high socio-economic stress. At both points of observation, significantly lower sensitivity was seen in the mothers from the mother–child institutions. The Care Index categories were, however, found to be too detailed for clinical use. It was, therefore, suggested that they should be divided into three: "good enough" interactions (more than eight points), "at-risk" interactions (7 to 5 points), and "maltreatment" interactions (4 to 0 points).

The main finding was that the use of the three classification categories could predict infant attachment at 1 year and therefore might be used to serve as a basis for selective and indicated prevention as well as early intervention.

Hospital Initiative, 2010, has stated guidelines and evaluation criteria that support breast-feeding, and nurses can encourage its adoption. Nurses can also encourage parents to get to know their infant using the sense of touch (Duhn & Ikuta, 2010; Karl, Beal, O'Hare, & Rissmiller, 2006). See Table 12.2 for expanded descriptions of Duhn's and Karl et al.'s recommendations and other specific examples of the theory used in practice with children, adults, and the elderly.

The Circle of Security International is a relationship-based early intervention program designed to enhance attachment security between parents and children. Decades of university-based research have confirmed that secure children exhibit increased empathy, greater self-esteem, better relationships with parents and peers, enhanced school readiness, and an increased capacity to handle emotions more effectively when compared with children who are not secure.

Attachment theory has been most frequently applied to work with children. The federal program in the United States, Early Head Start, is a visible example of a practice application of this theory (Boris & Zeanah, 2011). The Circle of Security International is a relationship-based intervention program based on attachment theory that is designed to help parents and even therapists help children become more secure in their relationships. Security is associated with increased empathy, school readiness, and the ability to manage

emotions more effectively (https://www.circleofsecurityinternational.com/).

The theory has also been used with children who have been mistreated (Allen, 2011) and children with disabilities (Howe, 2006; Wilkins, 2010). It has been found useful in situations where child custody was an issue (Garber, 2009; Marvin & Schutz, 2009), as well with children being adopted or in foster care (Walker, 2008) or placed in residential homes (News, 2014). Using Middle Range Theories in Practice 12.2 discusses the use of the theory by health care workers involved in adoption or foster care evaluations.

The use of attachment theory is not limited to involvement with children. It has been found useful by counselors and psychotherapists working with individuals with personality disorders (Fogany & Bateman, 2007; Van den Berg & Oei, 2009), depressed adolescents (Bowlby, 1979; Shaw, Dallos, & Shoebridge, 2009), and those suffering from addiction (Flores, 2006). The theory has also been applied to involvement with adult cancer patients and their partners (Burwell, Brucker, & Shields, 2006) and more recently as it relates to spiritual coping in older adults (Munnichs, Bowlby, & Miesen, 1986; Pickard & Nelson-Becker, 2011). There is also a growing interest in the use of attachment theory in nursing education, particularly as it relates to the mentor–mentee relationship (Miles, 2011). Table 12.1 provides additional examples of the theory's applications to practice.

**Table 12.2   Examples of Attachment Theory for Practice**

| Citation | Focus |
|---|---|
| Strachan, J. (2017). Psychological ideas in palliative care: Attachment theory. *European Journal of Palliative Care, 24*(1), 24–27 | Specific care behaviors are provided for the attachment styles: secure, avoidant, and ambivalent. In addition, the policies and services that promote secure relationships are contrasted with those that hinder. |
| Elliot, G., & Kelly, A. (2016). Doll therapy: An increasing popular intervention for those with dementia. *Canadian Nursing Home, 27*(1), 10–16 | Dolls or stuffed animals can help meet the connection or attachment needs of individuals with dementia. The WOW Model provides a framework for determining the appropriateness of therapeutic use of dolls or stuffed animals. It includes determining who the person is in relationship to past experiences with children or animals (W); observation of response to doll or stuffed animal (O); and what action to take, use or not use (W). |
| Chitty, A. (2015). Infant mental health: Health visitors as key partners. *Community Practitioner, 88*(10), 29–30 | In recognition of the importance of secure attachment relationships on the effect of babies' emotional and social well-being, resulting in fewer behavioral issues, healthier peer relationships, and fewer affective disorders, the city of Leeds developed a major project to promote infant mental health. It involved the development and distribution of a booklet, *Understanding Your Baby* by health visitors. In addition to support health visitors, they were provided with (a) training, (b) referral services to provide intensive counseling to families to improve the quality of parent–infant relationships, and (c) consultation to provide support to health visitors dealing with the emotional and practical issues they experience and reflective supervision using actual case studies. |
| Nicholls, W., Hulbert-Williams, N., & Bramwell, R. (2014). The role of relationship attachment in psychological adjustment to cancer in patients and caregivers: A systematic review of the literature. *Psycho-Oncology, 23*(10), 1083–1095. doi: 10.1002/pon.3664 | A systematic review of the literature was conducted to determine the role of attachment in psychological adjustment to cancer of patients and those close to them. In patients, an insecure attachment style was associated with poorer psychological adjustment to cancer and increased difficulty in accessing social support. In caregivers, insecure attachment style was associated with higher rates of depression, greater caregiver stress, less autonomous motivations for caregiving, and difficulties with caregiving. In patients, secure attachment style was associated with positive growth and well-being. Knowledge of attachment theory can help nurses become more aware of the impact of cancer on patients and their caregivers and better provide needed support. |
| Duhn, L., & Ikuta, L. (2010). The importance of touch in the development of attachment. *Advances in Neonatal Care, 10*(6), 294–300. doi: 10.1097/ANC.0b013e3181fd2263 | Based on a review of literature, which included evidence from experimental research, encouraging touch between parents and infants is important for developing secure attachment in children. This quality is associated with more adaptive, healthy development. Nursing approaches to promote this attachment include (a) encouraging and fostering nurturing touch during the immediate postpartum period, (b) promoting rooming in, (c) aiding parents who have infants in neonatal intensive care units to find ways to touch and care for their infants, and (d) educating parents on the importance of nurturing contact as part of daily interactions with their babies. |
| Karl, D. J., Beal, J. A., O'Hare, C. M., & Rissmiller, P. N. (2006). Reconceptualizing the nurse's role in the newborn period as an "attacher." *MCN: The American Journal of Maternal Child Nursing, 31*(4), 257–262 | Based on attachment theory and an understanding of the nurse–patient relationship, the role of "attacher" is described as a nurse as one in which (a) the nurse establishes a mutual and nurturing relationship with mothers that mirrors the mother–infant relationship, for example, respond to mother's needs; (b) maximize contact between mothers and their babies, for example, encourage rooming in, breast-feeding, and infant massage; and (c) facilitate mothers' availability and responsiveness to their infants, for example, model caregiving tasks (bathing, feeding, assessing). |
| Cookman, C. (2005). Attachment in older adulthood: Concept clarification. *Journal of Advanced Nursing, 50*(5), 528–535. doi: 10.1111/j.1365-2648.2005.03435.x | Concept analysis, using the Walker and Avant approach, was conducted to clarify antecedents, critical attributes, and consequences of attachment in adults, particularly older adults. Fear-provoking or challenging situations are antecedents of attachment behavior. Attachment behaviors are identified as (a) proximity, or keeping to one or more "preferred others," (b) protest following involuntary and perceived permanent separation from a preferred other, and (c) the presence of a secure base, viewed as necessary for developmental exploration and growth. Consequences, the persistence of a pattern throughout life, can be categorized as secure, anxious, or avoidant. Knowledge of attachment can alert nurses about the risks that the elderly experience at times of health transitions when attachment issues arise. "Nurses can use knowledge about attachment to search for ways to connect older people with others, and also to explore connections with other attachment figures such as pets, places, and cherished possessions. Reminiscence therapies may provide a rich source of insight into older people's previous attachments, the effect of those losses, and ways to move on" (p. 534). |

**USING MIDDLE RANGE THEORY IN PRACTICE    12.2**

**PROBLEM**

The selection of substitute caregivers and matching a child with a caregiver for children who are being adopted or placed in foster care is an important and challenging decision. Healthy adjustment is dependent on an appropriate placement.

**INTERVENTION**

Attachment theory provides a framework for assessing the qualities of potential caregivers and children. Assessment of the caregiver should include (a) the ability to manage a wide range of feelings of self and others, (b) the resolution of past personal losses or traumas, and (c) the ability to engage in reflection. The assessment of the child is also a critical consideration in placement decisions. A trained health professional can assess a child's attachment pattern during times of distress or fear. Of particular concern in placement is manifestation of disorganized attachment, in which children view caregivers as a source of danger and therefore must be controlled in some fashion. The involved adults' attachment pattern is also important and needs to be assessed, as does the dynamics of the couple relationship. A complementary attachment pattern in couples is considered most resilient. With these assessment data, decisions about appropriate placement of children can be more informed and hopefully result in a growth-producing environment for children.

## Further Research

There is a vast area of attachment research challenges and possibilities relevant to nursing. There are, for instance, strong warrants for further research regarding the role of attachment in the development of specific health conditions (McWilliams & Bailey, 2010). The study of attachment and comfort (Klette, 2007) also calls for further investigations. Other areas of importance are transgenerational continuities and discontinuities of attachment and the development of the earned secure status. Even though continuity seems to be a rule, there is much evidence of variety and change regarding the internal working models and patterns of attachment in adult attachment relationships. According to Bowlby, it is the quality of interpersonal communication that is the major factor in deciding whether a child or adult is in a secure, anxious, or distressed state (Kobac & Madsen, 2008). Further development of reliable measurements and programs for clinical intervention is also called for, especially with regard to school-age children and the very old.

## Summary

■ John Bowlby used knowledge from multiple disciplines to explain children's reactions to separations from their primary caregivers and develop attachment theory.

■ According to Bowlby, attachment theory is a theory about human development and the needs of people from the cradle to the grave.

■ A number of disciplines have included the theory of attachment in their body of knowledge and have contributed to its development as a theory (Cassidy & Shaver, 2008) with the discipline of nursing beginning to become more interested in research related to the theory and to make use of the theory in practice.

■ From a nursing point of view, there are many reasons for this increased interest; for instance, the theory can contribute to the clarification of many concepts/phenomena central to nursing, such as empathy, comfort, care, and health.

■ By taking a patient's attachment experiences and status into account, the nurse will be able to improve the understanding of individual possibilities and limitations, in particular with regard to the phenomenon of will.

■ Reflecting upon own attachment history with regard to attitudes, expectations, and patterns of self-protective behavior might also help nurses be more conscientious in their work.

■ Attachment theory highlights the importance of prevention, a traditionally central field of nursing. The importance of preventing child abuse and neglect cannot be overestimated.

■ While attachment theory and research are yielding an increasing amount of knowledge about the development of health and disease in humans, it is strongly recommended that the discipline of nursing start making more use of and contributing to this multidisciplinary and cross-cultural effort to improve human conditions.

## CRITICAL THINKING EXERCISES

1. One of the patterns of attachment is referred to as "earned secure." This pattern, characterized by coherence and balance, is achieved by adults who experienced unloving or harsh parenting. What individual characteristics or life experiences might contribute to achievement of this pattern?

2. Based on this theory, what behaviors would a nurse attempt to engender when working with parents to promote healthy attachment?

3. At times of threat, illness, or loss, self-protective behaviors in adults can emerge. How would adults manifest self-protective behaviors?

4. What is a research question that would provide validation of this theory?

## REFERENCES

Ainsworth, M. D. S., & Bell, S. M. (1970). Attachment, exploration and separation: Illustrated by the behaviour of one-year-olds in a strange situation. *Child Development, 41,* 49–65.

Ainsworth, M. S., & Bowlby, J. (1989). An ethological approach to personality development. *American Psychologist, 46*(4), 333–341.

Ainsworth, M. D. S., Blehar, M. C., Waters, E., & Wall, E. (1978). *Patterns of attachment. A psychological study of the strange situation.* Hillsdale, NJ: Erlbaum.

Allen, B. (2011). The use and abuse of attachment theory in clinical practice with maltreated children, Part II: Treatment. *Trauma, Violence & Abuse, 12*(1), 3–12.

Bar-On, I. K., & Scharf, M. (2016). The reconstruction of fatherhood across two generations: From experiences of deficiency, strictness, precocious maturity, and distance to indulgence, permissiveness, and intimacy. *Journal of Family Issues, 37*(5), 645–670. doi: 10.1177/0192513X14528712

Bartholomew, K., & Horowitz, L. M. (1991). Attachment styles among young adults: A test of a four category model. *Journal of Personality and Social Psychology, 61,* 226–244.

Behrens, K. Y., Haltigan, J. D., & Bahm, N. I. G. (2016). Infant attachment, adult attachment, and maternal sensitivity: Revisiting the intergenerational transmission gap. *Attachment & Human Development, 18*(4), 337–353. doi: 10.1080/1416734.2016.1167095

Boris, N. W., & Zeanah, C. H. (2011). Attachment research and Early Head Start: From data to practice. *Attachment & Human Development, 13*(1), 99–104.

Bowlby, J. (1958). The nature of the child's tie to his mother. *The International Journal of Psychoanalysis, 39,* 350–373.

Bowlby, J. (1960). Separation anxiety. *The International Journal of Psychoanalysis, XLI,* 89–113.

Bowlby, J. (1979). *The making & breaking of affectional bonds.* London, UK: Tavistock.

Bowlby, J. (1988). *A secure base: Clinical applications of attachment theory.* London, UK: Routledge.

Bretherton, I., & Munholland, K. A. (2008). Internal working models in attachment relationships: Elaborating a central construct in attachment theory. In J. Cassidy & P. R. Shaver (Eds.), *Handbook of attachment* (2nd ed., pp. 102–127). New York, NY: Guilford Press.

Burwell, S. R., Brucker, P. S., & Shields, C. G. (2006). Attachment behaviors and proximity-seeking in cancer patients and their partners. *Journal of Couple & Relationship Therapy, 5*(3), 1–16.

Cassibba, R., Coppola, G., Sette, G., Curci, A., & Costantini, A. (2017). The transmission of attachment across three generations: A study in adulthood. *Developmental Psychology, 53*(2), 396–405. doi: 10.1037/dev0000242

Cassibba, R., Granqvist, P., & Costantini, A. (2013). Mothers' attachment security predicts their children's sense of God's closeness. *Attachment & Human Development, 15*(1), 51–64. doi: 10.1080/14616734.2013.743253

Cassidy, J., & Shaver, P. R. (Eds.). (2008). *Handbook of attachment: Theory, research, and clinical applications* (2nd ed.). New York, NY: Guilford Press.

Cicirelli, V. G. (2010). Attachment relationships in old age. *Journal of Social and Personal Relationships, 27*(2), 191–199. doi: 10.1177/0265407509360984

Crittenden, P. M. (2000). *CARE-Index manual.* Miami, FL: Family Relations Institute.

Donovan, W. L., & Leavitt, L. A. (Eds.). (1985). Cardiac responses of mothers and infants in Ainsworth's strange situation. *The psychobiology of attachment and separation.* Orlando, FL: Academic Press.

Duhn, L., & Ikuta, L. (2010). The importance of touch in the development of attachment. *Advances in Neonatal Care, 10*(6), 294–300. doi: 10.1097/ANC.0b013e3181fd2263

Falk, H., Wijk, H., Persson, L. O., & Falk, K. (2013). A sense of home in residential care. *Scandinavian Journal of Caring Sciences, 27*(4), 999–1009. doi: 10.1111.scs.12011

Flores, P. J. (2006). Conflict and repair in addiction treatment: An attachment disorder perspective. *Journal of Groups in Addiction & Recovery, 1*(1), 5–26.

Fogany, P., & Bateman, A. W. (2007). Mentalizing and borderline personality disorder. *Journal of Mental Health, 16*(1), 83–101.

Fosse, R. (2009). Ingen gener for psykiske lidelser [No genes for psychiatric diseases]. *Tidsskrift for Norsk Psykologforening, 46*(6), 596–600.

Garber, B. D. (2009). Attachment methodology in custody evaluation: Four hurdles standing between developmental theory and forensic application. *Journal of Child Custody, 6*(1–2), 38–61.

Gathwala, G., Singh, B., & Balhara, B. (2008). KMC facilitates mother baby attachment in low birth weight infants. *Indian Journal of Pediatrics, 75*(1), 43–47.

Gemeay, E. M., Ahmed, E. S., Ahmad, E. R., & Al-Mahmoud, S. A. (2015). Effect of parents and peer attachment on academic achievement of late adolescent nursing students—A comparative study. *Journal of Nursing Education and Practice, 5*(6), 96–105. doi: 10.5430/jnep.v5n6p96

George, C., Kaplan, N., & Main, M. (1985). *Adult attachment interview.* Unpublished manuscript. Berkeley, CA: Department of Psychology, University of California.

George, C., & Solomon, J. (1996). Representational models of relationships: Links between caregiving and attachment. *Infant Mental Health Journal, 17*(3), 198–216.

George, C., & West, M. L. (2012). *The adult attachment projective picture system, attachment theory and assessment in adults.* New York, NY: The Guilford Press.

Gillath, O., Johnson, D. K., Selcuk, E., & Teel, C. (2011). Comparing old and young adults as they cope with life transitions: The links between social network management skills and attachment style to depression. *Clinical Gerontologist, 34*(3), 251–265. doi: 10.1080/07317115.2011.55434

Gojman, S., Millán, S., Carlson, E., Sánchez, G., Rodarte, A., González, P., & Hernández, G. (2012). Intergenerational relations of attachment: A research synthesis of urban/rural Mexican samples. *Attachment & Human Development, 14*(6), 553–566. doi: 10.1080/14616734.2012.727255

Habersaat, S., Monnier, M., Peter, C., Bolomey, L., Despars, J., Pierrhembert, B., … Hohlfeld, J. (2013). Early mother-child interaction and later quality of attachment in infants with orofacial cleft compared to infants without cleft. *Cleft Palate-Craniofacial Journal, 59*(6), 704–712. doi: 10.1597/12-094.1

Harlow, H. (1958). The nature of love. In J. M. Notterman (Ed.), *The evolution of psychology: Fifty years of the American psychologist* (pp. 41–64). Washington, DC: American Psychological Association.

Heim, C., Newport, D. J., Bonsall, R., Miller, A. H., & Nemeroff, C. B. (2003). Altered pituitary-adrenal axis responses to provocative challenge tests in adult survivors of childhood abuse. *American Journal of Psychiatry, 158*, 575–581.

Hesse, E. (2008). The adult attachment interview: Protocol, methods of analysis, and empirical studies. In J. Cassidy & P. R. Shaver (Eds.), *Handbook of attachment: Attachment theory, research and clinical applications* (2nd ed., pp. 552–599). New York, NY: Guilford Press.

Hofer, M. A. (1994). Hidden regulators in attachment, separation, and loss. *Monographs of the Society for Research in Child Development, 59*, 192–207.

Hofer, M. A. (2003). The emerging neurobiology of attachment and separation. In S. W. Coates, J. L. Rosenthal, & D. S. Schechter (Eds.), *September 11: Trauma and human bonds* (pp. 191–209). Hillsdale, NJ: Analytic Press.

Howe, D. (2006). Disabled children, parent–child interaction and attachment. *Child & Family Social Work, 11*(2), 95–106.

Karl, D. J., Beal, J. A., O'Hare, C. M., & Rissmiller, P. N. (2006). Reconceptualizing the nurse's role in the newborn period as an "attacher." *MCN: The American Journal of Maternal Child Nursing, 31*(4), 257–262.

Kaya, N. (2010). Attachment styles of nursing students: A cross-sectional and a longitudinal study. *Nurse Education Today, 30*(7):666–673. doi: 10.1016/j.nedt.2010.01.001

Killén, K., Klette, T., & Arenevik, E. (2006). Tidlig mor-barn samspill i norske familier [Early mother–child interaction in Norwegian families]. *Tidskift for Norsk Psykologforening, 43*, 694–701.

Klette, T. (2007). *Tid for trøst. En undersøkelse av sammenenger mellom trøst og trygghet over to generajsoner [Time for comfort. A study of connections between comfort and security across two generations].* In Nova Rapport 17/07. Oslo, Norway: Nova.

Klette, T. (2008). Omsorgssvikt og personlighetsforstyrrelser [Child maltreatment and personality disorders]. *Tidskrift for norsk legeforening, 128*, 1538–1540.

Kobac, R., & Madsen, S. (2008). Disruptions in attachment bonds: Implications for theory, research and clinical intervention. In J. Cassidy & P. R. Shaver (Eds.), *Handbook of attachment* (pp. 23–37). New York, NY: Guilford Press.

Kokkonen, T-M., Cheston, R. I. L., Dallos, R., & Smart, C. A. (2014). Attachment and coping of dementia care staff: The role of staff attachment style, geriatric nursing self-efficacy, and approaches to dementia in burnout. *Dementia 13*(4):544–568. doi: 10.1177/1471301213479469

Lee, G., McCreary, L., Breitmayer, B., Kim, M. J., & Yang, S. (2013). Promoting mother-infant interaction and infant mental health in low-income Korean families: Attachment-based cognitive behavioral approach. *Journal for Specialists in Pediatric Nursing, 18*(4), 265–276. doi: 10.1111/jspn.12034

Loetz, C., Müller, J., Frick, E., Petersen, Y., Hvidt, N. C., & Mauer, C. (2013). Attachment theory and spirituality: Two threads converging in palliative care? *Evidence-Based Complementary and Alternative Medicine, 2013*, 740291. doi: 10.1155/2013/740291

Luecken, L. J. (2000). Parental caring and loss during childhood and adult cortisol responses to stress. *Psychology and Health, 15*, 841–851.

Main, M., & Hesse, E. (1990). Parent's unresolved traumatic experiences are related to infant disorganized attachment status: Is frightened and/or frightening parental behaviour the linking mechanism? In M. T. Greenberg, D. Cicchetti, & E. M. Cummings (Eds.), *Attachment in the preschool years* (pp. 273–310). Chicago, IL: University of Chicago Press.

Main, M., & Solomon, J. (1990). Procedures for identifying infants as disorganized/disoriented during the Ainsworth strange situation. In M. Greenberg, D. Cicchetti, & E. M. Cummings (Eds.), *Attachment in the preschool years.* Chicago, IL: University of Chicago Press.

Marvin, R. S., & Schutz, B. M. (2009). One component of an evidence-based approach to the use of attachment research in child custody evaluations. *Journal of Child Custody, 6*(1–2), 1537–9418.

Maslow, A. (1999). *Toward a psychology of being* (3rd ed.). New York, NY: John Wiley & Sons.

May, R. (1969). *Love and will.* New York, NY: Norton.

McWilliams, J. A., & Bailey, S. J. (2010). Associations between adult attachment ratings and health conditions: Evidence from the National Comorbidity Survey Replication. *Health Psychology, 29*(4), 446–453.

Miles, K. (2011). Using attachment theory in mentoring. *Nursing Times, 10*(380), 23–25.

Munnichs, J., Bowlby, J., & Miesen, B. (1986). *Attachment, life-span and old-age.* Deventer, The Netherlands: Van Loghum Slaterus.

News. (2014). News: Fears for the children being placed in residential homes in 'dangerous areas'. *British Journal of School Nursing, 9*(3), 111.

Özcan, N. K., Boyacioğlu, N. E., Enginkaya, S., Bilgin, H., & Tomruk, N. B. (2016). The relationship between attachment styles and childhood trauma: A transgenerational perspective—A controlled study of patients with psychiatric disorders. *Journal of Clinical Nursing, 25*(15/16), 2357–2366. doi: 10.1111/jocn.13274

Pearson, J. L., Cohn, D. A., Cowan, P. H., & Cowan, C. P. (1994). Earned and continuous-security in adult attachment: Relation to depressive symptomatology and parenting style. *Development and Psychopathology, 6*(2), 359–373.

Penketh, V., Hare, D. J., Flood, A., & Walker, S. (2014). Attachment in adults with intellectual disabilities: Preliminary investigation of the psychometric properties of the Manchester Attachment Scale–Third Party Observational Measure. *Journal of Applied Research in Intellectual Disabilities, 27*(5), 458–470. doi: 10.1111/jar.12070

Pickard, J. G., & Nelson-Becker, H. (2011). Attachment and spiritual coping: Theory and practice with older adults. *Journal of Spirituality in Mental Health, 13*(2), 138–155.

Posada, G., Gao, Y., Wu, F., Posada, R., Tascon, M., Schöelmerich, A., … Synnevaag, B. (1995). The secure-base phenomenon across cultures: Children's behaviour, mother's preferences and experts concepts. *Monographs of the Society for Research in Child Development, 60*(2–3), 29–48. doi: 10.1111/j.1540-5834.1995.tb00202.x

Reite, M., & Field, T. (Eds.). (1985). *The psychobiology of attachment and separation.* Behavioral biology. Orlando, FL: Academic Press.

Roisman, G. I., Susman, E., Barnett-Walker, K., Booth-LaForce, C., Owen, M. T., Belsky, J., … Steinberg, L. (2009). Early family and child-care antecedents of awakening cortisol levels in adolescence. *Child Development, 80*(3), 907–992.

Schore, A. N. (1994). *Affect regulation and the origin of the self, the neurobiology of emotional development.* Hillsdale, NJ: Erlbaum.

Şen, S., & Kavlak, O. (2012). Transgenerational attachment in Manisa, Turkey. *Contemporary Nurse, 41*(1), 126–132.

Shaw, S. K., Dallos, R., & Shoebridge, P. (2009). Depression in female adolescents: An IP analysis. *Clinical Child Psychology and Psychiatry, 14*(2), 167–181.

Sherman, L. J., Stupica, B., Dykas, M. J., Ramos-Marcuse, F., & Cassidy, J. (2013). The development of negative reactivity in irritable newborns as a function of attachment. *Infant Behavior & Development, 36*(1), 139–146. doi: 10.1016/j.infbeh.2012.11.004

Simpson, J. A., & Belsky, J. (2008). Attachment theory within a modern evolutionary framework. In J. Cassidy & P. R. Shaver (Eds.), *Handbook of attachment* (pp. 131–157). New York, NY: Guilford Press.

Solomon, J., & George, C. (1996). Defining the care-giving system: Toward a theory of care-giving. *Infant Mental Health Journal, 17*(3), 183–197.

Spangler, G., Schieche, M., Ilg, U., Maier, U., & Ackerman, C. (1994). Maternal sensitivity as an external organizer for biobehavioural regulation in infancy. *Developmental Psychology, 27*(7), 425–437.

Szyf, M., McGowan, P., & Meaney, M. J. (2008). The social environment and the epigenome. *Environmental and Molecular Mutagenesis, 49*, 46–60.

Tilokskulchai, F., Phatthanasiriwethin, S., Vichitsukon, K., & Serisathien, Y. (2002). Attachment behaviors in mothers of premature infants: A descriptive study in Thai mothers. *The Journal of Perinatal & Neonatal Nursing, 16*(3), 69–83.

Van den Berg, A., & Oei, K. T. I. (2009). Attachment and psychotherapy in forensic patients. *Mental Health Review Journal, 14*(3), 40–51.

van Ijzendoorn, M. H., Goldberg, S., Koonenberg, P. M., & Frenkel, O. J. (1992). The relative effects of maternal and child problems on the quality of attachment: A meta-analysis of attachment in clinical samples. *Child Development, 63*, 840–858.

Verdecias, R., Jean-Louis, G., Zizi, F., Casimir, G. J., & Browne, R. C. (2009). Attachment styles and sleep measures in a community-based sample of older adults. *Sleep Medicine, 10*(6), 664–667. doi: 10.1016/j.sleep.2008.05.011

Viana Rêgo, R. M., Alves e. Souza, Â. M., Assis da Rocha, T. N., & Santos Alves, M. D. (2016). Paternity and breastfeeding: Mediation of nurses. *Acta Paulista de Enfermagem, 29*(4):374–380. doi: 10.1590/1982-0194201600052

Walker, J. (2008). The use of attachment theory in adoption and fostering. *Adoption and Fostering, 32*(1), 49–57.

Waters, E., & Deane, K. E. (1985). Defining and assessing individual differences in attachment relationships: Q-methodology and the organization of behavior in infancy and early childhood. In I. Bretherton & E. Waters (Eds.), *Growing points of attachment theory and research. Monographs of the society for research in child development* (50(1–2, Serial No. 209), pp. 41–65). Chicago, IL: University of Chicago Press.

Waters, H. S., & Rodrigues-Doolabh, L. (2004). *Manual for decoding secure base narratives.* Unpublished manuscript. State University of New York at Stony Brook.

Weinfeld, N. S., Sroufe, L. A., Egeland, B., & Carlson, E. (2008). Individual differences in infant-caregiver attachment: Conceptual and empirical aspect of security. In J. Cassidy & P. R. Shaver (Eds.), *Handbook of attachment* (pp. 880–905). New York, NY: Guilford Press.

Wilkins, D. (2010). I'm not sure what I want (and I don't know how to get it): How do social care workers perceive the parental relationships of children with autism spectrum conditions? *Journal of Social Work Practice, 24*(1), 89–101.

Wolke, D., Eryigit-Madzwamuse, S., & Gutbrod, T. (2014). Very preterm/very low birthweight infants' attachment: Infant and maternal characteristics. *Archives of Disease in Childhood-Fetal and Neonatal Edition, 99*(1), F70–F75. doi: 10.1136/archdischild-2013-303788

# 13 Comfort

Katherine Kolcaba and Cecelia L. Crawford

## Definition of Key Terms

| | |
|---|---|
| **Comfort** | The immediate experience of being strengthened by having needs for relief, ease, and transcendence met in four contexts (physical, psychospiritual, sociocultural, and environmental); much more than the absence of pain or other physical discomforts |
| **ComfortPlace™** | An institution practicing a philosophy of health care that focuses on addressing physical (including homeostatic mechanisms as well as sensations), psychospiritual, sociocultural, and environmental comfort needs of patients, families, and nurses. This type of health care has three components: (a) appropriate and timely comfort interventions, (b) delivery of comfort interventions that conveys caring and empathy, and (c) the intent to comfort. All components are based on an in-depth understanding of the patient's medical history and current medical problems, the family's needs for information or hope or a place to rest, and/or an institution's resolve to improve its working environment. |
| **Comfort interventions** | Skilled actions of the health care team intentionally designed to enhance patients' or families' comfort. Also, changes in the health care environment that enhance the comfort of nurses |
| **Comfort needs** | Patients' or families' desire for or deficit in relief/ease/transcendence in physical, psychospiritual, sociocultural, and environmental contexts of human experience |
| **Health-seeking behaviors (HSBs)** | Behaviors in which patients, families, or nurses engage consciously or subconsciously move them toward well-being; HSBs can be internal, external, or dying peacefully (when that is the most realistic option for patients). |
| **Institutional integrity (InI)** | The quality or state of health care organizations as complete, whole, sound, upright, professional, and ethical providers of health care |
| **Intervening variables** | Positive or negative factors over which the health care team has little control but which affect the direction and success of comfort care plans, comfort studies, or comfort interventions. Examples are presence or absence of social support, poverty, positive prognosis, concurrent medical or psychological conditions, health habits, environmental design, administrative philosophy, and so on. |

The concept of comfort has had a historic and consistent association with nursing. Nurses traditionally provide comfort to patients and their families through actions that, in this theory, are called comfort interventions. The theory of comfort, as applied in a *ComfortPlace™*, explicates a philosophy of care whereby holistic comfort needs of patients, families, and nurses are identified and addressed. Intervening variables are accounted for in planning and assessment. The desired and immediate outcome of this type of care is enhanced comfort, an altruistic and patient-centered goal. Later, Kolcaba expanded this desired outcome to apply to nurses and other members of health care teams. This application is useful when institutions are applying for national designations, such as achieving Magnet® recognition by the American Nurses Credentialing Center, the American Association of Critical-Care Nurses Beacon Award, or the Gold Seal of Approval® from the Joint Commission. In addition, enhanced comfort is related to subsequent desirable outcomes such as higher patient or nurse function, quicker discharge, fewer readmissions, increased satisfaction with care, longevity of employment, and stronger cost–benefit ratios for the institution. These subsequent outcomes provide additional rationale for health care leaders and teams to adopt a model of comfort as a unifying framework for care delivery.

## Historical Background

Nightingale was perhaps the first health care worker to recognize that comfort was essential for patients. She said, "It must never be lost sight of what observation is for. It is not for the sake of piling up miscellaneous information or curious facts, but for the sake of saving life and increasing health and comfort" (Nightingale, 1859, p. 70). In this quote, Nightingale implied that the relationship between health and comfort is strong and direct and that both are equally important.

At the beginning of the 20th century, the term *comfort* was used in a general sense, much as Nightingale had used it, and comfort was highly valued in nursing. Moreover, the ability to provide comfort determined, to a large degree, the nurse's skill and character.

At this time, nurses believed that the provision of comfort was their unique mission. Comfort was especially important because curative medical strategies were not yet developed. Enhancing patient comfort was seen as a positive nursing goal that also was strengthening and, in most cases, should entail an improvement from a previous state or condition. Comfort resulted from physical, emotional, and environmental interventions, but orders for specific comfort measures were under the physician's authority. Some common "comfort orders" in this period were for poultices, heat, and positioning of the patient in bed (McIlveen & Morse, 1995).

Although emotional care was not one of the specified roles of nurses, physical comfort interventions were intended to bring about mental comfort of patients, indicating that physical and mental comforts were closely related. In early nursing texts, the meaning of comfort was implicit, hidden in context, complex, and general. Many semantic variations, such as comforting, to comfort, in comfort, and comfortable, were used, and the term could be in the form of a verb, noun, adjective, or adverb. Comfort also referred to the process of comforting ("The nurse comforted the patient") or the outcome of comfort ("The patient was comforted by the nurse").

By the middle of the 20th century, comfort evolved to a less important nursing goal with a connotation more specific to the physical sense. In the 1950s, as analgesics became popular for pain control, few additional treatments for comfort were described (McIlveen & Morse, 1995). At this time, nurses took responsibility for patients' feelings, although nurses were told to refrain from discussing patients' medical conditions with them.

In the 1950s and 1960s, the term remained undefined for nursing, and it was narrowly interpreted, written about rarely, and, of course, not measured or documented. These conditions rendered comfort interventions by nurses, and the results on comfort of patients, invisible.

The 1980s saw many advances in medicine, and cures often resulted from surgery, antibiotics, radiation therapy (RT), and chemotherapy. Narcotics were used for treating severe pain. The importance of family comfort began to emerge at this time, and families were considered legitimate recipients of care and comfort interventions (McIlveen & Morse, 1995). Correlation between the comfort of patients and the comfort of their families was implied.

Also, during the 1980s, nurses promoted self-care for patients whenever possible. Comfort was the main goal of nursing only when patients were terminally ill, an observation that supported Glaser and Strauss' (1965) earlier suggestion that the goal of nursing reverted to comfort when there were no available cures. Where health care settings were less influenced by technology, such as hospice and long-term care, comfort was more important as a nursing goal. McIlveen and Morse (1995) suggested that this trend had broad implications for nursing in the twenty-first century, as demographics would shift to large numbers of elders who may wish for less technology and more comfort in their last years of life.

Much has been written about the turbulent managed care era of the 1990s (Bettelheim, 1999; Hall, 2004). Health maintenance organizations (HMOs) and other patient care organizations were criticized for focusing on the fiscal aspects of care rather than the human aspects. Consumers perceived compromised quality of care stemming from gatekeeping and other cost-containment efforts. Ultimately, the Congress enacted the Patient's Bill of Rights to address the public's backlash against managed care and restore consumer confidence, enhance clinician–patient relationships, and delineate a patient's right to safe and high-quality care (President's Advisory Commission on Consumer Protection and Quality in the Health Care Industry, 1997; Bettelheim, 1999; Hall, 2004). A multitude of gaps in meeting consumer/patient comfort needs can be extrapolated from the health care complexities of this decade.

The 2000s found nurses struggling with patients and families in addressing human pain, fear, loss, suffering, and, ultimately, quality of life (Malloch & Porter-O'Grady, 2010). Despite the managed care emphasis on cost containment, health care expenditures continued to rise. Consumers sought resources to address not only their fiscal needs but also their physiological, emotional, and spiritual needs. Nurses and consumers embraced the vast technological advances of the 21st century, including the digital revolution, and many became increasingly savvy in navigating and using these virtual resources and tools (Davidson, Weberg, Porter-O'Grady, & Malloch, 2017; Malloch & Porter-O'Grady, 2010). Nurses, patients, and families who were technically intuitive incorporated care-related software applications and smartphone technologies into their daily lives within and outside of clinical venues. However, an element of human connectedness was lost. Even while embracing these advances, people continued to rely on nurses to provide solace, guidance, ease, and relief during the human care experience (Kolcaba, 2003).

Comfort theory (CT) has evolved and thrived during the new millennium. Nurses and health care systems use this theory to assist in achieving patient, nursing, health, and financial goals (Kolcaba, 2003). The integration of Kolcaba's theory into the structures and processes of modern health care systems reduces human suffering and provides much satisfaction to nurses, patients, families, and the global community.

## Definitions of Theory Concepts

When a concept is germane to a discipline, as comfort is, but it has not yet been specifically defined, a concept analysis is necessary. Thus, in 1988, this task was undertaken by Kolcaba. It began with a study of several contemporary dictionaries, each of which contained six or eight definitions of comfort. Those meanings were compared to usages found in an extensive literature search in the journals and textbooks of several disciplines (nursing, medicine, theology, ergonomics, psychology, and psychiatry). From ergonomics came the insight that comfort of persons, for example, in their workplace or their cars, was important for optimum function or productivity (Kolcaba & Kolcaba, 1991). Kolcaba extended this insight to patients and their families.

Also consulted for the concept analysis were nursing history books and the Oxford English Dictionary (OED), which traces the origins and evolution of English words. In 1988, the nursing diagnosis (NANDA) for altered comfort was limited to specific physical discomforts such as pain, nausea, and itching. In nursing textbooks, comfort was discussed in terms of pain management. But the origins of comfort supported a significant association with strengthening, because the concept itself came from the Latin word *confortare*, which means "to strengthen greatly." That obsolete meaning of comfort, not included in modern dictionaries, was still very appropriate for nursing! From the OED, the following definitions of comfort were explicated: (a) strengthening, encouragement, incitement, aid, succor, and support and (b) physical refreshment or sustenance and refreshing or invigorating influence (Kolcaba & Kolcaba, 1991). These meanings, and the link to optimum function in the ergonomic literature, provide theoretical significance for comfort in nursing.

From this process, which took 2 years, three technical types of comfort were derived and labeled: relief, ease, and transcendence (Kolcaba & Kolcaba, 1991).

- *Relief* defined as the experience of a patient who has had a specific comfort need addressed; its theoretical background was consistent with Orlando's (1961/1990) need-based philosophy of nursing.
- *Ease* defined as a state of calm or contentment; its theoretical background was enriched by the writings of Henderson (1978) about 13 essential human requirements.
- *Transcendence* defined as the state in which one rises above problems or pain. Transcendence was a term previously used in the nursing literature by two psychiatric nurses to denote "more being" achieved through relationships with nurses (Paterson & Zderad, 1976/1988). More being was deemed important for "rising above" or "working through" difficult situations or symptoms.

The analysis was comprehensive but not particularly welcomed by American journals. After presenting these three types of comfort at a research conference, audience feedback was so stimulating that, in the middle of the night, Kolcaba awoke with the idea that the types of comfort (relief, ease, and transcendence) occurred physically and mentally. She sketched out a preliminary grid with the three types of comfort across the top and *physical* and *mental* down the side. Thus, there were six cells in this first grid. After presenting this preliminary grid to colleagues and professors at Case Western Reserve University (where she was a doctoral student), Kolcaba was advised that her "physical" and "mental" categories were not holistic, and to go back to the nursing literature to discover how holism was conceptualized. Doing so took another year.

Four contexts of holistic experience were subsequently derived from the literature and were labeled physical, psychospiritual, social, and environmental (Kolcaba, 1991):

- *Physical comfort* pertained to bodily sensations and homeostatic mechanisms.
- *Psychospiritual comfort* pertained to the internal awareness of self, including esteem, sexuality, and meaning in one's life; it also encompassed one's relationship to a higher order or being.
- *Social comfort* pertained to interpersonal, family, and societal relationships (later, this term was changed to *sociocultural comfort* and family/cultural traditions, and financial circumstances were added to the definition).
- *Environmental comfort* pertained to the external background of human experience; it encompassed light, noise, ambience, color, temperature, and natural versus synthetic elements. Environmental comfort did not include energy fields at this time.

When the three types of comfort were juxtaposed with the four contexts of experience, a 12-cell grid or taxonomic structure (TS) was created (Fig. 13.1) (Kolcaba, 1991). The grid depicted the defining attributes of comfort and was helpful for deriving the technical definition of comfort (provided at the beginning of this chapter). The technical definition of comfort is *the immediate experience of being strengthened by having needs for relief, ease, and transcendence met in four contexts (physical, psychospiritual, sociocultural, and environmental)* (Kolcaba, 1992). This grid has been useful for assessing comfort needs of patients, families, and nurses; planning interventions to address those needs; informally evaluating the effectiveness of those interventions to enhance comfort; and measuring the desired outcome of enhanced comfort for research and practice.

## Description of Theory: Major Components and Their Relationships

### ASSUMPTIONS

Assumptions are a theorist's point of view about reality, stated clearly so that future readers know where the theorist is "coming from." Kolcaba's (1994) assumptions are as follows:

|  | Relief | Ease | Transcendence |
|---|---|---|---|
| Physical |  |  |  |
| Psychospiritual |  |  |  |
| Environmental |  |  |  |
| Sociocultural |  |  |  |

**Figure 13.1**    Taxonomic structure of comfort.

- Human beings have holistic responses to complex stimuli.
- Comfort is an immediate and desirable holistic state of human beings that is germane to the discipline of nursing.
- Human beings strive to meet, or to have met, their basic comfort needs. It is an active endeavor.

## CONCEPTS

Concepts are ideas that make up the building blocks of specific theories. The concepts for the middle range theory of comfort are those listed and defined at the beginning of this chapter: comfort needs, comfort interventions, intervening variables, enhanced comfort, health-seeking behaviors (HSBs), and institutional integrity (InI). Consistent with middle range theories, these concepts are at a low level of abstraction (easily defined and measured) and are limited in number. All of these above concepts are relative to patients, families, and nurses; the term *family* encompasses significant others as determined by the patient (Kolcaba, 2003; Kolcaba, Tilton, & Drouin, 2006b).

Figure 13.2 is a diagram that shows three levels of abstraction from highest (at the top of the diagram) to lowest (at the bottom of the diagram)—a depiction called a substruction. This particular diagram served as the organizing framework for Kolcaba's dissertation study with women going through RT, discussed later in this chapter. Such diagrams are helpful for planning research studies; they are used in many of Kolcaba's articles and on her Web site (https://thecomfortline.com) (Kolcaba, 1997).

## PROPOSITIONS

Propositions are relational statements that link concepts together. At the middle range level (Fig. 13.2, Line 1), the following propositions link those respective variables (Kolcaba, 2001):

1. Nurses and other members of the health care team identify comfort needs of patients and their family members, especially those needs that have not been met by existing support systems. Nurses also identify their own comfort needs in their workplaces and work constructively for the fulfillment of these needs.
2. Comfort interventions are designed and coordinated to address those unmet comfort needs.
3. Intervening variables are taken into account in designing interventions and determining their probability for success.
4. When interventions are effective and delivered in a caring manner, the immediate outcome of enhanced comfort is attained.
5. Patients, nurses, and other members of the health care team agree upon desirable and realistic HSBs.
6. If enhanced comfort is achieved, patients, family members, and/or nurses are strengthened to engage in HSBs, which further enhance their comfort.
7. When patients and their family members engage in HSBs as a result of being strengthened by comfort interventions, patients, families, and nurses are more satisfied with health care and demonstrate better health-related and institutional outcomes.

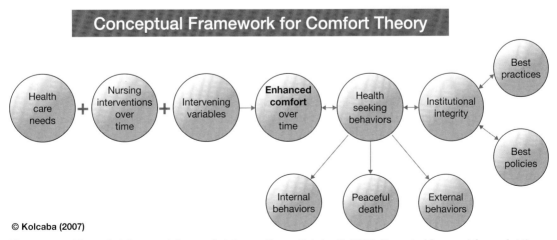

© Kolcaba (2007)

**Figure 13.2**  Theoretical framework for comfort theory. (*Source*: Kolcaba, K. (2002). *Conceptual framework for comfort theory.* Retrieved November 11, 2007 from http://thecomfortline.com/conceptualframework.html)

8. When patients, families, and nurses are satisfied with health care delivery in a specific institution, improved outcomes and public acknowledgment about the institutions' contributions to health will contribute to those institutions remaining successful.

Comfort theory (CT) can be adapted to any health care setting, health care discipline, or age group, whether in the home, hospital, or community, countries, and cultures (Bergström, Håkansson, Warrén Stomberg, & Bjerå, 2018; Ebrahimpour & Hoseini, 2018; Egger-Rainer, Trinka, Hofler, & Dieplinger, 2017; Ponte & da Silva, 2014). For research or practice, the concepts can be further defined, at a lower level of abstraction, in terms of specific patient populations as well as nurses and other health care professionals (Goodwin & Candela, 2013; Lima, Guedes, Silva, Freitas, & Fialho, 2017; Rondinelli, Long, Seelinger, Crawford, Valdez, 2015; Simes et al., 2018).

## PRACTICE APPLICATIONS

### Individuals

CT has been used to assess the comfort needs of patients and their families, to develop interventions to address those needs, and to evaluate their effectiveness for increasing recipients' comfort (Estridge, Morris, Kolcaba, & Winkelman, 2018; Kolcaba, 1997; Krinsky, Murillo, & Johnson, 2014; Parks, Morris, Kolcaba, & McDonald, 2017). It also provides an ethical perspective for decision-making in difficult health care situations. For example, when families are faced with difficult choices for their dying loved ones (Kolcaba, 2003) or when patients with epilepsy are admitted to an Epilepsy Monitoring Unit (Egger-Rainer, et al., 2017), it is helpful to consider what will make the *patient* more comfortable (Egger-Rainer et al., 2017; Kolcaba, 2003).

### Health Care Systems

CT can be adopted throughout an agency, health care system, private practice, or college of nursing to establish criteria for innovations in orientation for new employees, unified research programs, compassionate and value-based care, need assessment for patients or personnel, actions to take to improve quality, electronic documentation, evaluation of progress toward goals, and/or performance review. For instance, CT has been used by nurse educators as a framework to enhance learning environments for student nurses (Goodwin, Sener, & Steiner, 2007). The theory also has been used by nurse leaders to enhance working environments, especially for nurses, and for working toward national institutional recognitions (Kolcaba et al., 2006b). As a quality improvement initiative, CT has been utilized as a framework for raising patient satisfaction scores as developed by the Hospital Consumer Assessment of Healthcare Providers Service (HCAHPS). These scores are federally mandated from every hospital for the purpose of comparison on an open Web site. Using Middle Range Theory in Practice 13.1 provides an example of how the theory was used as a framework for raising retention rates and nurse satisfaction scores and patient satisfaction scores using the survey developed by the HCAHPS. Finally, the Veterans Health Administration (VHA) in the Midwestern United States recently used CT as the basis of team-driven comfort initiatives. A comfort center was designed for veterans' chronic pain needs, and CT concepts were integrated into the system's EHR (Boudiab & Kolcaba, 2015). The practical structures of CT elevated the VHA's proactive patient-centric activities to further enhance the health of veterans and their families.

### Other Disciplines

March and McCormack (2009) determined that slight modifications of CT could render it suitable for the thinking and work of other health care disciplines. For example, a comfort zone can provide a safe haven for health care teams to understand their coworkers' comfort needs and provide supportive encouragement (Boudiab & Kolcaba, 2015). Recommended modifications were primarily those of vocabulary inclusiveness, such as changing the words from "theory for nursing" to "theory for health care." Such changes were made on Kolcaba's Web site (https://thecomfortline.com), to facilitate coordinated usage of CT for interdisciplinary communication, assessment, planning, and evaluation throughout a given hospital, health system, or agency. Table 13.1 includes examples of research that supports the use of CT for different patient populations and practicing nurses throughout the world.

Ongoing work is occurring to provide evidence of the efficacy of applying CT in clinical practice situations. Table 13.2 identifies several examples of doctor of nursing practice projects using CT, and Table 13.3 provides evidence-based practice (EBP) and quality improvement projects that utilized CT in the intervention or found implications for CT in the outcomes. These examples demonstrate the usefulness of CT with a wide range of patient populations and in a variety of clinical settings.

**USING MIDDLE RANGE THEORY IN PRACTICE** 13.1

*Source: Kolcaba, K., Tilton, C., & Drouin, C. (2006). Comfort theory: A unifying framework to enhance the practice environment. The Journal of Nursing Administration, 36(11), 538–544.*

## PROBLEM

The hospital nursing leadership had as its goal enhancing the work environment, an all-important aspect in achieving Magnet© status.

## INTERVENTION

The intervention involved two consulting visits with Kolcaba. Prior to the consultations, efforts were made to promote the theory, primarily through education to the basic elements of comfort theory (CT) and its application to clinical practice. Among the actions taken were the following:

1. Dissemination of the book *Comfort Theory and Practice* to all units in the hospital
2. The use of a color theme for all communications that matched the cover of the book
3. Creation of bookmarks with the date of the workshop and brief excerpts from the book
4. Distribution of business-sized cards with a reminder of the workshop dates
5. Provision of pins for staff that stated, "Ask me about Comfort"
6. Invitation of faculty from area nursing schools and nursing leadership to attend a reception with the author
7. Collection of data from an informal survey of various personnel (health care and ancillary), asking how they brought comfort to patients and families
8. Inclusion of each person's name, picture, and their comments from the survey on large color-coordinated posters

The campaign spanned several months and reached all levels of the health care organization.

At both consultations during breakfast and lunch sessions, Kolcaba presented the clinical staff a brief overview of the theory, focusing on two major themes: (a) enhancing the comfort of nurses through environmental changes, which would encourage nurses and other valued employees to remain with the institution and participate in the entire culture, and (b) enhancing the comfort of patients and their families during hospital stays.

In addition, Kolcaba and the CNO conducted brainstorming session with clinical staff on each nursing unit. One goal of these meetings was to identify strategies for enhancing the nursing work environment. Nurses were encouraged to write down ideas for a "wish list" of changes that would create a more comfortable work environment. Another goal was to discuss comfort interventions to be used with patients to increase their comfort. Kolcaba emphasized the importance of assessment, and documentation before and after comforting interventions is essential to implementing CT. Documentation provides evidence of the effectiveness of the implementation of the theory. The theory Web site was identified as a resource for guidelines to document and assess the comfort needs of patients and families, design interventions to meet those needs, and evaluate their comfort postintervention for practice or research.

## OUTCOMES

Some specific organizational and unit-based initiatives resulted:

1. The nursing philosophy was modified to emphasize physical, environmental, sociocultural, and psychospiritual comfort for both patient/families and nurses. In addition, new objectives in the nursing strategic plan were specifically devoted to increasing the comfort of nurses through promoting a healthier, more comfortable work environment.
2. Orientation for new staff members was updated to integrate CT throughout the process. Core orientation competencies were included that used CT for assessment, intervention, and evaluation of patients' levels of comfort.
3. The theory was used as the foundation of clinical performance evaluation criteria of nurses.
4. Staffing patterns were reviewed and modified to further promote comfortable and safe work environments.
5. Comfort was considered when evaluating equipment for purchase.

The outcomes of these measures were encouraging, nursing turnover and vacancy rates declined and were significantly below state benchmarks, and nurse satisfaction rates increased.

In addition, to promote patient comfort, patient satisfaction surveys were administered. In response, the hospital expanded its service recovery program, involved consumers on committees, and revised the patient/family booklet. As a result, patient satisfaction scores rose.

**Table 13.1    Examples of Research for Application to Practice**

| Reference Country | Meta-Analysis/ Research Design | Clinical Issue/Research Question | Sample (n)/ Participants | Intervention | Outcome |
|---|---|---|---|---|---|
| Bergström, A., Håkansson, Å., Warrén Stomberg, M., & Bjerså, K. (2018). Comfort theory in practice—Nurse anesthetists' comfort measures and interventions in a preoperative context. *Journal of PeriAnesthesia Nursing*, 33(2), 162–171. doi: 10.1016/j.jopan.2016.07.004 Sweden | Qualitative observational study, with deductive thematic analysis | Describe the nurse anesthetist's comfort measures in the perioperative setting. | 12 general surgery patients 11 nurse anesthetists (NAs) | Observations lasting between 20 and 45 min, beginning at nurse–patient introduction in preop and ending in OR when patient was sedated | CT can be used as by NAs to gain a nursing perspective, assess patient needs, and determine interventions in the periop setting. |
| Dowd, T., Kolcaba, K., Steiner, R., & Fashinpaur, D. (2007). Comparison of a healing touch, coaching, and a combined intervention on comfort and stress in younger college students. *Holistic Nursing Practice*, 21(4), 194–202. United States | Experimental | Are levels of comfort and stress affected by healing touch, coaching, or a combination of the two treatments? | 58 college students, ages 18–24 | One group was exposed to a session of healing touch (HT), another was coached on stress reduction, a third was provided with both approaches, and a fourth was considered the waiting group and received no treatments. | Repeated measures revealed that HT had better immediate results on both outcomes, while coaching had better carryover effects. Findings for the combined treatment group were inconsistent, probably due to methodological issues |
| Ebrahimpour, F., & Hoseini A. S. S. (2018). Suggesting a practical theory to oncology nurses: Case report of a child in discomfort. *Journal of Palliative Care*, 33(4), 194–196. doi: 10.1177/0825859718763645 Iran | Case study | Apply CT for a child with cancer. | Young child with cancer needing an IV line | Playing, drawing, peer support, talking interactions between an older child and young child with cancer | Comfort food for the soul: satisfied child's need for relief and ease via peer interactions, emotional supports, and overcoming pain |
| Egger-Rainer, A., Trinka, E., Hofler, J., & Dieplinger, A. M. (2017). Epilepsy monitoring— The patients' views: A qualitative study based on Kolcaba's comfort theory. *Epilepsy & Behavior*, 68, 208–215. doi: 10.1016/j.yebeh.2016.11.005 Austria | Qualitative study with content analysis | Explore perceptions of personal comfort of patients during hospitalization on an Epilepsy Monitoring Unit. | Six women Six men | Problem-centered interviews | Comfort increasing factors: hope, support, intelligible information Comfort decreasing factors: bed rest, boredom, waiting for seizures |

| Reference | Design | Purpose | Sample | Measures | Findings |
|---|---|---|---|---|---|
| Estridge, K. M., Morris, D. L., Kolcaba, K., & Winkelman, C. (2018). Comfort and fluid retention in adult patients receiving hemodialysis. *Nephrology Nursing Journal, 45*(1), 25–60. United States | Descriptive correlational feasibility study | Determine potential relationship between comfort and fluid retention. | 51 adult patients with end-stage renal disease receiving dialysis | 48-item Adapted General Comfort Questionnaire | Association between comfort and fluid retention was not significant. Non-White patients receiving dialysis may need more education and self-management efforts to achieve clinical goals. |
| Goodwin, M., & Candela, L. (2013). Outcomes of newly practicing nurses who applied principles of holistic comfort theory during the transition from school to practice. *Nurse Education Today, 33,* 614–619 (qualitative, phenomenological design). doi:10.1016/j.nedt.2012.07.013 United States | Qualitative, phenomenological | Do newly practicing nurses benefit from learning holistic comfort theory during their baccalaureate education? In addition, the study had as its purpose providing a conceptual framework to support the transition from school to practice. | Nine graduates of a particular accelerated nursing program who graduated since 2006 and were practicing as registered nurses at a local hospital | Students were introduced to holistic comfort (HC) theory while assessing patients' needs and were then asked how they might apply the theory to their own needs as a nurse. | Kolcaba's HC principles were credited for easing nurses into the realities of work and advocating for best patient outcomes. The concept of transcendence helped new nurses rise above unavoidable difficulties during the transition from school to practice. |
| Krinsky, R., Murillo, I., & Johnson, J. (2014). A practical application of Katharine Kolcaba's comfort theory to cardiac patients. *Applied Nursing Research, 27*(2), 147–150. doi:10.1016/j.apnr.2014.02.004 United States | Case study | Describe CT as applied in care of cardiac patients. | Two patients with suspected acute coronary syndrome | "Quiet time" measures derived from CT versus lack of comfort measures | Improved standard of care and outcomes (reduced anxiety, resolved chest pain, sleep) specific to patient in CT case study, as well as other cardiac patients |
| Lima, J. V., Guedes, M. V., Silva, L. F., Freitas, M. C., & Fialho, A. V. (2016). Usefulness of the comfort theory in the clinical nursing care of new mothers: Critical analysis. *Revista Gaucha de Enfermagem, 37*(4), e65022. doi: 10.1590/1983-1447.2016.04.65022 Brazil | Reflexive–theoretical analysis study | Evaluate usefulness of CT for clinical nursing. | New mother | Verify the presence of characteristics related to CT usefulness, using a previously conducted 2014 study. | Applicable concepts facilitated nursing care of a postpartum woman and increased comfort levels; can be applied in different settings. |

*(Continued)*

**Table 13.1　Examples of Research for Application to Practice** (Continued)

| Reference Country | Meta-Analysis/ Research Design | Clinical Issue/Research Question | Sample (n)/ Participants | Intervention | Outcome |
|---|---|---|---|---|---|
| Parks, M. D., Morris, D. L., Kolcaba, K., & McDonald, P. E. (2017). An evaluation of patient comfort during acute psychiatric hospitalization. *Perspectives in Psychiatric Care, 53*(1), 29–37. doi: 10.1111/ppc.12134 United States | Descriptive pilot study | Assess comfort levels between patients receiving a warm blanket and those who did not. | 37 adult psychiatric patients | Warmed blankets | Comfort levels were lower for those who did not receive warm blankets. Warm blankets may increase patient comfort. |
| Ponte, K. M., & da Silva, L. (2014). Implementation of the care-research method based on the comfort theory: Experience report. *Ciencia, Cuidado e Saude, 13*(2), 388–393. doi: 10.4025/cienccuidsaude.v13i2.16439 Brazil | Qualitative observational study, with thematic analysis | Identify the technologies of clinical nursing care to promote comfort to women with acute myocardial infarction (AMI). | Women diagnosed with AMI | Interaction between care–research method and CT to identify and implement comfort needs | Appropriate care technologies and promotion of comfort implemented via relationships between caregiver researcher and cared–researched woman |
| Shu Hua, N. G. (2017). Application of Kolcaba's comfort theory to the management of a patient with hepatocellular carcinoma. *Singapore Nursing Journal, 44*(1), 16–23. Singapore | Case study | Application of CT for nursing care management | Patient with hepatocellular carcinoma | Enhance a patient-centric environment for persons needing end-of-life care. | Patient experienced positive outcomes for pain management, improved sodium and oxygen saturation levels, coping with anxiety, use of support services, and no falls during hospital stay |
| Simes, T., Roy, S., O'Neill, B., Ryan, C., Lapkin, S., & Curtis, E. (2018). Moving nurse educators towards transcendence in simulation comfort. *Nurse Education in Practice, 28*, 218–223. doi: 10.1016/j.nepr.2017.10.024 Australia | Qualitative research study | Identify factors influencing nurse educator comfort for medium- and high-fidelity simulation-based education. | Four university campus' schools of nursing 16 nursing education staff | Semistructured focus group interviews with thematic analysis | Four barrier themes: (a) educator intrinsic, (b) human resources, (c) structural, (d) suggestions Simulation comfort can be increased by: (a) central digital resource repository, (b) mentoring program, and (c) time for preparation and delivery to workload |

| Citation | Study type | Purpose | Sample | Intervention | Results |
|---|---|---|---|---|---|
| Stallings-Welden, L. M., Doerner, M., Ketchem, E. L., Benkert, L., Alka, S., & Stallings, J. D. (2018). A comparison of aromatherapy to standard care for relief of PONV and PDNV in ambulatory surgical patients. *Journal of PeriAnesthesia Nursing, 33*(2), 116–128. doi: 10.1016/j.jopan.2016.09.001 United States | Prospective randomized study | Determine effectiveness of aromatherapy (AT) in relieving postoperative or postdischarge nausea and vomiting (PONV or PDNV). | 211 surgical patients. 108 AT. 113 standard care (SC) | AT versus SC in postsurgical patients | For patients who had PDNV, AT was 100% effective versus 67% effective for SC group. Planning measures to avoid PDNV provide physical and psychological comfort. |
| Townsend, C., Bonham, E., Chase, L., Dunscomb, J., & McAlister, S. (2014). A comparison of still point induction to massage therapy in reducing pain and increasing comfort in chronic pain. *Holistic Nurse Practitioner, 28*(2), 78–84. United States | Randomized control trial (RCT) | Do specific complementary therapies provide pain relief and comfort for patients with chronic pain? | 22 participants, randomly, were assigned to massage or still point induction. | Each session was 30 min. The assigned 10-min technique (massage or still point induction) was administered 10 min into the session. At the end of the assigned protocol, the third spray of aromatherapy (diluted pure lavender essential oil) was delivered, and the subject continued to listen to the music (a CD of harp music) for the final 10 min of the session. | Statistically significant improvement in pain (numeric pain scale) and comfort (visual analog scale) was noted in both groups. The propositions of comfort theory are consistent with complementary therapies and guided the study. |
| Twohig, B., Manasia, A., Bassily-Marcus, A., Oropello, J., Gayton, M., Gaffney, C., & Kohli-Seth, R. (2015). Family experience survey in the surgical intensive care unit. *Applied Nursing Research, 28*(4), 281–284. doi: 10.1016/j.apnr.2015.02.009 United States | Descriptive survey study | Create a survey to assess family experiences in a SICU using CT. | 53 responses from SICU patients, spouses, or significant others | 12-item questionnaire with 2 opened-ended questions | Areas of improvement included spiritual life, cleaning and facilities, and physician communication. CT provided a basis for an enhanced "broad" approach to patient/family care. |

**Table 13.2** Examples of Doctor of Nursing Practice Projects for Application to Practice

| Reference Country | DNP Project Design | Clinical Issue/Problem | Sample (n)/ Subjects | Intervention | Outcome |
|---|---|---|---|---|---|
| Blackburn, K. J. (2014). Emergency nurses' knowledge of pediatric complaints. University of Kentucky, Doctor of Nursing Practice (DNP) Projects, Project 15. Retrieved November 6, 2018 from https://uknowledge.uky.edu/dnp_etds/15 United States | Quantitative descriptive survey design | Examine ER nurses' (a) recognition of pediatric pain, (b) barriers to pediatric pain assessment, and (c) possible relationship of educational preparation and ER experience on pediatric pain assessment knowledge. | 46 ER nurses | Pediatric Nurses Knowledge and Attitudes Survey (PNKAS), using comfort theory as a guide to improve practice in the pediatric setting | Additional education regarding pediatric pain assessment is needed. Areas of opportunity include knowledge of pharmacological treatments and drug side effects. Education and ER expertise did not impact knowledge scores. |
| LaFond, D. A. (2012). Promotion of comfort through early palliative care consultation for children and adolescents undergoing hematopoietic stem cell transplantation. University of Maryland Baltimore, School of Nursing, Doctor of Nursing Practice (DNP) Scholarly Projects. Retrieved November 1, 2018 from http://archive.hshsl.umaryland.edu/handle/10713/1722 or http://hdl.handle.net/10713/1722 United States | Single-site feasibility study | Examine (a) willingness of patients to receive palliative care, (b) willingness of health care team to refer families, (c) resource allocation, and (d) family and clinician satisfaction. | 12 eligible families | Early palliative care consultation for children and adolescents with advanced cancers and other life-limiting diseases undergoing stem cell transplantation | Top interventions were counseling, massage, aroma/play therapy, acupuncture or pressure, and integrative treatments. Comfort rated "very good." New care approach rated high satisfaction. |
| Marshall, A. M. (2016). Development of a practice guidelines for DNP prepared nurse practitioners working in long-term care facilities. Walden University, Walden Dissertation and Doctoral Studies, Doctor of Nursing Practice (DNP). Retrieved November 1, 2018 from https://scholarworks.waldenu.edu/dissertations/2093 United States | Literature review with expert synthesis and consensus | Frequently changing guidelines poses challenges for NP efforts to integrative EBP into daily patient care. | 34 articles examined 8 selected for final inclusion Clinical experts = 7 | Develop EBP guidelines for doctoral-prepared NPs in long-term care facilities. | DNP NP-focused practice guidelines based on current evidence and advisory committee of experts |
| Sartz, D. A. (2013). Screening for distress in ambulatory oncology patients: The cope project. Regis University, Doctor of Nursing Practice (DNP). Retrieved November 1, 2018 from Regis University ePublications: https://epublications.regis.edu/theses/205 United States | EBP project | Use the National Comprehensive Cancer Network Distress Thermometer to ceter-mine psychosocial distress levels in patients receiving chemotherapy. | 21 ambulatory oncology patients | Identify, assess, and refer cancer patients experiencing elevated distress levels measured by NCCN tool. | 57% reported moderate-to-severe distress, with physical ailments most frequent source. Guidelines integrated into routine assessment. |

**Table 13.3   Examples of Evidence-Based Practice/Quality Improvement Projects Applicable to Practice**

| Reference Country | QI/EBP Project Design | Clinical Issue/Problem | Sample (n)/Setting | Intervention | Outcome |
|---|---|---|---|---|---|
| Boudiab, L. D., & Kolcaba, K. (2015). Comfort theory: Unraveling the complexities of veterans' health care needs. *Advances in Nursing Science*, 38(4), 270–278. doi: 10.1097/ ANS.00000000000089 United States | Application of CT via case study and health care team–driven comfort initiatives | Complex health care needs of veterans and their families are interrelated and challenging | Midwestern VA system veteran population and health care team members | Implement the CT professional practice model and align with Blueprint for Excellence strategies. | Comfort center holistically addressed veterans' chronic pain and other needs. Concepts integrated into EHR Comfort open house and comfort for the staff sessions promoted a healing work environment. |
| Cordo, J., & Hill-Rodriguez, D. (2017). The evolution of a nursing professional practice model through leadership support of clinical nurse engagement, empowerment, and shared decision making. *Nurse Leader, 15*(5), 325–330. United States | Model development and enculturation with a case scenario | Move from professional care model to professional practice model (PPM) via joint decision-making and staff engagement and empowerment. | Freestanding pediatric hospital in Miami, FL | Create and adopt a multifaceted PPM using CT theoretical framework that is holistic and aligns with organizational mission and values. | Five key PPM components were identified with 27 related subcategories. Enculturation included education, training, comfort rounds, and shared leadership council oversight. |
| Ludington-Hoe, S. M. (2015). Skin-to-skin contact: A comforting place with comfort food. *MCN: The American Journal of Maternal/Child Nursing, 40*(6), 359–366; quiz E323–354. doi: 10.1097/ nmc.0000000000000178 United States | Review of empirical evidence for skin-to-skin contact (SSC) | Examine the effects and mechanisms of SSC related to the realms of newborn and infant comfort. | Database search of relevant SSC articles | Categorize review articles via physiologic, psychospiritual, and environmental realms. | Extrauterine life adaptation is optimized by maximizing comforts for physiologic (stability, warmth, sleep), psychospiritual (remove pain and stress), and environmental (breast milk) realms |

# Research Applications for the Theory of Comfort

Generally, in an experimental design, patients meeting inclusion criteria are randomly assigned to levels of intervention such as a usual care group, an intervention group, and/or an enhanced intervention group. Researchers use the General Comfort Questionnaire (GCQ) as a starting point, removing items that are not relevant to their research setting or population and adding items that are relevant. They plot all items on the TS, making sure that the content domain of comfort is evenly represented. Similar numbers of positive and negative items are utilized, unless patients are very frail cognitively. In that case, mostly positive items are used (Cohen & Mount, 1992). Kolcaba usually uses three measurement points, the first being baseline measures of the selected outcome(s). Power analysis is computed using a medium effect size, 0.80 power, and alpha of 0.10 for most interventions or protocols where known side effects are nonexistent, such as guided imagery (GI) or music therapy. The preferred test statistic is repeated measure multivariate analysis of variance (RM-MANOVA) (or if using a covariate, MANCOVA). These are appropriate statistics for comfort research because they capture holistically the interaction between time and intervention(s) (group assignment) and they have strong power (less subjects needed). Accounting for the impact of the interaction between time and intervention(s) (in other words, do any of the interventions increase comfort over time?) is congruent with CT. Although comfort is not a stable state from one moment to another, a trend for increased comfort over time can be demonstrated given effective comfort interventions.

All or parts of CT can be tested for research. The *first part* of the theory, Propositions 1 to 4, is the most frequently tested portion to date. An example of a test of these propositions was research by Manning (2016), which used multiple case studies to explore patient and clinician experiences in changing models of care. Manning compared patients with fall, back, or limb fracture injuries who were admitted for traditional hospitalization to patients referred to intermediate home care. Home care was effective for patients with limb fractures or falls with back injuries. Supportive care services allowed home care patients to remain independent without placing additional burdens on family members for health needs or activities of daily living. Patients admitted for hospitalization were either for pain management, immobility, and surgery or for an unconscious state. After interviewing all patients, intermediate care was determined to be not only cost-effective but also deemed a holistic alternative to hospital care.

The *second part* of the theory is represented by Propositions 5 and 6, relating comfort to selected HSBs. This part provides rationale for why nurses and other health care providers should focus on patient, family, and/or nurse comfort, beyond altruistic reasons. Because HSBs include internal and external behaviors, almost any health-related outcome that is deemed important by the patient or family in a given research setting can be classified as an HSB. The task for the investigator is to justify the choice of HSBs and discuss reasons that recipients would want to engage in those HSBs, whether consciously or unconsciously. Kolcaba et al. tested Propositions 5 and 6 in their studies with persons who have urinary incontinence (UI) (Dowd, Kolcaba, & Steiner, 2000, 2002, 2003). They found that people with higher comfort were more likely to engage in HSBs and be successful in increasing bladder function and management of UI. That is, comfort was a good predictor of the extent of engagement in HSBs.

The *third part* of CT is represented by Propositions 7 and 8, relating patients' comfort and their engagement in HSBs to InI. The concept of InI was added to the theory to provide direction for outcome research that would support the disciplines of nursing and other health professions. In addition, because institutions are driven by market competition to produce high patient satisfaction scores, those same institutions will be interested to know that patient and nurse comfort are strong predictors of patient satisfaction as well as other positive outcomes such as shorter lengths of stay, fewer hospital readmissions, and lower turnover of health care employees, especially nurses. Achieving sought-after national recognitions is another measure of InI. The practice example in Using Middle Range Theory in Practice 13.1 represents this type of comfort research.

The research examples in Using Middle Range Theories in Research 13.2 and 13.3 show how all two or three parts of CT were tested simultaneously. Effects of hand massage on patient comfort (immediate outcome) and satisfaction with care (institutional outcome) were measured in a population of long-term nursing home residents (Kolcaba, Schirm, & Steniner, 2006a). In a two-group design, those who received hand massage by their nursing assistants (NAs) as a part of their hygienic care were compared to residents who received usual care (no hand massage). The intervention was incorporated easily into the (NAs) routine, but lack of administrative encouragement

## USING MIDDLE RANGE THEORY IN RESEARCH    13.2

*Source: Kolcaba, K., & Fox, C. (1999). The effects of guided imagery on comfort of women with early stage breast cancer undergoing radiation therapy. Oncology Nursing Forum, 26(1), 67–72.*

### RESEARCH PURPOSE

The study was designed to answer the question: Will women who receive guided imagery (GI) while going through radiation therapy (RT) for early-stage breast cancer have greater comfort over time compared to a usual care group? (see Fig. 13.2). This question addressed Part 1 of *Comfort Theory*.

### RESEARCH DESIGN

The study was a randomized control trial (RCT).

### SAMPLE/PARTICIPANTS

There were 53 women (26 in the experimental group, 27 in the control group) aged 37 to 81.

### DATA COLLECTION

The audiotape developed for the study facilitated the delivery of the same holistic message every day to all women in the treatment group. In the script for GI, positive statements were directed to every cell in the TS of comfort known to be important for this population. Input for construction of the audiotape and design of the study was received from the RT nurses, technicians, and physicians.

The instruments used in this study were the Radiation Therapy Comfort Questionnaire (RTCQ), adapted from the GCQ, and four visual analog scales (one each for total comfort, relief, ease, and transcendence). During the pilot test for the methods, the women were asked specifically if there was anything left out of the questionnaire, anything that was forgotten or awkward in the audiotape, and if the instruments were easy to use. When everyone was satisfied with the protocol, the study began.

Nurses told the women who met the inclusion criteria about the study during their first appointment in the RT department. When the patients first heard about the study, about half the women burst into tears; the other half wanted to enroll. The nurses faxed to the data collectors the names and phone numbers of those who wanted to enroll, and the intake visit took place prior to the women's simulation visit. The women in the treatment group were asked to listen to the tape every day, in their own homes, with tape players that the study provided. They indicated in journals and during interviews that they complied with this request diligently for the first 3 weeks of RT, after which some were tired of the audiotape. When this occurred, they were encouraged to continue listening to the music side of the tape that would reinforce recall of the GI script. In this way, the script could be internalized.

Three complete data sets were collected (three visits for each woman) on 53 women, which took 1 year after IRB approvals were obtained. RM-MANOVA was used to test the hypotheses. Alpha was set at 0.10 because the intervention had no risks and the higher alpha reduced type II error (Lipsey, 1990).

### FINDINGS

Analysis of group differences at baseline on demographic data and comfort revealed that the groups were similar for all baseline variables. This was the desired result for Time 1 data. The result of the MANOVA, which analyzed data from all three time points simultaneously, was that the groups were significantly different on comfort at Times 2 and 3 ($p = 0.07$), a second desired result. Then, two posttests were conducted. The first was to determine which group had higher comfort (the treatment group did), and the second was to perform a trend analysis, looking at the "slopes" of the comfort data for both groups. This analysis revealed a linear slope over time, meaning that differences between the groups increased steadily over time. All of these results confirmed the efficacy of GI and supported the theory of comfort.

---

led to a decrease in interest in the study and performance of the intervention. Therefore, unlike other comfort studies, a trend toward gradually increasing comfort in a linear direction was not demonstrated. A systematic program of recognition of the NAs' work and contribution to science by the administrators might have resulted in positive findings.

For health care research, patient comfort can be correlated with institutional factors such as nurse–patient ratios, levels of nursing education, new hospital policies or protocols, strategies for nurse retention, and/or specific nursing interventions (especially those considered to be holistic or adjunctive to medical strategies). A full taxonomy of comfort measures is now available in the electronic

## USING MIDDLE RANGE THEORY IN RESEARCH | 13.3

*Source: Dowd, T., Kolcaba, K., & Steiner, R. (2000). Using cognitive strategies to enhance bladder control and comfort. Holistic Nursing Practice, 14(2), 91–103.*

### RESEARCH PURPOSE

The purpose of this study was to test the effectiveness of audiotaped cognitive strategies for improving comfort with innovative bladder management strategies and the HSB of actual bladder function, operationalized by incontinence and/or frequency. The research question was: Will the group practicing cognitive strategies have higher comfort and better bladder function compared to the usual care group over time?

### RESEARCH DESIGN

The study was a randomized control trial (RCT).

### SAMPLE/PARTICIPANTS

The sample was composed of 31 adults, ages 42 to 91, with incontinence and/or urinary frequency for at least 6 months, excluding symptoms related to urinary tract infections. Participants were randomly assigned to treatment group ($n = 21$) or control group ($n = 19$).

### DATA COLLECTION

A substructed diagram similar to the RT diagram was used to organize the study. Following this diagram, the known comfort needs of this population were targeted with cognitive strategies recorded on a new audiotape. The TS was used as a guide to cover the domain of comfort with the recorded statements. Possible covariates (intervening variables) were age, gender, and particulars of bladder health history. To measure comfort in this population, the UIFCQ was adapted from the GCQ and was pilot tested before using it in this study. The HSB was improved bladder function operationalized by the Bladder Function Questionnaire (researcher developed).

Both groups received basic information about bladder function and behavioral techniques to improve bladder health. In addition, the treatment group was provided with a tape recorder and audiotape of cognitive strategies to manage symptoms and was instructed to listen to the tape once a day at their convenience for 6 weeks. Persons in the control group were provided with a tape recorder and the audiotape and instructed to listen for a period of 3 weeks.

### FINDINGS

Results indicated that the treatment group had more comfort and improved bladder function over time compared with the usual care group. In addition, a crossover component was added when those in the original comparison group listened to the audiotape for 3 weeks, after which data were collected again from both groups. A significant improvement on bladder function was found in the crossover group, and their comfort had increased to the level of the treatment group after 3 weeks of the intervention.

Another interesting finding was that the UIFCQ predicted which participants ($N = 17$, or 90% of the treatment group) would demonstrate improvement in incontinence. Because comfort was a strong predictor of benefit from treatment for incontinence and frequency, these findings also supported the strengthening component of the theory of comfort.

---

NANDA database as nursing diagnoses, interventions, and outcome measures. The patient outcome of comfort can be added to other electronic databases or paper records as well. Identifying and tracking value-added nursing outcomes by staff nurses on their units and nursing leaders for the entire division, agency, or hospital are important for (a) earning recognition for one's sphere of influence, (b) elevating the specific contribution of nursing to health care of patients, and (c) counteracting the negative and dangerous reputations that have been created regarding hospital stays.

In addition, in a pay-for-performance reimbursement environment, comfort is a value-added and nursing-sensitive outcome. When patients and their families experience increased comfort, a benefit that they desire and need, through the direct actions and behaviors of a nurse, those actions and behaviors could be reimbursed separately. The credibility and validity of the GCQ and its modifications are ideally suited for this purpose. In 2003, the complete instrument was registered as a multidisciplinary outcome indicator by the National Quality Measures Clearinghouse (NQMC, 2013). This type of positive (value-added) patient/family measure is unusual because it is a *direct* indicator of quality, rather than an indirect indicator. Indirect indicators are actually indicators of *poor* quality such as "death among surgical patients," "prevalence of pressure ulcers," and "incidence of inpatient falls with injuries" (Dunton, Gonnerman, Montalvo, & Schumann, 2011). (Agency for Healthcare Research and Quality [AHRQ] housed this Web-based repository until it was shut down on July 16, 2018, as federal funding was no longer available to support the microsite.)

## Evidence-Based Nursing Practice Applications

Nurses have become well-versed in the concept and application of EBP, particularly those achieving masters or doctor of nursing practice (DNP) degrees. Nurses with DNPs are increasingly exploring institutional structures and nursing care processes using CT. An example of a DNP applying evidence to the clinical setting is Marshall's (2016) DNP clinical practice project that involved the development of EBP guidelines for nurse practitioners working in long-term care facilities. Frequent changes to care-related guidelines pose challenges for nurse practitioners (NPs) in integrating EBP into their daily workflow. CT was used as the guiding framework to not only improve resident outcomes but ultimately contribute to this vulnerable population's overall comfort. Using CT, expert synthesis, and consensus, a group of clinical experts examined the best available evidence and created NP-focused guidelines specific to long-term care settings.

Another DNP capstone project examined how to promote comfort via palliative care for children and adolescents undergoing hematopoietic stem cell transplantation (HSCT). This single-site feasibility study explored the willingness of patients and families to receive palliative care services, if the health care team was willing to refer these families, types of resources allocation, and family/staff satisfaction while also evaluating comfort needs of this pediatric population. Key comfort interventions included integrative techniques such as massage, aromatherapy, play therapy, acupuncture/pressure, and support counseling. Children and adolescents rated comfort as "very good," while families and clinicians reported high overall satisfaction rates.

## Quality Improvement/ Performance Improvement Applications

Comfort theory is notable for usefulness in guiding quality improvement (QI) and performance improvement (PI) projects (Boudiab & Kolcabe,

2015; Ludington-Hoe, 2015). This versatile theory can also be used to shape the health care environment itself, as seen by the development of a nursing professional practice model (PPM) in a pediatric hospital seeking to achieve Magnet® status (Cordo & Hill-Rodriguez, 2017). After examining three nursing theories, hospital nurse voted to use CTG due to ease of use and universal application to nurses, patients/families, and others on the health care team. Kolcaba interacted and consulted with the Nursing Shared Leadership Council during a focused visit that included CT educational sessions and unit rounding. CT facilitated the development of a PPM customized to fit the organization's unique environment and patient population, as well shared decision-making and leadership structure.

As the PPM and CT became embedded within the organizational and nursing environment, nurses increasing became empowered and engaged in their day-to-day care of patients and their families. Hourly rounding became comfort rounding, as advised by Dr. Kolcaba. Comfort calls were developed to meet the needs of family members unable to physically visit, which provided an update in the patient's current care plan/needs. The care experience was greatly enhanced not only for the patient and their significant others but also for the nurses and health care team. Cardo and Hill-Rodriguez included a case study of child who was admitted for a spinal fusion surgery. During this frightening surgical procedure, all four contexts of CT were used to successfully structure the age-appropriate preadmission, pre-, intra-, postoperative, and post-discharge care experiences for both the child and the family.

## Instruments Used in Empirical Testing

### GENERAL COMFORT QUESTIONNAIRE

If you want to do a comfort study yourself and a comfort instrument needs to be constructed for your unique population, you can start with the GCQ and adapt it using your knowledge of the population. Detailed instructions for doing so are on the Web (Kolcaba, 1997), and a full discussion of how the GCQ was developed is in Kolcaba (1992) and Kolcaba (2003).

As with the other comfort questionnaires available, the GCQ began with the TS. The GCQ contains 2 positive and 2 negative items for each of the 12 cells in the TS, resulting in 48 items. A four-response Likert-type scale was used for the pilot test, although subsequent questionnaires have six responses, which increase sensitivity of the instrument. An even number of responses also forces the responder to choose one side of the comfort fence or the other.

The GCQ was pilot tested in the community ($N = 30$) and several types of hospital units ($N = 226$). Results of this first instrumentation study were encouraging, as the Cronbach's alpha was 0.88, very high for a new instrument. (Perhaps, working from a theoretically driven map of the content domain helped!) Factor analysis, using principal components analysis, extracted 13 factors with eigenvalues above 1.0. The 13th factor had only one item and was collapsed into one of the other factors that was semantically similar, producing 12 factors consistent with the TS. In addition, factors were grouped together in three subscales on the screen plot that were semantically similar to the types of comfort (relief, ease, and transcendence). This factor structure accounted for 63.4% of the variance in the 48 items (Kolcaba, 1992).

Reliabilities for the subscales (factors) ranged from 0.66 to 0.80, which were lower than for the whole GCQ (0.88). This is because lower numbers of items generally decrease reliability scores. The GCQ revealed significant sensitivity in expected directions between several groups (construct validity). Findings were that (a) the community group had higher comfort than the hospital group and (b) people with higher comfort demonstrated a higher correlation with their own estimates of progress in rehabilitation.

When researchers adapt the GCQ to fit their population, they can use the psychometric properties and description of the instrumentation study (above) to support their choice of a comfort instrument. If appropriate, the number of items can be shortened or whole subscales that are not relevant can be removed. However, with each of those strategies, reliability scores may decrease. It is important, therefore, to pilot test adapted instruments with at least 15 subjects who are characteristic of those in the proposed study. A Cronbach's alpha of at least 0.70 is desirable for a new instrument. Kolcaba appreciates submission of your new instruments to her Web site (https://www.thecomfortline.com) (Kolcaba, 1997), so future researchers do not have to "reinvent the wheel" and the preliminary psychometric statistics that support the use of comfort instruments.

A recent psychometric systematic review examined current instruments used to measure patient comfort during hospitalization; the GCQ was one of 49 evaluated instruments. The authors determined that the GCQ reflected the patient hospitalization experience more closely than other tools.

Both the GCQ and their adaptations demonstrated strong methodological qualities; authors stated that they may be the best of the self-report instruments to determine patient comfort in various settings and conditions (Lorente, Losilola, & Vives, 2017).

## VERBAL RATING SCALES

For clinical research, patient comfort can be assessed with verbal ratings similar to those now conducted for pain. When a patient is asked to rate his/her comfort from 0 to 10, meaningful conversations can be initiated about detractors from comfort in the clinical setting and possible solutions. Findings from the use of verbal rating of either total comfort or discomfort can easily be added to documentation forms in health care settings. In a test of their reliability, verbal ratings of total comfort provided statistically significant data when comparing the effects of two comfort interventions, coaching and HT, for the goal of increasing comfort and decreasing stress of college students (Dowd et al., 2007).

Verbal ratings can be correlated with institutional factors such as nurse–patient ratios, levels of nursing education, new hospital policies or protocols, strategies for nurse retention, and specific nursing interventions (especially those considered to be holistic or adjunctive to medical strategies). A full taxonomy of comfort measures is now available in the electronic NANDA database as nursing diagnoses, interventions, and outcome measures. Identifying and tracking value-added nursing outcomes by nursing leaders are important for (a) earning recognition for one's unit, agency, or hospital, (b) elevating the contribution of nursing to health care in general, and (c) counteracting the negative and dangerous reputations that have been created regarding hospital stays.

## ADAPTED GENERAL COMFORT QUESTIONNAIRE FOR PATIENTS RECEIVING HEMODIALYSIS

This descriptive correlational cross-sectional research study examined a possible relationship between patient comfort and fluid retention for adults receiving hemodialysis (HD) for end-stage renal disease (ESRD). A literature review identified factors that could contribute to patient deviation from prescribed fluid regimes. Using these factors specific to patients receiving HD, the GCQ was adapted for use in this vulnerable patient population, seen in items such as "I am swollen right now" and "I am thirsty." The revised 48-item HD Questionnaire contained both positive and negative items for completeness and balance in this practice setting (Estridge et al., 2018).

Anticipating that patients receiving HD might need clinician support in completing the HD Questionnaire (HDQ) during their treatment session, a protocol was developed for bedside assistance, reading question items to patients, and providing a card with large print. The modified instrument performed well and yielded a Cronbach's alpha of 0.85 (Estridge et al., 2018), as compared to the original GCQ Cronbach's alpha of 0.88 (Kolcaba, 1992).

## POST HIP REPLACEMENT COMFORT SCALE

After a literature review revealed the lack of a scale specific to patient comfort after hip replacement surgery, Kilic and Tastan (2017) developed and tested the psychometric properties of the Post Hip Replacement Comfort Scale (PHRCS) to fill this gap in clinical practice. The modified scale evaluates medical interventions before and after hip replacement surgery, which contained 22 positive and 14 negative statements. This study employed internal reliability and test–retest methodology for tool evaluation. The final scale contained 26 items. Cronbach's alpha coefficient value was 0.758. Criterion validity revealed a positive relationship between the average PHRCS scores and the GCQ ($r = 0.701; p < 0.001$).

## HOSPICE COMFORT QUESTIONNAIRE (FAMILY AND PATIENT)

For this population, the GCQ was adapted again to create a 49-item Hospice Comfort Questionnaire (HCQ). Family members were asked to rate their own comfort, not that of their patient. The adapted instruments were tested in two phases (Novak, Kolcaba, Steiner, & Dowd, 2001). In phase I, patient and FM questionnaires had a six-item Likert scale response set, ranging from "strongly agree" to "strongly disagree," and higher scores indicated higher comfort. Each questionnaire took about 12 minutes for patients to complete and usually less time for FMs. Approximately equal numbers of positive and negative items were created for the FMs' EOL questionnaire; items were worded more simply and with less alternating between positive and negative orientations. This adaptation was necessary because of decreased mental agility in dying patients (Cohen & Mount, 1992).

In phase II, patient and caregiver questionnaires were reduced to a four-item Likert response set, because of concerns of the data collectors that six responses were too confusing. However, results showed that the instrument in phase I (six responses) had the strongest psychometric properties for both FMs and patients. Cronbach's alpha for the FM questionnaire was 0.89 ($N = 38$) and for the patient questionnaire was 0.83 ($N = 48$) (Novak et al., 2001).

In spite of these high reliability scores, nurse researchers working with this population a few years later thought that 49 items were too many, and they asked a panel of experts to prioritize the items that were most important. From that list of priority items, 24 of the highest items were plotted on the TS and balanced over the content domain. The result is a 24-item HCQ. This instrument was used in an experiment with hospice patients in which a hand massage protocol was tested with 31 patients over a 3-week period. Despite a lenient alpha of 0.10, the study did not yield significant results overall. However, of clinical significance is that comfort increased somewhat in the treatment group even as patients approached death, while, in the usual care group, comfort scores decreased steadily over the three weekly measurement points (Kolcaba, Dowd, Steiner, & Mitzel, 2004).

## PERINATAL BEREAVEMENT SCALE

The original Perinatal Bereavement Scale (PBS) was developed by Ligeikis-Clayton (2000) and has since been replicated in two additional studies (Rock, 2004; Rondinelli et al., 2015). Ligeikis-Clayton demonstrated PBS reliability of 0.97 through testing analysis of variance ($F = 14.26$, $p = 0.0000$). Rondinelli et al. (2015) conducted a cross-sectional online survey design study specific to the factors related to the nurses' comfort in fulfilling bereavement care interventions. The study also examined perinatal nurses' open-ended descriptions of facilitators and barriers while providing care to patients and families experiencing the death of a newborn baby. The 20-item scale contained 11 items assessing nurse comfort discussing bereavement components with parents and families, along with 9 items assessing nurse comfort while performing bereavement components during a loss event. The modified scale demonstrated acceptable reliability ($a = 0.98$). Total nurse comfort was significantly related to years of experience ($r = 0.346$, $p < 0.001$) and number of perinatal loss cases cared for ($r = 0.374$, $p < 0.001$).

Many of these instruments, and others under development or in different languages, are available on Kolcaba's Web site (http://www.thecomfortline.com) (Kolcaba, 1997).

Visit YouTube (https://www.youtube.com) for additional descriptions and example of using comfort theory.

# Summary

■ The theory of comfort provides a framework for research in any setting where patients have comfort needs and enhancing their comfort is valued.

■ The theory has been used to test the effectiveness of specific holistic interventions for increasing comfort, to demonstrate the correlation between comfort and subsequent HSBs, and to relate HSBs to desirable institutional outcomes.

■ It is important as a framework for interdisciplinary care and research because the focus is on the unifying and positive outcome of patient comfort. As such, CT has been used in many health care specialties, both nationally and internationally.

■ The comfort theory framework can be expanded for use in performance improvement, quality improvement, and evidence-based practice projects across the care continuum.

■ As a value-added indicator of improved quality, the desired outcome of comfort is used by nursing leaders for practice and research.

## CRITICAL THINKING EXERCISES

1. Nurse leaders attempt to advance practice one unit or agency at a time. In order to bring a philosophy of comfort management to your practice setting, rationale must be developed and presented. Compile logical and compelling rationale for implementing comfort management at your site and a brief proposal for how you would implement this model.

2. In order to practice comfort management, evidence must be collected about patients'/families' comfort needs, comfort interventions to address those needs, and assessment of baseline comfort compared to comfort after the intervention(s). Design appropriate comfort management documentation for your unit.

3. Research evidence suggests that patients do better when their expectations about specific benefits of nursing care are discussed and met. Design a "comfort contract" whereby patients or their surrogates designate an expected level of postsurgical overall comfort and also where they can specify chronic discomforts and interventions that they use at home for relief.

4. Twenty-first century health care requires using the best available evidence to create EBP and QI/PI projects that seek to deliver high-quality and safe care for patients and their families and meet organizational initiatives and goals. Outline how CT can be used to structure and guide these types of projects.

## REFERENCES

Bergström, A., Håkansson, Å., Warrén Stomberg, M., & Bjerså, K. (2018). Comfort theory in practice-nurse anesthetists' comfort measures and interventions in a preoperative context. *Journal of PeriAnesthesia Nursing, 33*(2), 162–171. doi: 10.1016/j.jopan.2016.07.004

Bettelheim, A. (1999). Managing managed care: Will reforms improve healthcare quality? *CQ Researcher, 9*(14), 305–328.

Blackburn, K. J. (2014). Emergency nurses' knowledge of pediatric complaints. University of Kentucky, Doctor of Nursing Practice (DNP) Projects, Project 15. Retrieved November 6, 2018 from https://uknowledge.uky.edu/dnp_etds/15

Boudiab, L. D., & Kolcaba, K. (2015). Comfort theory: Unraveling the complexities of veterans' health care needs. *Advances in Nursing Science, 38*(4), 270–278. doi: 10.1097/ANS.0000000000000089

Cohen, S., & Mount, B. (1992). Quality of life in terminal illness: Defining and measuring subjective well-being in the dying. *Journal of Palliative Care, 8*(3), 40–45.

Cordo, J., & Hill-Rodriguez, D. (2017). The evolution of a nursing professional practice model through leadership support of clinical nurse engagement, empowerment, and shared decision making. *Nurse Leader, 15*(5), 325–330.

Davidson, S., Weberg, D., Porter-O'Grady, T., & Malloch, K. (2017). *Leadership for evidence-based innovation in nursing and health professions.* Burlington, MA: Jones and Bartlett.

Dowd, T., Kolcaba, K., & Steiner, R. (2000). Using cognitive strategies to enhance bladder control and comfort. *Holistic Nursing Practice, 14*(2), 91–103.

Dowd, T., Kolcaba, K., & Steiner, R. (2002). Correlations among six measures of bladder function. *Journal of Nursing Measurement, 10*(1), 27–38.

Dowd, T., Kolcaba, K., & Steiner, R. (2003). The addition of coaching to cognitive strategies. *Journal of Ostomy and Wound Management, 30*(2), 90–99.

Dowd, T., Kolcaba, K., Steiner, R., & Fashinpaur, D. (2007). Comparison of a healing touch, coaching, and a combined intervention on comfort and stress in younger college students. *Holistic Nursing Practice, 21*(4), 194–202.

Dunton, N., Gonnerman, D., Montalvo, I., & Schumann, M. (2011). Incorporating nursing quality indicators in public reporting and value-based purchasing initiatives. *American Nurse Today, 6*(1), 14–17.

Ebrahimpour, F., & Hoseini, A. S. S. (2018). Suggesting a practical theory to oncology nurses: Case report of a child in discomfort. *Journal of Palliative Care, 33*(4), 194–196. doi: 10.1177/0825859718763645

Egger-Rainer, A., Trinka, E., Hofler, J., & Dieplinger, A. M. (2017). Epilepsy monitoring—The patients' views: A qualitative study based on Kolcaba's comfort theory. *Epilepsy & Behavior, 68*, 208–215. doi: 10.1016/j.yebeh.2016.11.005

Estridge, K. M., Morris, D. L., Kolcaba, K., & Winkelman, C. (2018). Comfort and fluid retention in adult patients receiving hemodialysis. *Nephrology Nursing Journal, 45*(1), 25–60.

Glaser, C., & Strauss, A. (1965). *Awareness of dying.* Chicago, IL: Aldine.

Goodwin, M., & Candela, L. (2013). Outcomes of newly practicing nurses who applied principles of holistic comfort theory during the transition from school to practice: A qualitative study. *Nurse Education Today, 33*(6), 614–619. doi: 10.1016/j.nedt.2012.07.013

Goodwin, M., Sener, I., & Steiner, S. H. (2007). A novel theory for nursing education: holistic comfort. *Journal of Holistic Nursing, 25*(4), 278–285.

Hall, M. A. (2004). Managed care patient protection or provider protection? A qualitative assessment. *American Journal of Medicine, 117*(12), 932–937.

Henderson, V. (1978). *Principals and practice of nursing.* New York, NY: Macmillan.

Kilic, H. S., & Tastan, S. (2017). Development of post hip replacement comfort scale. *Applied Nursing Research, 38*, 169–174.

Kolcaba, K. (1991). A taxonomic structure for the concept comfort. *Journal of Nursing Scholarship, 23*(4), 237–239.

Kolcaba, K. (1992). Holistic comfort: Operationalizing the construct as a nurse-sensitive outcome. *Advances in Nursing Science, 15*(1), 1–10.

Kolcaba, K. (1994). A theory of holistic comfort for nursing. *Journal of Advanced Nursing, 19*, 1178–1184.

Kolcaba, K. (1997). *The comfort line.* Retrieved October 7, 2011 from http://www.thecomfortline.com

Kolcaba, K. (2001). Evolution of the mid range theory of comfort for outcomes research. *Nursing Outlook, 49*(2), 86–92.

Kolcaba, K. (2003). *Comfort theory and practice: A vision for holistic health care and research.* New York, NY: Springer.

Kolcaba, K., Dowd, T., Steiner, R., & Mitzel, A. (2004). Efficacy of hand massage for enhancing comfort of Hospice patients. *Journal of Hospice & Palliative Nursing, 6*(2), 91–101.

Kolcaba, K., & Fox, C. (1999). The effects of guided imagery on comfort of women with early stage breast cancer undergoing radiation therapy. *Oncology Nursing Forum, 26*(1), 67–72.

Kolcaba, K., & Kolcaba, R. (1991). An analysis of the concept of comfort. *Journal of Advanced Nursing, 16*, 1301–1310.

Kolcaba, K., Schirm, V., & Steiner R. (2006). Effects of hand massage on comfort of nursing home residents. *Geriatric Nursing, 27*(2), 85–91.

Kolcaba, K., Tilton, C., & Drouin, C. (2006). Use of comfort theory to enhance the practice environment. *Journal of Nursing Administration, 36*(11), 538–544.

Krinsky, R., Murillo, I., & Johnson, J. (2014). A practical application of Katharine Kolcaba's comfort theory to cardiac patients. *Applied Nursing Research, 27*(2), 147–150. doi: 10.1016/j.apnr.2014.02.004

LaFond, D. A. (2012). Promotion of comfort through early palliative care consultation for children and adolescents undergoing hematopoietic stem cell transplantation. University of Maryland Baltimore, School of Nursing, Doctor of Nursing Practice (DNP) Scholarly Projects. Retrieved November 1, 2018 from http://archive.hshsl.umaryland.edu/handle/10713/1722 or http://hdl.handle.net/10713/1722

Ligeikis-Clayton, C. (2000). *Nurses' perceptions of their own comfort levels, abilities, and importance that they place on implementing RTS standards of care following the death of a stillborn infant* (Doctoral dissertation). Retrieved from Proquest Dissertations and Theses database (UMI Number 9958504).

Lima, J. V., Guedes, M. V., Silva, L. F., Freitas, M. C., & Fialho, A. V. (2017). Usefulness of the comfort theory in the clinical nursing care of new mothers: Critical analysis. *Revista Gaúcha de Enfermagem, 37*(4), e65022. doi: 10.1590/1983-1447.2016.04.65022

Lipsey, M. (1990). *Design sensitivity.* New Park, CA: Sage.

Lorente, S., Losilla, J. M., & Vives, J. (2017). Instruments to assess patient comfort during hospitalization: A psychometric review. *Journal of Advanced Nursing, 74*, 1001–1015.

Ludington-Hoe, S. M. (2015). Skin-to-skin contact: A comforting place with comfort food. *MCN: The American Journal of Maternal/Child Nursing, 40*(6), 359–366; quiz E323–354. doi: 10.1097/nmc.0000000000000178

Malloch, K., & Porter-O'Grady, T. (2010). *Introduction to evidence-based practice in nursing and health care* (2nd ed.). Sudbury, MA: Jones and Bartlett.

Manning, S. N. (2016). A multiple case study of patient journeys in Wales from A&E to a hospital ward or home. *British Journal of Community Nursing, 21*(10), 509–517.

March, A., & McCormack, D. (2009). Nursing theory-directed healthcare. *Holistic Nursing Practice, 23*(2), 75–80.

Marshall, A. M. (2016). Development of a practice guidelines for DNP prepared nurse practitioners working in long-term care facilities. Walden University, Walden Dissertation and Doctoral Studies, Doctor of Nursing Practice (DNP). Retrieved November 1, 2018 from https://scholarworks.waldenu.edu/dissertations/2093

McIlveen, K., & Morse, J. (1995). The role of comfort in nursing care: 1900–1980. *Clinical Nursing Research, 4*(2), 127–148.

Nightingale, F. (1859). *Notes on nursing.* London, UK: Harrison.

Novak, B., Kolcaba, K., Steiner, R., & Dowd, T. (2001). Measuring comfort in caregivers and patients during late end-of-life care. *American Journal of Hospice and Palliative Medicine, 18*(3), 170–180.

NQMC. (2003). *National Quality Measures Clearinghouse.* http://qualitymeasures.ahrq.gov/comfort (no longer supported by federal funding)

Orlando, I. (1961/1990). *The dynamic nurse–patient relationship.* New York, NY: National League for Nursing.

Parks, M. D., Morris, D. L., Kolcaba, K., & McDonald, P. E. (2017). An evaluation of patient comfort during acute psychiatric hospitalization. *Perspectives in Psychiatric Care, 53*(1), 29–37. doi: 10.1111/ppc.12134

Paterson, J., & Zderad, L. (1976/1988). *Humanistic nursing.* New York, NY: National League for Nursing.

Ponte, K. M., & da Silva, L. (2014). Implementation of the care-research method based on the comfort theory: Experience report. *Ciencia, Cuidado e Saude, 13*(2), 388–393. doi: 10.4025/cienccuidsaude.v13i2.16439

President's Advisory Commission on Consumer Protection and Quality in the Health Care Industry. (November 20, 1997). Consumer bill of rights. Retrieved from http://govinfo.library.unt.edu/hcquality/press/cbor.html

Rock, J. (2004). *Comfort levels of obstetric nurses caring for parents who have experienced a perinatal loss/stillborn infant* (Doctoral dissertation). Retrieved from ProQuest Dissertations and Theses database (UMI Number 3119159).

Rondinelli, J., Long, K., Seelinger, C., Crawford, C. L., & Valdez, R. (2015). Factors related to nurse comfort when caring for families experiencing perinatal loss. *Journal for Nurses in Professional Development, 31*(3), 158–163.

Sartz, D. A. (2013). Screening for distress in ambulatory oncology patients: The cope project. Regis University, Doctor of Nursing Practice (DNP). Retrieved November 1, 2018 from Regis University ePublications: https://epublications.regis.edu/theses/205

Shu Hua, N. G. (2017). Application of Kolcaba's comfort theory to the management of a patient with hepatocellular carcinoma. *Singapore Nursing Journal, 44*(1), 16–23.

Simes, T., Roy, S., O'Neill, B., Ryan, C., Lapkin, S., & Curtis, E. (2018). Moving nurse educators towards transcendence in simulation comfort. *Nurse Education in Practice, 28*, 218–223. doi: 10.1016/j.nepr.2017.10.024

Stallings-Welden, L. M., Doerner, M., Ketchem, E. L., Benkert, L., Alka, S., & Stallings, J. D. (2018). A comparison of aromatherapy to standard care for relief of PONV and PDNV in ambulatory surgical patients. *Journal of PeriAnesthesia Nursing, 33*(2), 116–128. doi: 10.1016/j.jopan.2016.09.001

Twohig, B., Manasia, A., Bassily-Marcus, A., Oropello, J., Gayton, M., Gaffney, C., & Kohli-Seth, R. (2015). Family experience survey in the surgical intensive care unit. *Applied Nursing Research, 28*(4), 281–284. doi: 10.1016/j.apnr.20l5.02.009

# 14 Health-Related Quality of Life

Kristin E. Sandau, Timothy S. Bredow, and Sandra J. Peterson

## Definition of Key Terms

| | |
|---|---|
| **Health-related quality of life (HRQOL)** | Subset of quality of life representing satisfaction in areas of life likely to be affected by health status; HRQOL is subjective, multidimensional, and temporal. |
| **Life domains** | Basic components of quality of life and HRQOL referring to specific aspects of life, most commonly physical, cognitive, socioeconomic, and psychological/spiritual |
| **Nursing interventions** | Although rarely included as a component in formal theoretical models of HRQOL, involve delivering specific care or treatments targeted for an individual or group who have deficits or potential deficits in an identified domain that may impact HRQOL. |
| **Quality of life** | Satisfaction in areas of life deemed important to the individual. |

Quality of life (QOL) has been a philosophical and sociopolitical phenomenon for hundreds, if not thousands, of years. Because QOL is not clearly identified with one theorist, it is difficult to define and describe. This lack of specificity has not diminished its popularity as an outcome measure among patients tested in thousands of studies published both nationally and internationally. QOL has been identified as a middle range theory (Meleis, 1997) representing a specific phenomenon, with a limited number of related concepts, that has obvious applications to practice. The more limited construct of health-related QOL in the context of health care (often referred to as HRQOL) may be even more fitted as a middle range theory because HRQOL is somewhat more limited in focus on areas of life most directly influenced by one's health.

## Historical Background

The concept of QOL, concerned with an individual's personal satisfaction with life, has its roots in classical Greek thought and religious teachings. Aristotle is credited with the initial conceptualization of QOL, defined as happiness, the good life, or the outcome of a life of virtue (Morgan, 1992). In the New Testament (John 10:10), Jesus stated that he came to give life and give it abundantly (Holman, 2017). The 10 stages of enlightenment in Buddhism start out with achieving joy in life (Stryk, 1968).

Pigou has been credited with modern introduction of the term in 1920 in his book on economics and welfare (Wood-Dauphinee, 1999). Politically, use of the concept, QOL, was limited until it was reintroduced in remarks made by Presidents Johnson and Nixon in speeches on environmental and social issues (Campbell, 1981; Dalkey, Rourke, Lewis, & Snyder, 1972). QOL has its academic roots in the disciplines of psychology and sociology (Spranger, 2001). In the 1970s, these disciplines began to consider the issue of QOL. In the 1970s, the business world adopted the term QOL to make claims about the ability of a product to enhance a person's life in the milieu of everyday living.

The WHO's more encompassing definition of health as physical, psychological, and social well-being, and not just the absence of illness or infirmity (World Health Organization, 1948), provided early impetus to the consideration of QOL as a relevant human experience for health care professionals. In 1978, the WHO provided a statement on the application of its definition of health, indicating that individuals have the right "to psychosocial care and adequate QOL in addition to physiologic care" (King & Hinds, 1998, p. xi). Nursing's interest in QOL is long-standing. Florence Nightingale's involvement with the British military provided multiple examples of how nurses can promote the QOL for individuals. This interest has intensified and become a focus of research for nurses.

HRQOL, a subcategory of global QOL, is a more recent concept. Health care trends have contributed to the emergence of HRQOL as an important phenomenon. In the past 15 to 20 years, the concern for patients has become more inclusive, focusing not just on the treatment of disease but also on the restoration and promotion of health (Read, 1993). With increased client longevity, health care professionals are attending to the lifestyle issues that accompany chronic disease and often affect QOL. The Food and Drug Administration (FDA) is reflecting this changing emphasis. It can require documentation of not only the safety and efficacy of new products but also their effect on a user's QOL (Spilker, 1996).

QOL has emerged as a concept of interest to many disciplines. This multiplicity of discipline-specific perspectives has led to little consensus on a definition. Philosophers consider the nature of existence and what is meant by the "good life." Ethicists are concerned with social utility. Economists pursue cost-effectiveness in producing the greatest good. Physicians focus on health- and illness-specific issues, while nurses may approach the issue of QOL more holistically (Anderson & Burckhardt, 1999).

## Definition of Theory Concepts

QOL and the subconstruct HRQOL have suffered from a lack of clarity for both conceptual and operational definitions in research studies. Regrettably, some researchers published results of HRQOL outcome studies without first stating their conceptual definition of HRQOL. Similarly, several researchers have not accurately matched their conceptual definition with their operational definition. For example, researchers have inaccurately stated that they are measuring the broad construct of QOL but have instead operationalized QOL as an objective measure, such as *length of time without return to surgery* (Elkins, Knott-Craif, McCue, & Lane, 1997).

In the 1980s and early 1990s, many researchers reported outcomes as QOL or HRQOL but had only measured one domain, such as physical functional status. However, functional status is not interchangeable with the construct HRQOL and is most appropriately considered only one of several components contributing to overall HRQOL. Functional status has traditionally been defined by degree of disability to perform standard activities in life (Stineman, Lollar, & Ustun, 2005). QOL is an even broader construct than is HRQOL: inclusive of all life domains important to a person. The construct HRQOL developed as

an entity separate from global QOL as a means of specifying health-related domains of particular interest to researchers (Wenger, Naughton, & Furberg, 1996).

Some authors have used the term *subjective health status* interchangeably with HRQOL, considering it a more accurate descriptor of the phenomenon (Staniszewska, 1998). However, Ferrans, Zerwic, Wilbur, and Larson (2005) categorized approaches to HRQOL measurement as *perceived status* or *evaluative* approaches to HRQOL. HRQOL-*perceived* status measures ask patients to rate their functional abilities, such as the commonly used SF-36 survey (Ware & Sherbourne, 1992) and the EORTC Quality of Life Questionnaire (Aaronson et al., 1993). Alternatively, HRQOL *evaluation* measures, such as the Ferrans and Powers' Quality of Life Index (Ferrans, 1990a) and the Quality of Life Scale for Cancer (Padilla et al., 1983), place less emphasis on the specific functional abilities and more emphasis on the patient's perception of how satisfied he or she is with his or her abilities or life domains. Both perceived status and evaluation measures have a purpose in research. Perceived status may be helpful in testing specific effects of an intervention, while evaluation measures may capture more personal judgments of life satisfaction based on internal expectations that are changeable within the individual. Some measures incorporate both perceived status and evaluative approaches. Such is the case with the WHO Quality of Life Assessment, which covers physical, psychological, social, and spiritual domains and as a result is quite lengthy (World Health Organization, 1995). The McGill Quality of Life Questionnaire uses evaluation approaches for its four domains, with additional status approaches for two of these domains (Cohen, Mount, Strobel, & Bui, 1995).

Despite significant confusion over related terminology, theorists and researchers have increasingly described the constructs of QOL and HRQOL as having three characteristics: HRQOL is *multidimensional*, *temporal*, and *subjective*. The multidimensional aspect of HRQOL (Aaronson et al., 1993; Faden & Leplege, 1992; Staniszewska, 1998) is reflected by the major life domains, commonly identified as physiological, psychological, and sociological (Padilla & Grant, 1985). Other investigators have stated that a spiritual domain is of importance (Cella & Tulsky, 1990; Ferrans & Powers, 1985). Recent publications have featured physical, psychosocial, spiritual, emotional, and cognitive/mental dimensions. Osoba (1994) has suggested that researchers can appropriately refer to their study as measuring HRQOL if at least three life domains received assessment.

HRQOL is temporal in nature; patients can change their self-perceptions as they experience events in everyday life and process what they feel are QOL priorities (Peplau, 1994; Sprangers & Schwartz, 1999). Some scholars state that HRQOL is primarily subjective in nature but may include objective assessments at times (Oleson, 1990; Zhan, 1992). However, most researchers now consider HRQOL as subjective in nature (Cella, 1992; Cooley, 1998; Harrison, Juniper, & Mitchell-DiCenso, 1996; Murdaugh, 1997). Further investigation is needed for practical considerations related to ethical implications of allowing those other than the patients to make treatment decisions based on assumed HRQOL when the patients are unable to speak for themselves, such as those in vegetative states. Work has been done to test the validity of parallel administration of subjective HRQOL with proxy health status measures completed for patients by health care providers or family members (Addington-Hall & Kalra, 2001). Measures obtained by others would be most accurately referred to as proxy subjective health status rather than HRQOL.

## Description of the Theory of Quality of Life and Health-Related Quality of Life

There are many models of QOL or HRQOL (Cowan, Young Graham, & Cochrane, 1992; Ferrans, 1990b; Ferrell, Grant, Dean, Funk, & Ly, 1996; Oleson, 1990; Padilla & Grant, 1985; Zhan, 1992), as found in King and Hinds (1998), most of which omit the relationship between specific interventions and the factors that affect HRQOL. Three seminal models of QOL were provided in the 1990s. Spilker (1996) provided an introductory framework for QOL in health care by illustrating QOL as a pyramid of three levels (Fig. 14.1). A model by Ferrans and Powers (1993) also identified QOL as a main outcome measure, rather than HRQOL (Fig. 14.2). However, HRQOL researchers have sometimes chosen to concentrate on specific parts of the model rather than the entire model. Researchers have adapted models for use according to the specific condition or population they wish to study (Sandau, Lindquist, Treat-Jacobson, & Savik, 2008). While technically a model may be designed to illustrate QOL, clinicians wishing to research the more limited construct of HRQOL have made adaptations. Researchers should provide clarity about how any adapted or abbreviated conceptual definition supports their selected operational measures.

Nurses Ferrans and Powers developed a theory in which they provided the seminal definition of QOL as a person's "sense of well-being that stems from satisfaction or dissatisfaction with the areas of life that are important to him/her" (Ferrans & Powers, 1992, p. 29). Because their model encompassed all major life domains, their resulting operational measure, the Ferrans and Powers QOL Index, is a global multidimensional measure designed to represent the comprehensive construct of QOL (Fig. 14.2). The listed domains are health and functioning, socioeconomic, psychological/spiritual, and family.

A commonly cited model in health care disciplines is that of Wilson and Cleary (1995). Although both authors were physicians, the model combines the "social" paradigm with the "medical" paradigm. This model represents the relationships among the basic concepts of HRQOL. The model identifies five determinants that exist on a "continuum of increasing biological, social, and psychological complexity" (p. 60). These leveled determinants of HRQOL are referred to as taxonomy and consist of

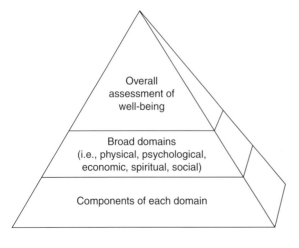

**Figure 14.1**   Three levels of quality of life. (From Spilker, B. (Ed.). (1996). *Quality of life and pharmacoeconomics in clinical trials* (2nd ed., p. 2). Philadelphia, PA: Lippincott-Raven Publishers.)

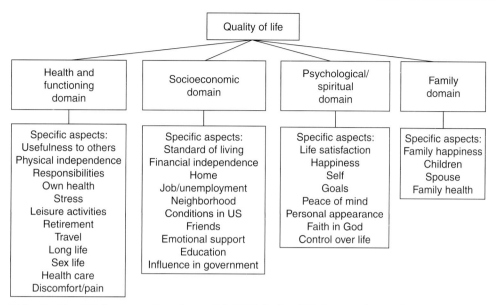

**Figure 14.2** Quality-of-life framework. (From Ferrans, C. E. (1990). Quality of life: Conceptual issues. *Seminars in Oncology Nursing,* 6(4), 248–254.)

biological factors, symptoms, functioning, general health perceptions, and overall HRQOL. They are in turn influenced by characteristics of the individual and environment.

Sousa and colleagues tested the Wilson and Cleary model, using multiple linear regression path analysis to evaluate the variables for empirical linkages to overall HRQOL (Sousa, Holzemer, Henry, & Slaughter, 1999). They reported that data were consistent with the theory and reported a 32% variance in overall QOL among their sample of persons with HIV. However, biological and physiological variables provided the weakest correlations with the other variables, suggesting little influence. The authors indicated that further research was necessary into areas such as other potential influences of personality, motivation, and social and economic supports, as well as the influences of time over the model (Sousa, 1999). Sousa and Chen (2002) continued work using structural equation modeling to address conceptual issues of HRQOL. The Wilson and Cleary model encompasses several large constructs as variables, so theory testing the model in its entirety is an intensive feat and is rarely done.

Anderson and Burckhardt (1999) suggested that a major limitation of the Wilson and Cleary model is that the medical factors seem central, rather than the nonmedical factors, to the overall HRQOL. Similarly, Murdaugh (1997) contended that the Wilson and Cleary model may be more accurately referred to as a taxonomy of patient outcomes due to its continuum of intuitively linked pathways with little empirical support. The majority of variance for overall HRQOL was unexplained, and many questions remain. Further study of relationships between other variables that can be affected by independent nursing interventions affecting QOL and HRQOL (such as interventions to support resiliency, self-efficacy, and hope) is encouraged.

Wilson and Cleary have described the arrows in the figure to represent the dominant causal relationships without excluding reciprocal connections between either adjacent or nonadjacent components of the model. Ferrans and nursing colleagues offered a revision to the Wilson and Cleary model (Ferrans et al., 2005), in which they made three major changes: They (a) added arrows to show that biological function is influenced by characteristics of the environment and individual, (b) deleted nonmedical factors, and (c) deleted labeling on arrows, which tends to restrict relationships.

Work by Padilla and Grant (1985) occurred as early as the above models but, aside from the oncology realm, appears to have been less recognized among health disciplines. Their work deserves discussion because it offered one of the first QOL models to specifically include independent nursing process interventions as a component in the formal model (Fig. 14.3). These include caring attitude, specific nursing interventions, and promotion of self-care. These interventions are perceived by the

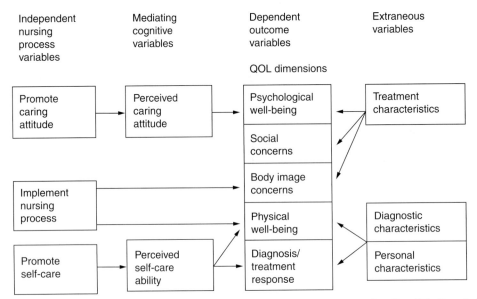

**Figure 14.3**    A model of the relationship between the nursing process and the dimensions of quality of life. (From Padilla, G. V., & Grant, M. M. (1985). Quality of life as a cancer nursing outcome variable. *Advances in Nursing Science, 8*(1), 45–60.)

patient and influence outcome variables that can be categorized by QOL dimensions. For example, the nursing interventions to promote healthy body image in a patient with a new colostomy can influence the patient's overall QOL by contributing to enhanced or maintained body image. Extraneous variables are recognized in the model, such as the individual's prognosis and personal characteristics, and whether the colostomy is temporary or permanent.

For their model, nurse researchers Stuifbergen, Seraphine, and Roberts (2000) used structural equation modeling to test the selected factors influencing health-promoting behavior or QOL in persons with chronic disabling conditions. QOL was defined as "an individual's overall sense of health, well-being, and satisfaction with life" (p. 124). A complex interaction of contextual factors (severity of illness being most dominant), antecedent variables, and health-promoting behaviors all contributed to QOL in their proposed model. Interventions to enhance mediating factors of social support, acceptance, decreased barriers to self-efficacy, and increased self-efficacy for health behavior can contribute to health-promoting factors and enhanced QOL. The purposeful use of concepts that are currently being tested in nursing makes this model unique to nursing and within the scope of independent nursing interventions. Additionally, Leplege and Hunt (1997) commended the authors for acknowledging the interconnectedness of QOL

with other aspects of existence such as changes in work, coping strategies, personal relationships, and self-image.

## Application of the Theory in Research

HRQOL measurement provides an understanding of the patient-perceived outcome experience of chronic illness, evaluation of a procedure, medication, or other intervention between groups, among individuals, or between populations. More recently, HRQOL measures have been used to evaluate efforts of health promotion, including independent nursing interventions such as education and counseling (see Using Middle Range Theory in Research 14.1). Use of formal HRQOL measures has not been routine in clinical practice. The gap between research and clinical practice was fed by the initial lack of understanding that HRQOL measures are not "soft" optional measures but determinates helpful in clinical practice (Rumsfeld, 2002). Rubenstein (1996) provided a table summary of recommendations for incorporating routine and symptom-specific HRQOL screenings into office practice. McClane (2006) recommended three specific HRQOL measures for use by clinical nurse specialists in routine clinical assessment of elderly persons.

## USING MIDDLE RANGE THEORY IN RESEARCH    14.1

*Source: Harrison, M. B., Browne, G. B., Roberts, J., Tugwell, P., Gafni, A., & Graham, A. D. (2002). QOL of individuals with heart failure: A randomized trial of the effectiveness of two models of hospital-to-home transition. Medical Care, 40(4), 271–282.*

### RESEARCH PURPOSE

Harrison and colleagues conducted a randomized controlled trial to evaluate the effect of transitional care on HRQOL, rates of readmission, and emergency room use of patients with heart failure.

### RESEARCH DESIGN

A 12-week, prospective, randomized controlled trial.

### SAMPLE/PARTICIPANTS

One hundred and fifty-seven adult hospitalized patients with heart failure.

### DATA COLLECTION

The nurse-led intervention included education and support for self-management for a period of 2 weeks after hospital discharge. HRQOL was operationalized by using both a generic health status (SF-36) and disease-specific QOL measure (Minnesota Living with Heart Failure Questionnaire [MLHFQ]).

### FINDINGS

At 6 weeks after hospital discharge, the overall MLHFQ score was better among the patients randomized to receive the nurse-led intervention than among the usual care patients. However, there was no significant difference in any of the subscales for the SF-36. At 12 weeks after discharge, more of the control group had been readmitted compared to the intervention group (31% versus 23%), and significantly, more of the usual care group visited the emergency department compared with the transitional group (46% versus 29%). This study provides evidence-based support for nurse-led interventions to successfully improve HRQOL.

The article, like many published in clinical journals, lacked a conceptual definition for HRQOL. However, the authors are to be commended for attempting to address whether or not the statistically significant improvements on the MLHFQ could be considered clinically significant. The authors added a "minimally clinical importance difference" (MCID) analysis, which they defined as a five-point or greater change in the total MLHFQ score. Relative changes in score between baseline and 12 weeks postdischarge were compared for both groups; the most contrast in scores was with the MLHFQ emotional dimension, where improvement was 36% for the transitional group (versus <1% for the control group). Finally, the fact that the generic SF-36 scores were not improved, while the MLHFQ scores were improved, highlights the importance of knowing one's sample and selecting a measure that will be sensitive to changes expected by a particular intervention in a select population.

## Instruments Used in Empirical Testing

### CATEGORIES OF MEASUREMENT

Measurement tools for HRQOL can be categorized in a variety of ways. For example, one category of measure is based on the number of life domains that are encompassed within the measure. If a tool is designed to examine a full spectrum of life domains, it may be considered *global*. Global tools are important because they may show QOL changes in all domains of life. Heart failure, for example, may have a pervasive effect on patients' ability to generate income, socialize, and be sexually intimate. The Minnesota Living with Heart Failure Questionnaire (Rector, Kubo, & Cohen, 1987) attempts to capture a global perspective of the impact of a specific disease on various domains of life. In contrast to global measures, another category is that of measures that target a single domain, such as psychological health, as is offered by the Hospital Anxiety and Depression Scale (Zigmond & Snaith, 1983).

Table 14.1 provides a method of categorizing types of tools commonly used to measure QOL and HRQOL. *Generic* tools, while not specific to disease or treatment, are helpful for making comparisons across studies and between populations (Guyatt, Feeny, & Patrick, 1993). The Nottingham Health Profile has been commonly used in the United Kingdom as a generic tool but is also considered global because of its broad coverage of various life domains (Hunt, McEwen, & McKenna, 1985). The SF-36, which is a generic measure of subjective health status, provides two main summary scores for self-perceived physical and mental functioning, as well as eight more specific health scales (Ware & Sherbourne, 1992).

| Table 14.1 | Measures Commonly Used to Assess HRQOL |
|---|---|
| **Type** | **Examples** |
| Generic measures | Ferrans & Powers Quality of Life Index (Ferrans & Powers, 1992)<br>WHOQOL Assessment Tool (World Health Organization, 1995)<br>Nottingham Health Profile (Hunt, McEwan, & McKenna, 1985)<br>SF-36 (Ware & Sherbourne, 1992)<br>EuroQOL (EuroQOL Group, 1990)<br>Sickness Impact Profile (Bergner, Bobbitt, Carter, & Gilson, 1981) |
| Disease-specific, condition-specific, and treatment-specific measures | Ferrans & Powers Quality of Life Index—Cancer Version (Ferrans, 1990a)<br>Minnesota Living With Heart Failure (Rector et al., 1987)<br>Seattle Angina Questionnaire (Spertus et al., 1995)<br>The Arthritis Impact Measurement Scales (Meenan, Mason, Anderson, Guccione, & Kazis, 1992)<br>Children's Health Survey for Asthma (Sullivan & Olson, 1995)<br>Quality of Life Index: Hemodialysis (Ferrans & Powers, 1993)<br>QLQ-C30 version 3.0 is the generic measure that can be supplemented with disease-specific modules (breast, lung, head and neck, esophageal, ovarian, gastric, and cervical cancers, and multiple myeloma) (Aaronson et al., 1993) |
| Symptom-specific measures | McGill Pain Questionnaire (Melzack, 1975)<br>Hospital Anxiety and Depression Scale (Zigmond & Snaith, 1983)<br>Patient Health Questionnaire (PHQ-9) is a screen for depression (Kroenke, Spitzer, & Williams, 2001) |
| Quality-adjusted life-year (QALY), health utilities, and time trade-off measures | EQ-5D (van Agt, Essink-Bot, Krabbe, & Bonsel, 1994)<br>Time Without Symptoms or Toxicity (Q-TWIST) (Gelber et al., 1996) |
| Qualitative measures | Interviews<br>Focus groups<br>Preference based on interview script |

Researchers have tended toward augmenting generic measures with *disease- or condition-specific measures* in order to capture both overall health status and perceived effects of a certain condition (Bliven, Green, & Spertus, 1998). Disease-, condition-, or symptom-specific tools provide more sensitivity than do generic tools for clinicians looking for changes in disease patterns, such as frequency of loose stools or angina. Similarly, use of treatment or therapy-specific tools is helpful to care providers in evaluating specific responses by individual patients to treatments or changes as a result of intervention (see Using Middle Range Theory in Research 14.1).

A *quality-adjusted life-year* (QALY) instrument is used by some researchers to measure the extent of health improvement due to an intervention combined with the costs associated with the intervention, resulting in a mathematical formula that is used to assess their relative worth of the intervention from an economic perspective (Phillips & Thompson, 2007). For example, a year of perfect health may be worth a score of 1, but a year of less than perfect health life expectancy may be worth −1 point, and death may be worth 0 point. These measures are somewhat controversial and limited in chronic illness, where QOL is more important than is survival, and limited by heterogeneity in the samples being measured (Phillips & Thompson, 2007). They are used most often in pharmacoeconomic studies.

Finally, *qualitative* measures are valuable for development of theoretical definitions and new HRQOL measures, as well as for validity testing of an existing tool in a new or changing population. Qualitative measures may be used to augment a quantitative measure. Typically, qualitative methodologies in HRQOL include personal interviews and focus groups, with possible open-ended questions.

## GUIDELINES FOR MEASUREMENT

Investigators selecting measures for HRQOL studies must make sure they have a clear conceptual definition of HRQOL, and their selection of operational measures should match. Unfortunately, this has not always been the case in the early surge of HRQOL studies. An investigator attempting to measure HRQOL among hospice patients should consider which domains are conceptually important, or have been shown in past research or through clinical experience, to be important in that population. For example, an HRQOL investigator wishing to assess HRQOL among hospice patients would appropriately select a measure that includes the spiritual domain or augment a generic measure with assessment of subjective spiritual status. Similarly, if an investigator plans to use a generic HRQOL measure among patients undergoing treatment for prostate cancer, this generic measure would most appropriately be augmented by a subjective measure that includes self-evaluation of the social and sexual dimensions.

Gill and Feinstein (1994) provided guidelines for proper measurement of HRQOL, including allowing patients to rate the importance of domains, as in the Ferrans and Powers QOL Index (1992). Gill and Feinstein also recommended allowing patients to supplement standardized measures. While supplementing quantitative measures with qualitative measures may not be feasible in every study, this practice may provide a test of content validity to the quantitative measure. Study participants may alert investigators of important concerns that were not addressed on the quantitative questionnaire. Similarly, qualitative research in HRQOL, such as interviews, focus groups, and journaling, may provide foundational information for researchers striving to measure HRQOL in a previously understudied population (Sandau, Hoglund, Weaver, Boisjolie, & Feldman, 2014). Although Gill and Feinstein encouraged HRQOL investigators to provide an aggregate score so that study results can be compared with others, some debate the conceptual clarity of mathematically combining several measures to produce an artificially aggregated score. However, obtaining a global satisfaction measure in addition to disease-specific measures may be helpful for comparing results for specific interventions in a discrete population.

Researchers studying HRQOL must be prepared to address challenges in psychometric properties among the vast variety of measures available. Challenges to reliability include aberrancies in data collection (such as one research assistant giving more extensive coaching to some participants than others), the absence of a baseline HRQOL measure, and the use of only pieces of HRQOL measures (unless they have been tested for reliability as a subset). Challenges to validity in HRQOL research include potential concurrent life changes. For example, an investigator wishing to study the effect of an intervention for back pain may have confounding results when a generic HRQOL measure is complicated by a life change in a participant (e.g., loss of spouse) that is unrelated to the treatment for back pain. Practical considerations in

use of HRQOL measures include timing of study measures. For example, if one is evaluating how a surgery such as mastectomy may affect HRQOL, it may not be appropriate to obtain measures while the patient is still recovering from postoperative incisional pain, unless the investigator's intention is a purposeful longitudinal assessment. Other practical considerations include subject burden (length of the survey) and clinical relevance (what degree of change in a score will be considered clinically significant). Further discussion of desired psychometric properties of HRQOL measures is provided by DeVon and Ferrans (2003). In summary, selection of a measure includes finding a good match with one's conceptual definition of HRQOL, identifying the life domains and concerns most important to the study population, being clear on the research purpose, investigating past performance of the measure for validity and reliability, and evaluating feasibility of the measure.

## Health-Related Quality of Life as an Outcome Measure in Nursing

The goal of nursing interventions in HRQOL research is to have a positive impact on a patient's perceived satisfaction with HRQOL (see Table 14.2 and Using Middle Range Theories in Practice: Student Project 14.2). This is a central component of HRQOL in that the patient provides a subjective and personal expression of both the level of satisfaction (Staniszewska, 1998) and the degree to which the specific nursing interventions contribute to that level (Robinson, Whyte, & Fidler, 1997). Thus, patient-perceived satisfaction with HRQOL becomes a significant indicator of the success of an intervention. Patient satisfaction is conceptualized as a mediating variable, based on the work of Donabedian (1980), who consistently regarded patient satisfaction as an outcome. He contended that satisfaction with care represents the patient's judgment of quality of care (Yang, Simms, & Yin, 1999, p. 3).

The Cochrane Database has reviews evaluating the effectiveness of specific nursing interventions on QOL or HRQOL. By reviewing results in the Cochrane Database for *nursing interventions* and *quality of life*, one can learn, for example, whether breast care nurses can improve QOL for patients (Cruickshank, Kennedy, Lockhart, Dosser, & Dallas, 2008). A more extensive review of Cochrane studies using the terms *nursing* and *quality of life* provides readers with a realistic and somewhat sobering overview of attempts by nurses to improve QOL. The reader is left with a sense that (a) comparatively few nursing interventional

**Table 14.2 Examples of Research for Application to Practice**

| Reference | Research Design/ Meta-Analysis | Clinical Issue/ Research Question | Sample (n)/ Participants | Intervention | Outcome |
|---|---|---|---|---|---|
| Penny, K. I., & Smith, G. D. (2012). The use of data mining to identify indicators of health-related quality of life in patients with irritable bowel syndrome. *Journal of Clinical Nursing, 21*, 2761–2771. doi: 10.1111/j.1365-2702.2011.03897 | Cross-sectional survey of patients with irritable bowel syndrome (IBS) | Examine health-related quality of life (HRQOL) in patients with IBS; to explore use of data mining methods to identify which sociodemographic and IBS symptoms have greatest association with HRQOL. | Convenience sample of 494 persons with IBS (United Kingdom) | Signs and symptoms of IBS; SF-36; five domains EuroQOL (EQ-5D) questionnaire | Patients with IBS reported impaired HRQOL compared to norma-tive values for the SF-36 in the SK population. Pain/discomfort and anxiety/depression were frequently reported per the EQ-5D. Authors noted that sociodemographic factors such as being employed, a daily social activity, and married status were associated with better HRQOL. None of the data mining models used in the study lead to a greatly accurate classification of HRQOL for the IBS patients. |
| Vogler, J., Klein, A., & Bender, A. (2014). Long-term health-related quality-of-life in patients with acquired brain injury and their caregivers. *Brain Injury, 28*(11), 1381–1388. doi: 10.3109/02699052.2014.919536 | Cross-sectional surveys | Assess long-term HRQOL in patients who had acute brain injury (ABI) and their caregivers. | Convenience sample of 104 caregivers; 30 patients with previous ABI (mean time postin-jury 18 y) (Germany) | Investigator-developed question-naires, Modified Caregiver Strain Index (MCSI), Burden Scale for Family Caregivers (BSFC), Beck Depression Inventory (BDI), WHO-Five Well-Being Index (WHO-5), EuroQOL-5 (EQ-5D), and single items of the Gross National Happiness (GNH) Index | After ABI, HRQOL and perceived health status (per EQ-5D) in caregiv-ers remained lower than did those in age-matched controls. HRQOL and perceived health status (per EQ-5D) were lower in patients than in caregivers; however, no differ-ences were noted between patients and caregivers for the GNH items for QOL, happiness, or enjoyment of life. Predictors for HRQOL in caregivers included well-being, caregiver strain, depressive symptoms, and caregiver age. Study supports the need for long-term support of caregivers. |

| Citation | Design | Purpose | Sample | Instruments | Findings |
|---|---|---|---|---|---|
| Chapa, D. W., Akintade, B., Schron, E., Friedmann, E., & Thomas, S. A. (2014). Is health-related quality of life a predictor of hospitalization and mortality among women or men with atrial fibrillation? *Journal of Cardiovascular Nursing, 29*(6), 555–564. doi: 10.1097/JCN.0000000000000095 | Secondary data analysis of limited-use data from the National Institutes of Health/National Heart, Lung, and Blood Institute Atrial Fibrillation Follow-up Investigation of Rhythm Management clinical trial | Examine clinical and HRQOL predictors of mortality and 1-year hospitalization in women compared with men with atrial fibrillation. | Patients with atrial fibrillation 262 female 431 male (United States) | SF-36, Quality of Life Index—Cardiac Version | Mortality did not differ according to gender. For women, clinical status (diabetes, stroke, age) predicted mortality. For men, clinical status (age), physical component scores of SF-36, and overall QOL (per Quality of Life Index—Cardiac Version) independently predicted mortality. For hospitalization, both HRQOL and clinical status were predictors for hospitalization among men and women. Nursing interventions have potential to modify predictors of mortality and hospitalization for women and men with atrial fibrillation. |
| Wong, F. M. F., Sit, J. W. H., Wong, E. M. L., & Choi, K. C. C. (2014). Factors associated with health-related quality of life among patients with implantable cardioverter defibrillator: Identification of foci for nursing intervention. *Journal of Advanced Nursing, 70*(12), 2821–2834. doi: 10.1111/jan.12434 | Descriptive design | Explore factors associated with HRQOL in patients with implantable cardioverter–defibrillators (ICDs). | Convenience sample of 139 adult Chinese outpatients with ICDs (Hong Kong) | Structured investigator-developed, face-to-face interviews; questionnaires; medical reviews; SF-36 for HRQOL; Hospital Anxiety and Depression Scale; Chinese (Hong Kong) version of the Social Support Questionnaire (short form) | Among patients with ICDs, the physical component summary (PCS) of the SF-36 was lower, but the mental component summary (MCS) was higher compared to the general Hong Kong Chinese population. Coexisting illnesses were associated with lower HRQOL. Factors negatively associated with PCS were female gender, self-care dependence, atrial fibrillation, diabetes mellitus, and depression, whereas anxiety and depression were negatively associated with MCS. Shock experience and social support were not found to be associated with HRQOL; however, lack of a measure to include ICD-specific concerns was a limitation. Nursing and pharmacologic interventions to improve HRQOL in patients with ICDs are needed. |

*(Continued)*

**Table 14.2   Examples of Research for Application to Practice** (Continued)

| Reference | Research Design/ Meta-Analysis | Clinical Issue/ Research Question | Sample (n)/ Participants | Intervention | Outcome |
|---|---|---|---|---|---|
| Bandayrel, K., & Johnston, B. C. (2014). Recent advances in patient and proxy-reported quality of life research. *Health and Quality of Life Outcomes, 12*(110), 1–9. doi: 10.1186/s12955-014-0110-7 | Review of literature | Identify and describe recent methodological advances and innovations in HRQOL. | Studies published in the *Health and Quality of Life Outcomes* journal in 2012–2013 were screened by title and abstract; 16 articles out of 358 screened were considered relevant to review. | Journal articles were summarized and grouped into thematic categories. | Several methodological advancements and innovations were described, including the PROMIS pediatric proxy-item bank and recommendations for creating patient-reported outcome (PRO) instruments. |
| Lim, J.-W., & Ashing-Giwa, K. T. (2013). Is family functioning and communication associated with health related quality of life for Chinese- and Korean-American breast cancer survivors? *Quality of Life Research, 22*(6), 1319–1329. doi: 10.1007/s11136-012-0247-y | Cross-sectional surveys | Investigate direct and indirect pathways of family flexibility, social support, and family communication on HRQOL for Chinese and Korean American breast cancer survivors (BCS) | Convenience sample of 86 Chinese and 71 Korean American BCS from Los Angeles area hospitals (United States) | Examination of the following: demographic and medical characteristics; SF-36; Family Adaptability and Cohesion Evaluation Scales (FACES IV), Family Communication Scale (general communication); Family Avoidance of Communication About Cancer (FACC) Scale (cancer-related communication); MOS Social Support Survey; Asian American Multidimensional Acculturation Scale (AAMAS), European American section; three-item investigator-developed items for shared decision-making | Family communication impacts HRQOL among Asian American BCS. Similarities in family characteristics exist between the two Asian American groups; however, specific ethnic variations also exist. Chinese Americans were more likely than were Korean Americans to have flexibility in the family functioning and to be acculturated. Specific cultural and familial contexts should be considered to better tailor interventions to enhance family communication and improve HRQOL. |
| Sandau, K. E., Hoglund, B. A., Weaver, C. E., Boisjolie, C., & Feldman, D. (2014). A conceptual definition of quality of life with a left ventricular assist device: Results from a qualitative study. *Heart Lung, 43*(1), 32–40. doi: 10.1016/j.hrtlng.2013.09.004 | Qualitative (grounded theory) | To develop a conceptual definition of quality of life (QOL) with a left ventricular assist device (LVAD) | Convenience sample of 11 outpatients with LVADs participated twice in interviews (United States) | Paired and individual semistructured interviews | A conceptual definition was established: "Being well enough to do and enjoy day-to-day activities that are important to me." Participants described five important life domains: physical, emotional, social, cognitive, and spiritual/meaning. However, participants identified unique concerns not addressed by generic or heart failure disease, specific measures typically used in the LVAD population. The conceptual definition and concerns provided a foundation for investigators to develop the QOLVAD, a disease-specific measure. |

---

**USING MIDDLE RANGE THEORIES IN PRACTICE :STUDENT PROJECT** | **14.2**

Source: Ahn, S., Chen, Y., Bredow, T., Cheung, C., & Yu, F. (2017). Effects of non-pharmacological treatments on quality of life in Parkinson's disease: A review. Journal of Parkinson's Disease and Alzheimer's Disease, 4(1).

### PROJECT PURPOSE

The purpose of this literature review was to analyze the state of the science on the effects of nonpharmacological treatments on quality of life in person's with Parkinson's disease.

### RESEARCH DESIGN

Systematic review of the literature. The literature search was conducted using keywords in electronic databases up to September 1, 2016, and cross-searching the references of identified articles. Of the 259 articles generated, 26 met the eligibility criteria and were included in this review. The majority of studies (77%) were Level I evidence and 23% level II evidence. The levels of study quality were strong (50%), moderate (15%), and weak (35%).

### FINDINGS

Parkinson's disease is a neurodegenerative chronic condition with a declining trajectory and lack of a cure, making quality of life an important aspect of care. The interventions varied across studies with 15 studies evaluating a similar intervention. About 58% of the studies showed that the interventions improved quality of life.

### CONCLUSION

A variety of nonpharmacological interventions have been increasingly studied for their effects on quality of life in Parkinson's disease, showing initial promising results. Interventions were effective in improving the participant's quality of life score while they were engaged in the trial, but declined when not involved with the intervention. Moreover, most interventions were only examined by a limited number of studies, and the minimal and optimal intervention doses needed for improving quality of life are yet unknown.

This project was done by Sangwoo Ahn as part of his doctoral work in the College of Nursing at the University of MN, under the guidance of Fang Yu, project advisor. It was supported in part by a grant from the Parkinson's Foundation.

---

studies with QOL as an outcome variable currently exist with randomized or comparison groups and (b) most nursing interventional studies may be better off avoiding a hypothesis that the outcome of global QOL will be an improved outcome based on a single nursing intervention.

What may be a realistic goal for nursing interventions is to make a clinically meaningful improvement in a particular domain, such as the social or mental domain, rather than expect changes to the huge construct of QOL (or even HRQOL), which are immense outcome variables potentially affected by a myriad of confounding factors. Life continues to present some complex conditions for which there is no simple cure. It is for these conditions (i.e., HIV, end of life, heart failure, diabetes, depression) that we should perhaps most energetically focus our efforts. Our work to identify, and combat alongside our patients, the persistent conditions of depression and anxiety, for example, that occur concomitant with chronic conditions, provides us with challenges for years to come.

Researchers wishing to evaluate the impact of specific nursing interventions on HRQOL should consider which specific domain or part of a domain their interventions will most likely impact. For example, though the Cochrane review of interventions by breast care nurses (Cruickshank et al., 2008) was unable to support a significant impact on overall QOL, the review reported early evidence (tempered by lack of large sample sizes) that interventions by breast care nurses significantly improved anxiety and helped early recognition of depressive symptoms (major factor in the psychosocial domain of HRQOL). Likewise, though a Cochrane review of structured nursing interventions among patients with lung cancer (Solà, Thompson, Subirana Casacuberta, Lopez, & Pascual, 2004) found no improvement in overall QOL, significant results were seen for symptom management of breathlessness as well as some improvements in emotional functioning. These are respectable and important contributions to people living with a complex and potentially isolating disease. Further, researchers have found depression to be an independent predictor for both physical and mental well-being (Mallik et al., 2005); thus, nursing interventions may have an effect difficult to measure but nonetheless contributory toward overall life quality.

Nursing researchers investigating HRQOL often use approaches and interventions from other models and theories, allowing connections to be made between HRQOL and these models or theories. For instance, Stuifbergen et al. (2000) related health-promoting behaviors from Pender's theory with HRQOL as an outcome. HRQOL as a middle range theory allows for concurrent application of theories that support health within illness, a concept thread that runs through the work of Peplau, Rogers, Parse, Newman, and others (Moch, 1989; Newman, 1984; Parse, 1994; Peplau, 1994; Rogers, 1970). As previously discussed, HRQOL is subjective, and therefore, we must listen to the patient's own summaries. As theorist and researcher Ferrans concludes, "A disability that makes life not worth living to one person may only be a nuisance to another" (Ferrans, 1990b, p. 252).

## Summary

- HRQOL is *subjective, multidimensional,* and *temporal.*

- Quality of life is a concept with a long history, which has become of interest to a number of disciplines.

- HRQOL is well matched to nursing because it involves variables that have traditionally been important to nursing.

- HRQOL often comprises three components: (a) *life domains,* (b) *interventions,* and (c) *perceived satisfaction.*

- Nurses can utilize the middle range theory of HRQOL to judge the effectiveness of an illness treatment and can make use of this middle range theory and the instruments designed to measure it.

## CRITICAL THINKING EXERCISES

1. Does HRQOL have subjective and objective components?

2. What are the underlying assumptions and potential ramifications of having proxy subjective health status or evaluation measures for children or those unable to speak for themselves?

3. Should further measurement tools only be accepted if based on commonly accepted conceptual definitions?

4. What are appropriate ways for researchers to test validity of HRQOL measures within their population? (Should an HRQOL measure be tested against an objective health status measure?)

## REFERENCES

Aaronson, N. K., Ahmedzai, S., Bergman, B., Bullinger, M., Cull, A., Duez, N. J., ..., de Haes, J. C. (1993). The European Organization for Research and Treatment of Cancer QLQ-C30: A quality-of-life instrument for use in international clinical trials in oncology. *Journal of the National Cancer Institute, 85,* 365–376.

Addington-Hall, J., & Kalra, J. (2001). Measuring quality of life: Who should measure quality of life? *British Medical Journal, 332,* 1417–1420.

Anderson, K. L., & Burckhardt, C. S. (1999). Conceptualization and measurement of quality of life as an outcomes variable for health care intervention and research. *Journal of Advanced Nursing, 29*(2), 298–306.

Bandayrel, K., & Johnston, B. C. (2014). Recent advances in patient and proxy-reported quality of life research. *Health and Quality of Life Outcomes, 12*(110), 1–9. doi: 10.1186/s12955-014-0110-7

Bergner, M., Bobbitt, R. A., Carter, W. B., & Gilson, B. S. (1981). The Sickness Impact Profile: Development and final revision of a health status measure. *Medical Care, 19,* 787–805.

Bliven, B. D., Green, P., & Spertus, J. A. (1998). Review of available instruments and methods for assessing QOL in anti-anginal trials. *Drugs and Aging, 13*(4), 311–320.

Campbell, A. (1981). *The sense of well being in America.* New York, NY: McGraw Hill.

Cella, D. F. (1992). Quality of life: The concept. *Journal of Palliative Care, 8*(3), 40–45.

Cella, D. F., & Tulsky, D. S. (1990). Measuring quality of life today: Methodological aspects. *Oncology, 4*(5), 29–38.

Chapa, D. W., Akintade, B., Schron, E., Friedmann, E., & Thomas, S. A. (2014). Is health-related quality of life a predictor of hospitalization and mortality among women or men with atrial fibrillation? *Journal of Cardiovascular Nursing, 29*(6), 555–564. doi: 10.1097/JCN.0000000000000095

Cohen, S. R., Mount, B. M., Strobel, M., & Bui, F. (1995). The McGill Quality of Life Questionnaire: A measure of quality of life appropriate for people with advanced disease. *Palliative Medicine, 9,* 207–291.

Cooley, M. E. (1998). Quality of life in persons with non-small cell lung cancer: A concept analysis. *Cancer Nursing, 21*(3), 151–161.

Cowan, M. J., Young Graham, K., & Cochrane, B. L. (1992). Comparison of a theory of quality of life between myocardial infarction and malignant melanoma: A pilot study. *Progress in Cardiovascular Nursing, 7*(1), 18–21.

Cruickshank, S., Kennedy, C., Lockhart, K., Dosser, I., & Dallas, L. (2008). Specialist breast care nurses for supportive care of women with breast cancer. *Cochrane Database of Systematic Reviews,* (1), CD005634. doi: 10.1002/14651858.CD005634.pub2

Dalkey, N. C., Rourke, D. L., Lewis, R., & Snyder, D. (1972). *Studies in the quality of life, delphi and decision making.* Toronto, ON: Lexington Books, D.C. Heath and Company.

DeVon, H. A., & Ferrans, C. E. (2003). The psychometric properties of four quality of life instruments used in cardiovascular populations. *Journal of Cardiopulmonary Rehabilitation, 23*(2), 122–138.

Donabedian, A. (1980). *The definition of quality and approaches to its assessment.* Ann Arbor, MI: Health Administration Press.

Elkins, R. C., Knott-Craif, C. J., McCue, C., & Lane, M. M. (1997). Congenital aortic valve disease: Improved survival and quality of life. *Annals of Surgery, 225*(5), 503–511.

EuroQol Group. (1990). EuroQol-A new facility for the measurement of health-related QOL. *Health Policy, 16,* 199–208.

Faden, R., & Leplege, A. (1992). Assessing quality of life, moral implications for clinical practice. *Medical Care, 30*(5 Suppl), 166–175.

Ferrans, C. E. (1990a). Development of a quality of life index for patients with cancer. *Oncology Nursing Forum, 17*, 15–19.

Ferrans, C. E. (1990b). Quality of life: Conceptual issues. *Seminars in Oncology Nursing, 6*(4), 248–254.

Ferrans, C., & Powers, M. (1985). Quality of Life Index: Development and psychometric properties. *Advances in Nursing Science, 8*, 15–24.

Ferrans, C., & Powers, M. (1992). Psychometric assessment of the Quality of Life Index. *Research in Nursing and Health, 15*, 29–38.

Ferrans, C. E., & Powers, M. J. (1993). QOL of hemodialysis patients. *ANNA Journal, 20*(5), 575–582.

Ferrans, C. E., Zerwic, J. J., Wilbur, J. E., & Larson, J. L. (2005). Conceptual model of health-related QOL. *Journal of Nursing Scholarship, 37*(4), 336–342.

Ferrell, B. R., Grant, M., Dean, G. E., Funk, B., & Ly, J. (1996). "Bone tired": The experience of fatigue and its impact on quality of life. *Oncology Nursing Forum, 23*, 1539–1547.

Gelber, R. D., Goldhirsch, A., Cole, B. F., Wieand, H. S., Schoeder, G., & Krrok, J. E. (1996). A quality-adjusted time without symptoms or toxicity (Q-TWiST) analysis of adjuvant radiation therapy and chemotherapy for resectable rectal cancer. *Journal of the National Cancer Institute, 88*(15), 1039–1045.

Gill, T., & Feinstein, A. (1994). A critical appraisal of the quality-of-life measurements. *JAMA, 272*, 619–620.

Guyatt, G. H., Feeny, D. H., & Patrick, D. L. (1993). Measuring health-related quality of life. *Annals of Internal Medicine, 118*, 622–628.

Harrison, M. B., Juniper, E. F., & Mitchell-DiCenso, A. (1996). Quality of life as an outcomes measure in nursing research: "May you have a long and healthy life." *Canadian Journal of Nursing Research, 28*(3), 49–68.

Holman. (2017). *The Holy Bible: Christian Standard Bible.* Nashville, TN: Holman Bible.

Hunt, S. M., McEwen, J., & McKenna, S. P. (1985). Measuring health status: A new tool for clinicians and epidemiologists. *The Journal of the Royal College of General Practitioners, 35*, 185–188.

King, C., & Hinds, P. (1998). *Quality of life.* Sudbury, MA: Jones & Bartlett Publishing.

Kroenke, K., Spitzer, R. L., Williams, J. B. W. (2001). The PHQ-9: Validity of a brief depression severity measure. *Journal of General Internal Medicine, 16*, 606–613.

Leplege, A., & Hunt, S. (1997). The problem of quality of life in medicine. *JAMA, 278*, 47–50.

Lim, J.-W., & Ashing-Giwa, K. T. (2013). Is family functioning and communication associated with health related quality of life for Chinese- and Korean-American breast cancer survivors? *Quality of Life Research, 22*(6), 1319–1329. doi: 10.1007/s11136-012-0247-y

Mallik, S., Krumholz, H. M., Lin, Z. Q., Kasl, S., Mattera, J. A., Roumains, S. A., & Vaccarino, V. (2005). Patients with depressive symptoms have lower health status benefits after coronary artery bypass surgery. *Circulation, 111*, 271–277.

McClane, K. S. (2006). Screening instruments for use in a complete geriatric assessment. *Clinical Nurse Specialist, 20*(4), 201–206.

Meenan, R. F., Mason, J. H., Anderson, J. J., Guccione, A. A., & Kazis, L. E. (1992). AIMS2. The content and properties of a revised and expanded Arthritis Impact Measurement Scales Health Status Questionnaire. *Arthritis and Rheumatism, 35*(1), 1–10.

Meleis, A. I. (1997). *Theoretical nursing: Development and progress* (3rd ed.). Philadelphia, PA: Lippincott-Raven.

Melzack, R. (1975). The McGill Pain Questionnaire: Major properties and scoring methods. *Pain, 1*, 277–299.

Moch, S. D. (1989). Health within illness: Conceptual evolution and practice possibilities. *Advances in Nursing Science, 11*(4), 23–31.

Morgan, M. L. (1992). *Classics of moral and political theory.* Indianapolis, IN: Hacket.

Murdaugh, C. R. (1997). Health-related quality of life as an outcome in organizational research. *Medical Care, 35*(11 Suppl), NS41–NS48.

Newman, M. A. (1984). Nursing diagnosis: Looking at the whole. *American Journal of Nursing, 85*, 1496–1499.

Oleson, M. (1990). Subjectively perceived quality of life. *Image: The Journal of Nursing Scholarship, 22*(3), 187–190.

Osoba, D. (1994). Lessons learned from measuring health-related quality of life in oncology. *Journal of Clinical Oncology, 12*, 199–220.

Padilla, G. V., & Grant, M. M. (1985). QOL as a cancer nursing outcome variable. *Advances in Nursing Science, 8*(1), 45–60.

Padilla, G. V., Presant, C., Grant, M. M., Metter, G., Lipselt, J., & Heide, F. (1983). Quality of life index for patients with cancer. *Research in Nursing and Health, 6*(3), 117–126.

Parse, R. R. (1994). Quality of life: Sciencing and living the art of human becoming. *Nursing Science Quarterly, 7*(1), 16–20.

Penny, K. I., & Smith, G. D. (2012). The use of data-mining to identify indicators of health-related quality of life in patients with irritable bowel syndrome. *Journal of Clinical Nursing, 21*, 2761–2771. doi: 10.1111/j.1365-2702. 2011. 03897

Peplau, H. E. (1994). Quality of life: An interpersonal perspective. *Nursing Science Quarterly, 7*(1), 10–15.

Phillips, C., & Thompson, G. (2007). What is a QALY? *Hayward Medical Communications, 1*(6). Retrieved January 22, 2007 from http://www.evidence-based-medicine.co.uk/what_is_series.html

Read, J. L. (1993). The new era of quality of life assessment. In S. R. Walker & R. M. Rosser (Eds.), *Quality of life assessment: Key issues in the 1990s* (pp. 3–10). London, UK: Kluwer Academic Publishers.

Rector, T. S., Kubo, S. H., & Cohen, J. N. (1987). Patients' self-assessment of their congestive heart failure. Part 2: Content, reliability and validity of a new measure, the Minnesota Living with Heart Failure questionnaire. *Heart Failure, 3*, 198–209.

Robinson, D., Whyte, L., & Fidler, I. (1997). Quality of life measures in a high security environment. *Nursing Standard, 11*(49), 34–37.

Rogers, M. E. (1970). *An introduction to the theoretical basis of nursing.* Philadelphia, PA: F.A. Davis Co.

Rubenstein, L. V. (1996). Using QOL tests for patient diagnosis or screening, or to evaluate treatment. In B. Spilker (Ed.), *QOL and pharmacoeconomics in clinical trials* (2nd ed., pp. 362–372). Philadelphia, PA: Lippincott-Raven Publishers.

Rumsfeld, J. S. (2002). Health status and clinical practice: when will they meet? (Editorial). *Circulation, 106*(1), 5–7.

Sandau, K. E., Hoglund, B. A., Weaver, C. E., Boisjolie, C., & Feldman, D. (2014). A conceptual definition of quality of life with a left ventricular assist device: Results from a qualitative study. *Heart and Lung, 43*(1), 32–40. doi: 10.1016/j.hrtlng.2013.09.004

Sandau, K. E., Lindquist, R. A., Treat-Jacobson, D., & Savik, K. (2008). Health-related quality of life and subjective neurocognitive function three months after coronary artery bypass graft surgery. *Heart and Lung, 37*(3), 161–172.

Solà, I., Thompson, E., Subirana Casacuberta, M., Lopez, C., & Pascual, A. (2004). Non-invasive interventions for improving well-being and quality of life in patients with lung cancer. *Cochrane Database of Systematic Reviews*, (4), CD004282. doi: 10.1002/14651858.CD004282.pub2

Sousa, K. H. (1999). Description of a health-related quality of life conceptual model. *Outcomes Management for Nursing Practice, 3*(2), 78–82.

Sousa, K. H., & Chen, F. F. (2002). A theoretical approach to measuring quality of life. *Journal of Nursing Measurement, 10*(1), 47–58.

Sousa, K. H., Holzemer, W. L., Henry, S. B., & Slaughter, R. (1999). Dimensions of health-related quality of life in persons living with HIV disease. *Journal of Advanced Nursing, 29*(1), 178–187.

Spertus, J. A., Winder, J. A., Dewhurts, T. A., Deyo, R. A., Prodzinski, J., McDonell, M., & Fihn, S. D. (1995). Development and evaluation of the Seattle Angina Questionnaire: A new functional status measure for coronary artery disease. *Journal of the American College of Cardiology, 25*(2), 333–341.

Spilker, B. (1996). *Quality of life and pharmacoeconomics in clinical trials* (2nd ed.). New York, NY: Lippincott-Raven.

Spranger, M. J. (2001). International Society of Quality of Life. *Newsletter, 6*(1). Retrieved June 15, 2001 from www.ISOQOL.org

Sprangers, M. A. G., & Schwartz, C. E. (1999). Integrating response shift into health-related quality of life research: A theoretical model. *Social Science and Medicine, 48*(11), 1507–1515.

Staniszewska, S. (1998). Measuring quality of life in the evaluation of health care. *Nursing Standard, 12*(17), 36–39.

Stineman, M. G., Lollar, D. J., & Ustun, T. B. (2005). International classification of functioning, disability, and health: ICF empowering rehabilitation through an operational bio-psycho-social model. In J. A. DeLisa (Ed.), *Physical medicine and rehabilitation principles and practice* (pp. 1099–1108). Philadelphia, PA: Lippincott Williams & Wilkins.

Stryk, L. (1968). *World of Budha: A reader*. Garden City, NY: Doubleday.

Stuifbergen, A. K., Seraphine, A., & Roberts, G. (2000). An explanatory model of health promotion and quality of life in chronic disabling conditions. *Nursing Research, 49*(3), 122–129.

Sullivan, S. A., & Olson, L. M. (1995). Developing condition-specific measures of functional status and well-being for children. *Clinical Performance and Quality Health Care, 3*, 132–138.

van Agt, H. M. V., Essink-Bot, M. L., Krabbe, P. F., & Bonsel, G. J. (1994). Test-retest reliability of health state valuations collected with the EuroQol questionnaire. *Social Science and Medicine, 39*(11), 1537–1544.

Vogler, J., Klein, A., & Bender, A. (2014). Long-term health—related quality-of- life in patients with acquired brain injury and their caregivers. *Brain Injury, 28*(11), 1381–1388. doi: 10.3109/02699052.2014.919536

Ware, J. E., & Sherbourne, C. D. (1992). The MOS 36-item short-form health survey (SF-36). *Medical Care, 20*, 473–483.

Wenger, N. K., Naughton, M. J., & Furberg, C. D. (1996). Cardiovascular disorders. In B. Spilker (Ed.), *Quality of life and pharmacoeconomics in clinical trials* (2nd ed., pp. 883–891). Philadelphia, PA: Lippincott-Raven.

Wilson, I. B., & Cleary, P. D. (1995). Linking clinical variables with health-related quality of life. *Journal of the American Medical Association, 273*(1), 59–65.

Wong, F. M. F., Sit, J. W. H., Wong, E. M. L., & Choi, K. C. C. (2014). Factors associated with health-related quality of life among patients with implantable cardioverter defibrillator: Identification of foci for nursing intervention. *Journal of Advanced Nursing, 70*(12), 2821–2834. doi: 10.1111/jan.12434

Wood-Dauphinee, S. (1999). Assessing quality of life in clinical research: From where have we come and where are we going? *Journal of Clinical Epidemiology, 55*, 355–363.

World Health Organization. (1948). Constitution of the World Health Organization. *Chronicle of the World Health Organization, 1*(1/2), 13.

World Health Organization. (1995). The World Health Organization Quality of Life Assessment (WHOQOL): Position paper from the World Health Organization. *Social Science and Medicine, 41*, 1403–1409.

Yang, K., Simms, L. M., & Yin, J. (1999). Factors influencing nursing-sensitive outcomes in Taiwanese nursing homes. *Online Journal of Issues in Nursing, 3*(2). Retrieved June 14, 2001 from www.nursingworld.org

Zhan, L. (1992). Quality of life: Conceptual and measurement issues. *Journal of Advanced Nursing, 17*(7), 795–800.

Zigmond, A. S., & Snaith, R. P. (1983). The hospital anxiety and depression scale. *Acta Psychiatrica Scandinavica, 67*, 361–370.

## BIBLIOGRAPHY

Ferrans, C. E. (1992). Conceptualizations of QOL in cardiovascular research. *Progress in Cardiovascular Nursing, 2*(7), 2–6.

King, C. R., & Hinds, P. S. (2003). QOL: *From nursing and patient perspective*. Sudbury, MA: Jones and Bartlett Publisher, Inc.

McDowell, I., & Newell, C. (1996). *Measuring health: A guide to rating scales and questionnaires* (2nd ed.). New York, NY: Oxford University Press, Inc.

# 15 Health Promotion

Marjorie C. McCullagh

## Definitions of Key Terms

| | |
|---|---|
| **Activity-related affect** | Subjective feelings associated with the health-promoting activity |
| **Commitment to a plan of action** | A commitment to carry out a health-promoting behavior. The plan should be specific to time and place and specify whether it will be with specified persons or alone |
| **Health-promoting behavior** | Behaviors or actions that people carry out with the intention of improving their health |
| **Immediate competing demands** | Distracting ideas about other things that must be done (e.g., childcare) immediately prior to their intention to carry out a health-promoting behavior |
| **Immediate competing preferences** | Distracting ideas about other attractive activities to engage in (e.g., shopping) immediately before engaging in a health-promoting behavior |
| **Interpersonal influences** | Beliefs concerning the behaviors, the beliefs, or the attitudes of others regarding a health-promoting behavior. Ideas include social norms, social support, and modeling |
| **Perceived barriers to action** | Beliefs about the unavailability, inconvenience, expense, difficulty, or time-consuming nature of a health-promoting behavior |
| **Perceived benefits of action** | Beliefs about the positive or reinforcing consequences of a health-promoting behavior |
| **Perceived self-efficacy** | A person's judgment of his or her own abilities to accomplish a health-promoting behavior |
| **Personal factors: biological, psychological, and sociocultural** | Factors about the person that influence health-promoting behavior. Examples of biologic factors are age, body mass index, and aerobic capacity. Examples of psychological factors are self-esteem, self-motivation, and perceived health status. Examples of sociocultural factors are race, ethnicity, acculturation, education, and socioeconomic status. The variables may be specific to each health-promoting activity, that is, factors influencing healthy dietary behaviors may not be the same as those affecting exercise behavior |
| **Prior related behavior** | Experience with the health-promoting behavior |
| **Situational influences** | Beliefs about the situation or context of the health-promoting behavior. These ideas may include perceptions of the available options, demand characteristics, and aesthetic features of the environment in which a given behavior is proposed to take place |

During the past century, the major cause of health problems has shifted from infectious diseases to chronic illnesses. Many chronic illnesses are closely related to lifestyle factors such as diet, exercise, and stress management. In order to improve the health of a population experiencing high rates of chronic illness, it is apparent that changes in lifestyle factors are required.

Nurses, as well as many other health professionals, are interested in learning more about how they can help their patients, families, and communities improve their lives. In seeking a way to promote greater longevity and a higher quality of life, nurses need to design interventions that enhance healthy lifestyles. The Health Promotion Model has achieved popularity among nurses as a model that can guide person-centered health counseling to improve a wide range of health behaviors.

Health promotion has many benefits. The benefits of living a healthier lifestyle exceed prevention of disease and include greater vigor and a subjective feeling of wellness. While these benefits can be enjoyed by the individual, society as a whole also profits from health promotion when people create personal and family lifestyles that are consistent with economic prosperity and interpersonal harmony. Health promotion can decrease social problems, such as violence, suicide, and sexually transmitted diseases. Further, health promotion has the potential to significantly decrease health care costs in the years ahead.

Health promotion is a concept well suited to the needs and interests of nurses and their clients. Nurses commonly work in schools, churches, homes, workplaces, and health care agencies. Many of these settings are ideal locations for the promotion of health. Nurses are skilled in many areas that are necessary for health promotion, such as education, counseling, and advocacy. For example, a parish nurse may offer classes to congregational members in a variety of health-related topics such as parenting and caring for aging family members. A school nurse may facilitate self-help group meetings for bereaved children. An occupational health nurse may advocate for inclusion of mental health services in employee health benefit packages. In addition, clients are likely to be receptive to nursing interventions to promote health, because they trust nurses and are accustomed to seeking assistance of these professionals in dealing with their health care needs.

## Historical Background

Nola Pender first published her Health Promotion Model in 1982. Some early study results (Garcia et al., 1995) suggested the need for addition of concepts to the model in order to increase its predictive power. Based on the analysis of the empirical support provided by each of the studies based on the model, Pender revised the model, retaining selected model concepts and deleting others. In addition, three new concepts and associated relationships were added to the model. The added concepts included prior related behavior, immediate competing demands and preferences, and commitment to a plan of action. These revisions to the model, based on both research and theoretical considerations, were made to increase its explanatory power and its potential for use in structuring health-promoting nursing interventions. The revised model was first published in 1996 and most recently in the seventh edition of *Health Promotion in Nursing Practice* (Pender, Murdaugh, & Parsons, 2015).

## Pender's Definition of Health

Nurses are accustomed to assessing their patients for evidence of disease or dysfunction. However, the assessment process commonly reflects a focus on illness, rather than health. This approach is limiting in several ways. First, it risks reducing the patient to a sum of his or her parts (e.g., respiratory, neurological, cardiovascular, etc.). Second, it fails to determine the meaning the client attaches to health and illness. This approach is a negative approach to health in that it views health as an absence of disease. Some consider health and illness to be opposite concepts. This way of thinking suggests that persons with disabilities and chronic illness and those who are near death cannot achieve health. However, many nurses experienced in working with these clients may oppose this view. Negative approaches to health as the absence of illness are inadequate for health professionals at a time that they are increasingly concerned with quality of life and healthy longevity.

Pender's (1996) definition of health is positive, comprehensive, unifying, and humanistic. She believes that health includes a disease component, but does not make disease its principal element. Her definition of health encompasses the whole person and their lifestyle and includes strengths, resiliencies, resources, potentials, and capabilities. Pender defines health as the actualization of inherent and acquired human potential through goal-directed behavior, competent self-care, and satisfying relationships with others, while adjustments are made as needed to maintain structural integrity and harmony with relevant environments.

A major strength of Pender's definition of health is that it offers an expanded view of health. This expanded view provides for greatly increased opportunities to improve client health, as it is not limited to absence of disease or even limitations in functioning or adaptation. For example, Pender's positive view of health permits the development of nursing interventions that are not limited to decreasing risks for disease, but also aimed at strengthening resources, potentials, and capabilities. This creates broader opportunities for nurses to assist individuals, families, and communities to achieve improved health, enhanced functional ability, and better quality of life.

### HEALTH PROMOTION

Health professionals have long recognized the benefits of early detection and treatment of illness, or secondary prevention. However, recently there has been increased appreciation for the role of primary prevention and health promotion in improving health and quality of life. Primary prevention involves activities aimed at the prevention of health problems before they occur and the avoidance of disease. An example of primary prevention is the administration of tetanus immunization to prevent tetanus infection. Health promotion is intended to increase the level of well-being and self-actualization of an individual or group. Examples of health promotion activities include physical activity and healthy nutrition.

While health promotion and primary prevention are distinct theoretical concepts, in practice they often overlap. Many activities directed toward health promotion will also have preventive effects. Indeed, many adults engage in healthy behaviors with the dual intent of increasing wellness and avoiding illness. For example, an adult may adopt a low-fat diet with two purposes in mind. One intention may be to lower blood cholesterol and, therefore, prevent future cardiovascular problems (primary prevention, also referred to by Pender as health protection). An accompanying intention may be to gain the benefits of weight loss, such as feeling more energetic (health promotion). Other examples of health behaviors that may have both health promotion and preventive benefits include physical activity, adequate rest, and management of stress.

Health promotion is activity directed toward actualization of human potential through goal-directed behavior, competent self-care, and satisfying relationships with others, while adjustments are made as needed to maintain structural integrity and harmony with relevant environments (Pender et al., 2015). The concept of health promotion is based on Pender's expanded definition of health that focuses on the whole person and promotes the positive aspects of health. This definition applies to all persons, including persons who are well and those who are experiencing an illness or disability.

Pender advocates the use of health promotion at a variety of levels and settings. Although health promotion is most commonly directed toward the individual, Pender suggests that interventions directed toward the family and community are most likely to be successful in creating a healthy society. Furthermore, Pender discusses health promotion in a variety of settings, including schools, workplaces, homes, and nurse-managed community health centers. In a broad sense, health promotion involves education, food production, housing, employment, and health care. It is multidimensional, encompassing individual, family, community, environmental, and societal health. This view of health promotion is consistent with an increasing global emphasis on creating a "culture of health" in all nations.

## Description of the Health Promotion Model

Pender's model is based on theories of human behavior. There is increased recognition of the role of behavior in primary prevention and health promotion, and there is increased attention among health professionals in helping clients adopt healthy behaviors. Motivation for healthy behavior may be based on a desire to prevent illness (primary prevention) or to achieve a higher level of well-being and self-actualization (health promotion). The Pender Health Promotion Model is primarily based on two theories of health behavior: expectancy-value theory and social–cognitive theory. The first, expectancy-value theory, is based on the work by Fishbein and Ajzen (Fishbein & Ajzen, 1975). The theory explains that people are more likely to work toward goals that are of value to them. This proposition by Fishbein and Ajzen relates to Pender's proposition that people will engage in "behaviors from which they anticipate deriving personally valued benefits" (Pender et al., 2015, p. 36). Expectancy-value theory also explains that people are more likely to invest their effort in goals that they believe are achievable and will result in the desired outcome.

The second parent theory is Bandura's (1986) social–cognitive theory. A major tenet of social–cognitive theory is self-efficacy. Self-efficacy is the confidence a person has in his or her ability to successfully carry out an action. Bandura's theory proposes that the greater a person's self-efficacy for a behavior, the more likely the person will engage in it, even when faced with obstacles. The concept of self-efficacy is one of the behavior-specific cognitions of Pender's model. Pender's belief is that when a person has high perceived competence or self-efficacy in a certain behavior, it results in a greater likelihood that the person will commit to action and actually perform the behavior.

Some have observed that the Health Promotion Model resembles the Health Belief Model. While it is true that the Health Promotion Model shares some concepts with the Health Belief Model, the Health Promotion Model differs from the Health Belief Model in at least one important way. The Health Promotion Model is a competence- or approach-oriented model that focuses on attainment of high-level wellness and self-actualization. This is contrasted with the Health Belief Model, which was intended for use in explaining patients' use of medical diagnosis and treatment of disease, such as tuberculosis. Further, the Health Belief Model incorporates fear or threat of disease as a motivation for action. While this perspective may be valid for diseases that have shorter prodromal periods, the Health Promotion Model does not consider fear or threat as a powerful motivation for distant threats to health.

The Health Promotion Model (Pender et al., 2015) consists of two major categories of predictors (individual characteristics and experiences, behavior-specific cognitions and affect) and the behavioral outcome. Pender identifies the behavior-specific cognitions and affect as the major motivational mechanisms for health promotion behavior. These include perceived benefits of action, perceived barriers to action, perceived self-efficacy, activity-related affect, interpersonal influences, and situational influences. Individual characteristics and experiences included in the

model are prior related behavior and personal factors. The model also includes additional concepts influencing the behavioral outcome, such as immediate competing demands and preferences, and commitment to a plan of action. These concepts are briefly described in Definitions of Key Concepts, which appears earlier in this chapter. The schematic representation of the model (Fig. 15.1) shows the relationship of model concepts to the behavioral outcome, health-promoting behavior.

The model includes multiple concepts and relationships, though some concepts and relationships may be more salient than others to a given health behavior. However, the model does not provide assistance in selecting which concepts and relationships are appropriate for specific

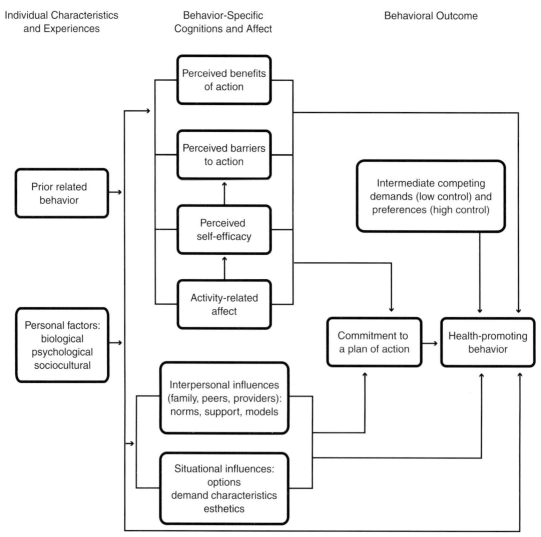

**Figure 15.1**    **Health Promotion Model.** (*Source*: Pender, N., Murdaugh, C., & Parsons, M. (2015). *Health promotion in nursing practice* (7th ed.). © Reprinted by permission of Pearson Education, Inc., Upper Saddle River, NJ.)

behaviors. Therefore, the researcher who seeks to use the model should select concepts and relationships based on previous research, theoretical foundations, clinical experience, and practical limitations in regard to a specific behavior. Indeed, extant research using the Health Promotion Model shows the selectivity of researchers in determining which model concepts to include in their study designs.

## Measurement of Model Concepts

Instruments have been developed to measure a variety of concepts related to the Health Promotion Model. Primary of these is the HPLP-II (Susan Walker, personal communication, June 24, 2002). Due to the broad nature of the model, many instruments have been developed to measure behavior-specific attitudes and beliefs. A sample of these is described in Table 15.1.

## Implications of the Model for Clinical Practice

The Health Promotion Model offers a conceptual framework for the provision of effective nursing care directed at improved health and functional ability. First, the model provides a method for the assessment of client's health-promoting behaviors. The model directs nurses to systematically assess clients for their perceived self-efficacy, perceived barriers, perceived benefits, interpersonal influences, and situational influences that are relevant to the selected health behavior.

Second, the model identifies several additional client characteristics as targets for assessment. These client characteristics include prior behavior, demographic characteristics, and perceived health status. While these characteristics are not amenable to alteration, they offer a basis for tailoring of nursing interventions, as discussed below.

Third, the model suggests that nursing interventions can be designed to alter clients' perceptions

**Table 15.1    Health Promotion Model Instruments**

| Instrument | First Author, Date | Description |
|---|---|---|
| Health-Promoting Lifestyle Profile II (HPLP-II) | Susan Walker, personal communication, June 24, 2002 | 52-item questionnaire in a four-point response format measures the frequency of health-promoting behaviors in six domains (health responsibility, physical activity, nutrition, spiritual growth, interpersonal relations, and stress management). |
| HPLP Spanish Language Version | Walker, Sechrist, and Pender (1997) | This instrument provides a Spanish language version of the HPLP. |
| HPLP—Japanese Version | Wei et al. (2000) | This instrument provides a Japanese language version of the HPLP. |
| Exercise Benefits/ Barriers Scale (EBBS) | Sechrist, Walker, and Pender (1987) | This Likert scale measures the person's "perceived benefits to undertaking preventive behaviors that reduce risk factors in coronary artery disease." |
| Perceived Self-Efficacy of Hearing Protector Use Scale | Lusk, Ronis, and Hogan (1997) | This 10-item scale asks respondents to rate the extent to which they have confidence in their ability to use hearing protection. An example of an item from this scale is, "I am sure I can use my hearing protection so it works effectively." |
| Perception of Accessibility and Availability of Hearing Protectors Scale | Lusk et al. (1997) | This nine-item scale asks respondents to report on this dimension of situational factors influencing this health behavior. A sample item from this scale is, "Ear plugs are available to pick up at my job sites." |
| Interpersonal Influences on Hearing Protector Use Scale | Lusk et al. (1997) | This scale includes three subscales measuring dimensions of this variable: interpersonal norms, interpersonal modeling, and interpersonal support. The Interpersonal Norms Subscale includes four items that query respondents about their beliefs about how much others (family members, friends, supervisor, and coworkers) think they should wear hearing protection. The Interpersonal Support Subscale measures encouragement or praise from family, friends, coworkers, and supervisors about the respondent's use of hearing protection. The Interpersonal Modeling Subscale measures how much they believe others use hearing protection when exposed to noise. |

in these areas. Success in these interventions is expected to result in more frequent health behaviors and resultant improved wellness.

Although the model identifies foci for nursing interventions, it does not explicitly describe how nurses can effect changes in client perceptions. While these nursing interventions directed at changing client perceptions are proposed by the Health Promotion Model, few studies that test the effectiveness of these proposed interventions have been completed. Also, the model is designed for use with individual clients; it is not designed for use with groups/aggregates/populations, although some researchers have developed interventions for groups based on model concepts.

Pender prescribes the use of the nursing process as the method of producing behavior change. She emphasizes nursing assessment of health, health beliefs, and health behavior using established frameworks, such as North American Nursing Diagnosis Association (NANDA) and Gordon's functional health patterns. In addition, she recommends the use of model-based assessments such as the Health-Promoting Lifestyle Profile II (HPLP-II). Pender emphasizes use of the nursing process in empowering self-care across the life span. She outlines a multistep process for health planning that includes reinforcing client strengths, developing a plan based on client preferences and Prochaska et al.'s (1994) stages of change, addressing facilitators and barriers, and committing to goals.

Areas of intervention for health promotion include exercise, nutrition, stress management, and social support. Pender (1996) reviews several interventions in each of these areas, based on a variety of models, and many of which are research based. These are directed toward increasing the client's capacity for a vigorous and productive life.

## USE OF THE HEALTH PROMOTION MODEL IN TAILORING NURSING INTERVENTIONS

Model variables, such as client characteristics, cognitions, and affect, may be used to tailor or target nursing interventions to clients. Tailoring of interventions involves shaping of health messages based on characteristics unique to that person. Several comparison studies have found tailoring interventions to increase intervention effectiveness (Kroeze, Werkman, & Brug, 2006; Neville, O'Hara, & Milat, 2009; Velicer, Prochaska, & Redding, 2006). This innovative intervention strategy offers exciting possibilities for designing health promotion interventions to meet the unique needs of each individual client. Once the nurse assesses the client on each of the relevant factors of the model, this information can be used to custom-design a health promotion program for that individual client. Recent applications of the Health Promotion Model have used computers to quickly and accurately assess the health of the client on model-based variables. With the help of computer technology, nurses have used this information to design a health promotion intervention that is unique to the needs of this individual (Kerr, Savik, Monsen, & Lusk, 2007). This computer-assisted approach offers nurses the opportunity to provide interventions that are more appropriate to the individual and may, as a result, enhance intervention effectiveness. In a similar manner, model variables may be used to design interventions for groups of clients who share characteristics.

## SELECTING THE HEALTH PROMOTION MODEL

Nurses are faced with selecting among a variety of models for use in clinical practice and research. This selection may be based on a variety of factors, including philosophy, research, clarity, and utility.

The Health Promotion Model is appealing to many nurses because it offers a view of health consistent with their motivation for pursuing the profession of nursing. Its holistic and humanistic view is congruent with many nurses' own personal philosophy of health and nursing. The model reflects a belief that persons are capable of introspection and are capable of personal change. In turn, the model proposes that health care is more than treatment and prevention of disease, but involves creating conditions where clients can express their unique human potential. The nurse is presented as an agent for creating behavioral and environmental changes.

The Health Promotion Model has been used successfully in several research studies, as discussed earlier in this chapter. While some models have been tested more extensively, the Health Promotion Model does have a body of extant literature that provides support for its use. A more thorough discussion of studies using the Health Promotion Model is presented in Pender's seventh edition (Pender et al., 2015). Examples of research applications of the Health Promotion Model are presented in Using Middle Range Theory in Research 15.1 and Using Middle Range Theories in Practice 15.2.

Most nurses will find that the Health Promotion Model is straightforward and easy to understand. It uses terms that are readily comprehended, and its propositional statements are presented clearly. The phenomena addressed by the model are familiar to nurses, and most nurses will require minimal learning of new terms and concepts in order to use and understand the model. The model is clearly presented in graphic form.

## USING MIDDLE RANGE THEORY IN RESEARCH  15.1

*Source: Walker, S. N., Pullen, C. H., Hageman, P. A., Boeckner, L. S., Hertzog, M., Oberdorfer, M. K., & Rutledge, M. J. (2010). Maintenance of activity and eating change after a clinical trial of tailored newsletters with older rural women. Nursing Research, 59(5), 311–321.*

Midlife and older rural women are at increased risk for chronic illness, functional limitations, and disability and experience lower access to health care and are less likely to receive preventive services. The purpose of this study was to compare the maintenance of change in healthy eating and physical activity following generic mailed newsletter interventions versus newsletters tailored on Health Promotion Model behavior-specific cognitions, eating behavior, and activity behavior. In the Wellness for Women Project, a randomized controlled clinical trial, outcomes for 225 women aged 50 to 69 years were compared at 18 and 24 months. At 18 months, the tailored group maintained levels of all eating and activity behaviors, whereas the generic group maintained levels of selected behaviors (e.g., fruit and vegetable servings, activity, stretching exercise, lower body strength and flexibility), but increased saturated fat intake and declined in weekly strength exercise and cardiorespiratory fitness. At 24 months, the tailored group maintained levels of strength exercise and lower body strength, whereas the generic group decreased in both. A greater proportion of women who received tailored newsletters achieved most Healthy People 2010 criteria for eating and activity. Results demonstrated that tailored newsletters were more effective than generic newsletters in facilitating change in eating and activity for 6 months post intervention and in maintaining change in strength exercise for 12 months post intervention

The Health Promotion Model has been used in a variety of settings, including schools, workplaces, ambulatory treatment facilities, a rehabilitation center, and a prison. Its use has been with a wide variety of health behaviors, including exercise, nutrition, and use of hearing protection. The studies have involved diverse clients in regard to gender and age. The model has a limited history of application in culturally diverse groups. However, samples of Korean, Taiwanese, Thai, and Japanese individuals have participated in prior studies. It is noteworthy that persons included as study participants have been well or experiencing chronic illness, such as HIV infection.

The Health Promotion Model has been used by nurses working in a variety of community-based settings, such as occupational health and public health. The model is well suited to clients whose

## USING MIDDLE RANGE THEORIES IN PRACTICE  15.2

Josephina, age 52, is diagnosed with diabetes, hypertension, and hyperlipidemia, which are not well controlled. In addition to prescription medication, her physician has recommended using physical activity to manage her condition.

The outpatient clinic nurse assessed Josephina for the importance (value) of physical activity in her life; the extent to which she feels capable of physical activity (self-efficacy); her goals for a work, family, and personal life (definition of health); her perceived benefits and barriers to physical activity; access and availability of facilities for physical activity; the presence of other persons in her life who may serve as physical activity role models; social support for physical activity; and her use of reminders (cues) for engaging in physical activity.

Based on the assessment, the nurse learns that the cost of a gym membership (barrier) and child care and other family responsibilities (immediate competing demands) frequently interfere with her engaging in physical activity. In addition, the nurse learns that Josephina lives in a cold climate, which limits her opportunities to engage in physical activity outdoors (situational influences), and feels that even if she engages in physical activity, she will continue to experience diabetes, hypertension, and hyperlipidemia (self-efficacy).

The nurse initiates several interventions on behalf of Josephina based on the assessment. First, with Josephina's consent, the nurse connects her with a middle-aged woman from her practice who has made significant gains in her disease management through self-care activities, including physical activity and diet (addressing her self-efficacy). Through a series of questions, the nurse also helps Josephina identify several physical activities in which Josephina feels she could engage with her children, such as playing ball and walking the dog (addressing a barrier and immediate competing demands). Working together, the nurse and Josephina identify ways to incorporate physical activity into her day (e.g., climbing stairs, parking a distance from work), thereby addressing her situational influences. They also develop a goal for minutes of exercise each week and a log for tracking her exercise and plan to meet again in a few weeks to monitor the success of her plan (addressing her self-efficacy).

## USING MIDDLE RANGE THEORIES IN PRACTICE AND PROJECTS    15.3

*Source: Khodaveisi, M., Omidi, A., Farokhi, S., & Soltanian, A. R. (2017). The effect of Pender's health promotion model in improving the nutritional behavior of overweight and obese women. International Journal of Community Based Nursing and Midwifery, 5(2), 165–174.*

### PROJECT PURPOSE:

The purpose of this study was to test the effectiveness of an intervention in improving the nutritional behavior of overweight and obese women in a clinic setting in Iran.

### RESEARCH DESIGN:

In this quasi-experimental study, 108 women aged 18 to 60 years with BMI > 25 were recruited from a clinic practice and randomly assigned to two groups: experimental and control. The experimental group participated in three 30-minute group education sessions over 2 weeks where lectures, Q and A, and group discussions in three 30-minute sessions over 2 weeks focused on Pender Model–based constructs related to nutrition: benefits of healthy nutrition, practical skills to promote nutrition, barriers and strategies to promote healthy nutrition, and nutritional self-efficacy.

### FINDINGS:

Mean scores for several nutrition-related behaviors and attitudes were significantly improved among participants in the experimental group after receiving the intervention based on the Pender Health Promotion Model (e.g., nutritional behavior, perceived benefits, perceived self-efficacy, commitment to action, interpersonal and situational influences, behavior-related affect, and perceived barriers).

### CONCLUSION:

The results of this study suggest that an educational intervention based on the Pender Health Promotion Model aimed at nutrition-related behaviors and attitudes may be effective in promoting improved nutritional behavior among obese women in Iran.

This report is based on an MSc thesis study conducted by the author (SF), "Use of Pender's Health Promotion Model for Improvement of Nutritional Behaviors in Overweight Women admitted to Clinics of Fatemiyeh Hospital in Hamadan." *The project was* funded by Hamadan University of Medical Sciences (Grant No. 6228).

health status is stable and whose basic needs are met. Although Pender's definition of health is broad and encompasses persons who are experiencing illness, application of the Health Promotion Model is untested in acute care settings and with clients whose health concerns are urgent or living conditions are unstable.

See Using Middle Range Theories in Practice and Projects 15.3 for an example project.

## Summary

■ The HPM is designed to guide nurses in helping clients achieve improved health, enhanced functional ability, and better quality of life.

■ The model encompasses both behavioral and environmental changes to effect improvements in a society where lifestyle factors account for a large proportion of health problems.

■ The model is based on established theories of human behavior, including expectancy-value theory and social–cognitive theory.

■ The HPM claims that a variety of client characteristics and cognitive–affective factors combine with competing demands and preferences as well as commitment to a plan of action to explain the likelihood of health-promoting behavior.

■ The model has been tested in several clinical studies using a variety of settings, health behaviors, and client characteristics. It presents exciting possibilities for the creation of interventions that are tailored to the unique characteristics and needs of individual clients.

■ The model was last revised in 1996 based on review and analysis of results of model testing and intervention effectiveness research. Future development is needed in measures of model concepts that fit specific target populations and design of robust interventions that can change model beliefs and, subsequently, health outcomes. Interventions that address not only individuals but families and communities in creating multilevel interventions employing the HPM in combination with community action models are most likely to achieve success.

## CRITICAL THINKING EXERCISES

1. The Pender Health Promotion Model identifies benefits and barriers as factors influencing health behavior. Respond to the following items, considering clients from your own clinical practice. What are the barriers to and the benefits of adopting a selected healthy behavior, such as exercise? Why might this information be important to collect?

2. Generate several questions designed to elicit specific information about your clients' perceptions of their barriers and benefits.

3. How can you use this information to improve the effectiveness of your efforts to influence your clients' adaptation of healthy behaviors?

## REFERENCES

Bandura, A. (1986). *Social foundations of thought and action: A social cognitive theory*. Englewood Cliffs, NJ: Prentice-Hall.

Fishbein, M., & Ajzen, I. (1975). *Belief, attitude, intention and behavior: An introduction to theory and research*. Reading, MA: Addison-Wesley.

Garcia, A. W., Broda, M. A., Frenn, M., Coviak, M., Pender, N. J., & Ronis, D. L. (1995). Gender and developmental differences in exercise beliefs among youth and their prediction of their exercise behavior. *Journal of School Health, 65*, 213–219.

Kerr, M. J., Savik, K., Monsen, K. A., & Lusk, S. L. (2007). Effectiveness of computer-based tailoring versus targeting to promote use of hearing protection. *The Canadian Journal of Nursing Research = Revue Canadienne De Recherche En Sciences Infirmieres, 39*, 80–97.

Kroeze, W., Werkman, A., & Brug, J. (2006). A systematic review of randomized trials on the effectiveness of computer-tailored education on physical activity and dietary behaviors. *Annals of Behavioral Medicine: A Publication of the Society of Behavioral Medicine, 31*, 205–223. doi: 10.1207/s15324796abm3103_2

Lusk, S. L., Ronis, D. L., & Hogan, M. M. (1997). Test of the health promotion model as a causal model of construction workers' use of hearing protection. *Research in Nursing & Health, 20*, 183–194.

Neville, L. M., O'Hara, B., & Milat, A. J. (2009). Computer-tailored dietary behaviour change interventions: a systematic review. *Health Education Research, 24*, 699–720.

Pender, N. (1996). *Health promotion in nursing practice* (3rd ed.). Stamford, CT: Appleton & Lange.

Pender, N., Murdaugh, C., & Parsons, M. A. (2015). *Health promotion in nursing practice* (7th ed.). Upper Saddle River, NJ: Prentice Hall.

Prochaska, J., Velicer, W., Rossi, J., Goldstein, M., Marcus, B., Rakowski, W., … Rosenbloom, D. (1994). Stages of change and decisional balance for 12 problem behaviors. *Health Psychology, 13*, 39–46.

Sechrist, K., Walker, W., & Pender, N. (1987). Development and psychometric evaluation of the exercise benefits/barriers scale. *Research in Nursing & Health, 10*, 357–365.

Velicer, W. F., Prochaska, J. O., & Redding, C. A. (2006). Tailored communications for smoking cessations: Past successes and future directions. *Drug and Alcohol Review, 25*, 49–57.

Walker, S., Sechrist, K., & Pender, N. (1997). The health-promoting lifestyle profile: Development and psychometric characteristics. *Nursing Research, 39*, 268–273.

Wei, C. N., Yonemitsu, H., Harada, K., Miyakita, T., Omori, S., Miyabayashi, T., … Ueda, A. A. (2000). Japanese language version of the health-promoting lifestyle profile. *Nippon-Eiseigaku-Zasshi, 54*, 597–606.

# 16 Deliberative Nursing Process

Mertie L. Potter

## Definition of Key Terms

| | |
|---|---|
| **Automatic nursing process** | Actions (visible behaviors) the nurse takes based on reasons other than the patient's immediate needs |
| **Deliberative Nursing Process** | Means by which the professional nurse purposefully explores with the patient the nurse's perceptions (stimulation of any one of the five senses), thoughts, and/or feelings related to the patient's immediate need for help |
| **Dynamic nurse–patient relationship** | Interactive contact/connection between nurse and patient, when the nurse begins to explore the meaning behind the patient's verbal and nonverbal behaviors |
| **Immediate need for help** | Requirement of the patient in a specific situation. Providing help for the identified need relieves or diminishes the patient's immediate distress and/or improves the patient's immediate sense of adequacy or well-being |
| **Nursing situation** | Circumstance that involves a patient's behavior, the nurse's reaction (perceptions, thoughts, and feelings combined together), and the nurse's action (activity the nurse completes with or for the patient) |
| **Patient distress** | Feeling experienced by a patient when the patient cannot meet certain needs and is not helped in meeting such needs |
| **Patient outcomes/ product** | Improved verbal and nonverbal patient behaviors that can result from the nurse's deliberative and effective action(s) with the patient |
| **Validation** | Ongoing process of exploring and determining with a patient if the nursing reaction was accurate and if the nursing action was helpful |

The birthing of Deliberative Nursing Process by Ida J. Orlando culminated in 1961, after a number of years laboring to define both the function and the product of professional nursing (Orlando, 1961). The theory began to take shape through Orlando's experiences within nursing practice and nurse education. She reviewed more than 2,000 anecdotal recordings of faculty, students, and nurses related to their interactions with patients and began to see patterns of effective and ineffective nursing process in various nurse–patient situations (Pelletier, 1976). Emerging from these early experiences, Deliberative Nursing Process since has matured into a significant, enduring, and practical nursing theory.

As a middle range theory, Deliberative Nursing Process has a limited number of variables and is limited in scope (McEwan, 2002; Walker & Avant, 1995). However, it is specific and adequate enough to apply and test in research and practice. Although categorized as a grand theory by some (Walker &

Avant, 1995; Wills, 2002), Deliberative Nursing Process demonstrates the following middle range theory characteristics: comprehensive yet focused, generalizable, restricted in its concepts, clear in its propositions, and conducive to testable hypotheses (McEwan, 2002).

An unusual paradox within Deliberative Nursing Process is its proclivity toward both simplicity and complexity as a theory. This paradox partially explains the attractiveness of using this theory. Generally, it is straightforward in its presentation while being multifaceted in its applications. For example, developing a nurse–patient relationship that is dynamic and unique is not complicated. However, the dynamics of the nurse–patient relationship itself may be very complex (Orlando, 1961).

A unique feature related to the development of this theory is the inductive manner in which Orlando defined effective nursing (Schmieding, 2002). Orlando determined effective and ineffective nursing from her observations of "good" and "bad" nursing practice (Orlando, 1961, 1972; Pelletier, 1976; Schmieding, 1993a). From her observations of specific phenomena (nurse–patient interactions), she identified relationships with other phenomena to develop propositions that led to the development of larger concepts and, ultimately, the theory (Johnson & Webber, 2001).

Orlando desired that nurses become educated to assist patients to express what help they actually need (Pelletier, 1967). Another distinctive feature of Deliberative Nursing Process is that patient input is critical. It is the nurse's professional responsibility to involve the patient in the process of identifying and meeting the patient's immediate needs for help (Orlando, 1961, 1972, 1990).

## Historical Background

The need for nurses to have a distinct body of knowledge to direct and enhance nursing practice and the movement of nursing toward becoming a profession were beginning to take place at the turn of the 20th century (Alligood, 2002). Orlando's Deliberative Nursing Process evolved during an era when nurses were attempting to distinguish nursing from other disciplines and when psychiatric–mental health nurses were determining their place among nurses of other specialties. Deliberative Nursing Process came into being as Orlando realized that nursing needed to address three areas: "nurse–patient relationships, the nurse's professional role and identity, and the development of knowledge which is distinctly nursing" (Orlando, 1961, p. viii).

Orlando first published work related to this theory after she examined what made nursing interventions effective or ineffective. She asserted early on that effective nursing was "good nursing" and ineffective nursing was "bad nursing" (Orlando, 1976; Schmieding, 1993a). Although this terminology might not be acceptable during today's trend of political correctness and relativity, Orlando was bold in her assertion that nursing was either "good" or "bad." She also stressed that nursing needed to define exactly what "nursing" was and contended that nursing could not be a profession unless it was able to distinguish that which nurses did as unique (Orlando, 1961).

Orlando was asked to determine what mental health principles were needed in a nursing curriculum. However, she became acutely aware during the project that professional nursing did not have a clear function or product. Nursing was at a crossroads. Orlando (1961) understood that nurses were unclear in their attempts to define what nursing was. For someone concerned with meeting patients' immediate needs, here were immediate needs for nurses—to define and to distinguish nursing's function and product. She recognized that the patient and the patient's needs were getting lost in nurses' assumptions of what those needs were. During a project funded by the National Institute of Mental Health, Orlando began to examine nurses' interactions with patients.

## DEFINING NURSING AND OUTCOME VARIABLES

Resolute in her mission, Orlando set forth in her later work to assist nurses further in defining what nursing is and what it should entail to distinguish it from other disciplines. Key goals became the following: to define the distinct professional function of nurses, to encourage nurses to assume authority to carry out that function, and to educate nurses to use process discipline (Deliberative Nursing Process) to assure that the product of nursing function involves the patient and others who impact the patient's care (Orlando, 1972). She developed a user-friendly theory that was readily understandable and broadly applicable.

Orlando held that "to nurse" and "nursing" were very different from "to doctor" and "doctoring" (Orlando, 1961, 1972; Orlando & Dugan, 1989). She asserted that doctors' orders are designed for patients, not nurses, and that nurses keep themselves on a dependent path when they focus on following doctors' orders rather than assisting patients to meet their needs for help, which may include the patient's needing to comply with doctors' orders (Orlando, 1987). Orlando contended that licensure authorizes nurses to fulfill a professional role, but authority is only implicit until the nurse engages in a process with the patient to meet the function of nursing, namely, to help the patient meet immediate needs for help that the patient is unable to meet on his or her own (Orlando, 1972).

Orlando suggested that the concept of "nursing" derives its meaning from the nursing of infants and the need to have someone nurture and assist infants in obtaining what they need from the environment to survive. She postulated that, at times, individuals might need assistance from others to obtain what is needed from the environment to meet their needs when they are unable to nurse themselves (Orlando, 1961, p. 4; Orlando &Dugan, 1989). Orlando (1972, 1987) distinguished the difference between lay and professional nursing by stating that a professional nurse is needed when a layperson cannot assure that the patient's distress will be identified or relieved.

In some of her works, she questioned whether or not expanded roles of nursing should be considered in the realm of nursing or that of doctoring at a lower cost (Orlando & Dugan, 1989). She used straightforward and uncomplicated language. She contemplated and encouraged nurses to discern what the words "to nurse" meant and referred to a dictionary to emphasize her point of what nursing should entail. She accepted Funk and Wagnall's definition of "to nurse" to mean: "to encourage, to look after; to nourish, protect, and nurture; to give curative care to an ailment" (Orlando, 1987, p. 408).

The conceptual framework of nursing proposed by Orlando identified promotion of "comfort," or the relieving of distress, as crucial to the task of nursing. Orlando's work contributed to the evolution of the concept of comfort by subsequent nursing theorists (Tutton & Seers, 2003). In particular, she designated the nursing role as addressing matters prohibiting a client's "mental and physical comfort" (Orlando, 1961, p. 23). In a review of the development of the concept of comfort in nursing, Tutton and Seers (2003) note that while Orlando does not define the "exact nature of comfort," her promotion of Deliberative Nursing Process to enhance patients' perceived needs makes comfort "pivotal" to her definition of nursing, as it relates to both physical and psychological care (p. 691).

Notably, Orlando was ahead of her time in her concern for and measurement of outcome variables. She promoted progressive ideas, such as defining professional nursing, employing critical thinking within the nursing process, involving the patient in the nursing process, and measuring patient outcomes. Orlando was aware that ineffective nursing activities impacted areas, such as nursing care costs, patient progress, material costs, and medication costs. She was concerned that nursing was acquiring too many nonprofessional tasks that would take the nurse away from helping the patient (Orlando, 1961). Always seeking patient involvement in the provision of nursing care, Orlando looked for a "helpful outcome" as validated with the patient to include "change in the behavior of the object indicating either relief from distress or that a solution to a living or work problem had been found" (Orlando, 1972, p. 61). She addressed work problems involving staff members, as well as patient problems in her 1972 reported studies.

## ORLANDO'S LEGACY

Work on Deliberative Nursing Process theory has spanned more than a half century. Orlando's initial development on this theory began in the early 1950s, and work on the theory's development continues. Her early works referred to the "Deliberative Nursing Process." Orlando began using the term

"Nursing Process Discipline" in 1972 because she asserted that nursing process was a discipline that could be learned (Orlando, 1972, p. 2). The term "Deliberative Nursing Process" will be used throughout this chapter for consistency.

It is obvious in both her published and unpublished writings that Orlando not only was intensely passionate about nursing as an individual but also was a determined advocate for nursing (Orlando, 1961, 1972, 1976, 1983, 1987). Several basic tenets come through strongly in her work, primarily (a) that the function of nursing is to meet the patient's immediate need for help when the patient is unable to do so without the nurse's help and (b) that the product of nursing is to relieve the patient's distress caused by the immediate need for help and to be able to observe improvement either verbally or nonverbally (Orlando, 1961, 1972). Furthermore, her theory promotes the uniqueness of nurses and maintains that patients must be involved in the identification and determination of their immediate needs for help (Orlando, 1961). Orlando was not hesitant to express her grave concern with the definition of nursing promoted in the American Nurses Association Social Policy Statement of 1980—she found "no operational meaning" in it and no differentiation between professional and lay nursing (Orlando, 1983, p. 2). Her passion for nursing clearly was evident throughout her life, accompanied by her assertion that the profession needed to define nursing (I. J. Orlando, personal communication, June 24, 2002).

Ida Jean Orlando Pelletier continues as a symbol of nursing leadership and theory development, having taught and implemented her theory at some of the nation's most respected academic institutions; she was formally recognized as a "Nursing Living Legend" by the Massachusetts Registered Nurse Association in 2006—the year prior to her death (Tyra, 2008).

## Definition of Theory Concepts

### DELIBERATIVE NURSING PROCESS

Deliberative Nursing Process remains relevant and significant as a nursing theory due to its patient-focused approach; nurse exploration of nurse perceptions, thoughts, and feelings with patients; and effective outcomes that result from its use. Orlando (1961) proposes a practical approach, with a broad application within nursing education, practice, and research. She focuses on the nurse's unique and deliberative response to the patient who has expressed an immediate need for help. This is accomplished by the nurse's exploration and validation of the nurse's perceptions, thoughts, and feelings about the patient's behavior with the patient. Furthermore, it is the nurse's responsibility in deliberative nursing to see to it that the patient's need for immediate help is met either by the nurse's own activity or by eliciting the help of others (Orlando, 1961).

Orlando acknowledges and affirms the nurse's distinctive interpretation and validation of observations made. Furthermore, she stresses the independent function performed during a deliberative nursing interaction. She recognizes that what makes nurse–patient relationships dynamic is nurses continually sharing their unique perceptions, thoughts, and feelings (i.e., their immediate reaction) about patients' unique behaviors within a deliberative process with patients (Orlando, 1961, 1972).

Orlando asserts that good nursing initially involves a nurse determining with the patient a number of elements: (a) What does the patient think is occurring? (b) What does the patient define as the immediate distress? (c) Is the patient's distress related to an immediate need for help? (d) Is the nurse's help needed for the patient to obtain relief? She also observed that nurse–patient interactions involving Deliberative Nursing Process resulted in positive outcomes, namely, both verbal and nonverbal positive changes within the patient (Pelletier, 1976).

Deliberative Nursing Process was renamed Nursing Process Discipline by Orlando (1972). She also refers to Deliberative Nursing Process as effective nursing (Orlando, 1961, 1972) or good nursing (Orlando, 1976). She analyzed nurse–patient interactions and determined that effective interactions involved open disclosure of the nurse of perceptions, thoughts, and feelings and validation of the same with the patient. After implementing a

nursing action, the nurse validates with the patient if the nursing action met the patient's immediate need for help (Fig. 16.1; Orlando, 1961).

Orlando also noted that ineffective interactions often involved a more secretive style. Both patient and nurse were not aware of each other's perceptions, thoughts, and feelings in such interactions (Fig. 16.2).

Orlando (1972, p. 28) developed a nursing process record to assist in learning Deliberative Nursing Process (process discipline) and to be better able to discern nursing process done in secret or using open disclosure (Fig. 16.3). Orlando referred to the nurse's perceptions, thoughts, and feelings as part of the nurse's reaction and whatever the nurse said and/or did to, with, or for the patient as the nurse's action (see Fig. 16.3; [Orlando, 1972], p. 56).

## AUTOMATIC NURSING PROCESS

Automatic nursing process refers to any actions or interventions a nurse takes to help a patient that may not be related to the process of helping the patient. Automatic nursing process may be impacted by other influences, such as nursing care costs, patient progress, or additional expenses. Automatic nursing process also is referred to as nursing process without discipline (Orlando, 1972), ineffective nursing (Orlando, 1961, 1972), and bad nursing (Orlando, 1976).

Orlando asserted that automatic nursing process activities were ineffective when they (a) involved nursing action without determining the meaning of the patient's behavior to the patient or the need that caused the behavior, (b) did not assist the patient to inform the nurse how the activity influenced the patient, (c) did not connect the nursing activity to the patient's need, (d) were

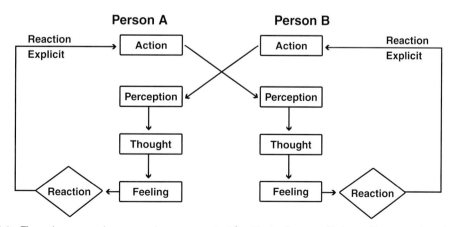

**Figure 16.1**   The action process in a person-to-person contact functioning by open disclosure. The perceptions, thoughts, and feelings of each individual through the observable action. (Used with permission from Orlando, I. J. (1972). *The discipline and teaching of nursing process: An evaluative study* (p. 26). New York, NY: Putnam.)

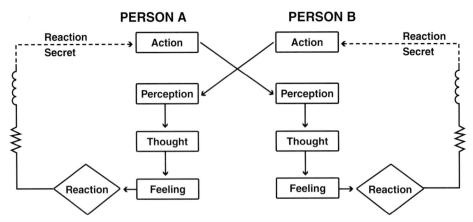

**Figure 16.2**    The action process in a person-to-person contact functioning in secret. The perceptions, thoughts, and feelings of each individual are not directly available to the perception of the other individual through the observable action. (Used with permission from Orlando, I. J. (1972). *The discipline and teaching of nursing process. In an evaluative study* (p. 26). New York, NY: Putnam.)

**Nursing Process Record**

| Perception of or About the Patient | Thought and/or Feeling About the Perception | Said and/or Did to, With, or for the Patient |
|---|---|---|
| **PROCESS A**<br>Mr. G walking back and forth; face red | Looks angry; something must have happened. I'm afraid to ask because he might hit me. | "Good morning, Mr. G." |
| **PROCESS B**<br>Mr. G walking back and forth; face red | Looks angry; something must have happened. I'm afraid to ask because he might hit me. | "I'm afraid you will hit me if I ask a question. Should I be afraid?" |

**Figure 16.3**    Process A illustrates the nursing process functioning in secrecy. Process B illustrates the nursing process functioning by open disclosure. (Used with permission from Orlando, I. J. (1972). *The discipline and teaching of nursing process: An evaluative study* (p. 28). New York, NY: Putnam.)

implemented because of the nurse's inability to explore the nurse's reaction to the patient's behavior, or (e) did not indicate that the nurse was attuned to how the nursing activity influenced the patient (Orlando, 1961, p. 65). Such activities are not necessarily wrong or negative, but they do not determine if the activity is perceived as helpful in relieving the patient's immediate needs. Furthermore, automatic nursing activities indicated to Orlando that nursing care had been given without a disciplined or deliberative professional process (Orlando, 1976).

An example of the difference between the use of an automatic nursing process, which involves nurses' assumptions, and a Deliberative Nursing Process, which involves nurses' exploration of the patients' immediate needs for help, is demonstrated in a study by Bochnak, Rhymes, and Leonard (1962). When two different types of nursing activities to address patients' complaints of pain were examined, statistically significant results occurred at the 0.05 level. In the control group, it was assumed that any complaint of pain indicated a need for pain-relieving medication, and when patients complained of pain, they were given pain-relieving medication. Relief was variable and slow. However, in the experimental group, nurses who used a deliberative approach to determine more accurately what the patients' complaints of pain were about did not automatically administer pain-relieving medication. Their explorations with the patients led to various interventions that provided more extensive relief and quicker relief for the patients (Bochnak et al., 1962).

## DYNAMIC NURSE–PATIENT RELATIONSHIP

According to a recent study, patients are most concerned with personal care issues related to five essential themes: having their needs met, being treated pleasantly, being cared for, having competent nurses, and having care provided promptly (Bolden & Larrabee, 2001). These areas relate to meeting patients' immediate needs for help, which are foundational in Orlando's theory of Deliberative Nursing Process. Orlando (1961) based her ideas about a dynamic nurse–patient relationship on principles from other theories, such as behavioral theory, which postulates that humans are living and behaving organisms who interact continually with one another and within the environment.

Defining the function and product of nursing is explicit in Orlando's definition of the dynamic nurse–patient relationship. Orlando fervently strove to have nurses define the unique function and product of nursing. She defined nursing function as helping the patient and defined nursing product as the improvement or helpful result in the patient's behavior, observable both verbally and nonverbally (Orlando, 1961, 1972, 1983).

## IMMEDIATE NEED FOR HELP

Immediate need for help refers to the patient's inability to fulfill a need for help; the patient may or may not need assistance identifying and/or communicating what the actual need for help is (Orlando, 1961). The observed behavior of the patient is assumed until the meaning behind the behavior is explored (1961, p. 23). Behaviors observed by the nurse may be nonverbal or verbal. Nonverbal behaviors include motor activity, physiological manifestations, and vocalizations. Verbal behaviors take into account complaints, requests, questions, refusals, demands, comments, and statements (1961, pp. 36, 37). Immediate needs for help also are referred to simply as "need" in earlier writings (1961).

Therefore, an immediate need for help is any condition in which patients need to have immediate distress relieved or diminished or their sense of sufficiency or welfare improved (Orlando, 1961, p. 5). Immediate need for help definitely implies that the patient cannot meet the need without professional help.

## PATIENT DISTRESS

Patient distress occurs when a patient's immediate needs are unmet. It is a sense of discomfort that arises when a patient is unable to communicate his or her needs adequately or clearly. Orlando cited physical challenges, unfavorable reactions to the environment, and unfavorable occurrences as examples of circumstances that keep the patient from being able to meet immediate needs (Orlando, 1961, p. 11).

Patient distress is what the patient perceives to be stressful. Orlando holds that behavior has meaning and that nurses cannot assume what the behavior means without exploring with the patient what the behavior and accompanying distress mean to the patient.

## NURSING SITUATION

According to Orlando (1961, p. 36), a nursing situation encompasses three elements and is dependent upon the nurse's use of them: (a) the patient's behavior, (b) the nurse's reaction, and (c) the nurse's actions intended for the patient's benefit. The interaction of these three elements comprises nursing process.

## VALIDATION

Validation is an ongoing nursing action within the Deliberative Nursing Process. It involves checking with the patient if the nurse's perceptions, thoughts, and/or feelings were accurate in relation to the patient's behavior and if the nurse's interventions were "correct, helpful, or appropriate" (Orlando, 1961, p. 56). In addition, Orlando sees the nurse as primarily responsible for initiating the process of exploration and discovery in relation to how the patient is responding to any nursing action (1961). The presence or absence of validation in the nurse–patient relationship and subsequent actions differentiates the deliberative process (with patient validation) from the automatic response (without patient validation), as visualized in Figure 16.4 (Aponte, 2009).

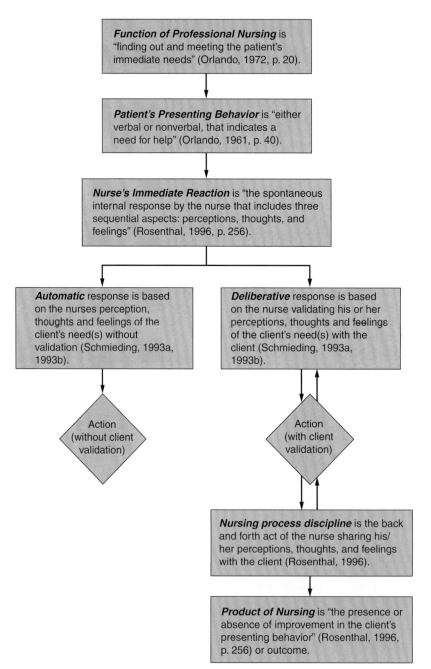

**Figure 16.4**    Orlando's *Dynamic Nurse–Patient Relationship Nursing Framework.* (From Aponte, J. (2009). Meeting the linguistic needs of urban communities. *Home Healthcare Nurse, 27*(5), 327. Copyright © 2009 by Wolters Kluwer Health. Reprinted with permission.)

## PATIENT OUTCOMES/PRODUCT

The end result of a nursing action is to "bring about improvement" (Orlando, 1961, p. 6). That improvement should be observable both verbally and nonverbally in the patient's behavior (Orlando, 1972, p. 21). Patient outcomes also should be both "predictable and helpful" and may include such outcomes as "avoidance, relief or diminution of helplessness suffered or anticipated by the individual in an immediate experience" (Orlando, 1972, p. 9). The nurse's activity may result in help, no help, or be unknown (Orlando, 1961, p. 67). If the outcome does not transpire as predicted, then the nurse must continue to explore what else may be needed to meet the patient's immediate need for help.

# Description of the Theory of Deliberative Nursing Process

## SIMPLE YET COMPLEX THEORY

Deliberative Nursing Process is a theory that is readily understood, has a specific focus (i.e., meeting patients' immediate needs for help), addresses patient problems and probable outcomes (felt distress and lowered distress, respectively), and is explicit to nursing. Its concepts and their relationships are testable, and they answer questions about nursing, which are indicators of a middle range nursing theory (Marriner-Tomey, 1998). Orlando's work helped refocus nurses on patients rather than on tasks and on an active, rather than passive, role of patients in their own care.

Complexity refers to the "richness" of a theory to elucidate more variables and their interrelationships (Stevens-Barnum, 1990, p. 97). Part of the theory's complexity involves learning how to use it. Becoming proficient in the use of Deliberative Nursing Process necessitates time, practice, and self-reflection, often in the form of a supervisory experience. The use of nursing process recordings (see Fig. 16.3) helps the nurse distinguish perceptions, thoughts, and feelings—no small task in itself. Learning Deliberative Nursing Process often involves a close supervisory experience in which the learner reconstructs and examines interactions. The process of becoming comfortable in owning one's perceptions, thoughts, and feelings and sharing them with patients is at times difficult and complex.

## FUNCTION OF NURSING

Orlando observed patients in distress and asserted that it was professional nursing's role to determine and meet their immediate needs for help

by exploring with the patient the nurse's unique thoughts and feelings, resulting from perceptions related to the observed patient behaviors (Orlando, 1961, 1972, 1990). When the nurse shares perceptions, thoughts, and/or feelings, it is considered to involve open disclosure; by not sharing, the patient is unaware of the nurse's reaction (Orlando, 1972, p. 26). Nurses must not make assumptions but must explore their perceptions, thoughts, and feelings about the patient's behavior with patients. Orlando's (1961) incorporation of nurses' exploration of their thoughts with patients as part of a deliberative process indicates how critical thinking is an essential part of the Deliberative Nursing Process (Schmieding, 2002).

## MAJOR COMPONENTS AND THEIR RELATIONSHIPS

Nursing is independent, has its own unique professional function, and has its own distinct product (Pelletier, 1976, p. 17). The dynamic nurse–patient relationship involves reciprocity between the nurse and patient; each is influenced by what the other does and says (Marriner-Tomey, 1998). It is dependent upon a nurse-initiated exploration of perceptions, thoughts, and feelings about the patient's behavior and validation that the nurse's perceptions, thoughts, and feelings are accurate.

The nurse initiates the deliberative process to determine the immediate need for help by helping the patient identify and express the meaning of his or her behavior (Orlando, 1961). Further, the nurse helps the patient explore distress related to the immediate need for help to determine the help needed (p. 29). Within the dynamic nurse–patient relationship, the nurse observes a patient whom the nurse thinks is in distress. This dynamic relationship is dependent upon "what the nurse and patient start with, to the length of their contact and to what they are able to accomplish" (Orlando, 1961, p. 91).

As Schmieding points out, nurses using Deliberative Nursing Process realize "that the patient is the source of the nurse's power" (Schmieding, 2002, p. 327). The nurse uses reflection as part of a critical thinking process to help ascertain the meaning of the patient's behavior according to the patient and to determine how the behavior relates to the nurse's assumption that an immediate need exists, which is leading to distress for the patient. Nurses obtain information either directly from the patient or indirectly from other sources, such as family, friends, and nursing staff. Orlando considers that nurses have access to a tremendous amount of information about the patient (Orlando, 1961).

The nurse using a deliberative process will check what the meaning of the information is with the patient. In an automatic process, the nurse assumes what the information means. Most likely, the outcomes would be significantly different, depending upon which process the nurse uses. Using the deliberative process, the patient partners with the nurse to identify the need, and a successful outcome is more likely. When an automatic process is used, the patient is not included in the assessment or decision-making processes, making a successful outcome less likely (Orlando, 1961, 1972).

Deliberative Nursing Process is a learned and practiced process (Orlando, 1972). The nurse validates with the patient that the patient has an immediate need for help and that the immediate need for help cannot be met without a professional nurse's help. The nurse intervenes, after exploring with the patient what meaning the patient ascribes to behaviors related to the situation that resulted in an immediate need for help. The nursing situation involves (a) the patient's behavior, (b) the nurse's reaction, and (c) the nurse's activity or actions to assist the patient. Nursing process is the interaction of the three elements contained within a nursing situation (Orlando, 1961, p. 36).

The nurse validates that the immediate need for help has been met by asking the patient and evaluating if the anticipated product or patient outcome of the nursing action, namely, improvement and relief of distress, has occurred. If the nursing action has resulted in the patient's relief, the nursing action has been effective in achieving the desired and predicted patient outcome or product. As mentioned, Orlando used nursing process recordings to study nursing process and to educate nurses in Deliberative Nursing Process.

Assumptions and propositions will be described, based upon Johnson and Webber's (2001) definitions. Assumptions are assumed truths that are associated with the relationships (p. 15). Patients' becoming distressed when they cannot meet their own needs is an example of an assumption within Deliberative Nursing Process (Orlando, 1961). A more complete listing of assumptions implied within Orlando's Deliberative Nursing Process theory can be found in Table 16.1.

Propositions direct the relationship between concepts and provide a description of the relationship between concepts (Johnson & Webber, 2001, p. 15). An example that Orlando cited was that "the professional function of nursing is distinct and of central importance to patients in any treatment setting" (Pelletier, 1967, p. 30). Implied propositions within Orlando's Deliberative Nursing Process theory are also listed in Table 16.1.

**Table 16.1    Assumptions and Propositions Within Orlando's (1961) Deliberative Nursing Process**

| Assumptions | Propositions |
|---|---|
| Patients require the expertise of professional nurses to meet certain immediate needs for help. | Nurses can determine patients' immediate needs for help by using a Deliberative Nursing Process to ascertain with the patient what the immediate need is. |
| Patients experience distress when they cannot meet their own needs. | Nurses can help alleviate patients' distress most effectively when implementing actions based upon a Deliberative Nursing Process because the actions will be designed to meet the need causing distress. |
| Nursing can be evaluated as either good or bad. | Good nursing involves open disclosure of and validation with the patient of the nurse's perceptions, thoughts, and/or feelings related to the patient's behavior and validation with the patient that the nursing action taken met the patient's immediate need for help. |
| It is the responsibility of professional nurses to meet patients' immediate needs for help or to assure that those needs are met by someone else. | Professional nurses using a Deliberative Nursing Process function differently than lay nurses because they are trained in a process whereby they validate with patients (a) what the patients' needs are and (b) if the needs have been met effectively by the nursing actions implemented. |
| Each nursing situation with a patient is unique and dynamic. | Patients' individualized needs and nurses' distinctive styles create individually unique nursing situations, and each nursing situation is dynamic because it involves ongoing deliberation by the nurse. |
| The desired outcome of good nursing is that the patient reports or demonstrates (a) relief from distress, (b) experience of less distress, or (c) improvement in "adequacy or well-being" (p. 5). | The nurse can determine with the patient if nursing actions based on the Deliberative Nursing Process alleviated or decreased the distress or helped the patient gain a sense of improved "adequacy or well-being" (p. 5). |

# Applications of the Theory

Deliberative Nursing Practice has been applied to a broad range of practice settings, including inpatient and acute nursing settings, residential care facilities, as well as in outpatient or community settings by advanced practice nurses. Deliberative Nursing Process application and outcome measures may be utilized to validate clients' needs and perceived outcomes to improve nursing care. Furthermore, it may lead to professionalization of nursing's role in any of these practice settings, as it demonstrates efficacy and potential impact of nursing. The following examples represent a sampling of contexts in which Deliberative Nursing Practice has been incorporated.

## DELIBERATIVE NURSING PROCESS IN THEORY DEVELOPMENT

Deliberative Nursing Process has been linked with recent models of social information processing to develop a new nursing theory. Sheldon and Ellington (2008) applied the Crick and Dodge model of social information processing to interactions within nursing responses to patient behaviors. By evaluating interviews with experienced nurses, nursing scholars identified Deliberative Nursing Process as foundational for understanding nurse–patient relationships. They concluded that social information processing theory was instrumental to further describe how nurses learn to effectively respond to patients' social cues and environmental factors (Sheldon & Ellington, 2008). Their research suggests that the coupling of Deliberative Nursing Process and social information processing may contribute to new nursing theory and curriculum development, in order to enhance nursing training programs and communication skills and improve patient care.

## PRACTICE APPLICATIONS

### Deliberative Nursing Process in a Group Context

The author supervised nurses in 12-week group leadership training. Nurses received contact hours for coleading a weekly patient group session for 12 weeks, completing written assignments and readings, and participating actively in supervision throughout the group experience (Potter, Williams, & Costanzo, 2004). Each group focused upon the following:
- Meeting patients' immediate needs for help
- Validating that nurse coleaders understood what group members stated was their immediate need for help
- Sharing nurse coleaders' perceptions with patient group members, thoughts, and/or

feelings in response to behaviors (verbal or nonverbal) that group members presented within the group

Group members often commented, either during or at completion of group sessions, how helpful they felt the group had been and frequently commented that they felt better. Group members found that check-ins and check-outs were extremely helpful in addressing patients' immediate needs for help and decreasing patient distress. Positive feedback was given on postgroup surveys as well.

Nurses were educated to use Deliberative Nursing Process within a nursing situation (involving the patient's behavior, the nurse's reaction, and the nurse's action) to identify with the patient what the meaning of the patient's behavior is, so that the patient's immediate need for help could be met and distress relieved. Involvement of the patient in discerning the meaning of his or her behavior was found to effectively promote a dynamic nurse–patient relationship. Validation with the patient that the need had been correctly identified and met resulted in positive patient outcomes (Potter et al., 2004).

### Deliberative Nursing Process With Prospective Nursing Students

Nursing Camp 2002 was a 2-week camp for 8th grade students that ran during the summer at Saint Anselm College in Manchester, New Hampshire. Nursing Camp 2002 was a partnership between the Manchester School-to-Careers Partnership, Saint Anselm College, Elliot Hospital, Hanover Hill Health Care Center, New Hampshire Hospital (NHH), and Visiting Nurses Association Childcare Center. Sylvia Durette, camp director, and this writer introduced 27 students to Orlando's Deliberative Nursing Process as part of their overview of the nursing profession. Students also participated in an interactive experience related to Deliberative Nursing Process.

### Deliberative Nursing Process in Clinical Practice

Deliberative Nursing Process can be applied within a variety of practice settings. See Table 16.2 for examples of Deliberative Nursing Process in practice.

Nursing staff at an extended care facility requested assistance from their nursing supervisor regarding problematic night behaviors of two older adult patients (Faust, 2002). The supervisor incorporated Deliberative Nursing Process to determine apparent unmet needs of the patients. She met with staff and formulated a plan of action. She assigned an additional nursing assistant to that wing, assumed responsibility for the two patients, observed the patients' behaviors, and validated her perceptions with these patients. Both patients

| Table 16.2 | Examples of Theory in Practice |
|---|---|
| **Citation** | **Focus** |
| Abraham, S. (2011). Fall prevention conceptual framework. *The Health Care Manager, 30*(2), 179–184. doi: 10.1097/HCM.0b013e31826fb74 | Deliberative Nursing Process is used as a conceptual framework for fall risk prevention in hospitals. |
| Dufault, M., Duquette, C. E., Ehmann, J., Hehl, R., Lavin, M., Martin, V., …, Wiley, C. (2010). Translating an evidence-based protocol for nurse-to-nurse shift handoffs. *Worldviews on Evidence-Based Nursing, 7*(2), 59–75 | Deliberative Nursing Process is used as evidence of best practice protocol to create a standardized "SBARP" (Situation, Background, Assessment, Recommendation, Patient) format for nursing shift handoffs. |
| Dye, M. C. (2013). *Assumptions can mislead: Failures in health care and elsewhere.* Bloomington, IN: Trafford Publishing | The use of one's perceptions, thoughts, and/or feelings to validate patient needs is applied in a variety of settings. Multiple examples illustrate that Deliberative Nursing Process can be used to avoid making assumptions and poor patient outcomes. |
| Faust, C. (2002). Orlando's deliberative nursing process theory: A practice application in an extended care facility. *Journal of Gerontological Nursing, 28*(7), 14–18 | Deliberative Nursing Process is used in an extended care facility to meet patient's unmet needs and reduce unwanted night behaviors. |
| Potter, M. L., & Moller, M. D. (2016). *Psychiatric-mental health nursing: From suffering to hope.* Boston, MA: Pearson Education, Inc. | Deliberative Nursing Process is used throughout a textbook to assist nursing students in using their perceptions, thoughts, and/or feelings to validate patient needs. |

demonstrated less distress and increased sleep during the nights.

Dye (2013) ascertains that Deliberative Nursing Process can be applied in multiple practice settings. Dye (2013) provides numerous examples to establish that one's perceptions, thoughts, and/or feelings can be used in situations to assess patient's needs. Dye (2013) further asserts that one needs to use one's perceptions, thoughts, and/or feelings to seek validation from the patient and use this validation to take further action. Dye (2013) concludes that when this is not done, assumptions often are made, which lead to poor patient outcomes. Dye (2013) also provides multiple examples to affirm that Deliberative Nursing Process can be applied to settings beyond nursing.

Yekefallah et al. (2017) reported on an Orlando nursing intervention what they did with 60 male and female endoscopy patients ranging from 20 to 70 years. In this study, they assigned half of the patients to a control group and half to an intervention group. Both groups received standard hospital intervention including music. The intervention group received Orlando nursing process for 10 to 15 minutes including provision about the nature and sequence of the examination, information about the endoscopy unit, and description and discussion of relaxation strategies. The females were more anxious than the males prior to the intervention. There was a significant difference ($p < 0.001$) between the groups with the intervention group demonstrating less anxiety postintervention.

Bezanson (2002) proposed a theoretical application of Deliberative Nursing Process for an outpatient surgery center of an acute care, community-based hospital. Bezanson asserts that implementation of Deliberative Nursing Process could provide opportunities to improve nursing practice, increase patient satisfaction, and enhance staff satisfaction with their nurse–patient interactions. Bezanson also suggests that mechanisms of evaluation might include patient-focused satisfaction surveys, staff self-reports of satisfaction in practice, and improved patient outcomes.

### Deliberative Nursing Process in Education Applications

Potter and Moller (2016) apply the Deliberative Nursing Process in their textbook to assist nursing students in learning the deliberative process of communicating with patients. Throughout the textbook, a variety of case examples are employed to assist students in using their perceptions, thoughts, and feelings to validate patient needs with patients (see Using Middle Range Theory in Practice 16.1).

With the increased emphasis on communication technologies being used in patient care, there is also an increased need to teach nursing students to communicate more directly and effectively with patients. Gaudet and Howett (2018) used the Deliberative Nursing Process as a model to improve nurse–patient interactions, teaching students this approach to analyze communication. The theory was used during role-playing, scenarios, simulation debriefings, and pre- and postclinical conferences for the purpose of analysis. The theory was also used for evaluation of students' communication techniques (p. 372).

---

## USING MIDDLE RANGE THEORY IN PRACTICE   16.1

Deliberative Nursing Process is being used in educational settings to assist nursing students to communicate effectively with patients to meet patient needs. Potter and Moller (2016) included examples of Orlando's Deliberative Nursing Process in their psychiatric–mental health nursing textbook to enhance student nurse communication skills.

*Source: Potter, M. L., & Moller, M. D. (2016). Psychiatric-mental health nursing: From suffering to hope. Boston, MA: Pearson Education, Inc.*

### PROBLEM

Nursing students may have a difficult time communicating with patients. They may be unsure of what to say or do to best help a patient in distress, especially in short interactions with patients.

### INTERVENTION

Throughout the Potter and Moller textbook, case study inserts model Orlando's Deliberative Nursing Process to help nursing students be more effective in communicating with patients. In each case study, the patient's behavior (actions and words) is shown. Following that are the nurse's perceptions, thoughts, and/or feelings of the patient behavior. Each case study then shows the nurse's exploration of their perceptions, thoughts, and/or feelings of the behavior, that is, what the nurse says to the patient. The nurse's perceptions, thoughts, and/or feelings of the patient's behavior are then validated to help the nurse best meet the patient's need for immediate help and relieve patient distress.

---

## DELIBERATIVE NURSING PROCESS IN MEASURING NURSING OUTCOMES

The nursing executive leadership at NHH established Orlando's dynamic nursing process theory as a foundation for practice in 1996 and utilized Deliberative Nursing Process as a driving principle in the formation and functioning of a Nursing Practice Enhancement Project (NPEP) (Allen, Bockenhauer, Egan, & Kinnaird, 2006). The NPEP was instituted with the purpose of "redesign[ing] a model" to apply in psychiatric nursing care at NHH. The nursing leadership at NHH identified the interpersonal nurse–client professional relationship as key to healing and psychiatric care. In the process of developing the NPEP, Deliberative Nursing Process was instrumental in helping nurse staff to find a "common approach" to a broad range of clients; furthermore, affirmation of the nursing role as described in the Deliberative Nursing Process became "one of the cornerstones of empowered nursing practice" (Allen et al., 2006, p. 141). A Nursing Practice Outcomes Committee was formed to measure the effectiveness of the redesigned nursing model of psychiatric care at NHH and found that the revised model of care was effective in reducing the occurrence of seclusion–restraint, improving both patient satisfaction and nurses' job satisfaction (Allen et al., 2006).

An example of how Deliberative Nursing Theory can be used in a practice project can be found in Using Middle Range Theory in Practice Projects 16.2

## RESEARCH APPLICATIONS

Deliberative Nursing Process has been categorized as a nursing process theory (Orlando, 1990), a prescriptive theory (Wooldridge, Skipper, & Leonard, 1968), and a reflective practice theory (Schmieding, 2002). The inductive, research-based approach Orlando used to develop Deliberative Nursing Process as a theory was unique. Meleis (1997, p. 348) points out that Orlando used field methodology before it became widely accepted in research use.

### Diverse Range of Research Applications

Orlando's theory has been widely used as a framework for numerous studies in a variety of settings. Areas studied encompass nursing theory, practice, education, and administration. Both qualitative and quantitative approaches have been employed.

Deliberative Nursing Process has been applied in theory analysis (Alligood & Choi, 1998; Andrews, 1989; Walker & Avant, 1995). A number of patient outcomes have been studied using Deliberative Nursing Process including but not limited to pain (Barron, 1966; Bochnak, 1963; Bochnak et al., 1962), postoperative recovery (Eisler, Wolfer, & Diers, 1972), blood pressure and pulse rates (Mertz, 1963), vomiting (Dumas & Leonard, 1963), and levels of distress (Potter & Bockenhauer, 2000). Additional areas explored using Deliberative Nursing Process include spousal grieving (Dracup & Breu, 1978), breastfeeding (Clausen, 1983), and

## USING MIDDLE RANGE THEORY IN PRACTICE PROJECTS    16.2

*Source: LiVolsi, K. (2018). Improving neonatal outcomes through the implementation of a delayed bathing program (Doctor of Nursing Process Project). Seton Hall University, South Orange, NJ. UMI: AAI10823295.*

### SUMMARY OF THE PROJECT

**Purpose**

To improve the overall outcomes of neonates by delaying their first baths from 2 hours after birth to 24 hours.

**Methods**

Staff and parent education took place to present the change in bath schedule. Implementation followed with first baths of neonates took place 24 hours after birth.

### HOW THE THEORY WAS USED

Orlando's nursing theory was the theoretical framework for need assessment and effective communication in presenting the project.

### OUTCOME OF THE PROJECT

A number of positive outcomes were observed: (a) breastfeeding rates improved by 10%, (b) supplemental formula feeding rates decreased by 10%, (c) hypoglycemia decreased by 2%, and (d) hypothermia in infants at risk decreased by 4%.

### CONCLUSIONS AND RECOMMENDATIONS

There was an overall improvement in infant health and observed increased parent participation in infant care. The project outcomes provide evidence for a change in practice.

---

cancer (Reid-Ponte, 1988). Nursing education (Abdoli & Safavi, 2010; Haggerty, 1987; Orlando, 1972) and nursing administration (Schmieding, 1984, 1992) also have been examined using the Deliberative Nursing Process. (For additional studies using Deliberative Nursing Process, refer to the Bibliography.)

Potter, Vitale-Nolen, and Dawson (2005) designed a study to determine if implementation of a safety agreement tool made a difference in the rate of patient self-harm incidents and in nurses' feeling more comfortable interacting with patients at risk for self-harm. A safety agreement was designed to assist nurses in incorporating Deliberative Nursing Process when interacting with patients at risk for self-harm (see Using Middle Range Theory in Research 16.3).

Deliberative Nursing Process can be used as a framework to design research in various settings and to examine specific patient outcomes. The study illustrated in Using Middle Range Theory in Research 16.4 demonstrates patient outcomes related to reduction in levels of distress when Deliberative Nursing Process was implemented in an acute care psychiatric hospital setting.

Olson and Hanchett (1997) carried out a study examining Orlando's assertion that relationships exist between nurse-expressed empathy and several patient outcomes. They used a descriptive,

correlational format, described in Using Middle Range Theory in Research 16.5.

### Delivering Culturally Competent Care

Recently, Deliberative Nursing Process was used in the formation and implementation of the Influenza Initiative in New York City—a collaborative nursing effort to meet linguistic needs and provide culturally competent care. This project involved delivering education and immunizations for influenza prevention to an urban population (Aponte, 2009). In this program, bilingual nursing students were paired with nursing providers from a home health care agency to translate for non–English-speaking Spanish, Chinese, Russian, and Ukrainian residents participating in the New York City Influenza Initiative in Fall 2006 and Fall 2007. With Deliberative Nursing Process as a nursing framework for providing care, nursing students were able to confirm and validate clients' needs, ensure accurate understanding of information, confirm consent for treatment, and direct RNs to administer immunizations in a safe and culturally competent manner (Aponte, 2009).

### Ethical Values in Caring for Older Adults

In a study by Jonasson (2009), the dynamic nurse–patient relationship is presented as crucial to the

## USING MIDDLE RANGE THEORY IN RESEARCH    16.3

*Source: Potter, M. L., Vitale-Nolen, R., & Dawson, A. M. (2005). Implementation of safety agreements in an acute psychiatric facility. Journal of the American Psychiatric Association, 11(3), 144–155.*

Nurses at New Hampshire Hospital (NHH), a university-affiliated, state psychiatric facility, were interested in determining if implementation of safety agreements would affect patient outcomes and nursing comfort levels when working with patients at risk for self-harm (Potter et al., 2005). Registered nurses (RNs) serving on a Continuous Quality Improvement (CQI) Committee had examined the use of safety contracts by nurses at the facility and developed a safety agreement tool that they thought would facilitate incorporating Orlando's Deliberative Nursing Process when assessing patients at risk for self-harm.

Validity of safety contracts in general has not been tested. Confusion and controversy exist in relation to the definition and the use of safety contracts with patients who are suicidal (Potter & Dawson, 2001). It is suspected that these confusion and controversy lead to a discomfort and a lack of direction when nurses "contract" with patients for safety.

It has been demonstrated by nurses at NHH that Deliberative Nursing Process can make a difference in patient outcomes (Potter & Bockenhauer, 2000).

### PURPOSE

The purpose of the study was to determine if a more standardized process, using Orlando's Deliberative Nursing Process to enhance communication, would promote patients' agreeing to be safe and, in turn, decrease the rate of self-harm incidents and increase RNs' comfort levels when working with patients at risk for self-harm.

### RESEARCH DESIGN

The researchers used quasi-experimental methods.

### PARTICIPANTS

There were 44 RNs who responded to the initial survey and 49 who responded to the follow-up survey.

### DATA COLLECTION

Safety agreements were implemented as the standard of care on all units in acute psychiatric services (APS). Incidents of self-harm were collected via the organizational-wide data collection system pre- and postimplementation. Instruction for RNs in the use of safety agreements occurred the month before implementation of safety agreements. RNs already used Deliberative Nursing Process as a framework for nursing care. The RNs were invited to complete two different surveys on the use of safety agreement—first was offered at the end of the first 3-month period and the second was offered at the end of 12 months. There were two convenience sample databases: (a) anonymous lists of self-harm incidents (only chart numbers used, not patient names) and (b) all RNs who performed direct patient care.

The investigators used $t$-tests to detect differences in pre- and postintervention outcomes and Stat Pac Gold computer software to analyze data for statistical differences.

### FINDINGS

The mean rate of self-harming incidents did not change significantly pre- and postimplementation of safety agreements. RNs were equally divided in relation to thinking that safety agreements enhanced or did not enhance nurse–patient interactions. However, RNs did report improvement in the following areas related to the use of safety agreements: patient responsibility, nurse contact with patients, guidance for safety concerns, discussions with patients related to safety, and time guidelines around issues of safety.

---

process of determining the ethical care of older adults. In her study of nurse–patient interactions between nurses, older adults, and their next of kin, Jonasson points to the processes of validation and evaluation as crucial to providing true benefit to the patient and their family. Through observation and interview data collection, she found that body language, elements of respect, and behavior elements of the initial approach of a nurse with an older adult client are crucial in developing a therapeutic nursing relationship. Moreover, the patient and next of kin's perceptions of the nurses' availability and approachability led to improved patient and family feelings of being valued and acknowledged. Jonasson challenges nurses to recognize the extent to which their approach to patients impacts

## USING MIDDLE RANGE THEORY IN RESEARCH    16.4

*Source: Potter, M. L., & Bockenhauer, B. J. (2000). Implementing Orlando's nursing theory: A pilot study. Journal of Psychosocial Nursing and Mental Health Services, 38, 14–21.*

### PURPOSE

The study's purpose was to determine if within a large, university-affiliated state psychiatric facility implementation of Orlando's nursing theory-based practice (Deliberative Nursing Practice) made a difference in patient outcomes when compared with patient outcomes resulting from interventions using nonspecified nursing practice.

### RESEARCH DESIGN

This was a quasi-experimental pilot study.

### PARTICIPANTS

Two inpatient units were selected that matched most closely in staffing patterns, patient census, and acuity levels. Ten RNs participated—six in the experimental group and four in the control group. The experimental and control groups of RNs had no significant differences in their demographic composition. Thirty patients were involved in the study—19 in the experimental group and 11 in the control group. Patient experimental and control groups were statistically similar.

### DATA COLLECTION

The RNs were educated in the use of the Bockenhauer-Potter Scale of Immediate Distress (BPSID), a five-point Likert-scaled instrument that quantifies the level of patient-demonstrated distress. The BPSID was developed to control for subjectivity when assessing patients' levels of distress. The two investigators, a consultant in Orlando's theory, and three hospital RN specialists reviewed and enhanced reference points on the scale. Videotaped simulated interactions helped nurses to learn how to use the BPSID, thus increasing interrater reliability. RNs in the experimental group received instruction in Deliberative Nursing Process. Data collection took place over a 12-week time frame. Distress levels of patients were measured before and after RN interventions.

### FINDINGS

A greater reduction ($p = 0.04$) in patients' levels of distress occurred in the group in which RNs used the Deliberative Nursing Process. Interestingly, RNs who used the Deliberative Nursing Process reported that having a "road map" helped them feel more effective in their nursing interventions. Further research is suggested to control the possible "halo effect" of additional attention provided to the experimental group of RNs via weekly support and education and to obtain verbal feedback from patients who experience nursing interventions that incorporate Deliberative Nursing Process.

---

patients' feelings and outcomes, as dependent upon nurse "attitude and actions" (Jonasson, 2009, p. 26).

### Nursing Informatics

In a paper regarding nursing process theory and the development of nursing information systems to improve care delivery in the future, Alexander (2007) highlights the role of Orlando's prescribed elements of nursing process: observations, actions, reporting, and recording. In particular, Alexander proposes a nursing informatics model, called the nurse–patient trajectory framework. This trajectory incorporates both patient and provider inputs to coordinate patient care and nursing process elements with human–computer interaction to direct the overall plan of care (Alexander, 2007).

In comparison with other models of nursing informatics to determine the plan of care, this model would uniquely involve patient input. This would ensure inclusion of validation and evaluation of the client's needs and perceived sources of distress and comfort, rather than promoting an automatic nursing process through technology-guided information processing.

---

## Instruments Used in Empirical Testing

There are no set means or tools to measure Deliberative Nursing Process. This is indicative of the nature of the theory because Orlando emphasized that Deliberative Nursing Process

## USING MIDDLE RANGE THEORY IN RESEARCH    16.5

Source: Olson, J., & Hanchett, E. (1997). Nurse-expressed empathy, patient outcomes, and development of a middle-range theory. Image: Journal of Nursing Scholarship, 29, 71–76.

### PURPOSE

The purpose of the study was to explore the relationships between nurse-expressed empathy and two patient outcomes (patient-perceived empathy and patient distress). The hypotheses were as follows: (a) A negative relationship will exist between measures of nurse-expressed empathy and measures of patient distress; (b) a positive relationship will exist between measures of nurse-expressed empathy and patient-perceived empathy; and (c) a negative relationship will exist between patient-perceived empathy and measures of patient distress.

### RESEARCH DESIGN

A descriptive, correlational research design was used to test the hypotheses.

### PARTICIPANTS

One hundred and forty subjects comprised the sample. Seventy staff RNs were selected from a pool of 50% of all eligible nurses who were invited. Seventy patients for whom the nurses cared during a day shift were randomly selected to participate.

### DATA COLLECTION

Nurse participants completed the Staff–Patient Interaction Response Scale (SPIRS) and the Behavioral Test of Interpersonal Skills (BTIS). Both measure nurse-expressed empathy. Patient participants completed the Empathy Subscale of the Barrett-Lennard Relationship Inventory (BLRI) to determine patient-perceived empathy measures; their patient distress scores were measured using the Profile of Mood States (POMS) and the Multiple Affect Adjective Checklist (MAACL).

Testing of hypothesis was as follows: (a) Hypotheses one and three were tested together by means of one canonical correlation, and (b) hypothesis three was tested by means of multiple regression analysis.

### RESULTS

All three hypotheses received statistically significant support with the BTIS measurement. A fuller description of methodology and findings are recorded in a report by Olson (1995). This study supported Orlando's (1961, 1972) assertion that relationships exist between accurate perceptions of patients' needs (nurse-expressed empathy and patient-expressed empathy) and patient distress.

---

involves a nursing situation in which the uniqueness of the nurse is brought to the experience to meet the immediate needs for help, as expressed by the patient, explored by the nurse and the patient, and validated by the nurse with the patient. Each circumstance or nursing situation will be unique and different, because each nurse perceives, feels, and thinks differently than any other nurse entering the same nursing situation.

Different tools have been developed and/or used to measure different aspects of Deliberative Nursing Process. These tools facilitate examination of such factors as patient outcomes, nursing process, nurse empathy, and patient-perceived empathy. The instruments have been developed and/or used to test Deliberative Nursing Process qualitatively and quantitatively. Instruments used in different studies explore different aspects of the Deliberative Nursing Process, such as theory description and analysis, use in research, use in clinical practice, and use in administrative practice.

Much of the testing done with Deliberative Nursing Process involves questionnaires and surveys. Examples of tools that have been used for studies involving Orlando's Deliberative Nursing Process are listed in Table 16.3.

### SAFETY AGREEMENT INSTRUMENT

One instrument used in the study of Deliberative Nursing Process has been the safety agreement. The safety agreement instrument, developed by nurses at NHH, was designed to measure patients' risk for self-harm and willingness and the ability to agree to remain safe (see Table 16.3). Most of the agreements are designed in Likert-style format. A question related to a patient's perceived ability to remain safe requires a "yes" or "no" response. In addition, a question seeking to determine how the patient and RN might work together to manage the current risk for self-harm elicits a response from a number of given choices with an "other" option

**Table 16.3    Deliberative Nursing Process Tools**

| Category | Abbreviation | Example |
|---|---|---|
| Anxiety | | State Anxiety Inventory (Spielberger, Gorsuch, & Lushene, 1970) |
| Attitude change | | Spouse Questionnaire (Silva, 1979)<br>Spouses' Perception Scale (Silva, 1979) |
| Emotional state | WI | Welfare Inventory (Eisler et al., 1972) |
| Nurse-expressed empathy | BTIS | Behavioral Test of Interpersonal Skills (Gerrard & Buzzell, 1980) |
| | SPIRS | Staff–Patient Interaction Response Scale (Gallop, Lancee, & Garfinkel, 1989) |
| Patient-perceived empathy | BLRI | Barrett-Lennard Relationship Inventory (Barrett-Lennard, 1962) |
| Patient distress | POMS | Profile of Mood States (McNair, Lorr, & Droppleman, 1971) |
| | MAACL | Multiple Affect Adjective Checklist (Zuckerman & Lubin, 1965) |
| | BPSID | Bockenhauer-Potter Scale of Immediate Distress (Potter & Bockenhauer, 2000)<br>Pain and distress questionnaire (Hall-Lord & Larsson, 2006) |
| Patient's self-harm incidents | SA | Safety agreement (Potter et al., 2005) |
| Nurse-perceived comfort with the use of safety agreements | | Registered Nurses Evaluation Survey (Potter et al., 2005) |
| Therapeutic effectiveness | EPPS | Edwards Personal Preference Schedule (Edwards, 1959) |
| | SII | Social Interaction Inventory (Methven & Schlotfeldt, 1962) |
| Postoperative physical recovery | RI | Recovery Inventory (Eisler et al., 1972) |
| Social approval | SD Scale | Social Desirability Scale (Crowne & Marlowe, 1964) |

included. The intent of the safety agreement is to assist the RN in a deliberative process of determining with the patient the patient's risk for self-harm.

A safety agreement was implemented by Potter et al. (2005) at NHH; the agreement was used in a convenience sample, with all patients admitted or considered at risk for self-harm. Patients were asked to self-rate the following areas with the RN: (a) their current harm level, (b) the likelihood of their acting on their thoughts of self-harm, (c) their thoughts about managing the risk with the RN, (d) their willingness to enter an agreement for safety with the RN, and (e) their thoughts about how long they think they can remain safe.

In the context of this study, RNs were given the Registered Nurses Evaluation Survey, which also was in Likert-type format, except one question. RNs were asked to evaluate (a) the number of times they used the safety agreement in a 3-month period, (b) if the safety agreement assisted them in feeling more comfortable while helping patients at risk for self-harm, (c) if they thought self-harming incidents decreased since implementation of safety agreements, and (d) if they had any other comments to share related to use of safety agreements. With the use of safety agreements, RNs reported improvement in patient responsibility, nurse

contact with patients, guidance for safety concerns, discussions with patients related to safety, and time guidelines around issues of safety. Using Middle Range Theory in Research 16.2 describes the design and outcome of this research study implementing safety agreements at NHH (Potter et al., 2005).

## PAIN AND DISTRESS INSTRUMENT

A study of nursing caregivers (RNs and nursing students) revealed associations between nursing assessments of patient distress according to particular patient and caregiver characteristics (Hall-Lord & Larsson, 2006). The investigators measured patients' pain and distress with a 13-item pain and distress questionnaire to evaluate sensory, emotional, and existential dimensions of distress (see Table 16.3). Caregiver characteristics were assessed using the sense of coherence (SOC) scale, five-factor personality inventory (FFPI), and their degree of experience in nursing. When given the same patient scenarios, Hall-Lord and Larsson (2006) refer to Orlando's assertion that nurses' personality factors contribute to their automatic responses, which is supported in their research. They report that nursing experience and personality factors apparently impacted their assessments and ability to empathize with patients in distress, along with factors of patient age and illness type and severity. Their study supports the need for more reliable pain and distress instruments and improved self-awareness among nurses, to diminish biases and variability in assessments of patient comfort.

## Conclusion

Ida Jean Orlando developed Deliberative Nursing Process theory at a time of great need and growth within the nursing profession, and as demonstrated in the recent examples, her work continues to be relevant to improving patient outcomes and advancing the nursing profession. Soon after Orlando's original publication, Gowan and Morris (1964) speculated that the nursing shortage of that era and the increased expectations upon nurses led to nurses spending more time designing care than providing care. Results from their study indicated that patients experienced undue delays in receiving care and withheld requests that involved their well-being due to patient perceptions that the nurses were too busy, would disapprove, would not like to be interrupted, or would think the request was not helpful to the patient. Might this same scenario be repeating itself today?

In 1990, the National League for Nursing honored Orlando by reprinting *The Dynamic Nurse–Patient Relationship*. Orlando noted in the Preface to that edition that interest in the United States using her theory had waned (Orlando, 1990, p. viii). Interest and use of the theory may have subsided temporarily, but it never ceased. As noted by Orlando herself, her work has been published in five foreign countries, and there have been numerous publications in recent years related to Deliberative Nursing Process (Potter & Bockenhauer, 2000; Potter & Dawson, 2001; Potter & Tinker, 2000; Rosenthal, 1996; Schmieding, 1993b, 1999, 2002). Many changes have occurred in nursing. However, the essence of nursing, described so simply yet eloquently by Orlando, has not changed—namely, that the nurse–patient relationship involves a dynamic and unique process that evolves between nurse and patient when approached deliberatively and validated with the patient on an ongoing basis.

Deliberative Nursing Process is a nursing theory for all times. The use of Deliberative Nursing Process helps nurses maintain a patient-centered approach when providing nursing care amidst additional and varied expectations of the nurse. Orlando has kept the message of Deliberative Nursing Process clear throughout the years: "It is the nurse's direct responsibility to see to it that the patient's needs for help are met, either directly by her own activity or indirectly by calling in the help of others" (Orlando, 1961, p. 29). Adopting such a clear function promotes effective and efficient nursing practice as has been demonstrated through empirical studies on Deliberative Nursing Process for more than 40 years.

## Summary

- The Deliberative Nursing Process was developed by Ida Orlando based upon her observations of many nurse–patient interactions.

- Deliberative Nursing Process is classified as a middle range theory; it is both a simple and complex theory.

- Deliberative Nursing Process (DNP) is relevant for all times, places, and persons and can be applied in education, practice, and research.

- Orlando asserts that it is the nurse's responsibility, directly or indirectly, to see that patient needs are met.

- Nurses should never assume they know what the patient's needs are.

- Nurse–patient interactions are unique for that nurse and patient in that moment in time.

- Deliberative Nursing Process involves nurses using their perceptions, thoughts, and feelings related to the patient's behavior to identify a patient's need for immediate help.

- Nurses need to validate with patients that their needs have been identified and met.

- According to Orlando, automatic nursing process is "bad" or ineffective nursing, and Deliberative Nursing Process is "good" or effective nursing.

### CRITICAL THINKING EXERCISES

1. Scenario: Upon entering a patient's room on the medical unit, the nurse notices the patient's right hand over her heart. The patient has her head down and is sobbing. Give examples of how you, as the nurse, might share each of the following:
   a. Your perceptions
   b. Your thoughts
   c. Your feelings

2. What is the function of "validation" in Deliberative Nursing Process?

(Continued)

3. State three ways that using Deliberative Nursing Process is more beneficial in the nurse–patient relationship than using automatic nursing process.

4. Compare and contrast the concept and definition of comfort in Deliberative Nursing Process with the concept of comfort according to other nursing theorists, such as Kolcaba or Leininger.

5. Discuss if/how Deliberative Nursing Process could benefit nursing practice in an intensive care setting, even if patients were unconscious or unable to communicate verbally.

6. Consider Orlando's distinction between the roles of "nursing" and "doctoring" in patient care. Discuss how the same roles do/do not apply to physicians and nurses today.

7. Do you agree with Orlando's assertion that nursing is either "good" or "bad"? If so, why? If not, how would you define excellence in nursing?

## Acknowledgments

Much appreciation is expressed to Mimi Dye, MSN, ARNP, who completed the critique on Deliberative Nursing Process in the Appendix A and studied Deliberative Nursing Process as a student with the theorist, Ida J. Orlando, MS, RN; Joy L. Potter, who served as research assistant in the second edition; Dorothy Y. Kameoka, MLS, MSW, RN, who sought out materials for the first and second editions; Rebecca E. Andersen, RN, MSN, who served as research assistant in the third edition; and Sarah Ames, RN, MS, who served as research assistant on this fourth edition—thank you and may you enjoy the deep satisfaction nursing offers.

## REFERENCES

Abdoli, S., & Safavi, S. S. (2010). Nursing students' immediate responses to distressed clients based on Orlando's theory. *Iranian Journal of Nursing and Midwifery Research, 15*(4), 178–184.

Alexander, G. L. (2007). The nurse–patient trajectory framework. In K. Kuhn, et al. (Eds.), *MEDINFO 2007.* Amsterdam, The Netherlands: IOS Press.

Allen, D. E., Bockenhauer, B., Egan, C., & Kinnaird, L. S. (2006). Relating outcomes to excellent nursing practice. *Journal of Nursing Administration, 26*(3), 140–147. doi: 10.1097/00005110-200603000-00008

Alligood, M. R. (2002). The nature of knowledge needed for nursing practice. In M. R. Alligood & A. Marriner-Tomey (Eds.), *Nursing theory—Utilization & application* (2nd ed., pp. 3–14). St. Louis, MO: Mosby.

Alligood, M. R., & Choi, E. C. (1998). Evolution of nursing theory development. In A. Marriner Tomey & M. R. Alligood

(Eds.), *Nursing theorists and their work* (4th ed., pp. 55–66). St Louis, MO: Mosby.

Andrews, C. M. (1989). Ida Orlando's model of nursing practice. In J. J. Fitzpatrick & A. L. Whall (Eds.), *Conceptual models of nursing: Analysis & application* (2nd ed., pp. 69–87). Norwalk, CT: Appleton & Lange.

Aponte, J. (2009). Meeting the linguistic needs of urban communities. *Home Healthcare Nurse, 27*(5), 324–329. doi: 10.1097/01.NHH.0000356786.85750.e9

Barrett-Lennard, G. T. (1962). Dimensions of therapist response as casual factors in therapeutic change. *Psychological Monographs: General and Applied, 76*(43), 1–36.

Barron, M. A. (1966). The effects varied nursing approaches have on patients' complaints of pain. *Nursing Research, 15*, 90–91. doi: 10.1097/00006199-196601510-00053

Bezanson, A. (2002). *Theoretical application of Orlando's theory of deliberate nursing process in an outpatient surgery center.* Unpublished manuscript.

Bochnak, M. A. (1963). The effect of an automatic and deliberative process of nursing activity on the relief of patients' pain: A clinical experiment. *Nursing Research, 12*, 191–192.

Bochnak, M. A., Rhymes, J. P., & Leonard, R. C. (1962). The comparison of two types of nursing activity on the relief of pain. *Innovations in nurse–patient relationships: Automatic or reasoned nurse action* (Clinical Paper No. 6). New York, NY: American Nurses Association.

Bolden, L. V., & Larrabee, J. H. (2001). Defining patient-perceived quality of nursing care. *Journal of Nursing Care Quality, 16*, 34–60.

Clausen [Cameron], J. C. (1983). Clinical nursing research on the science and art of breastfeeding using a deliberative nursing care approach. *Western Journal of Nursing Research, 5*, 29.

Crowne, D. P., & Marlowe, D. (1964). *The approval motive.* New York, NY: John Wiley & Sons.

Dracup, K. A., & Breu, C. S. (1978). Using nursing research findings to meet the needs of grieving spouses. *Nursing Research, 27*, 212–216.

Dumas, R. G., & Leonard, R. C. (1963). The effect of nursing on the incidence of postoperative vomiting. *Nursing Research, 12*, 12–15. doi: 10.1097/00006199-196301210-00005

Dye, M. C. (2013). *Assumptions can mislead: Failures in health care and elsewhere.* Bloomington, IN: Trafford Publishing.

Eisler, J., Wolfer, J. A., & Diers, D. (1972). Relationship between need for social approval and postoperative recovery and welfare. *Nursing Research, 21*, 520–525. doi: 10.1097/00006199-197211000-00013

Faust, C. (2002). Orlando's deliberative nursing process theory: A practice application in an extended care facility. *Journal of Gerontological Nursing, 28*(7), 14–18.

Gallop, R., Lancee, W. J., & Garfinkel, P. (1989). How nursing staff respond to the label "borderline personality disorder." *Hospital and Community Psychiatry, 40*(8), 815–819.

Gaudet, C., & Howett, M. (2018). Communication and technology: Ida Orlando's theory applied. *Nursing Science Quarterly, 31*(4), 369–373. doi: 10.1177/0894318418792891

Gerrard, B., & Buzzell, M. (1980). *User's manual for the behavioral test of impersonal skills for health professionals.* Reston, VA: Reston Publishing.

Gowan, N. I., & Morris, M. (1964). Nurses' responses to expressed patient needs. *Nursing Research, 13*, 68–71. doi: 10.1097/00006199-196401310-00023

Haggerty, L. A. (1987). An analysis of senior nursing students' immediate responses to distressed patients. *Journal of Advanced Nursing, 12*, 451–461. doi: 10.1111/j.1365-2648.1987.tb01354.x

Hall-Lord, M. L., & Larsson, B. W. (2006). Registered nurses' and student nurses' assessment of pain and distress related to specific patient and nurse characteristics. *Nurse Education Today, 20*, 377–387. doi: 10.1016/j.nedt.2005.11.007

Johnson, B. M., & Webber, P. B. (2001). *Theory and reasoning in nursing*. New York, NY: Lippincott Williams & Wilkins.

Jonasson, L. (2009). *Ethical values in caring encounters from elderly patients" and next of kin's perspective* (Thesis No. 107). Linköping University Studies in Health Sciences, Linköping, Sweden.

Marriner-Tomey, A. (1998). Introduction to analysis of nursing theories. In A. Marriner-Tomey & M. R. Alligood (Eds.), *Nursing theorists and their work* (4th ed., pp. 3–15). St. Louis, MO: Mosby.

McEwan, M. (2002). Middle-range nursing theories. In M. McEwan & E. M. Wills (Eds.), *Theoretical basis for nursing* (pp. 202–225). Philadelphia, PA: Lippincott Williams & Wilkins.

McNair, D. M., Lorr, M., & Droppleman, L. F. (1971). *Manual for the profile of mood states*. San Diego, CA: Educational and Industrial Testing Services.

Meleis, A. I. (1997). *Theoretical nursing: Development & progress* (3rd ed., pp. 343–353). Philadelphia, PA: Lippincott-Raven.

Mertz, H. (1963). A study of the process of the nurse's activity as it affects the blood pressure readings and pulse rate of patients admitted to the emergency room. *Nursing Research, 12*, 197–198.

Olson, J. K. (1995). Relationships between nurse expressed empathy, patient perceived empathy, and patient distress. *Image: Journal of Nursing Scholarship, 27*, 323–328. doi: 10.1111/j.1547-5069.1995.tb00895.x

Olson, J., & Hanchett, E. (1997). Nurse-expressed empathy, patient outcomes, and development of a middle-range theory. *Image: The Journal of Nursing Scholarship, 29*, 71–76. doi: 10.1111/j.1547-5069.1997.tb01143.x

Orlando, I. J. (1961). *The dynamic nurse patient relationship*. New York, NY: Putnam.

Orlando, I. J. (1972). *The discipline and teaching of nursing process: An evaluative study*. New York, NY: Putnam.

Orlando, I. J. (1976, August). The fundamental issue in professional nursing. Paper presented at the University of Tulsa College of Nursing, Tulsa, OK.

Orlando [Pelletier], I. J. (1983, October). Comments on ANA's social policy statement of 1980. Paper presented at Southeastern Massachusetts University, College of Nursing, Honor Society, South Dartmouth, MA.

Orlando, I. J. (1987). Nursing in the 21st century: Alternate paths. *Journal of Advanced Nursing, 12*, 405–412. doi: 10.1111/j.1365-2648.1987.tb01349.x

Orlando, I. J. (1990, reissue). *The dynamic nurse–patient relationship*. New York, NY: National League for Nursing.

Orlando, I. J., & Dugan, A. B. (1989). Independent and dependent paths: The fundamental issue for the nursing profession. *Nursing and Health Care, 10*, 77–80.

Pelletier, I. O. (1967). The patient's predicament and nursing function. *Psychiatric Opinion, 4*, 25–30.

Pelletier, I. O. (1976). *The fundamental issue in professional nursing* (pp. 1–22). Unpublished manuscript.

Potter, M. L., & Bockenhauer, B. J. (2000). Implementing Orlando's nursing theory: A pilot study. *Journal of Psychosocial Nursing and Mental Health Services, 38*, 14–21.

Potter, M. L., & Dawson, A. M. (2001). From safety contract to safety agreement. *Journal of Psychosocial Nursing and Mental Health Services, 39*, 38–45.

Potter, M. L., & Moller, M. D. (2016). *Psychiatric-mental health nursing: From suffering to hope*. Boston, MA: Pearson Education, Inc.

Potter, M. L., & Tinker, S. W. (2000). Put power in nurses' hands: Orlando's nursing theory supports nurses—Simply. *Nursing Management, 31*, 40–41.

Potter, M. L., Vitale-Nolen, R., & Dawson, A. M. (2005). Implementation of safety agreements in an acute psychiatric facility. *Journal of the American Psychiatric Nurses Association, 11*(3), 144–155. doi: 10.1177/1078390305277443

Potter, M. L., Williams, R. B., & Costanzo, R. (2004). Using nursing theory and a structured psychoeducational curriculum with inpatient groups. *Journal of the American Psychiatric Nurses Association, 10*(3), 122–128. doi: 10.1177/1078390304265212

Reid-Ponte, P. (1988). *The relationship among empathy and the use of Orlando's deliberative process by the primary nurse and the distress of the adult cancer patient* (Doctoral dissertation). Boston University, Boston, MA.

Rosenthal, B. C. (1996). An interactionist's approach to perioperative nursing. *AORN Journal, 64*, 254–260.

Schmieding, N. J. (1984). Putting Orlando's theory into practice. *American Journal of Nursing, 84*, 759–761. doi: 10.2307/3463720

Schmieding, N. J. (1992). Relationship between head nurse responses to staff nurses and staff nurse response to patients. *Western Journal of Nursing Research, 13*, 746–760. doi: 10.1177/019394599101300606

Schmieding, N. J. (1993a). *Ida Jean Orlando: A nursing process theory*. London, UK: Sage.

Schmieding, N. J. (1993b). Successful superior–subordinate relationships require mutual management. *The Health Care Supervisor, 11*, 52–63.

Schmieding, N. J. (1999). Reflective inquiry framework for nurse administrators. *Journal of Advanced Nursing, 30*, 631–639. doi: 10.1046/j.1365-2648.1999.01134.x

Schmieding, N. J. (2002). Orlando's nursing process theory. In M. R. Alligood & A. Marriner Tomey (Eds.), *Nursing theory utilization & application* (2nd ed., pp. 315–337). St. Louis, MO: Mosby.

Sheldon, L. K., & Ellington, L. (2008). Application of a model of social information processing to nursing theory: How nurses respond to patients. *Journal of Advanced Nursing, 64*(4), 344–398. doi: 10.1111/j.1365-2648.2008.04795.x

Silva, M. C. (1979). Effects of orientation information on spouses' anxieties and attitudes toward hospitalization and surgery. *Research in Nursing and Health, 2*, 127–136. doi: 10.1002/nur.4770020308

Spielberger, C. D., Gorsuch, R. L., & Lushene, R. E. (1970). *Manual for the state-trait anxiety inventory*. Palo Alto, CA: Consulting Psychologists Press.

Stevens-Barnum, B. J. (1990). *Nursing theory: Analysis, application, evaluation*. Glenview, IL: Scott Foresman/Little & Brown.

Tutton, E., & Seers, K. (2003). The concept of comfort. *Journal of Clinical Nursing, 12*, 689–696. doi: 10.1046/j.1365-2702.2003.00775.x

Tyra, P. A. (2008). In memoriam: Ida Jean Orlando Pelletier. *Journal of the American Psychiatric Nurses Association, 14*, 231–232. doi: 10.1177/1078390308321092

Walker, L. O., & Avant, K. C. (1995). *Strategies for theory construction in nursing* (3rd ed.). Norwalk, CT: Appleton & Lange.

Wills, E. M. (2002). Overview of grand nursing theories. In M. McEwan & E. M. Wills (Eds.), *Theoretical basis for nursing* (pp. 111–124). Philadelphia, PA: Lippincott Wilkins & Williams.

Wooldridge, P. J., Skipper, J. K. Jr, & Leonard, R. C. (1968). *Behavioral science, social practice, and the nursing profession*. Cleveland, OH: Case Western Reserve University.

Yekefallah, L., Ashktorab, T., Ghorbani, A., Pazokian, M., Azimian, J., & Samimi, R. (2017). Orlando's nursing process application on anxiety levels of patients undergoing endoscopy examination. *International Journal of Epidemiologic Research, 4*(1): 53–60.

Zuckerman, M., & Lubin, B. (1965). *Manual for the multiple affect adjective check list*. San Diego, CA: Educational and Industrial Testing Service.

## BIBLIOGRAPHY

Abraham, S. (2011). Fall prevention conceptual frame-work. *Health Care Manager*, *30*(2), 179–184. doi: 10.1097/HCM.0b013e318216fb74

Cameron, J. (1963). An exploratory study of the verbal responses of the nurse–patient interactions. *Nursing Research*, *12*, 192.

Chapman, J. S. (1969). *Effects of different nursing approaches upon psychological and physiological responses of patients* (Unpublished doctoral dissertation). Case Western Reserve University, Frances Payne Bolton School of Nursing, Cleveland, OH.

Dufault, M., Duquette, C. E., Ehmann, J., Hehl, R., Lavin, M., Martin, V., …, Willey, C. (2010). Translating an evidence-based protocol for nurse-to-nurse shift handoffs. *Worldviews on Evidence-Based Nursing*, *7*(2), 59–75.

Dumas, R. G., & Johnson [Anderson], B. A. (1972). Research in nursing practice: A review of five clinical experiments. *International Journal of Nursing Studies*, *9*, 137–149. doi: 10.1016/0020-7489(72)90040-5

Dye, M. C. (1963a). Clarifying patients' communication. *The American Journal of Nursing*, *63*, 56–59. doi: 10.2307/3452729

Dye, M. C. (1963b). A descriptive study of conditions conducive to an effective process of nursing activity. *Nursing Research*, *12*, 194.

Edwards, A. L. (1959). *Edwards personal preference schedule: Manual*. New York, NY: Psychological Corporation.

Elms, R. R., & Leonard, R. C. (1966). Effects of nursing approaches during admission. *Nursing Research*, *15*, 39–48.

Farrell, G. A. (1991). How accurately do nurses perceive patients' needs? A comparison of general and psychiatric settings. *Journal of Advanced Nursing*, *16*, 1062–1070. doi: 10.1111/j.1365-2648.1991.tb03367.x

Faulkner, S. A. (1963). A descriptive study of needs communicated to the nurse by some mothers on a postpartum service. *Nursing Research*, *4*, 260. doi: 10.1097/00006199-196301240-00037

Fawcett, J., & Garity, J. (2009). Evaluation of middle-range theories. In J. Fawcett & J. Garity (Eds.), *Evaluating research for evidence-based nursing practice* (pp. 73–88). Philadelphia, PA: F.A. Davis.

Forchuck, C. (1991). A comparison of the works of Peplau and Orlando. *Archives of Psychiatric Nursing*, *5*, 38–45. doi: 10.1016/0883-9417(91)90008-S

Gillis, S. L. (1976). Sleeplessness: Can you help? *The Canadian Nurse*, *72*, 32–34.

Hampe, S. O. (1975). Needs of grieving spouses in a hospital etting. *Nursing Research*, *24*, 113. doi: 10.1097/00006199-197503000-00009

Kokuyama, T., & Schmieding, N. J. (1995). Responses staff nurses prefer compared with their perception of head nurse responses. *Japanese Journal of Nursing Administration*, *5*, 33–38.

Laurent, C. L. (1999). A nursing theory for nursing leadership. *Journal of Nursing Management*, *8*, 83–87. doi: 10.1046/j.1365-2834.2000.00161.x

Mahaffy, P. P. (1965). The effects of hospitalization on children admitted for tonsillectomy and adenoidectomy. *Nursing Research*, *14*, 12–19. doi: 10.1097/00006199-196501410-00005

Methven, D., & Schlotfeldt, R. M. (1962). The social interaction inventory. *Nursing Research*, *11*, 83–88.

Nelson, B. (1978). A practical application of nursing theory. *Nursing Clinics of North America*, *13*, 157–169.

Peitchinis, J. A. (1972). Therapeutic effectiveness of counseling by nursing personnel. *Nursing Research*, *21*, 138–148.

Pride, L. F. (1968). An adrenal stress index as a criterion measure of nursing. *Nursing Research*, *17*, 292–303. doi: 10.1097/00006199-196807000-00002

Rittman, M. R. (2001). Ida Jean Orlando (Pelletier): The dynamic nurse–patient relationship. In M. E. Parker (Ed.), *Nursing theories and nursing practice* (pp. 125–130). Philadelphia, PA: Davis.

Schmieding, N. J. (1987a). Analyzing managerial responses in face-to-face contacts. *Journal of Advanced Nursing*, *12*, 357–365. doi: 10.1111/j.1365-2648.1987.tb01342.x

Schmieding, N. J. (1987b). Face-to-face contacts: Exploring their meaning. *Nursing Management*, *12*, 82–86.

Schmieding, N. J. (1987c). Problematic situations in nursing: Analysis of Orlando's theory based on Dewey's theory of inquiry. *Journal of Advanced Nursing*, *12*, 431–440. doi: 10.1111/j.1365-2648.1987.tb01352.x

Schmieding, N. J. (1988). Action process of nurse administrators to problematic situations based on Orlando's theory. *Journal of Advanced Nursing*, *13*, 99–107. doi: 10.1111/j.1365-2648.1988.tb01396.x

Schmieding, N. J. (1990a). A model for assessing nurse administrator's actions. *Western Journal of Nursing Research*, *12*, 293–306. doi: 10.1177/019394599001200303

Schmieding, N. J. (1990b). Do head nurses include staff nurses in problem solving? *Nursing Management*, *21*, 58–60. doi: 10.1097/00006247-199003000-00016

Schmieding, N. J. (2006). Ida Jean Orlando (Pelletier): Nursing process theory. In A. M. Tomey & M. R. Alligood (Eds.), *Nursing theorists and their work* (6th ed., pp. 431–451). St. Louis, MO: Mosby.

Sitzman, K., & Eichelberger, L. W. (2004). *Understanding the work of nurse theorists: A creative beginning*. Sudbury, MA: Jones & Bartlett.

Tarasuk [Bochnak], M. B., Rhymes, J., & Leonard, R. C. (1965). An experimental test of the importance of communication skills for effective nursing. In J. K. Skipper Jr & R. C. Leonard (Eds.), *Social interaction and patient care* (pp. 110–120). Philadelphia, PA: Lippincott Williams & Wilkins.

Tryon, P. A. (1966). Use of comfort measures as support during labor. *Nursing Research*, *15*, 109–118. doi: 10.1097/00006199-196601520-00003

Tryon, P. A., & Leonard, R. C. (1964). The effect of patients' participation on the outcome of a nursing procedure. *Nursing Forum*, *3*, 79–89. doi: 10.1111/j.1744-6198.1964.tb00273.x

Vanda Hey, S. A. (2009). *The routine screening practices of nurse practitioners for autism in children* (Unpublished master's thesis). University of Wisconsin, Oshkosh, WI.

Williamson, Y. M. (1978). Methodologic dilemmas in tapping the concept of patient needs. *Nursing Research*, *27*, 172–177. doi: 10.1097/00006199-197805000-00023

# 17 Resilience

Joan E. Haase and Celeste R. Phillips

## Definition of Key Terms

| | |
|---|---|
| **Boundaries of resilience** | The contextual influences, dimensions, and assumptions that are considered in determining the attributes of resilience |
| **Meaning-based models** | Explanatory models focused on the patterns and experiences of illness from a subjective and holistic perspective |
| **Mixed-methods research** | Use of a combination of quantitative and qualitative research approaches either sequentially or simultaneously to answer research questions and to refine, evaluate, and/or extend theory |
| **Person-focused resilience research** | Research to identify the patterns of variables in which resilience naturally occurs in individuals and then examining what might contribute to these outcomes, or using cutoff scores on selected variables to categorize adversity subgroups and then examining outcomes in these groups |
| **Positive health research** | Efforts to gain understanding of ways individuals sustain or regain optimal health |
| **Protective factors** | The individual, family, social, or other contextual factors that enhance resilience processes and outcomes |
| **Quality of life** | A sense of well-being |
| **Resilience** | General definition: positive adjustment in the face of adversity. Illness context definition: the degree to which individuals identify, develop, and/or engage protective resources to flexibly manage illness-related stressors in order to achieve the outcomes of resilience resolution, self-transcendence, and sense of well-being |
| **Risk factors** | The individual, family, social, or other contextual factors that impede development of resilience processes and outcomes |
| **Strengths-based research** | Research that focuses on positive health concepts (e.g., hope, optimism, resilience, spirituality) rather than on risks within the individual, family, or community |
| **Variable-focused approaches** | Use of multivariate statistics to test for linkages to resilience among measures of adversity, outcomes, and environmental or individual qualities that may protect from, or compensate for, negative consequences |

Researchers have long sought answers to questions about the psychosocial impact of illness, especially chronic conditions. Much of this research was guided by pathology and deficit-based models that examined risks, adjustment problems, and developmental delays (Hymovich & Roehnert, 1989). In the 1970s, researchers in nursing and other disciplines began to recognize the importance of understanding why some individuals do well in the face of adversity (Antonovsky, 1979; Masten, 2007). Theories of resilience (Rutter, 1979, 1987), hardiness (Kobasa, 1982), self-efficacy, and learned resourcefulness (Bandura, 1977; Rosenbaum, 1983) were developed to explain positive adjustment to illness, based on the belief that such theories may yield information about effective interventions (Forsyth, Delaney, & Gresham, 1984; Garmezy, 1991; Kadner, 1989; Sinnema, 1991). In 2001, the Committee on Future Direction for Behavioral and Social Sciences highlighted the significance of behavioral and psychosocial processes in disease etiology, well-being, and health promotion (Singer & Ryff, 2001). The committee identified resilience as a research priority for the National Institutes of

Health and recommended increased study of the protective factors that are correlates of resilience. These factors included optimism, meaning and purpose, social and emotional support, and related neurobiological mechanisms that promote recovery and increased survival rates (Singer & Ryff, 2001). The rapidly increasing number of theory and research reports in the literature indicates strong uptake of the recommendations. Nurses recognize the importance of positive health concepts and are increasingly seeking understanding of resilience as a potentially useful way to (a) guide development of interventions to enhance positive outcomes; (b) improve outcomes for at-risk populations; (c) prevent poor outcomes; (d) influence public policy related to individuals, families, and communities; and (e) prevent nurse burnout.

## Historical Background and Current Perspectives

Historically, resilience was consistently and broadly defined as a phenomenon of positive adjustment in the face of adversity. Resilience was first studied in children and adolescents and was characterized by attributes usually identified as positive in the presence of adversity. After describing children who thrived despite adversity, subsequent studies were directed to understanding attributes to explain individual differences in response to adversity. Examples of such individual protective factors found in early research on resilience include the following:

- Competence (Garmezy, Masten, & Tellegen, 1984; Rutter, 1979)
- Self-esteem (Garmezy, 1981)
- Superior coping (Garmezy, 1991; Murphy & Moriarty, 1976)
- Advanced self-help, communication, and problem-solving skills (Garmezy, 1981; Hauser, Vieyra, Jacobson, & Wertlieb, 1985)
- Tendency to perceive experiences constructively (Werner & Smith, 1982)
- Ability to use spirituality to maintain a positive vision of a meaningful life (Rutter, 1979; Wells & Schwebel, 1987)

Resilience researchers gradually began to recognize family and social protective factors as influencing resilience development (Rutter, 1987). This expanded view of protective factors, studied as processes occurring over time, included research on childhood exposure to adverse conditions of socioeconomic adversity (Rutter, 1979), abuse (Henry, 2001), urban poverty and community

violence (Luthar, Cicchetti, & Becker, 2000), and chronic illness (Wells & Schwebel, 1987). In addition to continuing to describe protective factors, researchers sought to understand the underlying mechanisms or processes of interaction between risk and protective factors and their influence on resilience outcomes (Luthar et al., 2000).

Since 2000, when researchers increasingly viewed resilience from a multilevel—society to cell— perspective and when multidimensional analysis strategies (e.g., latent variable structural equation modeling) improved, research on resilience gained much attention and significantly advanced the understanding of resilience (Cicchetti, 2011; Cicchetti & Blender, 2006; Masten, 2007). The recognition that resilience occurs at multiple levels fostered interdisciplinary research to simultaneously examine psychological, biological, and environmental–contextual processes (Cicchetti & Blender, 2006). Theoretical models were also developed and tested (Mullins et al., 2015).

## Definition of Resilience and Concepts

There is now widespread agreement that resilience is a complex, multidimensional construct. Largely because of the complexity of the construct, there is a lack of consensus regarding (a) terminology, (b) characteristics, and (c) boundaries of resilience. The following sections examine the various perspectives within these three areas from both the general and the nursing literature.

### PERSPECTIVES ON RESILIENCE

#### Terminology and Attributes of Resilience

To adequately define a construct, terminology needs to be consistently used. In the case of resilience, even the labels for the construct are inconsistently used (e.g., resilience, resiliency, and ego-resilience). The term *resilience*, rather than *resiliency*, is favored to describe positive adjustment in the face of adversity (Luthar et al., 2000). "Resiliency" is not recommended because the word implies a personality trait that is difficult to alter, much like hardiness. The term *ego-resilience* characterizes resilience as a distinct personality trait. Hence, ego-resilience decreases the options for intervention and increases the danger of labeling individuals as innately "inadequate."

There are two generally recognized essential attributes of resilience present in most definitions.

These are the presence of (a) "good" or positive adaptation that (b) occurs in spite of the adversity associated with adjustment difficulties (Fletcher & Sarkar, 2013).

**Good Outcomes.** "Good" or positive outcomes are not consistently theoretically or operationally defined in the literature. Debate centers on what constitutes "good" outcomes and who decides. Additional questions include whether external criteria (e.g., academic achievement), intrapersonal characteristics (e.g., sense of well-being, self-esteem), or a combination of both is a defining characteristic of positive outcomes (Masten, 2001).

Paradigmatic approaches also contributed to differences in ways positive outcomes are defined. A pathology-based worldview often defines positive outcomes as the absence of psychopathology or low levels of symptoms or impairments (Masten & Coatsworth, 1998). Developmental and life span perspectives usually define positive outcomes as those that meet or exceed expectations. The emerging perspective emphasizes dynamic ecosystems influenced by complex, ever-changing, and interacting forces (Richardson, 2002; Waller, 2001) and by the notion that resilience is possibly a common human characteristic—"ordinary magic" (Masten, 2001).

**Adverse Conditions.** The theoretical and operational definitions of "adverse conditions" are also inconsistent in the literature. Frequently, definitions imply threats or risk factors that occur in contexts such as war, illness, community deficits, or family adversity. Beyond the requirement that such factors negatively affect resilience outcomes, there is no agreement regarding how such risks should be operationalized. Options include (a) current or past occurrence, (b) predictors of poor outcomes or status (moderating) variables such as low socioeconomic status, or (c) single-exposure variables or cumulative combinations of factors. Adding to the inconsistency of defining characteristics, risk factors can be continuous bipolar variables classified as either less or more aversive (e.g., mild to severe symptoms) or as negative to positive assets (e.g., low to high economic status and negative to positive coping) (Masten, 2001). In general, much research indicates that risk factors, however operationalized, often co-occur (Masten, 2001). Adding to the confusion, the term adversity is value-laden and implies events that are exclusively negative when, indeed, there are also positive events that may have potentially poor outcomes, such as job promotion or marriage (Fletcher & Sarkar, 2013).

## Boundaries of Resilience

Boundaries are the contextual influences (i.e., conditions under which resilience exists/varies/disappears), dimensions (e.g., objective/subjective and physiological/psychological), and underlying assumptions (e.g., growth versus stability and state versus trait) that are considered in determining the attributes of resilience. Some boundaries of resilience that need careful explication in theory and research include (a) state/trait/process/outcome, (b) psychological/physiological, (c) individual/aggregate, and (d) objective/subjective perspective. Within each of these boundaries, the cross-cultural implications also need thoughtful examination and further research. Resilience may also vary in relation to contextual severity, ranging from everyday hassles to extensively stressful experiences (e.g., loss of a child) (Fletcher & Sarkar, 2013).

**Trait/State/Process/Outcome.** Although the definition of resilience as the presence of "good" outcomes that occur in the face of adverse conditions implies a process, there is no consensus on the issue of whether resilience is a trait, state, process, or outcome. Again, the confusion is exacerbated by inconsistent terminology and the inability to draw conclusions of causality (Pettit, 2000). For example, as indicated above, the term *ego-resiliency* is frequently used interchangeably with resilience, but the former refers to a set of personal characteristics (traits) that may or may not be specifically linked to adversity (Luthar et al., 2000). In addition, terms such as *resilient children* cause confusion. Although this term implies that resilience is a trait, it is used most often in conjunction with the two coexisting conditions of adversity and positive adaptation, with adaptation usually conceptualized as a process. When researchers do not clearly specify a model of resilience that stipulates how the underlying mechanisms in a resilience process may result in specific resilience outcomes, even terms such as *outcome* and *process* contribute to the confusion. Researchers should clearly specify the context in which resilience outcomes apply and delineate the outcomes by using terms such as *emotional resilience*, *behavioral resilience*, or *educational resilience*. It would also be helpful, through staged model specification, to distinguish proximal resilience outcomes, such as self-transcendence and confidence/mastery, from more distal outcomes, such as sense of well-being or quality of life, which results from the resilience process and resilience outcomes.

**Psychological/Physiological.** Psychological concepts associated with resilience are more widely studied than physiological concepts. Concepts such as self-esteem, self-perception, personality, temperament, intellect, coping, and problem-solving skills are just a few of the psychological concepts that have been studied as correlates of resilience. With advances in statistical modeling and computer science, it is now possible to examine resilience on multiple levels, such as gene–environment interactions (Masten, 2007). Singer and Ryff (2001) identified several positive physiological mechanisms, including those that involve the hypothalamic–pituitary–adrenal (HPA) axis and the autonomic nervous system, which may be linked to positive health and resilience. They further argue for integrative levels of analysis that include the physiological, behavioral, environmental, and psychosocial systems to better understand how each contributes individually and interactively to resilience. Curtis and Cicchetti (2003) provided a thoughtful perspective of the theoretical and methodological considerations for examining the biological contributors to resilience. Specifically, they discuss a transactional organizational theoretical perspective as a framework for including biological considerations. The recent advances in neurosciences and related technology, such as functional magnetic resonance imaging (fMRI), are highly promising avenues of investigation.

**Individual/Aggregate.** Resilience is most often studied in individuals, but to avoid confusion about yet another boundary, it is important for researchers to specify levels of analysis. For example, Haase's Resilience in Illness Model (RIM) identifies family environment as a protective factor (composed of family, adaptability, cohesion, communication, and perceived strengths) that influences the individual child, adolescent, and young adult resilience outcomes (Haase et al., 2014). Other models of resilience for children with chronic illness characterize the child and family's adjustment as a transactional process occurring over time (Mullins et al., 2015). The social ecological model (Kazak, 2006; Kazak, Segal-Andrews, & Johnson, 1995) is one example that identifies many systems—child, family, social group, school, community, and culture—all interacting to influence the child and family outcomes. In nursing, the Children's Oncology Group adapted Haase's RIM as the guiding framework for research proposed by the Nursing Discipline Committee; they expanded it to include family and culture, as well as the individual and family ages, development levels, and genetic characteristics (Kelly, Hooke, Ruccione, Landier, & Haase, 2014).

**Objective/Subjective.** The issue of which perspective—objective or subjective—to value is another area of inconsistency. For example, in a qualitative study of homeless adolescents, the sample included adolescents who considered themselves resilient (Hunter & Chandler, 1999). According to the adolescents, being resilient was "surviving." The self-assigned attribute of resilience by the adolescents is quite different from the characteristics of resilience found in other literature. Hunter and Chandler's research indicated that resilience in homeless adolescents may be a "process of defense using such tactics as insulation, isolation, disconnecting, denial, and aggression or a process of survival by using responses such as violence" (p. 246). These findings indicate that self-attributed resilience in homeless adolescents lacks a positive or good outcome, a key characteristic of resilience in the literature. These findings were further supported in a subsequent study by Hunter (2001) that examined cross-cultural perspectives of resilience in adolescents from New England and Ghana, wherein all the adolescents viewed themselves as resilient, regardless of age, gender, culture, or socioeconomic status. Yet, depending on the presence or absence of consistent, loving, caring, and mentoring adults, there were qualitative differences in how the adolescents overcame adversities. Hunter classified these as two different "forms of resilience:" self-protective survival resilience or connected resilience.

Hunter and Chandler's findings illustrate how, if the objective and subjective dimensions of resilience are not carefully delineated, much of what determines the process and outcomes of resilience will be difficult to ascertain. For example, the cognitive appraisal of the adversity, the actions that are taken to deal with the adversity, and subsequent evaluation of how one dealt with the adversity can all influence how resilience as a process proceeds (Fine, 1991). Further, if the objective and subjective appraisal, actions, and evaluation differ, then evaluation of outcomes and development of interventions will be more complex.

One potentially helpful way to delineate the objective/subjective dimensions of resilience is to consider whether resilience may be interpersonally assigned to an individual, much like courage is interpersonally assigned (Haase, 1987). Research indicates that individuals usually do not attribute courage to themselves, unless someone else initially indicates that their behavior could be interpreted as courageous (Haase, 1987). Likewise, it is possible that individuals require time to reflect on the meaning of their actions before seeing themselves as resilient. That is, resilience may occur through a process that includes deriving meaning from the experience through interaction with others (Haase, Heiney, Ruccione, & Stutzer, 1999). After interviews were conducted, Hunter and Chandler's findings supported this perspective in that the adolescents' resilience scores increased from baseline measures (Hunter, 2001). A second consideration regarding the subjective perspective is the social desirability of being labeled "resilient." It is possible that a label of being resilient parallels a label such as "honest" in that, when asked, one is not likely to readily deny having such a characteristic.

**Cross-Cultural Considerations Related to Boundaries.** In the midst of adversity, individuals are especially likely to return to cultural tradition to seek solutions (Hwang, 2006, p. 90). Hence, a full understanding of resilience needs to include cultural considerations. Few studies have explicitly examined the cultural boundaries of resilience, and resilience models need to be carefully evaluated cross-culturally prior to use. Following are two examples of potential differences in factors influencing resilience between Eastern and Western culture.

In Western society, interpersonal interactions have an assumption of respect for the principles of egalitarianism and independence (Triandis, Bontempo, Villareal, Asai, & Lucca, 1988). Thus, interpersonal relationships are based on a decisional choice. In Chinese culture, interpersonal relationships are composed of horizontal and vertical relationships. Horizontal relationships are constructed according to intimacy/distance, and vertical relationships are built according to superiority/inferiority (Hwang, 1997). Horizontal relationship indicates interaction within equal family or social positions, such as sibling or peer relationships. Vertical relationship means interaction among hierarchal family or social positions, such as child–parent or student–teacher relationships. The vertical relationship is less emphasized in Western society.

Since sense of self is also culturally different in Western and Chinese societies, how sense of self and interpersonal relationships work to foster resilience is also likely to be different. In Western society, the presentation of self is based on one's interpretation of interactions in specific social situations (Charon, 1998; Mead, 1952). In contrast, in Chinese society, the self is defined not by any situational interpretation but by person-in-relation status, which is called the "relational self" (Ho, Chen, & Chiu, 1991). In Chinese society, based on relational self, personal coping strategies, purpose in life, and interpersonal interactions may be more driven by status concerns in social relationships compared to Western cultures.

In a comparison of Haase's RIM with qualitative findings from interviews with Taiwanese adolescent survivors of brain cancer, data indicated that fatalistic coping, a risk factor component of defensive coping in Haase's RIM (i.e., avoidant, fatalistic), may have a positive influence on survivorship in Taiwan (Chen, Chen, & Haase, 2007; Chen, Chen, & Wong, 2014). The adolescents used fatalistic coping, accepting that there was nothing one could do but accept the cancer experiences based on tenets of one's sense of relational self, wherein individuals have greater obligations to family, including those who have died, than to "small self" (personal self). In a quantitative study with the same population, findings indicate that adolescent survivors of brain cancer have greater problems than do well adolescents. In the Chinese culture, family or community protective factors may have greater influence as pathways to resilience, and individual protective factors, such as positive coping, may require alignment with family goals to actually serve a protective function. Clearly, a full understanding of resilience needs to include cultural considerations.

## RESILIENCE PERSPECTIVES IN NURSING

Not surprisingly, information in Table 17.1 indicates the nursing literature on resilience parallels that of the general literature in that there is no greater consensus on definitions, characteristics, or boundaries of resilience in the nursing literature. Although nurses historically focused more extensively on individual and family strengths than many disciplines, systematic study of resilience by nurses only began in the mid to late 1980s. A major contribution to understanding resilience from the nursing literature is the focus on resilience in the context of health, as well as a more recent focus on understanding resilience in nurses. Articles included in Table 17.1 provide a representative sample of both theoretical and empirical efforts to understand resilience by nurses, including varied populations and approaches to knowledge development.

### Terminology and Attributes of Resilience

Most definitions in Table 17.1 include the characteristic of adversity. Some definitions specifically describe the adversity as stress, loss, or illness, whereas others use more global terms, such as "challenging life condition" (Drummond, Kysela, McDonald, & Query, 2002) or a "traumatic event" (Garcia-Dia et al., 2013). The "good" varies considerably in the definitions as well. Although several of the definitions use vague terminology, such as "maintenance of positive adjustment" (Drummond et al., 2002) or "spring back" (Mandleco & Peery, 2000), other definitions indicate the "good" is reflected in processes of adaptation, positive health, and/or

**Table 17.1    Nursing Literature on Resilience**

| Source | Methods of Knowledge Development | Populations Studied | Definition of Resilience | Primary Boundaries | Components: Antecedents/ Exogenous Variables | Components: Attributes/ Processes | Components: Outcomes | Key Relational Statements/ Findings |
|---|---|---|---|---|---|---|---|---|
| Bekhet, Johnson, and Zauszniewski (2012) | Review of literature | Family members of a person with autism spectrum disorder (ASD) | (Borrowed) Dynamic process encompassing positive adaption within the context of significant adversity | Individual process determined by balancing risk and protective factors in the face of adversity | *Risk factors:* Symptom severity, marital quality, parents' anger, and number of children with ASD  *Protective factors:* Social support, age of the child, time since diagnosis, locus of control, cognitive appraisal, religious beliefs/spirituality | Self-efficacy Acceptance Sense of coherence Optimism Positive family functioning Enrichment | Positive mental health Better marital quality Greater psychological well-being Greater life satisfaction | Parents of children with ASD who possess indicators of resilience are better able to manage the adversity associated with caring for children with ASD |
| Garcia-Dia, DiNapoli, Garcia-Ona, Jakubowski, and O'Flaherty (2013) | Concept analysis | HIV/AIDS | One's ability of bounce back or recover from adversity | A dynamic process that can be influenced by the environmental, the external, and/or the individual and the outcome | Presence of an adverse/traumatic event  Event interpreted as being physically and/ or psychologically traumatic  Response—development of protective factors or maladaptive practices | Rebounding Determination Social support Self-efficacy | Integration Effective coping | Individuals have personality traits, protective factors, and experiences accumulated through life that precipitates resilience to surface from within as a process and/ or develops as an outcome. Protective factors can be either internal or external, which can either predispose to "protect" or place individuals "at risk," leading to resilience or maladaptation |

| | | | | | | | |
|---|---|---|---|---|---|---|---|
| Grafton, Gillespie, and Henders (2010) | Review of literature | Nurses | Dynamic process used by individuals to access resources to cope with and recover from adversity; and, therefore, can be learned and taught | Dynamic process and an innate energy or life force (i.e., internal resources used to cope and learn from experience in order to positively transform) | Adverse or stressful event(s) | Self-awareness; Self-efficacy; Confidence; Sense of purpose and meaning | Positive adaptation; Cognitive transformation (i.e., effective coping, strengthen biopsychosocial spiritual well-being of self and personal growth) | Conceptualization of resilience as an innate resource increases understanding that is a valuable stress management resource and is potentially available to every individual |
| Haase (2004); Haase et al. (1999, 2014, 2017) | Triangulation using qualitative model and instrument generation, quantitative exploratory and confirmatory model-evaluating studies | Adolescents/ young adults with chronic illness, primarily cancer | Process of identifying or developing resources and strengths to manage stressors flexibly and gain a positive outcome (i.e., a sense of confidence or mastery, self-transcendence, and self-esteem) | Individual psychosocial process, resulting in specific outcomes | Integration: connectedness with friends, community, and health care providers; Family protective: family atmosphere; Family support/ resources; Illness-related risk: illness perspective; Illness-related distress | Individual risk: defensive coping (sustained over time); Individual protective: derived meaning; Courageous coping | Resilience resolution, self-transcendence, confidence/ mastery; Quality of life/ well-being | Illness-related risk and social and family protective factors directly affect individual risk and protective factors. All these factors directly or indirectly affect outcomes |
| Hart, Brannan, and De Chesney (2014) | Integrative review | Nurses | (Borrowed) Ability to bounce back or to cope successfully despite adverse circumstances | | Challenging workplaces; Psychological emptiness; Diminishing inner balance; Sense of dissonance | Hope; Self-efficacy; Coping; Competence; Control; Flexibility; Adaptability | Increased quality of life; Better health; Effective use of adaptive coping strategies | Individuals can strengthen their resilience by participating in cognitive reframing practices and developing connections with others |

*(Continued)*

**Table 17.1    Nursing Literature on Resilience (Continued)**

| Source | Methods of Knowledge Development | Populations Studied | Definition of Resilience | Primary Boundaries | Components: Antecedents/ Exogenous Variables | Components: Attributes/ Processes | Components: Outcomes | Key Relational Statements/ Findings |
|---|---|---|---|---|---|---|---|---|
| van Kessel (2013) | Review of literature | Older adults | Ability to bounce back and recover physical and psychological health in the face of adversity | Dynamic process | Adversity related to ongoing life experiences rather than specific event (i.e., being old, suffering poor health, or process of dying) | Internal factors: Self-efficacy Spirituality Hope Meaning and purpose Acceptance External factors: social support Connectedness | Maintenance of normal development or functioning or better than expected functioning, given exposure to the specific adversity | Older people who have a sense of their own abilities, in particular, exhibit the ability to manage their emotions, solve problems, draw on spirituality, accept their circumstances, look to the future, or care for others are more likely to demonstrate resilience |
| Windle (2011) | Synthesis of methodological approaches: concept analysis, literature review using systematic principles, and stakeholder consultation | Not limited | Process of effectively negotiating, adapting to, or managing significant sources of stress or trauma (p. 152) | Individual psychosocial processes influenced by family, community, and political factors | Biological, psychological, economic, or social stressors. Not if a majority of people would experience no adaptive response, leading to negative consequence | Protective factors: (a) individual (e.g., psychological, neurobiological), (b) social (e.g., family cohesion, parental support), (c) community/society (e.g., political capital, institutional, and community factors). Competence seen as essential component (p. 157) | | Resilience experience varies throughout the life span, with different vulnerabilities and strengths emerging from changing life events |

| | | | | | | | | |
|---|---|---|---|---|---|---|---|---|
| Delgado, Upton, Ranse, Furness, and Foster (2017) | Integrative review | Nurses | (Borrowed) Trait, process, or outcome depending on which context the concept is applied | Overarching protective process that can enable and build nurses' capacity to deal with and adapt to the risk of emotional dissonance in nursing work | Relational, situational, and emotional demands within the nurse–patient, nurse–family, and collegial interactions | Emotional intelligence | Well-being Psychological health Improved work relationships Professional quality of life Increased job satisfaction | Resilience may mitigate stress and burnout related to the emotional labor of nursing work; however, more research is needed |
| Reyes, Kearney, Lee, Isla, and Estrada (2018) | Integrative review | Individuals exposed to psychological trauma, traumatic events, and those at risk of developing posttraumatic stress disorder (PTSD), including those with PTSD symptoms | (Borrowed) A process that allows individuals to adapt positively in the face of stress or trauma | Positive outcomes in the midst of stressful and traumatic experiences | Psychological trauma and/or traumatic events | None reported | Reduced PTSD Resilience | Research on trauma-focused interventions aimed at improving resilience is still in its infancy. Research in this area is challenging because there is a lack of consistency in the definition of resilience |

well-being (Ahern, 2006; Bekhet et al., 2012; Haase, 2004; Vinson, 2002). Only a few definitions of resilience provide clear descriptions of outcome variables associated with resilience.

Regarding the antecedents of resilience, there is some consensus that there are both risk and protective factors related to resilience. Risk factors are internal and external characteristics that hinder the individual's ability to cope or thrive during adversity. Protective factors "assist individuals to recover from and thrive despite adversity" (Grafton et al., 2010). However, there is the same inconsistency in the nursing literature as was found in the general resilience literature. Risk factors are believed to have the potential to hinder the development of protective factors identified as enhancing resilience. In some cases, both risk and protective factors were listed together. In these cases, one is forced to assume either that the risk factor is the absence of the protective factor identified or that resilience occurs on a continuum of risk to protection. Examples of the risk factors identified in the nursing literature include (a) presence of an adverse or traumatic event (Garcia-Dia et al., 2013), (b) symptom severity (Bekhet et al., 2012; Haase, 2004), (c) challenging workplaces (Hart et al., 2014), and (d) ongoing challenging life experiences such as aging (van Kessel, 2013). Few models specify the mechanisms by which the adversity itself may influence and even contribute to resilience.

The positive factors of resilience reflected in Table 17.1 are numerous. In many cases, where resilience models were specified based on literature synthesis and/or qualitative research, the relationship to and among positive factors is clearly described. Taken as a whole, this literature set provides an emerging pattern that may help distinguish the attributes of resilience from the consequences (i.e., outcomes) of resilience. However, there appears to be some confusion on whether some of the concepts are actually attributes or consequences of resilience.

The most common attributes of resilience include the following:

- Self-efficacy (Bekhet et al., 2012; Earvolino-Ramirez, 2007; Garcia-Dia et al., 2013; Gillespie, Chaboyer, & Wallis, 2007; Grafton et al., 2010; Hart et al., 2014)
- Positive coping (Ahern, 2006; Drummond et al., 2002; Gillespie et al., 2007; Haase, 2014; Hart et al., 2014; Vinson, 2002)
- Hope (Gillespie et al., 2007; Hart et al., 2014)
- Spirituality/meaning and purpose (Grafton et al., 2010; Haase, 2014; van Kessel, 2013; Windle, 2011)

- Connectedness and social support (Ahern, 2006; Earvolino-Ramirez, 2007; Garcia-Dia et al., 2013)
- Positive family functioning (Drummond et al., 2002; Windle, 2011)
- Sense of humor (Ahern, 2006; Earvolino-Ramirez, 2007)

Consequences of resilience include the following:

- Enhanced quality of life/well-being (Bekhet et al., 2012; Haase, 2014; Hart et al., 2014; Vinson, 2002)
- Positive adaptation (Drummond et al., 2002; Earvolino-Ramirez, 2007)
- Effective coping (Garcia-Dia et al., 2013; Gillespie et al., 2007; Grafton et al., 2010; Hart et al., 2014)
- Confidence/mastery (Earvolino-Ramirez, 2007; Haase, 2014)

### Boundaries of Resilience

With the exception of the psychological dimension identified by all authors, all the other boundaries of resilience, either explicit or implied, are inconsistent. There appears to be an emerging consensus that resilience is a dynamic process; however, some authors refer to it as a trait or state (Felten, 2000; Hunter, 2001; Mandleco & Peery, 2000). Most definitions imply that a change occurs, but there is inconsistency as to whether the resilience change is a return to a steady state or is part of a growth producing process. Only one definition explicitly addresses a time frame (Hunter, 2001; Hunter & Chandler, 1999).

The existence of biological contributions to resilience remains strikingly missing from most of the nursing literature. This gap is reflective of the general state of the science on resilience on biological dimensions. This situation may improve with the advancing technologies that have resulted in a rapidly developing knowledge base in neuroscience (Curtis & Cicchetti, 2003). Mandleco and Peery (2000) are among the few who consider biological contributions to resilience. They identified four biological factors as possibly affecting resilience: general health, genetic predisposition, temperament, and gender. Research supports that children with resilience are usually quite healthy and have little hereditary or chronic illness. However, hypotheses about gender and temperament need further exploration. Evidence that temperament is a factor of resilience is derived from studies examining infant temperament; however, it is not clear that temperament is biologically based. Regarding gender, although males are more vulnerable to all risk factors, one cannot assume that more vulnerability equates to less resilience.

Resilience was most frequently studied as an individual dimension rather than as a family or community aggregate. In studies focused on individuals, the family or community variables were often included as protective factors that influence outcomes for the individual. In some ways, the state of knowledge on family resilience is further along than individually focused research in that the limited number of proposed models is more consistently being used and evaluated, and there is more consistency in the ways that family-level measures are used.

Nurses studying resilience seem to agree about the importance of obtaining subjective indicators. Subjective indicators were obtained as narratives and as self-reported quantitative measures of resilience-related concepts. As indicated in section on "methods," nurse researchers have also developed creative methods for obtaining the personal meanings associated with resilience. Ways of making sense of simultaneously objective, physiological measures as they relate to subjective ratings are not addressed well in either the nursing or the general literature. Since nurses focus on both physiological and psychosocial aspects of health, it would seem logical that nurse researchers would be well positioned to provide leadership in this area.

## Description of Resilience in Theories and Models

There is agreement that models of resilience should include factors generally characterized as "protective." In addition, "risk" factors are also generally identified as influencing resilience processes and outcomes. A major problem in developing theory about resilience is that these protective and risk factors frequently resemble "laundry lists." That is, they lack an explicit description of underlying assumptions or an explicit theoretical framework that describes the mechanisms by which the protective and risk factors are linked to outcomes. Especially lacking are hypothesized paths and the magnitude of their influence on development of resilience. In addition, much confusion relates to whether these protective and risk factors are direct ameliorative effects or if they are interactive effects reserved for individuals who have a particular attribute and who have been relatively unaffected by high or low levels of adversity (Luthar & Cicchetti, 2000). Without guiding theories of resilience, the mechanisms by which interventions influence resilience outcomes remain elusive. Three recent systematic reviews of resilience interventions (Chmitorz, Kunzler, & Helmreich, 2018; Eicher, Matzka, Dubey, & White, 2015; Joyce et al.,

2018) indicate the definitions, concepts, research designs, and methods used are of limited use to assess the efficacy of interventions.

The important elements that should be considered in all resilience modeling efforts are contexts, including culture; psychological and physiological mediating units; and the patterns of mediators in relation to the context (Coyne & Downey, 1991; Freitas & Downey, 1998). Further, there is value in interventions that manipulate mediating variables such as coping and hope, since they both influence resilience outcomes (Singer & Ryff, 2001). Masten (2001) provides a useful distinction between variable- and person-focused approaches to model development. In variable-focused approaches, multivariate statistics are used to test for linkages among measures of adversity, outcomes, and environmental or individual qualities that may protect or compensate for negative consequences. Models may examine direct, indirect, and interaction effects (Luthar et al., 2000; Masten, 2001). Direct-effects models hypothesize direct effects in multivariate correlational analyses. Two direct-effects examples are (a) when the relationship of high and low scores to outcomes is directly related to high and low scores on measures of adversity or (b) when a path diagram directly links specific variables with an outcome. Figure 17.1A,B illustrates the direct-effects model. Indirect-effect models are those that hypothesize that the effect of variables, such as adversity or personal characteristics, is mediated by another variable, such as parental styles, as seen in Figure 17.1C. Interaction models hypothesize that the effects of adversity can be modified by individual characteristics or the environment. In general, variable-focused research indicates that adversity does not result in lasting or major effects unless moderating and mediating systems, such as parent or social protective factors, are compromised (Masten, 2001).

Person-focused research attempts to identify and describe the patterns of variables that naturally occur. This process often involves identifying persons with either positive or poor functioning and then examining what might contribute to these outcomes, or using cutoff scores on selected variables to categorize adversity subgroups and then examining outcomes in these groups. These types of person-focused designs often lack comparison low-risk groups, which are important to answering the question: *Do resilient children differ from children who are doing well but do not have high-risk characteristics*? Masten (2001) also argues for more complex person-oriented models that include both health and maladaptive pathways of development in lives studied over time, giving special attention to turning points. These pathway models have a greater potential for providing intervention frameworks.

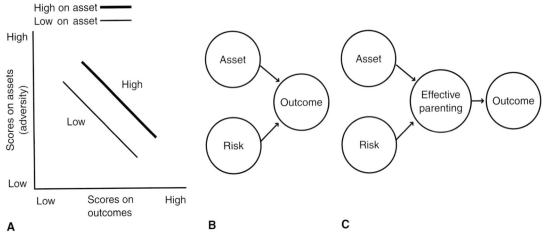

**Figure 17.1**　Variable-focused research models: (A) main, (B) direct, and (C) indirect effects.

## APPROACHES TO RESILIENCE KNOWLEDGE DEVELOPMENT IN NURSING LITERATURE

Resilience research in the nursing literature reflects a variety of approaches. The articles in Table 17.1 used concept analysis, integrative literature reviews, model development and testing, and methodological (measurement) synthesis to further knowledge of resilience. Some of the reviewed articles also proposed models of resilience in specific health contexts. For example, Bekhet et al. (2012) reviewed literature to consider resilience in family members of individuals with autism spectrum disorder, and Garcia-Dia et al. (2013) used concept analysis to consider resilience in individuals with HIV/AIDS. Haase and colleagues used a sequential mixed-methods approach to develop and test the Adolescent Resilience Model (ARM), renamed the Resilience in Illness Model (RIM) (Haase, 1987, 2004; Haase, Britt, Coward, Leidy, & Penn, 1992; Haase et al., 1999, 2014).

The data-based nursing studies fall into two categories of design. First are studies describing characteristics of participants who were designated, a priori, as having resilience. Such studies examined resilience in women older than 85 experiencing illness or loss (Felten, 2000; Felten & Hall, 2001), resilience in homeless adolescents (Hunter, 2001; Hunter & Chandler, 1999), and resilience in adult daughters of battered women (Humphreys, 2001). Second are studies of resilience conducted with a specific population but without a priori designation of participants as being resilient. Examples include resilience studies of adolescents with cancer (Haase et al., 1999) and resilience in children with asthma (Vinson, 2002). Although these studies fit into Masten's description of variable- and person-focused research, they do not reflect the complexity of design recommended by Masten. He recommended including both healthy and maladaptive pathways of development in lives studied over time and giving special attention to turning points (Masten, 2001). By their creative approaches to clarifying the patterns/processes/components of resilience, it is clear that studies conducted by nurses are increasingly adding to the knowledge base on resilience. More complex designs and interventions to address resilience are recommended.

### Specific Models of Resilience

The articles in Table 17.1 that describe literature synthesis and concept analysis of resilience indicate the value that nurse scientists place on carefully developed theory. Models or theories of resilience have been increasing. Szanton and colleagues linked society to cellular levels of coping in older adults (Szanton & Gill, 2010; Szanton, Gill, & Thorpe, 2010). Individual-level resilience models include the following:

- Mastery of chronic illness with resilience as an emergent outcome (White, 1995)
- A "CARE" framework (containment, awareness, resilience, and engagement) for guiding mental health practice (McAllister & Walsh, 2003)
- The RIM developed in the context of adolescents/young adults with cancer and other chronic conditions (Haase, 1999; Haase et al., 2014, 2017)
- The Inner Core Child Resilience Model for children with asthma (Vinson, 2002)
- A model of resilience in community-dwelling women older than 85 overcoming adversity from illness or loss (Felten, 2000; Felten & Hall, 2001)

In addition, a model of resilience in adolescents was proposed by Rew and Horner (2003), adapted by Ahern (2006), and used to guide clinicians who work with high-risk teens (Halloran, 2011). Some models propose a continuum of risk and protective factors. Other models were constructed with consideration of the perspectives of those experiencing the adversity. Interventions to enhance resilience are proposed on the basis of three models (Ahern, 2006; Haase, 2004; Rew & Horner, 2003). These models differ in the specificity of targeted factors and in potential timing of interventions. Although there is less nursing literature on family or community resilience models, these models are being developed and used in practice with increasing frequency. The Family Resilience Model developed by McCubbin and McCubbin (1996) is supported in the literature on family resilience (Board & Ryan-Wenger, 2000; Svavarsdottir, McCubbin, & Kane, 2000; White, Bichter, Koeckeritz, Lee, & Munch, 2002). This model was suggested as a framework for caring for those with chronic pain (West, Usher, & Foster, 2011). Other family models are also being proposed. Drummond et al. (2002) proposed and tested a model of family adaptation that identified family protective factors of appraisal, support, and coping as mediators of adaptation. Appraisal was a key variable predicting adaptation. Community-based models have been considered for drug education of adolescents (Brown, Jean-Marie, & Beck, 2010) and mental health promotion and mental illness prevention (Power, 2010).

Across the models of resilience, many adversity and positive concepts were inconsistently identified as antecedents, critical components, and outcomes of resilience. Antecedents usually included adversity (e.g., death, loss, illness, stressor[s], and homelessness). Protective factors were modeled as antecedents in only a few studies (Haase et al., 1999; Hunter & Chandler, 1999). Across several studies, especially those that viewed resilience as a trait, it was difficult to discern the role (e.g., mediator, moderator) of resilience-related concepts such as coping, hope, or mastery. These concepts were alternatively viewed as antecedent and critical component protective factors or as outcomes of resilience. For example, in some articles, coping is viewed as a mediating protective factor, whereas in others it is an outcome of resilience. Reflective of the general literature, many protective factors fall into broad categories of factors classified as individual, social, or family.

It is clear that more work needs to be done to clarify the relationship among concepts that are correlated with resilience and those that influence resilience outcomes. To increase explanatory power, this work will most productively be done in longitudinal studies, with models that attempt to capture the full, integrative perspective of resilience.

# Application of a Theory: The Resilience in Illness Model

## RESEARCH TO DEVELOP THE MODEL

The RIM provides one example of how a theoretical model built on experiences of the population of interest can be useful to guide interventions. The context for the RIM was chronic illness in adolescents. Most of the research was derived from the perspective of adolescents with cancer; however, some studies included parent and health care provider perspectives.

To develop the RIM, two series of studies were conducted: (a) model generation studies, using inductive approaches, and (b) model evaluation studies, involving instrumentation and exploratory and confirmatory model testing (Haase et al., 1999, 2014, 2017). The qualitative, model-generating studies provided a basis for the development of the RIM through the identification and clarification of salient concepts to be included in the model and through the use of the model as a qualitative means of evaluating subsequent model-testing results. These studies were also guided by the Haase Decision-Making Process for Model and Instrument Development (Haase et al., 1999).

Both protective and risk factors are included in the RIM. Three classes of RIM protective factors are hypothesized to positively affect resilience outcomes:

- Class I, Individual Protective Factors, includes courageous or positive coping and derived meaning.
- Class II, Family Protective Factors, includes family adaptability, cohesion, communication, and perceived strengths.
- Class III, Social Protective Factors, includes connectedness with health care providers and social integration.

Two classes of RIM risk factors are hypothesized to negatively affect resilience:

- Class IV: Individual Risk Factor, sustained defensive coping.
- Class V, Illness-Related Factors, includes illness perspective and illness distress.

The RIM outcome, resilience resolution includes self-esteem as a sense of mastery/confidence, and self-transcendence, as well as quality of life, defined as a sense of well-being. Figure 17.2

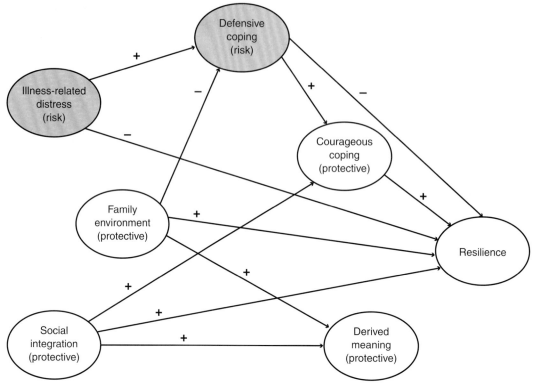

**Figure 17.2**   The resilience in illness model.

shows the relationship between the protective and risk factors of the RIM, and these factors are related to specific variables as found in Table 17.2.

### RESEARCH TO EVALUATE RIM: INSTRUMENTATION, MODEL EVALUATION, MODEL-FOCUSED INTERVENTIONS, AND CULTURAL ADEQUACY

The quantitative studies of the RIM for instrumentation model were done using latent variable structural equation modeling approaches. The first studies were done to evaluate the psychometric properties of the instruments used to measure each latent variable and to develop the measurement model. Based on the exploratory studies of the theoretical model, factors were identified that affect the development of resilience, and the RIM was then confirmed using baseline data from a multisite randomized controlled trial (RCT). Based on the findings, researchers are now using RIM to address knowledge gaps related to individual factors in the model, gaps in knowledge regarding the relationships between factors, and guide intervention research with the benefit of a full set of measures to evaluate outcomes of these interventions.

To explore cultural differences in RIM, in 2018, Haase began working with colleagues in/from Taiwan, Korea, China, and Japan to establish the Asian Resilience Enhancement for Adolescents/ Young Adults (AREA) Cooperative Group. The goals of the group are to compare the fit of RIM to the confirmed RIM and of RIM across these four countries. The first AREA task is to ascertain which RIM measures are already translated into Chinese Mandarin, Taiwanese Mandarin, Korean, and Japanese and to then translate/back translate prior to recruiting adolescent and young adult (AYA) with cancer and other chronic illness to complete the measures.

### RESEARCH USING A MODEL TO GUIDE THE INTERVENTION

Once the RIM was validated, it effectively guided evaluation in a multisite RCT of a therapeutic music video intervention for adolescents/young adults undergoing a stem cell transplant (Robb et al., 2014). These findings are described in Using Middle Range Theory in Research 17.1. Based on findings from the therapeutic music study findings, a second RCT evaluated a parent communication intervention targeting the family environment factor in RIM. In 2011,

**Table 17.2    Adolescent Resilience Model Latent and Manifest Variables**

| Latent Factor | Manifest Variables |
|---|---|
| **I. Individual Protective** | |
| Courageous coping | Confrontive coping |
| | Optimistic coping |
| | Supportant coping |
| Derived meaning | Hope |
| | Spiritual perspective |
| **II. Family Protective** | |
| Family atmosphere | Adaptability and cohesion |
| | Parent–adolescent communication |
| | Perceived social support—family |
| Family support/ resources | Family strengths |
| | Socioeconomic status variables |
| **III. Social Protective** | |
| Social integration | Perceived social support—health care provider |
| | Perceived social support—friends |
| **IV. Individual Risk** | |
| Defensive coping | Evasive coping |
| | Emotive coping |
| **V. Illness-Related Risk** | |
| Illness perspective | Uncertainty in illness |
| Illness distress | Symptom distress |
| | Severity of illness |
| **VI. Resilience** | |
| | Confidence/mastery |
| | Self-transcendence |
| | Self-esteem |
| Quality of life | Sense of well-being |

the RIM was adopted by the Children's Oncology Group—Nursing Discipline Committee—as the organizing framework to guide all the clinical trials sponsored by the committee (Landier, Leonard, & Ruccione, 2013; Kelly et al., 2014).

## OTHER PRACTICE APPLICATIONS OF THE THEORY

Much of the nursing literature on resilience focuses on research that examines the correlations between resilience and health outcomes in a variety of populations. The articles that address how resilience can be promoted are more frequently found in educational and public health peer-reviewed journals than in nursing journals. Research focused on resilience in health care providers, including clinicians, students, and educators, is a relatively new and growing focus. See Using Middle Range Theory in Practice 17.2 for a description of a resilience training program for ICU nurses.

Several articles encourage health care workers to reinforce the resilience strategies of others. Ward et al. (2011) explored the additive and subtractive processes used by nonsmokers to never smoke and by smokers to quit smoking. Herrick et al. (2011) described strength-based approaches to prevent HIV in gay men. Other articles simply provide a description of recommended behaviors to promote resilience, for instance, in high-risk teens (Halloran, 2011) and social workers involved in the community (Megele, 2011). In addition to Megele's article identifying strategies to promote resilience in social workers, Aiello et al. (2011) discussed an intervention to build resilience in health care workers who would be required to deal with a viral pandemic, and Delport, Strydom, Theron, and Geyer (2011) described a support program for educators working with HIV/AIDS. This program, referred to as Resilient Educators (REd), included nine modules that consider health promotion, psychosocial impact of the pandemic, stigma, health care, and resilience while providing background information and interactive activities.

There are also examples of substantial projects developed to apply a resilience framework for promoting healthy behavior. One such project is an "international and prospective application of resilience in school-based drug education, Project REBOUND [resilience-bound]" (Brown et al., 2010, p. 331). The approach was based on an analysis of literature that found (a) risk-based education was basically ineffective; (b) protective factors and risk factors are independent phenomena; and (c) resilience is a normative process that can be predicted in relation to caring connected relationships, opportunities for participation and contribution, and high expectations of self (p. 337). The education program developed to influence drug use behavior of young people was based on these three predictors. This drug education model included a Resilience Education (focused more on protective factors) with Risk Competence informational orientation (focused more specifically on the topic of drug use). Both were used in processional development for educators, counselors, and administrators, which involved six 1.5-day workshops. The workshops were designed to not only introduce them to the curriculum but also assist them to integrate the lessons to be taught into their own lives.

## USING MIDDLE RANGE THEORY IN RESEARCH    17.1

Source: Robb, S., Burns, D., Stegenga, K., Haut, P., Monahan, P., Meza, J., ..., Haase, J. E. (2014) Randomized clinical trial of therapeutic music video intervention for resilience outcomes in adolescents/young adults undergoing hematopoietic stem cell transplant: A report from the Children's Oncology Group. Cancer, 120, 909–917. doi: 10.1002/cncr.28355

### RESEARCH PURPOSE

Adolescents/young adults often experience high distress during hematopoietic stem cell transplant (HSCT). The purpose of this study was to test the hypotheses that therapeutic music videos would "(a) increase protective factors of spiritual perspective, social integration, family environment ..., courageous coping, and hope-derived meaning ...; (b) decrease risk factors of illness related distress ... and defensive coping; and (c) increase outcomes of self-transcendence and resilience" (p. 910).

### RESEARCH DESIGN

The study was an RCT.

### SAMPLE/PARTICIPANTS

Participants were recruited from eight Children's Oncology Group institutions. To be eligible, the participants needed to be aged 11 to 24 years, undergoing myeloablative HSCT for cancer, and able to read and speak English. The target number of participants was 130 adolescents/young adults but was not achieved.

### DATA COLLECTION

Participants were randomly assigned to the music video or low-dose (audiobook), control group using 24 strata (eight different sites and three age groups: 11 to 14, 15 to 18, and 19 to 24 years). Both groups received six sessions (two per week) during the acute HSCT phase. For the treatment group, sessions 1 to 3 included singing, brainstorming, lyric writing, discussion, and song recording. Sessions 4 and 5 involved selecting the visual content for the video based on the previously developed song lyrics. In session 6, the treatment group participants viewed their videos. The control group selected an audiobook from a list of 15 that were determined to be age appropriate. They listened to and discussed the books during sessions. Evaluations were completed after the sixth session and 100 days posttransplant. Sixteen different instruments were used to measure the variables: illness-related distress, social integration, spiritual perspective, family environment, coping, hope-derived meaning, and resilience. To determine statistically significant differences between the two groups, a two-sided $t$ test was used.

### FINDINGS

The treatment group experienced improved courageous coping immediately after the sixth session and improved social integration and family environment 100 days after transplant. It was concluded that improved coping during treatment would likely result in better long-term adjustment. Based on findings, a second RCT was developed to target the family environment through a parent/AYA communication intervention.

## USING MIDDLE RANGE THEORY IN PRACTICE    17.2

Source: Mealer, M., Conrad, D., Evans, J., Jooste, K., Solyntjes, J., Rothbaum, B., & Moss, M. (2014). Feasibility and acceptability of a resilience training program for intensive care unit nurses. American Journal of Critical Care, 23(6), e97–e105. doi: 10.4037/ajcc201447

### PROBLEM

ICU nurses work in a stressful environment and often experience psychological issues such as anxiety, depression, burnout syndrome, and posttraumatic stress. This distress may help explain the high turnover rate of ICU nurses, which has been reported to be 25% to 60% annually.

### INTERVENTION

Thirteen ICU nurses were randomly assigned to an intervention group with 14 ICU from the same clinical academic institution randomly assigned to the control group. The 12-week intervention included the following:

1. Two-day educational workshop. This provided an introduction to resilience training and the types of psychological distress experienced by ICU nurses. The participants were provided with instruction on self-care and cognitive behavioral therapy. An expert conducted a 2-hour guided mindfulness exercise session and provided a compact disc that could be used during the intervention period. A 4-hour session on written exposure was also included.

**USING MIDDLE RANGE THEORY IN PRACTICE**    **17.2** (CONTINUED)

2. Written exposure therapy. E-mailed prompts were provided to which participants were asked to write twelve 30-minute sessions. Topics that were suggested included challenges at work, feeling conflicted, and ruminating about sensitive issues.

3. Mindfulness practices. Each participant was to use the mindfulness activities for 15 minutes three times per week. Body scan and sitting meditation were the techniques to be used by the nurses.

4. Exercise. Membership to the wellness center was provided, and participants were asked to engage in aerobic exercise for 30 to 45 minutes at least three times per week.

5. Event-triggered counseling sessions. Events that triggered the sessions were a patient's death, participating in end-of-life discussion with family members, performing cardiopulmonary resuscitation, performing futile care for a terminally ill patient, and caring for a patient with massive bleeding or traumatic injuries. Each session was 30 to 60 minutes and focused on cognitive behavioral approaches to challenge negative thoughts and promote resilience.

Members of the control group were not involved in any of the interventions but were asked to provide a record of their exercise.

**OUTCOME**

All the nurses in the intervention group attended the workshop and completed all the weekly writing sessions. The participation rates were slightly less for mindfulness exercises (66%) and physical exercise (88%). The average number of event-triggered counseling sessions was two. The participants rated their level of satisfaction with the activities high. Four main themes emerged from the written exposure exercises: (a) patient centricity, (b) cognitive processing, (c) work structure, and (d) workplace relationships. Nurses in the intervention group had statistically significant lower levels of depression when compared to the control group. Both the intervention and control groups experienced a statistically significant reduction in PTSD symptoms and improved resilience scores. Resilience training was considered both feasible and acceptable to ICU nurses.

The curriculum was delivered in 90-minute lessons over a 16-week period. One of the first issues introduced was the necessity for authentic presence and openness to learn. Most of the Resilience Education was devoted to protective factors, addressing the importance of connection, participation and contribution, and high expectations for self. Finally, these topics were linked to decisions related to drug behavior. Following the focus on Resilience Education, the remaining sessions were devoted to Risk Competence. In those sessions, individual risk is explored, drug information is provided, critical thinking is facilitated, and self-awareness with special emphasis on strengths is encouraged. Project REBOUND has been supported by the Mentor Foundation and the European Union. It was developed to be first implemented in Germany and then be adopted throughout Europe and the United States. As it is implemented, evaluation will occur at each step of the program.

Several other examples of implementation strategies to promote resilience are found in Table 17.3 and the project described in Using Middle Range Theory in Practice Projects 17.3. These studies demonstrate the usefulness of the theory for patient populations and health care professionals.

# Instruments Used in Empirical Testing of Resilience

Measurement is an approach to knowledge development for resilience that is gaining more attention (Ahern, Kiehl, Sole, & Byers, 2006). Windle, Bennett, and Noyes (2011) screened close to 3,000 peer-reviewed articles, published from 1989 to September 2009 to identify published resilience scales. They conducted a systematic methodological review of these scales, applying established quality assessment criteria to evaluate their psychometric properties. Windle et al. identified 15 scales, some with refinements and all self-report instruments; the earliest was published in 1989 and the most recent in 2008. These scales provided measurements for all population age groups, children through older adults. Three scales, all developed for use with adults, were determined to have the best psychometric properties: (a) the Connor-Davidson Resilience Scale, (b) the Resilience Scale for Adults, and (c) the Brief Resilience Scale. At best, the quality of these questionnaires would be considered moderate. All 15 scales are described by target population, mode of completion, number of items, purpose, and quality assessment. In addition, complete references and

| Table 17.3 | Examples of Theory in Practice |

| Citation | Focus |
| --- | --- |
| Foureur, M., Besley, K., Burton, G., Yu, N., & Crisp, J. (2013). Enhancing the resilience of nurses and midwives: Pilot of a mindfulness-based program for increased health, sense of coherence and decreased depression, anxiety and stress. *Contemporary Nurse, 45*(1), 114–125 | Mindfulness-based stress reduction (MBSR) was considered integral to resilience development. Its effectiveness was tested in a randomized controlled trial. The intervention consisted of a 1-d workshop focused on teaching MBSR techniques and a CD to guide practice sessions. The goal was that participants would engage in daily 20-min practice sessions over a period of 8 wk. Results provide support for this approach. |
| McDonald, G., Jackson, D., Wilkes, L., & Vickers, M. H. (2013). Personal resilience in nurses and midwives: Effects of a work-based educational intervention. *Contemporary Nurse, 45*(1), 134–143 | In this study, participants participated in six resilience workshops and a mentoring program over a 6-mo period. In each of the workshops, issues associated with resilience were considered: positive and nurturing relationships, mentoring, positive outlook, intellectual flexibility, emotional intelligence, life balance, spirituality, reflection, and critical thinking. Assertive communication, spirituality, and creative movement were considered. The participants experienced enhanced confidence, self-awareness, assertiveness, and self-care related to personal and professional resilience. |
| Sanders, E. D. (2015). Nursing resilience: A nursing opportunity. *Nursing Administration Quarterly, 39*(2), 132–136. doi: 10.1097/NAQ.0000000000000091 | Resilience can be fostered in self and promoted in others. Self-reflection and finding greater meaning in one's lives are associated with greater personal resilience. Relationships are also key in the development of resilience. By role-modeling healthy behaviors, nurses can help build resilience in their patients and colleagues. They can promote self-care and self-development. Mindfulness meditation was described in some detail as a tool to promote resilience. |
| Eicher, M., Ribi, K., Senn-Dubey, C., Senn, S., Ballabeni, P., & Betticher, D. (2018). Interprofessional, psycho-social intervention to facilitate resilience and reduce supportive care needs for patients with cancer: Results of a noncomparative, randomized phase II trial. *Psycho-Oncology, 27*(7), 1833–1839. doi: 10.1002/pon.4734 | Evaluated the feasibility, acceptability, and preliminary effectiveness of two interventions for interprofessional supportive care in cancer (IPSC-C) to facilitate resilience and reduce unmet supportive care needs of newly diagnosed patients. *Intervention 1* (low-intensity interprofessional supportive care in cancer [LI-IPSC-C]) consisted of three electronic assessments of resilience, unmet supportive care needs, mood, and coping effort over 16 wk with an immediate feedback to clinicians including tailored intervention recommendations to facilitate resilience and supportive care. *Intervention 2* (high-intensity interprofessional supportive care in cancer [HI-IPSC-C]) added five structured consultations (face-to-face and telephone) provided by specialized nurses. Results showed that resilience scores increased slightly in both arms. Relatively more patients unmet needs were decreased in HI-IPSC-C arm. Feasibility was limited for the LI-IPSC-C arm, mainly due to lack of time; acceptability was high in both arms. The HI-IPSC-C showed more positive effects on secondary outcomes and was feasible. |

comments on theoretical background are provided. It was noted that different approaches to measuring resilience have resulted in lack of clarity related to potential risk factors and protective processes and a number of the scales are in early stages of development and require further validation.

The resilience scale with the widest application is the Resilience Scale (Wagnild & Young, 1993). This scale designed with a two-factor structure, involving personal competence and acceptance of self and life, has been used in studies that represent different cultural and age samples.

Most quantitative studies of resilience used existing instruments or developed instruments to measure numerous variables in proposed models. However, in many cases, it is not clear whether the instruments were derived from theories that are congruent with the conceptual frameworks or the philosophical approaches that were being used in the studies. Haase et al. (1999) describe one approach to identifying and/or developing instruments that is clearly linked to the Resilience in Illness Model (RIM). Mixed methods were done in a series of studies to develop and test the RIM and to identify or develop the instruments used to evaluate the model (Haase, 1987; Haase & Rostad, 1994; Haase et al., 1992, 1999). Decision trees were used to decide on labels and definitions for each model factor and to decide whether to use existing instruments or ones developed to measure the model factors. This iterative process of decision-making sought to retain the inductively derived meanings from the qualitative studies while taking advantage of existing theory and instruments. The result was a set of 15 instruments to measure manifest variables—8 existing instruments meeting established criteria for reliability and validity and 7 new instruments. To test the RIM and instruments, latent variable instrument and model-testing studies were done (Haase et al., 1999, 2014).

## USING MIDDLE RANGE THEORY IN PRACTICE PROJECTS    17.3

### OVERVIEW
**Problem:**

Adolescents and young adults (AYAs) with cancer have more psychosocial challenges than do younger children or older adults. Health care providers (nurses, physicians, and social workers) struggle to assess and address their needs, especially at diagnosis.

**Members of Project Team:**

Nurses, physicians, and social workers

**Expected Outcome:**

Improve resilience outcomes by enhancing AYA RIM protective factors and minimizing risk factors.

### INTEGRATION OF THEORY

The authors developed and pilot tested the *Resilience Enhancement for AYA with Cancer and their Healthcare Providers* (REACH) intervention. REACH systematically assesses each of the RIM protective and risk factors. AYA and parent scores are then summarized in a user-friendly fashion that can be used by the health care team to guide discussions regarding the AYA's RIM protective and risk factors at diagnosis.

### OUTCOMES

The REACH intervention was pilot tested with six AYA–parent dyads. One hundred percent of approached dyads agreed to participate and completed all measures within the time frame and with no missing data. AYAs and parents actively engaged in the focused conversations. They were highly satisfied with REACH content, the time commitment required, and helpfulness for gaining insight into their protective strengths to build on and identifying areas where they needed additional support.

### CONCLUSION/OUTCOMES

With high feasibility, acceptability, and usefulness, our next steps are to conduct a pilot study to estimate effect sizes of REACH on QoL outcomes and to develop feasible strategies for health care providers' use of the REACH profile for routine assessment and care planning.

Project leasers: Phillips, C. R., & Haase, J. E. (2018). *Feasibility, acceptability, and usefulness of the resilience enhancement for adolescents and young adults with cancer and healthcare providers (REACH) intervention.* Podium presentation at the International Society of Paediatric Oncology, Kyoto, Japan.

---

It is clear that additional measurement work is needed to further the science of resilience from a nursing perspective. Cultural considerations in measurement are not well addressed. Measurement in nursing research on resilience needs to consider the issues of boundaries, including trait/process and physiological/psychological. Measurement also needs to focus on differences in resilience based on developmental factors, including age.

## Summary

■ The work that nurse scientists have accomplished to add to the body of knowledge on resilience is considerable, but much work still needs to be done.

■ Areas of strength within the nursing literature include the following:

■ Careful attention to theory, both by clarifying concepts through literature analysis and synthesis and by use of qualitative methods that explore experiences of resilience from the perspectives of those who have experienced adversity

■ The recognition of resilience as a positive health concept and the recognition of resilience as a dynamic process

■ Research on resilience in the workforce

■ To advance the science, much work remains for nurses in collaboration with scientists from other disciplines. Some specific recommendations are:

■ Continue efforts on measurement issues, to ensure that instruments are context and culturally sensitive, meaning-based, and time sensitive.

■ Conduct longitudinal, prospective studies of resilience to test integrative models.

■ Develop and test interventions planned to manipulate targeted variables that have promising evidence of their ability to influence resilience outcomes.

■ Take advantage of the rapid advancements in neurocognitive sciences to include biological markers that may contribute to the existing knowledge of resilience.

## CRITICAL THINKING EXERCISES

1. The RIM was primarily developed for use in adolescents/young adults with cancer. Identify other populations where this model could be used to guide further research. What issues would you need to consider before applying the model to another population?

2. Develop a potential intervention targeted at one or more of the protective factors in the RIM that may influence resilience and quality of life in adolescents and young adults (AYAs).

3. Describe how the middle range theory described in this chapter helps refine your previous conceptualization of resilience.

4. Describe the benefits of meaning-based models or strengths-based research in your area of interest.

## REFERENCES

Ahern, N. R. (2006). Adolescent resilience: An evolutionary concept analysis. *Journal of Pediatric Nursing*, *21*(3), 175–185.

Ahern, N. R., Kiehl, E. M., Sole, M. L., & Byers, J. (2006). A review of instruments measuring resilience. *Issues in Comprehensive Pediatric Nursing*, *29*(2), 103–125.

Aiello, A., Khayeri, M. Y., Raja, S., Peladeau, N., Romano, D., Maunder, R. G., … Schulman, R. B. (2011). Resilience training for hospital workers in anticipation of an influenza pandemic. *Journal of Continuing Education in the Health Professions*, *31*(1), 15–20. doi: 10.1002/chp.20096

Antonovsky, A. (1979). *Health, stress, and coping*. San Francisco, CA: Jossey-Bass.

Bandura, A. (1977). Self-efficacy: Toward a unifying theory of behavioral change. *Psychological Review*, *84*, 191–215.

Bekhet, A. K., Johnson, N. L., & Zauszniewski, J. A. (2012). Resilience in family members of persons with autism spectrum disorder: A review of the literature. *Issues in Mental Health Nursing*, *33*, 650–656. doi: 10.3109/01612840.2012.671441

Board, R., & Ryan-Wenger, N. (2000). State of the science on parental stress and family functioning in pediatric intensive care units. *American Journal of Critical Care*, *9*(2), 106–122; quiz 123–124.

Brown, J. H., Jean-Marie, G., & Beck, J. (2010). Resilience and risk competence in schools: Theory/knowledge and international application in Project REBOUND. *Journal of Drug Education*, *40*(4), 331–359. doi: 10.2190DE.40.4.b

Charon, J. M. (1998). The nature of the self. In J. M. Charon (Ed.), *Symbolic interactionism: An introduction, an interpretation, an integration* (6th ed., pp. 72–97). Upper Saddle River, NJ: Prentice-Hall.

Chen, C. M., Chen, Y. C., & Haase, J. E. (2007). The game of lives in surviving childhood brain tumors. *Western Journal of Nursing Research*, *30*(4), 435–457. doi: 10.1177/0193945907303050

Chen, C. M., Chen, Y. C., & Wong, T. T. (2014). Comparison of resilience in adolescent survivors of brain tumors and healthy adolescents. *Cancer Nursing*, *37*(5), 373–381. doi: 10.1097/NCC.0000000000000094

Chmitorz, A., Kunzler, A., Helmreich, I., et al. (2018). Intervention studies to foster resilience—A systematic review and proposal for a resilience framework in future intervention studies. *Clinical Psychology Review*, *59*, 78–100.

Cicchetti, D. (2011). Resilience under conditions of extreme stress: A multilevel perspective. *World Psychiatry*, *9*, 145–154.

Cicchetti, D., & Blender, J. A. (2006). A multiple-levels-of-analysis perspective on resilience: Implications for the developing brain, neural plasticity, and preventive interventions. *Annals of the New York Academy of Sciences*, *1094*, 248–258.

Coyne, J. C., & Downey, G. (1991). Social factors and psychopathology: Stress, social support, and coping processes. *Annual Review of Psychology*, *42*, 401–425.

Curtis, W. J., & Cicchetti, D. (2003). Moving research on resilience into the 21st century: Theoretical and methodological considerations in examining the biological contributors to resilience. *Development and Psychopathology*, *15*(3), 773–810.

Delgado, C., Upton, D., Ranse, K., Furness, T., & Foster, K. (2017). Nurses' resilience and the emotional labour of nursing work: An integrative review of empirical literature. *International Journal of Nursing Studies*, *70*, 71–88.

Delport, R., Strydom, H., Theron, L., & Geyer, S. (2011). Voices of HIV&AIDS-affected educators: How they are psychosocially affected and how REds enabled their resilience. *AIDS Care*, *23*(1), 121–126. doi: 10.1080/09540121.2010.498857

Drummond, J., Kysela, G. M., McDonald, L., & Query, B. (2002). The family adaptation model: Examination of dimensions and relations. *Canadian Journal of Nursing Research*, *34*(1), 29–46.

Earvolino-Ramirez, M. (2007). Resilience: A concept analysis. *Nursing Forum*, *42*(2), 73–82.

Eicher, M., Matzka, M., Dubey, C., & White, K. (2015). Resilience in adult cancer care: An integrative literature review. *Oncology Nursing Forum*, *42*(1):E3–E16.

Eicher, M., Ribi, K., Senn-Dubey, C., Senn, S., Ballabeni, P., & Betticher, D. (2018). Interprofessional, psycho-social intervention to facilitate resilience and reduce supportive care needs for patients with cancer: Results of a noncomparative, randomized phase II trial. *Psycho-Oncology*, *27*(7), 1833–1839. doi:10.1002/pon.4734

Felten, B. S. (2000). Resilience in a multicultural sample of community-dwelling women older than age 85. *Clinical Nursing Research*, *9*(2), 102–123.

Felten, B. S., & Hall, J. M. (2001). Conceptualizing resilience in women older than 85: Overcoming adversity from illness or loss. *Journal of Gerontological Nursing*, *27*(11), 46–53.

Fine, S. B. (1991). Resilience and human adaptability: Who rises above adversity? 1990 Eleanor Clarke Slagle Lecture. *American Journal of Occupational Therapy*, *45*(6), 493–503.

Fletcher, D., & Sarkar, M. (2013). Psychological resilience: A review and critique of definitions, concepts, and theory. *European Psychologist*, *18*(1), 12–23.

Forsyth, G. L., Delaney, K. D., & Gresham, M. L. (1984). Vying for a winning position: Management style of the chronically ill. *Research in Nursing & Health*, *7*(3), 181–188.

Foureur, M., Besley, K., Burton, G., Yu, N., & Crisp, J. (2013). Enhancing the resilience of nurses and midwives: Pilot of mindfulness-based program for increased health, sense of coherence, and decreased depression, anxiety, and stress. *Contemporary Nurse*, *45*(1), 114–125.

Freitas, A. L., & Downey, G. (1998). Resilience: A dynamic perspective. *International Journal of Behavioral Development*, *22*(2), 263–285.

Garcia-Dia, M. J., DiNapoli, J. M., Garcia-Ona, L., Jakubowski, R., & O'Flaherty, D. (2013). Concept analysis: Resilience. *Archives of Psychiatric Nursing*, *27*, 264–270. doi: 10.1016/j.apnu.2013.07.003

Garmezy, N. (1981). *Children under stress: Perspectives on antecedents and correlates of vulnerability and resistance to psychopathology*. New York, NY: Wiley.

Garmezy, N. (1991). Resilience in children's adaptation to negative life events and stressed environments. *Pediatric Annals*, *20*, 459–466.

Garmezy, N., Masten, A. S., & Tellegen, A. (1984). The study of stress and competence in children: A building block for developmental psychopathology. *Child Development*, *55*(1), 97–111.

Gillespie, B. M., Chaboyer, W., & Wallis, M. (2007). Development of a theoretically derived model of resilience through concept analysis. *Contemporary Nurse*, *25*(1–2), 124–135.

Grafton, E., Gillespie, B., & Henderson, S. (2010). Resilience: The power within. *Oncology Nursing Forum*, *37*(6), 698–705.

Haase, J. (1987). The components of courage in chronically ill adolescents. *Advances in Nursing Science*, *9*(2), 64–80.

Haase, J. (2004). The Adolescent Resilience Model as a guide to interventions. Special section: Proceedings from the 5th annual state of the science workshop on resilience and quality of life in adolescents. *Journal of Pediatric Oncology Nursing*, *21*(5), 289–299.

Haase, J. E., & Rostad, M. (1994). Experiences of completing cancer therapy: Children's perspectives. *Oncology Nursing Forum*, *21*(9), 1483–1492; discussion 1493–1494.

Haase, J. E., Britt, T., Coward, D. D., Leidy, N. K., & Penn, P. E. (1992). Simultaneous concept analysis of spiritual perspective, hope, acceptance and self-transcendence. *Image: The Journal of Nursing Scholarship*, *24*(2), 141–147.

Haase, J. E., Heiney, S. P., Ruccione, K. S., & Stutzer, C. (1999). Research triangulation to derive meaning-based quality-of-life theory: Adolescent resilience model and instrument development. *International Journal of Cancer. Supplement*, *12*, 125–131.

Haase, J. E., Kintner, E. K., Robb, S. L., Stump, T. E., Monahan, P. O., Phillips, C., … Burns, D. S. (2017). The resilience in illness model part 2: Confirmatory evaluation in adolescents and young adults with cancer. *Cancer Nursing*, *40*(6), 454–463.

Haase, J. E., Robb, S., Kintner, E. K., Monahan, P. O., Stump, T., Burns, D. S., … Haut, P. R. (2014). The resilience in illness model, part 1: Exploratory evaluation in adolescents and young adults with cancer. *Cancer Nursing*, *37*(3), E1–E12. doi: 10.1097/NCC.0b013e31828941bb

Halloran, L. (2011). Risky business: Working with high-risk teens to foster resilience. *The Journal for Nurse Practitioners*, *7*(5), 426–427. doi: 10.1016/j.nurpra.2011.02.004

Hart, P. L., Brannan, J. D., & De Chesnay, M. (2014). Resilience in nurses: An integrative review. *Journal of Nursing Management*, *22*, 720–734.

Hauser, S. T., Vieyra, M. A., Jacobson, A. M., & Wertlieb, D. (1985). Vulnerability and resilience in adolescence: Views from the family. *Journal of Early Adolescence*, *5*, 81–100.

Henry, D. L. (2001). Resilient children: What they tell us about coping with maltreatment. *Social Work in Health Care*, *34* (3–4), 283–298.

Herrick, A. L., Lim, S. H., Wei, C., Smith, H., Guadamuz, T., Friedman, M. D., & Stall, R. (2011). Resilience as an untapped resource in behavioral intervention design for gay men. *AIDS and Behavior*, *15*(Suppl. 1), S25–S29. doi: 10.1007/s10461-011-9895-0

Ho, D. Y. F., Chen, S. G., & Chiu, C. Y. (1991). Relational orientation: To find an answer for the methodology of Chinese social psychology. In K. S. Yang & K. K. Hwang (Eds.), *The psychology and behavior of Chinese people (in Chinese)*. Taipei, Taiwan: Gui-Guan.

Humphreys, J. C. (2001). Turnings and adaptations in resilient daughters of battered women. *Image: The Journal of Nursing Scholarship*, *33*(3), 245–251.

Hunter, A. J. (2001). A cross-cultural comparison of resilience in adolescents. *Journal of Pediatric Nursing*, *16*(3), 172–179.

Hunter, A. J., & Chandler, G. E. (1999). Adolescent resilience. *Image: The Journal of Nursing Scholarship*, *31*(3), 243–247.

Hwang, K. K. (1997). Guanxi and mientze: Conflict resolution in Chinese Society. *Intercultural Communication Studies*, *7*(1), 17–42.

Hwang, K. K. (2006). Constructive realism and confucian relationalism: An epistemological strategy for the development of indigenous psychology. In U. Kim, K. S. Yang, & K. K. Hwang (Eds.), *Indigenous and cultural psychology: Understanding people in context*. New York, NY: Springer.

Hymovich, D. P., & Roehnert, J. E. (1989). Psychosocial consequences of childhood cancer. *Seminars in Oncology Nursing*, *5*(1), 56–62.

Joyce, S., Shand, F., Tighe, J., Laurent, S. J., Bryant, R. A., & Harvey, S. B. (2018). Road to resilience: A systematic review and meta-analysis of resilience training programmes and interventions. *BMJ Open*, *8*(6), e017858. doi: 10.1136/bmjopen-2017-017858

Kadner, K. D. (1989). Resilience. Responding to adversity. *Journal of Psychosocial Nursing and Mental Health Services*, *27*(7), 20–25.

Kazak, A. E. (2006). Pediatric psychosocial preventative health model (PPPHM): Research, practice, and collaboration in pediatric family systems medicine. *Families, Systems & Health*, *24*, 381–395. doi: 10.1037/1091-7527.24.4.381

Kazak, A. E., Segal-Andrews, A. M., & Johnson, K. (1995). Pediatric psychology research and practice: A family/systems approach. In M. C. Roberts (Ed.), *Handbook of pediatric psychology* (2nd ed., pp. 84–104). New York, NY: Guilford.

Kelly, K. P., Hooke, M. C., Ruccione, K., Landier, W., & Haase, J. E. (2014). Developing an organizing framework to guide nursing research in the Children's Oncology Group (COG). *Seminars in Oncology Nursing*, *1*, 17–25. doi: 10.1016/j.soncn.2013.12.004

Kobasa, S. C. (1982). Commitment and coping in stress resistance among lawyers. *Journal of Personality and Social Psychology*, *42*(4), 707–717. doi: 10.1037/0022-3514.42.4.707

Landier, W., Leonard, M., & Ruccione, K. S. (2013). Children's Oncology Group's 2013 blueprint for research: Nursing discipline. *Pediatric Blood & Cancer*, *60*(6), 1031–1036.

Luthar, S. S., & Cicchetti, D. (2000). The construct of resilience: Implications for interventions and social policies. *Development and Psychopathology*, *12*(4), 857–885.

Luthar, S. S., Cicchetti, D., & Becker, B. (2000). The construct of resilience: A critical evaluation and guidelines for future work. *Child Development*, *71*(3), 543–562.

Mandleco, B. L., & Peery, J. C. (2000). An organizational framework for conceptualizing resilience in children. *Journal of Child and Adolescent Psychiatric Nursing*, *13*(3), 99–111.

Masten, A. S. (2001). Ordinary magic. Resilience processes in development. *American Psychologist*, *56*(3), 227–238.

Masten, A. S. (2007). Resilience in developing systems: Progress and promise as the fourth wave rises. *Development and Psychopathology*, *19*, 921–930.

Masten, A. S., & Coatsworth, J. D. (1998). The development of competence in favorable and unfavorable environments. Lessons from research on successful children. *American Psychologist*, *53*(2), 205–220.

McAllister, M., & Walsh, K. (2003). CARE: A framework for mental health practice. *Journal of Psychiatric and Mental Health Nursing*, *10*(1), 39–48.

McCubbin, H., & McCubbin, M. (1996). Resiliency in families: A conceptual model of family adjustment and adaptation in response to stress and crisis. In H. I. McCubbin, A. I. Thompson, & M. A. McCubbin (Eds.), *Family assessment: Resiliency, coping and adaptation—Inventories for research and practice* (pp. 1–64). Madison, WI: University of Wisconsin System.

McDonald, G., Jackson, D., Wilkes, L., & Vickers, M. H. (2013). Personal resilience in nurses and midwives: Effects of work-based educational intervention. *Contemporary Nurse*, *45*(1), 134–143.

Mead, G. H. (1952). Mind, self and society. In C. W. Morris (Ed.), *Mind, self and society*. Chicago, IL: University of Chicago Press.

Mealer, M., Hodapp, R., Conrad, D., Dimidjian, S., Rothbaum, B. O., & Moss, M. (2017). Designing a resilience program for critical care nurses. *AACN Advanced Critical Care, 28*(4), 359–365.

Megele, C. (2011). How to … develop emotional resilience. *Community Care, 17*(1857), 30.

Mullins, L. L., Molzon, E. S., Suorsa, K. I., Tackett, A. P., Pai, A. L. H., & Chaney, J. M. (2015). Models of resilience: Developing psychosocial interventions for parents of children with chronic health conditions. *Family Relations, 64*(1), 176–189. doi: 10.1111/fare.12104

Murphy, L., & Moriarty, A. (1976). *Vulnerability, coping and growth from infancy to adolescence*. New Haven, CT: Yale University Press.

Pettit, G. S. (2000). Mechanisms in the cycle of maladaptation: The life-course perspective. *Prevention and Treatment, 3*(35), 1–8.

Phillips, C. R., & Haase, J. E. (2018). *Feasibility, acceptability, and usefulness of the resilience enhancement for adolescents and young adults with cancer and healthcare providers (REACH) intervention*. Podium presentation at the International Society of Paediatric Oncology, Kyoto, Japan.

Power, A. K. (2010). Transforming the nation's health: Next steps in mental health promotion. *American Journal of Public Health, 100*(12), 2343–2346.

Rew, L., & Horner, S. D. (2003). Youth Resilience Framework for reducing health-risk behaviors in adolescents. *Journal of Pediatric Nursing, 18*(6), 379–388.

Reyes, A. T., Kearney, C. A., Lee, H., Isla, K., & Estrada, J. (2018). Interventions for posttraumatic stress with resilience as outcome: an integrative review. *Issues in Mental Health Nursing, 39*(2), 166–178.

Richardson, G. E. (2002). The metatheory of resilience and resiliency. *Journal of Clinical Psychology, 58*(3), 307–321.

Robb, S., Burns, D., Stegenga, K., Haut, P., Monahan, P., Meza, J., … Haase, J. E. (2014). Randomized clinical trial of therapeutic music video intervention for resilience outcomes in adolescents/young adults undergoing hematopoietic stem cell transplant: A report from the Children's Oncology Group. *Cancer, 120*, 909–917. doi: 10.1002/cncr.28355

Rosenbaum, M. (1983). Learned resourcefulness as a behavioral repertoire for the self-regulation of internal events. In M. Rosenbaum, C. M. Franks, & Y. Jaffe (Eds.), *Perspectives on behavior therapy in the eighties* (pp. 54–73). New York, NY: Springer.

Rutter, M. (1979). Protective factors in children's responses to stress and disadvantage. *Annals of the Academy of Medicine, Singapore, 8*(3), 324–338.

Rutter, M. (1987). Psychosocial resilience and protective mechanisms. *American Journal of Orthopsychiatry, 57*(3), 316–331.

Sanders, E. D. (2015). Nursing resilience: A nursing opportunity. *Nursing Administration Quarterly, 39*(2), 132–136. doi: 10.1097/NAQ.000000000000091

Singer, B. H., & Ryff, C. (2001). *New horizons in health: An integrative approach*. Washington, DC: National Academy Press.

Sinnema, G. (1991). Resilience among children with special health-care needs and among their families. *Pediatric Annals, 20*(9), 483–486.

Svavarsdottir, E. K., McCubbin, M. A., & Kane, J. H. (2000). Well-being of parents of young children with asthma. *Research in Nursing & Health, 23*(5), 346–358.

Szanton, S. L., & Gill, J. M. (2010). Facilitating resilience using a society-to-cells framework: A theory of nursing essentials applied to research and practice. *Advances in Nursing Science, 33*(4), 329–343. doi: 10.1097/ANS.013e3181fb2ea2

Szanton, S. L., Gill, J. M., & Thorpe, R. J. (2010). The society-to-cells model of resilience in older adults. *Annual Review of Gerontology and Geriatrics, 30*(1), 5–34. doi: 10.1891/0198-8794.30.5

Triandis, H. C., Bontempo, R., Villareal, M. J., Asai, M., & Lucca, N. (1988). Individualism and collectivism: Cross-culture perspectives on self-in-group relationships. *Journal of Personality and Social Psychology, 54*(2), 323–338.

van Kessel, G. (2013). The ability of older people to overcome adversity: A review of the resilience concept. *Geriatric Nursing, 34*, 122–127.

Vinson, J. A. (2002). Children with asthma: Initial development of the child resilience model. *Pediatric Nursing, 28*(2), 149–158.

Wagnild, G. M., & Young, H. M. (1993). Development and psychometric evaluation of the Resilience Scale. *Journal of Nursing Measurement, 1*(2), 165–178.

Waller, M. A. (2001). Resilience in ecosystemic context: Evolution of the concept. *American Journal of Orthopsychiatry, 71*(3), 290–297.

Ward, P. R., Muller, R., Tsourtos, G., Hersh, D., Lawn, S., Winefield, A. H., & Coveney, J. (2011). Additive and subtractive resilience strategies as enablers of biographical reinvention: A qualitative study of ex-smokers and never-smokers. *Social Science and Medicine, 72*, 1140–1148. doi: 10.1016/j.socscimed.2011.01.023

Wells, R., & Schwebel, A. (1987). Chronically ill children and their mothers: Predictors of resilience and vulnerability to hospitalization and surgical stress. *Journal of Developmental and Behavioral Pediatrics, 2*(2), 83–89.

Werner, E., & Smith, R. (1982). *Vulnerable but invincible: A longitudinal study of resilient children and youth*. New York, NY: McGraw-Hill.

West, C., Usher, K., & Foster, K. (2011). Family resilience: Towards a new model of chronic pain management. *Collegian, 18*, 3–10. doi: 10.1016/jcolegn.2010.004

White, K. R. (1995). The transition from victim to victor: Application of the theory of mastery. *Journal of Psychosocial Nursing and Mental Health Services, 33*(8), 41–44.

White, N., Bichter, J., Koeckeritz, J., Lee, Y. A., & Munch, K. L. (2002). A cross-cultural comparison of family resiliency in hemodialysis patients. *Journal of Transcultural Nursing, 13*(3), 218–227.

Windle, G. (2011). What is resilience? A review and concept analysis. *Reviews in Clinical Gerontology, 21*, 152–169. doi: 10.1017/S09592598110000420

Windle, G., Bennett, K. M., & Noyes, J. (2011). A methodological review of measurement scales. *Health and Quality of Life Outcomes, 33*(4), 329–343. doi: 10.1186/1477-7525-9-8

# 18 Planned Change

Timothy S. Bredow and Kennith Culp

## Definition of Key Terms

| | |
|---|---|
| **Change agent** | As in chemistry where a catalyst helps a reaction to proceed, a change agent is a person or event that aids or promotes a change to take place in a person or an organization. |
| **Change process** | The change process is the series of events that occur over a period of time to bring a person or an organization to a different place or level of operation that they have not been at, as evidenced by either a shift in behavior or a new and different processes for carrying out business operations. This process is impacted by both internal and external people and/or events. |
| **Planned change** | Change may occur randomly or as part of natural evolution. However, planned change as reviewed here implies a deliberative process. Such a process is controlled and suggests a conscious process undertaken to alter the status quo. |

One of the challenges of nursing is the rapid pace of change as it relates to knowledge development, health science technology, and the economics of health care delivery. Clinical practice is changing constantly and there are many challenges related to translating evidence into practice, but inevitably some notion of change will be involved. Change theory is well-developed historically (Marris, 2014), but casual pathways to motivating clinicians and/or patients to change their behavior or way of thinking are evolving. Why does change come so hard for people? Why are attitudes so critical to change and why is it frightening? Attempts to change attitudes and behavior are extremely complex, and oftentimes it begins with being unhappy or discontent with the status quo (Vogel & Wanke, 2016).

Change theory is a component of many aspects of nursing. Advances in medical technology and nursing science necessitate change, clinicians who remain static in their treatment approaches and assessment techniques will not succeed in their careers, and, most likely, patients will not benefit from the advancements of lower cost and better care offered by the change. Indeed, some clinicians and patients can engage in fake behavior under forced-change conditions or in an extremely regulated environment (Fisher, Robie, Christiansen, & Komar, 2018), but it is better to adopt change theory when introducing change in either individual clients or organizations (Deci & Ryan, 2000).

Advanced nursing practice role competencies underscore expertise in being a change agent leader in all types of settings; some examples are school nursing (Davis, 2018), inpatient mental health care (Wyder et al., 2017), outpatient clinics (Padilha, Sousa, & Pereira, 2018), and inpatient quality improvement initiatives (Repique, Vernig, Lowe, Thompson, & Yap, 2016). Also, planned organizational change is a component of the midrange theory spectrum of change. For example, complex curriculum reorganization in nursing schools (Ferguson, DiGiacomo, Gholizadeh, Ferguson, & Hickman, 2017), policy, and procedure change in hospitals related to accreditation standards (Tuck & Hough, 2017) involve changing the entire departments or work sections. In the area of professional development, change can seem more invasive if we want to modify the procedure for evaluating peers for clinical practice proficiencies (DiLibero, DeSanto-Madyea, & O'Dongohue, 2016). Interdisciplinary care may involve change theory, for example, fragmented care or lack of communication between clinical specialists may require modifications in how care is delivered so that interdisciplinary teams can work together to solve patient problems (Suva et al., 2018).

Change theory is often used as either a standalone model or as a synchronous conceptual framework in many capstone experiences for the Doctor of Nursing Practice (DNP) degree (Campbell, Gilbert, & Laustsen, 2014) and clinical nurse leader (CNL) program implementation projects (Harris, Roussel, & Thomas, 2014). Nursing student projects have occasionally been critiqued for not refining the theoretical framework to the issue/research question or selecting an overly generic change model when planning clinical initiatives (McEwen, 2018). Thus, the relationship between change theory, research, and practice is reciprocal in nature and is mutually beneficial if incorporated into the practice problem even if "change" is not the key emphasis or theoretical approach in these student projects.

Nurses often borrow theories from the social sciences to guide interventions aimed at individual and community behavior change (Henry, 2018). Indeed, evidence supports positive outcomes when using the Lewin's change model in health care organizations (Shirey, 2013), but does Lewin really explain all of the factors involved in changed behavior when applied in the personal health? Would intentional change theory (ITC) and interactive health coaching be more appropriate (Boyatzis & Jack, 2018)? In the area of organizational change, stakeholder analysis (Godakandage et al., 2017) is another tool to develop collaborations and identify key individuals who may adopt or impede transitions initiated by the change agent (Mazur & Pisarski, 2015; Sucala, Nilsen, & Muench, 2017). Additionally, the use of the aware, desire, knowledge, ability, and reinforcement (ADKAR) change management model can be used to guide the process principles (Pawl & Anderson, 2017). This ADKAR is also useful in identifying stakeholders.

One might wonder why using a process implementation theory might be needed. After all, don't we have the patient's best interest at heart in our change and isn't that the most important thing? Implementation theories provide the overall guidelines for all aspects of planned practice change including assessment, implementation, and evaluation. For too long, nurses have identified issues in practice and tried to implement changes to affect health outcomes based on best intentions and a desire to provide "good care." However, without a systematic approach based on implantation theory, the change planner may not have included all stakeholders, nor worked to engage buy-in, nor fully assessed the individual's and organization's readiness for change. This attempt at practice change would certainly be more likely to fail.

This chapter reviews three common theories aimed at affecting individual health behavior: (a) the Health Belief Model (HBM), (b) the Theory of Planned Behavior (TPB), and (c) the Self-Determination Theory (SDT). Two additional theories aimed at system or community implementation of change reviewed include Lewin's Theory of Change and Roger's Diffusion of Innovations Theory.

## Historical Background

The practice discipline of nursing has a long history of examining how we might affect change on an individual level related to improving health choices and the use of planned change theories to change practice on an organizational level. Lewin (1947) was one of the first to take the concept of change and propose a model to try to explain the relationship of the concepts. Throughout his career, Lewin was interested in resolving social conflict, which he felt was the only way to improve the human condition (Burnes, 2004). His change theory was influenced by his earlier work in field theory, group dynamics, and action research. His work in group dynamics, with his emphasis on focusing on group change instead of individual change, was an integral component of his three-step model of planned change (Burnes & Cooke, 2013). Other attempts to identify additional factors that affect change built upon Lewin's groundbreaking work. The HBM was first presented in 1975 along with the theory of reasoned action in that same year. The theory of reasoned action preceded and gave rise to the TPB in 1991. All of these theories are considered as borrowed theories for nursing purposes because they are authored by nonnurses, but can readily be used by nursing professional to help describe, explain, or predict change that happens in a variety of nursing situations in clinical practice. The health promotion model published by Pender in 1982 is a nurse authored middle range theory that is covered in Chapter 13 of this text. SDT revolutionized the psychology of human motivation for change and was developed by Ryan and Deci in 2000. Since then, much work has been done to determine the strength of the relationships between the factors and concepts proposed by each of these three theories and will be presented in this chapter.

## The Health Belief Model

The HBM was developed by social psychologists (Becker & Maiman, 1975) and the United States Public Health Service in an effort to explain why healthy people did not engage in programs to prevent or detect illness. During the ensuing years, the model has been modified (Rosenstock, Strecher, & Becker, 1988) to include behavior in response to diagnosed illness, especially with one's ability to adhere to medical regimens and to apply to people's beliefs regarding symptoms (Clark & Janevic, 2014).

The model is premised on the belief that people will take action to prevent or screen for illness if they perceive themselves to be susceptible to the condition, believe that occurrence of the condition has serious consequences, believe that the course of action they may take will ameliorate or prevent the condition, and believe that the benefits of taking action outweigh the barriers to behavior change (Champion & Skinner, 2008). These dimensions make up the structure of the HBM and define factors that influence the individual's likelihood of engaging in the recommended behavior change.

## DESCRIPTION OF THE THEORY

Perceived susceptibility represents the individual's subjective perception of his or her own risk of contracting a health condition (Fig. 18.1). In individuals with an already diagnosed illness, this component encompasses one's acceptance of the diagnosis, beliefs of disease progression, and susceptibility to illness in general.

Perceived severity addresses one's beliefs regarding the seriousness of contracting an illness or leaving it untreated. Both medical and clinical consequences affect this dimension and include such factors as death, disability, pain, and other symptoms. Additionally, social factors related to illness such as effects of contracting the illness on family, work, and social relationships are included here (Pender, 2011). Perceived benefit is also important as it applies to change; this helps to internalize motivation. An example of this would be the perceived treatment benefits of controlling

anxiety symptoms in clients with socially stigmatizing symptoms from a chronic anxiety disorder (Langley, Wootton, & Grieve, 2017).

The combination of susceptibility and severity has been labeled as perceived threat. As depicted in the model, susceptibility to a perceived threat of disease, illness progression, or adverse symptom affects the individual's likelihood of making a healthy behavior change, but is not the only intervening factor.

Likelihood of action is also affected by perceived benefits and perceived barriers to behavior change. Perceived benefits of behavior change may be health related (decreased symptoms, decreased morbidity and mortality) and nonhealth related (make a loved one happy and save money). A belief that the action taken will be efficacious in preventing or reducing disease effects is necessary, in addition to perceived susceptibility and severity behavior change, for healthy behavior action.

Potentially negative aspects of a health action are the perceived barriers. These barriers include such factors as expense, level of danger (i.e., negative side effects or iatrogenic outcomes), unpleasantness, inconvenience, and length of time for treatment. Although not presented in the early model, the concept of self-efficacy, or the belief in one's ability to take health action, is now postulated as part of the HBM. Rosenstock et al. (1988) suggest that the lack of self-efficacy is perceived as a barrier to successful health behavior change. Janz and Becker (1984) offer that a subconscious cost–benefit analysis of the benefits versus the barriers occurs. In the end, the perceived benefits minus the perceived barriers

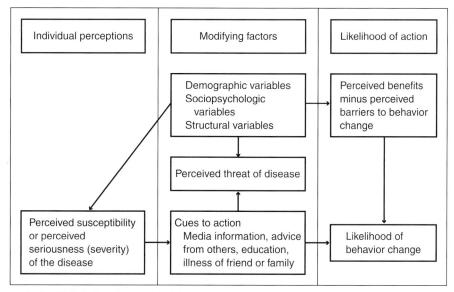

**Figure 18.1**    The health belief model. (Modified from Pender, N. J. (2011). *Health promotion in nursing practice* (6th ed., p. 36). Stamford, CT: Appleton & Lange.)

to behavior change affect an individual's likelihood of action.

ITC and the HBM might be helpful in some projects for building a theoretical framework for changing personal health behavior. For example, ITC proposes that changing a person's perception of perceived benefit could be enhanced by arousing positive emotions to the desired positive behavior via a personal health coach (Boyatzis & Jack, 2018). Since perceived vulnerability in the HBM is somewhat self-regulating as a motivator as it is a negative emotion, a positive emotion for change can be a stabilizing factor. In the ITC model, vision-focused coaching with compassion creates a motivation to change as the person envisions enhanced health and well-being (Howard, 2015). Nurses are skilled at health coaching and empathy, yet ITC is seldom mentioned outside the field of psychology.

## APPLICATION OF THE HBM IN PRACTICE

Social marketing of an intervention program (SIMP) to influence Ghana women to participate in a breast cancer screening campaign was initiated using a HBM approach with $N = 363$ participants in this West African study (Tweneboah-Koduah, 2018). Ghana has limited resources for tertiary care of breast cancer patients, so primary prevention is of great importance and changing breast cancer prevention behavior to include breast self-exams is somewhat novel in this region given the tribal and cultural norms. Researchers performed an extensive cross-sectional survey of the Ghanaian middle-class women and assessed their willingness to engage in a healthy behavior related to cancer screening based on cues to action, self-efficacy, and perceived susceptibility.

The participants had interesting views on the disease: 26.2% of the respondents identified environmental factors as the major cause of breast cancer and 44.9% attributed breast cancer to such factors as spiritual beliefs and too much breast-feeding. Researchers found that 25.1% were convinced that breast cancer disease could be best prevented through prayer. Based on these results, the investigators felt that designing and implementing an intervention based on HBM could result in changing behavior toward breast cancer prevention. The component of perceived susceptibility was the most powerful single predictor changing these West African women's behavior related to breast cancer screening. The study recommended that to change the breast cancer–protective behavior of these Ghanaian women, SMIP should raise the susceptibility levels of women in Ghana with a social campaign that addresses vulnerability and also addresses the erroneous and superstitions causes identified.

# Theory of Planned Behavior

TPB evolved from the reasoned action model in the social sciences (Montano, Kasprzyk, & Taplin, 1997) and morphed over time to its application related to health behavior (Fishbein, Ajzen, Albarracin, & Hornik, 2007). The TPB approach examines the relationships between beliefs, attitudes, intentions, and behavior (Fishbein & Ajzen, 2010). Analytical persuasion is more powerful in changing health behavior as opposed to simply being authoritative and instructing a patient on healthy habits as a health care provider. The theory recognizes social norms, but also encourages analytical reasoning when applied to health behavior. For example, childhood sun exposure and parental adoption of sun-protective behavior are enhanced by reasoning with parents on other types of childhood-protective behavior and appealing to their perception of the normative pattern of other parents on the beach (Hamilton, Kirkpatrick, Rebar, & Hagger, 2017).

## DESCRIPTION OF THE THEORY

The TPB asserts that the most important predictor of behavior is an individual's behavioral intention as seen in Figure 18.2. Behavioral intention is an important concept in TPB; it's the perceived likelihood of performing a behavior. Intentions are the most prominent and important predictor of behavior and capture the psychology of motivation to engage in changed behavior (Montanaro, Kershaw, & Bryan, 2018). Intention is affected by three types of beliefs including behavioral beliefs, normative beliefs, and control beliefs. Planned behavior theory blends social phenomena and the scientific knowledge of social sciences in an analytical manner that is applicable to understanding change in health behavior (Scalco, Ceschi, & Sartori, 2018). For example, TPB has been used as a theoretical framework for change in how to recruit new donors to a bone marrow registry by campaigns that dealt with both good intentions and the normative beliefs of young college students (Hyde, McLaren, & White, 2014).

Intention is directly determined through one's attitude toward performing the behavior and subjective norm. Each dimension consists of two determining factors. Attitude toward the behavior is determined through behavioral beliefs (beliefs about the outcomes or attributes of performing the behavior) weighted by evaluations of those outcomes or attributes. Therefore, an individual with strong beliefs that mostly positive outcomes will result from performing a behavior will have a positive attitude toward that behavior. A person

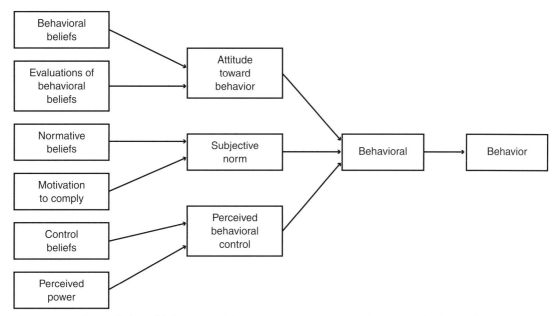

**Figure 18.2**  Theory of planned behavior (TPB). (From Montano, D. E., & Kasprzyk, D. (2008). The theory of reasoned action, theory of planned behavior, and the integrated behavioral model. In K. Glanz, B. K. Rimber, & K. Viswanath (Eds.), *Health behavior and health education: Theory, research, and practice* (4th ed., pp. 67–96). San Francisco, CA: Jossey Bass.)

with mostly negative beliefs of the outcome of a behavior will have a negative attitude toward that behavior.

Subjective norms are determined through an individual's perceptions of whether or not other individuals important to them approve or disapprove of the behavior (normative beliefs) weighted by the individual's motivation to comply with those referent others. Thus, a person who believes that others think a behavior should be performed, and who is motivated to comply with those expectations, will have a positive subjective norm. A negative subjective norm is a result of an individual's belief that important referents believe he or she should not undertake the behavior.

**APPLICATION OF THE THEORY IN PRACTICE**

Smokers who attended a smoking cessation clinic in a community hospital in southern Taiwan ($N = 148$) were randomly selected to analyze the contribution of TPB in predicting actual quitting behavior 6 months after the clinic ended (Tseng et al., 2018). This study suggested that it was easier to quit smoking in those participants who scored higher on the intention subscales. They found that individuals' social norms about smoking and verbalizing the considerable time effort in trying to quit, then relapsing, and then attempting again were "more intentioned" in their smoking cessation.

# Self-Determination Theory

Self-Determination Theory (SDT) is based on the central idea that if a person establishes major goals, their activities are internal and autonomous rather than controlled by external forces (Deci & Ryan, 2002). The premise of the theory is on "internalized" social acceptance and emerges in a context that supports individual autonomy, relatedness, and competence (Assor, Feinberg, Kanat-Maymon, & Kaplan, 2018). This model is in contrast to some of the other change theory approaches that imply suppressing personal autonomy (Deci & Ryan, 2000). One notion of SDT is that changes in behavior are a cyclical process; change comes with clear limits and structure, but comes from self-adoption rather than external influences (Ryan & Deci, 2000). Intrinsic motivation contrasts with extrinsic motivation where an individual is compelled to change.

**DESCRIPTION OF THE THEORY**

Every human being has three basic needs: autonomy, competence, and relatedness. A person can change their behavior when they learn from negative experiences (personal growth) and enact intentions to change (Koole, Schlinkert, Maldei, & Baumann, 2019). Being "intentioned" means a person must be internally motivated to change;

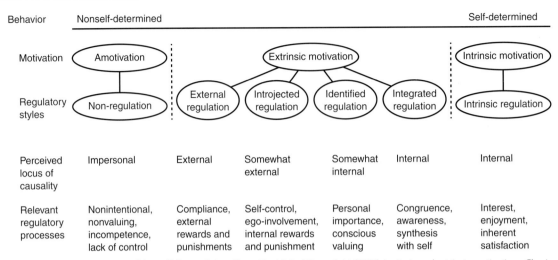

**Figure 18.3**    Components of the self-determinism. (From Deci, E. L., & Ryan, R. M. (2000). Intrinsic and extrinsic motivations: Classic definition and new directions. *Contemporary Educational Psychology, 25*(1), 54–67.)

otherwise, there is no inspiration to do so. Human motivation in SDT actually contains a taxonomy organized into three regulatory styles: amotivation, extrinsic motivation, and intrinsic motivation (see Fig. 18.3). These three classifications of motivation are inherent to understanding SDT: (a) in contrast to external motivation, internal SDT motivation is invigorating, (b) internal motivation divorces itself cognitively from amotivation and external pressures because it is based on an attitude of self-willingness to change, and (c) goals for change are self-endorsed and occur more rapidly than the cognitive process of adopting external norms established by others (Koole et al., 2019). Understanding these three differences embraces the self-determination model.

Amotivation is perceived as impersonal. External or extrinsic motivation is a slow cognitive process where change is integrated into a hierarchical synthesis of goals or achievements (Lemos & Veríssimo, 2014). Extrinsic motivation is unidimensional, a thought process related to endorsing goals initiated by one's social network powerful others. Intrinsic motivation or self-determination as described in SDT is described more as change resulting from different reasons and goals because it is inherently enjoyable or interesting to the individual.

In Self-Determination Theory, the need for competence means the desire is to be self-controlling but also to be connected to caring others (relatedness). Autonomy means knowing how things will turn out and that these outcomes or goals are the results are of self-initiated actions. The need for autonomy does not mean to be independent but rather a sense

of free will when acting in harmony with an integrated self. This is often a challenge, for example, in new spinal cord injury patients who may struggle with autonomy and relatedness in their rehabilitation (Sweet et al., 2018). An individual is intrinsically motivated to change their behavior when they are motivated to do something they enjoy or find some benefit from their own actions.

## APPLICATION OF THE THEORY IN PRACTICE

Self-Determination Theory has implications for helping individuals accomplish positive change related to their health. The strategies and techniques used to help internalize and modify behaviors relate to a variety of behaviors. These include pain management (Brooks et al., 2017), management of depression symptoms (Cecchini, Fernandez-Rio, Mendez-Gimenez, Carriedo, & Arruza, 2017), compulsive behavior like gambling (Kushnir, Godinho, Hodgins, Hendershot, & Cunningham, 2016), and weight loss or obesity self-management (Guertin, Barbeau, Pelletier, & Martinelli, 2017; Trief, Cibula, Delahanty, & Weinstock, 2017). Strategies may be well-thought out, subtle, and ingrained in nature and self-empowering for health outcomes to be positively changed (Garces-Ozanne, Kalu, & Audas, 2016).

Low-income women of color (WOC) with human immunodeficiency virus (HIV) frequently encounter barriers to care, are subject to ridicule and harassment from their partner, and are psychologically depressed (Quinlivan, Messer, Roytburd, & Blickman, 2017). These researchers examined levels of satisfaction and core self-determination and found that violence and addiction were common co-occurring illnesses and experiences. These WOC needed social support as they felt helpless and a loss of autonomy when they learned of their diagnosis. Quinlivan and colleagues used that Basic Needs Satisfaction in General (BNSG) Scale with subscales that measured autonomy, relatedness, and competency in $N = 189$ participants. Their average age was 46 years and 28% had less than high school education. The researchers found that alcohol and drug use was strongly associated with loss of relatedness (alcohol $\beta = -1.93$, 95% CI = $-3.27$ to $-0.60$ and a similar result was found for drug use $\beta = -1.65$; 95% CI = $-2.89$ to $-0.41$). In these HIV-infected WOC, reductions in all three subscales revealed more affective depression symptoms. For these women to change their outlook related to HIV and move forward with positive health choices, the researchers recommended a supportive social network and activities that facilitated a greater sense of competency (e.g., completing their high school education).

## Organizational Change Theories

### LEWIN'S THEORY OF CHANGE

Kurt Lewin wrote "Change and constancy are relative concepts: group life is never without change, merely differences in the amount and type of change exist" (Lewin, 1947, p. 13). The "differences in the amount and type of change" are ever-present in the field of health care. There is no health care system in the United States that is not constantly in a state of equilibrium with driving and restraining forces. The prominence of change in the field of nursing is so great that nurses have established a new doctoral degree, the doctorate of nursing practice (DNP), in part to implement change. The main goal of the role of the DNP is translation of research or changing practice to reflect the current level of evidence.

### Description of the Theory

Lewin's theory appears deceptively simple with only three components to planned change: unfreezing, moving, and refreezing (Lewin, 1947). The difficult part of this theory involves identifying and understanding driving forces and restraining forces of the planned change. The first step of the theory, unfreezing, involves destabilizing the "quasi-stationary equilibrium" (Burnes, 2004) is seen in Figure 18.4. The individual, group, and/or institution must come to recognize that the current pattern of behavior is no longer the best way of doing things. This is where the driving forces and restraining forces are in play.

Driving forces are the events or circumstances that make the change at best appealing and at worst at least necessary. Restraining forces are the events or circumstances that inhibit change. For the change process to begin, the driving forces must be larger than the restraining forces. Although driving forces and restraining forces are easily defined, they are not always easily identified in an institutional setting. Many factors such as group norms, psychological safety, and individual and group beliefs are a part of the forces. The change agent must take time to reflect on as many restraining forces as possible, since they can be difficult to overcome.

Once unfreezing has occurred, the moving step can follow. Moving is where the actual change takes place. This step should be easier than unfreezing because once the process has come to this point, the driving forces were able to overcome the restraining forces. Moving, however, is not the end of the process. The next step is refreezing or ensuring that the changed way of operating is a part of the new "quasi-stationary equilibrium." The new quasi-stationary equilibrium becomes the

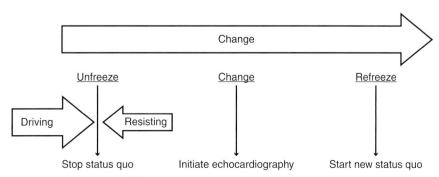

**Figure 18.4**  Lewin's force field analysis.

## USING MIDDLE RANGE THEORIES IN PRACTICE PROJECTS     18.1

**Project Title:** Development of a Protocol for Safety and Role Responsibilities for Care of Patients Requiring Emergent Hyperbaric Therapy.

**Project Purpose:** Inconsistencies in the team approach to preparing patients requiring emergent hyperbaric therapy were identified as a patient safety and quality issue that poses a potential threat to patients. A uniform safety checklist was developed using the current best evidence to help improve and ensure consistent delivery of care.

**Theoretical Perspective Used in the Project:** Kurt Lewin's theory of planned change provided guidance to the change project as the best practice safety checklist was developed for use for the unique needs of the hyperbaric environment.

**Project Team and Work Plan:** All members of the interdisciplinary team working the hyperbaric unit met to complete and evaluate a systematic review of the literature applicable to patients requiring hyperbaric therapy. Gaps in quality were identified and opportunities with an effective method of quality improvement were implemented. A best practice safety checklist was developed and put into practice in the hyperbaric unit.

**Project Outcomes:** Evaluation of outcomes on every checklist used for every patient admitted to the unit was performed. The date from this review demonstrated that there was an improvement of start times by 10 to 15 minutes after the new checklist was implemented. Additionally, all team members felt an improvement in communication, and cohesive teamwork had occurred with the implementation of the new checklist.

**Conclusions:** The change project was completed on time and team moral was enhanced. A safety checklist is an efficient tool to use in the hyperbaric unit.

*Author: Omodt, S. M. (2015). Unpublished Masters Project, Bethel University.*

status quo and, technically speaking, the new environment for the next process of change. (See Using Middle Range Theories in Practice Projects 18.1.)

## ROGERS' DIFFUSION OF INNOVATIONS THEORY

Everett Rogers' (2003) *Diffusion of Innovations* Theory for new knowledge dissemination and adoption has in the past several years become more widely cited in the health care change literature. Rogers defines diffusion as a special type of communication concerned with new knowledge diffusion. This communication is a process in which participants create and share information with one another in order to reach a mutual understanding. Because the process involves new information, there is a degree of uncertainty on the part of the receivers or people or social systems in which adoption of the innovation is expected to occur. The innovator utilizes the innovation-development process and the innovation-decision process to implement new knowledge or behavior and utilizes information in hopes of ameliorating uncertainty among adopters. Central to the Rogers model is consideration of characteristics of the innovation itself and attributes of the adopters that can affect success of the innovation diffusion across the group. Rogers defines the process of diffusion that includes an innovation, communication, time, and social systems. Rogers connects these concepts to one another noting that "The main elements in the diffusion of new ideas

are: (a) an *innovation* (b) that is *communicated* through certain *channels* (c) over *time* (d) among the members of a *social system*" (p. 36).

### Description of the theory

The innovation-development process is the entire time and activities that occur between one person becoming aware of the need for change through adoption and diffusion. Rogers (2003) defined five steps in this process: (a) awareness, (b) interest, (c) evaluation, (d), trial, and (e) adoption. Mitchell (2013) described how these stages have been compared to the three stages of the Lewin change model as well. Awareness as defined by Rogers is when disequilibrium is introduced into the system, creating a need for change. This is analogous to Lewin's "unfreezing" category. Interest, evaluation, and trial are stages in which change planners gather all available information and solve any problems, develop a detailed plan of change, and test the innovation. Mitchell noted the consistency with those three stages in Diffusion of Innovations with the "moving" stage in Lewin's theory. Finally, adoption occurs and is maintained in the system. This is also similar to the "refreezing" stage in the Lewin theory.

The innovation-decision process is the procedure through which an individual, group, or institution passes while considering and then implementing a new idea or innovation. This five-stage process includes knowledge, persuasion, decision, implementation, and confirmation (Rogers, 2003).

Rogers (2003) described knowledge as the first stage in the sequential process of innovation decision-making. Knowledge occurs when a person (or other decision-making party) becomes aware of the innovation and gains understanding of its function and potential use. DiCenso, Guyatt, and Ciliska (2005) noted that the innovation adoption process begins with identification of the most current and highest level literature available. Furthermore, DiCenso et al. suggested that there is a hierarchy of preprocessed sources that includes the following levels from highest to lowest: (a) systems level includes practice guidelines, clinical pathways, or evidence-based textbook summaries, (b) synopses of syntheses level include synopses of systematic reviews, (c) syntheses level is a systematic review of all the evidence addressing a clinical area, (d) synopses of single studies, and (e) single studies. When finding or developing knowledge for evidence-based innovation, one should search for the highest level and most current information available. It is only after identifying this literature that one may move to the next stage.

DiCenso et al. (2005) suggested that during the persuasion stage, decision-makers and other practitioners form opinions about the innovation and consider its consequences. Characteristics of the innovation, organization, environment, and individuals involved need to be assessed for influence on the decision to adopt or reject an innovation.

Rogers (2003) noted that the characteristics specific to the innovation include its perceived relative advantage compared to current practice and compatibility with the existing values, beliefs, and needs of the organization. Also important is the extent of the innovation and if it can be adopted in segments or on a small scale in which adopter may "try out" the innovation to determine its advantages and disadvantages. It is also critical that the benefits of the innovation be observable to the adopters. The measurable outcomes should be indicators valued in the organization or unit. Finally, the innovation is more likely to be adopted if adopters perceive advantages and that the innovation has low levels of complexity.

Individual characteristics assessed include opinion leadership or the level of influence one unit of change has on others. Innovativeness or the degree to which an individual is relatively earlier in adopting new ideas than other members of the social system and likely rate of adoption is also important. Rogers (2003) defines adopter categories or classifications of the members of the social system based on their innovativeness. These categories include innovators, early adopters, early majority, late majority, and laggards. Haider and Kreps (2004) note the importance of finding innovators and working to make them champions for the innova-

tion as well as the early inclusion of those laggards who have high levels of organizational influence.

Environmental characteristics important in assessment include decision-making autonomy, urban or rural nature, prestige, competition, and peer pressure. Environments that have more autonomy are urban, understand the prestige in providing innovative care, and engage in a sense of competition with other care systems are more likely to adopt innovations supported by current and high-level literature.

Important organizational characteristics include structural influences such as complexity and functional differentiation. Also, workplace culture, communication systems, leadership support, and resources for innovation are important in assessment. Rogers (2003) distinguished the notion that organizations with greater complexity and functional divisions have higher rates of innovation adoption. Also, workplace culture that values use of research evidence has functional communication systems, decision-making that is decentralized, and whose leaders value the change is more likely to successfully adopt new ideas.

Key stakeholders are those individuals or groups that can directly or indirectly affect the decision to adopt an innovation (DiCenso et al., 2005). It is important to have the early involvement and support of those identified as key stakeholders. A stakeholder analysis will help determine the values, beliefs, and interests of the key decision-makers. Through this analysis, champions of the innovation are identified. Additionally, the decision is made to either adopt or refuse to adopt the innovation.

Rogers (2004) described implementation as the new idea or innovation being put to use in the social system. DiCenso et al. (2005) offered several strategies to promote implementation of an innovation. Those methods most likely to result in adoption of the innovation are multifaceted in nature. DiCenso suggests that education conducted by a peer with individuals in their own practice settings is the most effective with changing provider prescribing and ordering practice. Additionally, reminders provide reinforcement of the innovation. Technology should also be used as appropriate. Rogers (2003) noted that in the confirmation stage, evidence of adoption is examined. Additionally, the adopter seeks reinforcement for the innovation decision that has already been made. Reinforcement needs to occur or the adopter may discontinue the use of the innovation.

The process of diffusion of innovation through communication channels over time in a social system can be influenced by members of the social system. Potential for innovation adoption may be assessed using the innovation-decision model. The first three stages of the five-stage model include thinking and decision-making processes. The decision of key stakeholders to adopt an innovation is dependent on the level of knowledge and current nature of the evidence or research supporting the innovation. Additionally, factors related to the innovation itself, organization, environment, and individuals expected to change all must be assessed in the persuasion stage. If the decision has been made to adopt an innovation, confirmation of the adoption and the benefits of the adoption must be relayed to those involved to reinforce continued innovation use.

## Process-Oriented Change Concepts

### SWOT

The challenge of adopting innovation into complex health care networks is daunting. Many nurses use the strength, weakness, opportunities, and threat (SWOT) analysis approach. While of some value, SWOT has historically been articulated with the diffusion of innovation framework as described above, but eventually all innovations lose the novelty (Peng & Vlas, 2017). Has SWOT exhausted its usefulness in nursing and health care as some have suggested (Meeks, 2017)? Shin and Dess argue that SWOT may be a good first step to organizational change as it helps to persuade change agents to compile lists (Shin & Dess, 2017). This can be done via public forums or small group discussions, listening campaigns, and informational interviews with stakeholders. Data collection will help inform the community members and workers when developing the SWOT analysis.

### ADKAR

Systematic change in an organization means identifying the roles of key players who may be involved in the change process. Hiatt's five elements of ADKAR change can be used to develop sequential approach to organizational change (Hiatt & Creasey, 2003). These elements are described in Using Middle Range Theories in Practice Projects 18.1. As a change agent, the nurse can use the ADKAR model to identify resistance in specific individuals and to formulate a successful action for organizational change in a logical and sequential manner. The ADKAR model was used in moving a community hospital to the American Nurses Credentialing Center's Magnet Recognition Program (Arthurs et al., 2017) and also in merging nursing curriculum from two institutions (Pawl & Anderson, 2017). For nurses, the organizational

| BOX 18.2 | **Five Sequential Elements in the Adkar Change Model** |
|---|---|
| **Element** | **Characteristic** |
| Awareness | A person's view of the current state; how a person perceives problems, credibility and trust of the leader, misinformation, and rumors that circulate, disagreement of the need to change |
| Desire | The nature of change (incremental or large transformation), "What's in it for me?" An individual's personal life, intrinsic motivation—what motivates them? |
| Knowledge | The current knowledge base of an individual, the capacity and capability of the individual to gain additional knowledge, resources available for education, the access to expertise, and this knowledge for learning |
| Ability | Psychological blocks and fear, physical ability to work the new way, intellectual capability, the time available to develop the new skills, the availability of resources to develop those skills |
| Reinforcement | How meaningful to the individual is this change? Is the progress demonstrated and reinforced? Is there a no blame culture? Are there accountability systems in place? |

ADKAR change model offers sequential stages for implementing an evidenced-based practice change related to pulmonary care (Patton, Lim, Ramlow, & White, 2015). While ADKAR model is instrumental and helps to move individuals in an organization to adoption, it is also useful in helping to identify stakeholders in the organization and conducting a stakeholder analysis. (See Five Sequential Elements in the ADKAR Change Model 18.2.)

### STAKEHOLDER ANALYSIS

A stakeholder is a person, group, or organization that has an interest or concern in an organizational actions, objectives, and policies (Powers, Knapp, Powers, & Edd, 2010). Stakeholder analysis is a way to delineate the interests of others, identify potential issues that could disrupt project implementation, and as a last resort manage those who are negative toward the project and simply must be "pulled along" in order to introduce change into the organizational environment. It's best to start by constructing a list of stakeholders (Bullen & Brack, 2015) and recording a few perceptions about the change project after

| BOX 18.3 | **Stakeholder Template** | | | | | | |
|---|---|---|---|---|---|---|---|
| **Stakeholder Name/Title** | **Contact Person** *Phone, e-mail, and address* | **Importance** *How impor- tant is the project to them? (low, medium, high)* | **Influence** *How much influence do they have over the project? (low, medium, high)* | **What Is Im- portant to the Stake- holder?** | **How could the Stake- holder Con- tribute to the Project?** | **How Could the Stake- holder Block the Project?** | **Strategy for Engag- ing the Stake- holder** |
| This is a modified template from Bullen and Brack (2015), and their tools4dev blog is licensed under a Creative Commons Attribution from https://creativecommons.org/licenses/by-sa/3.0/deed.en_US | | | | | | | |

talking with them about the project (see Box 18.3). It is sometimes difficult to determine the importance of both internal and external stakeholders (Mazur & Pisarski, 2015). Internal stakeholders could include project managers, executives, project sponsors, or other departments in the organization, which may play a vital role in executing or implementing a proj- ect (Sucala et al., 2017). External stakeholders could include clients, suppliers, and governing and/or accrediting agencies. Ideally, the stakeholder analy- sis should occur at the beginning of or at the stage of planning; this means some environmental assess- ment must be made as to the identification of the

stakeholders as to the impact and influence change process; the scope can be project or activity.

For the change agent to be effective, conducting a stakeholder matrix (Fig. 18.5) is critical and will help to develop change agent strategies for several key groups based on their influence over the project and by their perception of importance of the project (Brouwer & Brouwers, 2017). Inevitably, some stake- holders will view the change as "wicked" in nature and a threat to either themselves or the organiza- tional structure (Dentoni, Bitzer, & Schouten, 2019).

Bringing different individuals together in a "managed" strategy format for the stakeholder

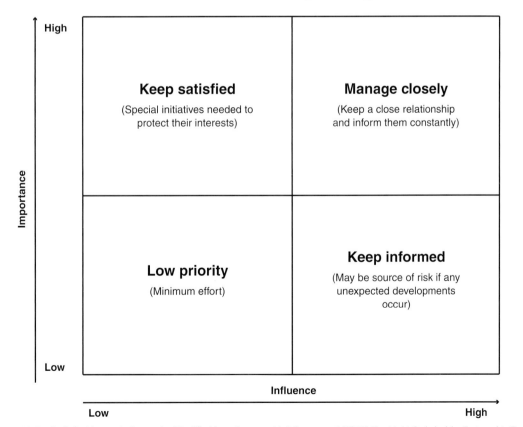

**Figure 18.5**    Stakeholder analysis matrix. (Modified from Brouwer, H., & Brouwers, J. (2017). The Multi-Stakeholder Partnership Tool Guide. In Wageningen University (Ed.), The Netherlands: Wageningen Research Centre for Development Innovation.)

by classifying them means the change agent can predict their behavior somewhat and successfully move toward project objectives and tasks.

## Summary

Change is one of the most common elements in many DNP capstone projects and for CNLs in many specialty settings. If change is not the lead theory, it certainly is a secondary consideration even if one of the major frameworks is selected from a different chapter in this book. One of the key tasks is that the change agent must establish multiple goals that are appropriate to the project and identify environmental and developmental benchmarks for successful adoption.

■ Examine multiple middle range theories to guide the development of evidence-based practice.

■ Utilize appropriate theories to obtain higher-quality planned change project outcomes.

■ Use middle range planned changed theories as they study the best ways to implement, manage, and evaluate change in our ever increasingly complex health system.

■ Disseminate new practice knowledge widely to increase nursing's practice knowledge base.

■ New practice knowledge from planned change projects can improve the quality of nursing services provided to the public and may lead to improved population and individual health outcomes.

This chapter has reviewed three change theories that are commonly used in practice change application as well as two frequently used theories for increasing the likelihood of successful change implantation across complex health systems.

■ There is no question that nurses currently are and will continue to be called upon to participate and sometimes lead the efforts for planned change and practice improvement. This fact is especially true for nurses prepared at the graduate level, a priority of today's expectations being practice change leadership and evaluation. Nurses can use midrange planned changed theories as they study the best ways to implement, manage, and evaluate change in our ever increasingly complex health system. Utilization of appropriate theories will lead to higher-quality planned change project outcomes, a more likely successful implementation, and data useable to generate practice knowledge for dissemination. Dissemination of new practice knowledge widely will increase out practice knowledge base. Ultimately, this practice knowledge can improve the quality of nursing services provided to the public and may lead to improved population health outcomes.

## CRITICAL THINKING EXERCISES

Use the following case study to answer the critical thinking questions.

Andrea, a 16-year-old white, high school student from an upper middle-class family, is ambivalent about getting the Gardasil vaccine. She is interested in boys but does not date anyone in particular and has never been sexually active. She is a cheerleader and plays tennis at her high school where she excels in her class work. She is a Christian and active in the local Young Life group at her school and attends an evangelical free church. Her parents are not encouraging her to get the shots, as they think it will promote promiscuity, but one of her friends' mothers is very vocal about "all of the girls" getting the vaccine. Andrea's mother has a history of breast cancer but not cervical cancer. She does have an aunt with a history of cervical cancer. As far as she knows, no close relatives have ever had a case of venereal warts. She has little information about HPV or cervical cancer, except that she is basically afraid of cancer as she saw its effects on her grandfather when he slowly died of lung cancer. She has seen several commercials about getting the Gardasil shots while searching the web. She has communicated with her Christian and secular friends who are talking about or have gotten the Gardasil shots to protect against HPV. Her nurse practitioner recommended it the last time she was in the clinic for her annual exam.

1. Choose one of the change theories presented in the chapter to help you analyze the case study:
   a. What is the likelihood that Andrea will opt for the Gardasil series of shots?
   b. How could you, as a nurse, influence Andrea's behavior?
   c. How could you change Andrea's behavior and also help change the behavior of her friends?

2. Use the individual concepts within the change theory you chose to predict what will happen if all conditions remain the same in the scenario.

3. Choose another change theory that was presented in the chapter, and prescribe a planned change project that could affect not only an individual behavioral change but a population-based change in the target population.

# REFERENCES

Arthurs, K., Bell-Gordon, C., Chalupa, B., Rose, A. L., Martinez, D., Watson, J. A., & Bernard, D. P. (2017). A culture of nursing excellence: A community hospital's journey from Pathway to Excellence® to Magnet® recognition. *Journal of Nursing Education and Practice*, 8(5), 26.

Assor, A., Feinberg, O., Kanat-Maymon, Y., & Kaplan, H. (2018). Reducing violence in non-controlling ways: A change program based on self determination theory. *The Journal of Experimental Education*, 86(2), 195–213. doi: 10.1080/00220973.2016.1277336

Becker, M. H., & Maiman, L. A. (1975). Sociobehavioral determinants of compliance with health and medical care recommendations. *Medical Care*, 13(1), 10–24.

Boyatzis, R. E., & Jack, A. I. (2018). The neuroscience of coaching. *Consulting Psychology Journal: Practice and Research*, 70(1), 11–27. doi: 10.1037/cpb0000095

Brooks, J. M., Iwanaga, K., Chiu, C. Y., Cotton, B. P., Deiches, J., Morrison, B.,…, Chan, F. (2017). Relationships between self-determination theory and theory of planned behavior applied to physical activity and exercise behavior in chronic pain. *Psychology, Health & Medicine*, 22(7), 814–822. doi: 10.1080/13548506.2017.1282161

Brouwer, H., & Brouwers, J. (2017). The Multi-Stakeholder Partnership Tool Guide. In Wageningen University (Ed.), The Netherlands: Wageningen Research Centre for Development Innovation. Retrieved from https://library.wur.nl/WebQuery/wurpubs/fulltext/409844

Bullen, P., & Brack, T. (2015). Stakeholder analysis matrix template. Retrieved April 28, 2018 from http://www.tools4dev.org/resources/stakeholder-analysis-matrix-template/

Burnes, B. (2004). Kurt Lewin and complexity theories: Back to the future? *Journal of Change Management*, 4, 309–325.

Burnes, B., & Cooke, B. (2013). Kurt Lewin's field theory: A review and reevaluation. *International Journal of Management Review*, 15, 408–425.

Campbell, L., Gilbert, M. A., & Laustsen, G. R. (2014). *Capstone coach for nursing excellence* (2nd ed.). Philadelphia, PA: F.A. Davis Company.

Cecchini, J. A., Fernandez-Rio, J., Mendez-Gimenez, A., Carriedo, A., & Arruza, J. A. (2017). A self-determination approach to the understanding of the impact of physical activity on depressive symptoms. *Stress and Health*, 33(5), 600–607. doi: 10.1002/smi.2744

Champion, V. L., & Skinner, C. S. (2008). The health belief model. In K. Glanz, B. K. Rimer, & K. Viswanath (Eds.), *Health behavior and health education: Theory, research and practice* (4th ed., pp. 45–65). San Francisco, CA: Josey-Bass.

Clark, N. M., & Janevic, M. R. ( 2014). Theoretical models of health behavior change: Individual theories. In K. A. Riekert, K. J. Ockene, & L. Pbert (Eds.), *The handbook of health behavior change* (4th ed., pp. 3–27). New York, NY: Springer.

Davis, C. R. (2018). Administrator leadership styles and their impact on school nursing. *NASN School Nurse*, 33(1), 36–39. doi: 10.1177/1942602X17714202

Deci, E. L., & Ryan, R. M. (2000). Intrinsic and extrinsic motivations: Classic definition and new directions. *Contemporary Educational Psychology*, 25, 54–67. doi: 10.1006/ceps.1999.1020

Deci, E. L., & Ryan, R. M. (2002). *Handbook of self-determination research*. Rochester, NY: University of Rochester Press.

Dentoni, D., Bitzer, V., & Schouten, G. (2019). Harnessing wicked problems in multi-stakeholder partnerships. *Journal of Business Ethics*, 150(2), 333–356. doi: 10.1007/s10551-018-3858-6

DiCenso, A., Guyatt, G., & Ciliska, D. (2005). *Evidence-based nursing: A guide to clinical practice*. St. Louis, MO: Elsevier Mosby.

DiLibero, J., DeSanto-Madyea, S., & O'Dongohue, S. (2016). Improving accuracy of cardiac electrode placement: Outcomes of clinical nurse specialist practice. *Clinical Nurse Specialist*, 30(1), 45–50. doi: 10.1097/NUR.0000000000000172

Ferguson, C., DiGiacomo, M., Gholizadeh, L., Ferguson, L. E., & Hickman, L. D. (2017). The integration and evaluation of a social-media facilitated journal club to enhance the student learning experience of evidence-based practice: A case study. *Nurse Education Today*, 48, 123–128. doi: 10.1016/j.nedt.2016.10.002

Fishbein, M., & Ajzen, I. (2010). *Predicting and changing behavior : The reasoned action approach*. New York, NY: Psychology Press.

Fishbein, M., Ajzen, I., Albarracin, D., & Hornik, R. C. (2007). *Prediction and change of health behavior: Applying the reasoned action approach*. Mahwah, NJ: Lawrence Erlbaum Associates.

Fisher, P. A., Robie, C., Christiansen, N. D., & Komar, S. (2018). The impact of psychopathy and warnings on faking behavior: A multisaturation perspective. *Personality and Individual Differences*, 127, 39–43. doi: 10.1016/j.paid.2018.01.033

Garces-Ozanne, A., Kalu, E. I., & Audas, R. (2016). The effect of empowerment and self-determination on health outcomes. *Health Education & Behavior*, 43(6), 623–631. doi: 10.1177/1090198116667665

Godakandage, S. S., Senarath, U., Jayawickrama, H. S., Siriwardena, I., Wickramasinghe, S., Arumapperuma, P., …, Umesh, C. (2017). Policy and stakeholder analysis of infant and young child feeding programmes in Sri Lanka. *BMC Public Health*, 17(2), 522.

Guertin, C., Barbeau, K., Pelletier, L., & Martinelli, G. (2017). Why do women engage in fat talk? Examining fat talk using self-determination theory as an explanatory framework. *Body Image*, 20, 7–15. doi: 10.1016/j.bodyim.2016.10.008

Haider, M., & Kreps, G. L. (2004). Forty years of diffusion of innovations: Utility and value in public health. *Journal of Health Communication*, 9, 3–11.

Hamilton, K., Kirkpatrick, A., Rebar, A., & Hagger, M. S. (2017). Child sun safety: Application of an integrated behavior change model. *Health Psychology*, 36(9), 916–926. doi: 10.1037/hea0000533

Harris, J. L., Roussel, L., & Thomas, P. (2014). *Initiating and sustaining the clinical nurse leader role : A practical guide* (2nd ed.). Burlington, MA: Jones & Bartlett Learning.

Henry, K. (2018). Frameworks for behavioral change. In R. A. Utley, K. Henry, & L. Smith (Eds.), *Frameworks for advanced nursing practice and research : Philosophies, theories, models, and taxonomies*. New York, NY: Springer Publishing Company, LLC.

Hiatt, J., & Creasey, T. J. (2003). *Change management: The people side of change*. Ft Collins, CO: Prosci.

Howard, A. R. (2015). Coaching to vision versus coaching to improvement needs: A preliminary investigation on the differential impacts of fostering positive and negative emotion during real time executive coaching sessions. *Frontiers in Psychology*, 6, 455. doi: 10.3389/fpsyg.2015.00455

Hyde, M. K., McLaren, P. J., & White, K. M. (2014). Identifying belief targets to increase bone marrow registry participation among students who have never donated blood. *Psychology, Health & Medicine*, 19(1), 115–125. doi: 10.1080/13548506.2013.775467

Janz, N. K., & Becker, M. H. (1984). The health belief model: A decade later. *Health Education Quarterly*, 11(1), 1–47.

Koole, L., Schlinkert, C., Maldei, T., & Baumann, N. (2019). Becoming who you are: An integrative review of self-determination theory and personality systems Interactions theory. *Journal of Personality*, 87(1), 15–36. doi: 10.1111/jopy.12380

Kushnir, V., Godinho, A., Hodgins, D. C., Hendershot, C. S., & Cunningham, J. A. (2016). Motivation to quit or reduce gambling: Associations between self-determination theory and the transtheoretical model of change. *Journal of Addictive Diseases*, 35(1), 58–65. doi: 10.1080/10550887.2016.1107315

Langley, E. L., Wootton, B. M., & Grieve, R. (2017). The utility of the health belief model variables in predicting help-seeking intention for anxiety disorders. *Australian Psychologist*, 53(4), 291–301. doi: 10.1111/ap.12334

Lemos, M. S., & Veríssimo, L. (2014). The relationships between intrinsic motivation, extrinsic motivation, and achievement, along elementary school. *Procedia—Social and Behavioral Sciences*, 112, 930–938. doi: 10.1016/j.sbspro.2014.01.1251

Lewin, K. (1947). Frontiers in group dynamics: Concept, method, and reality in social science, social equilibria, and social change. *Human Relations*, 1(1), 5–41.

Marris, P. (2014). *Loss and change (Psychology revivals): Revised edition*. New York, NY: Routledge.

Mazur, A. K., & Pisarski, A. (2015). Major project managers' internal and external stakeholder relationships: The development and validation of measurement scales. *International Journal of Project Management*, 33(8), 1680–1691. doi: 10.1016/j.ijproman.2015.07.008

McEwen, M. (2018). Application of theory in nursing. In M. McEwen, & E. M. Wills (Eds.), *Theoretical basis for nursing* (5th ed., pp. 377–380). Philadelphia, PA: Wolters Kluwer.

Meeks, D. (2017). Has SWOT outlived its usefulness. *Academy of Strategic Management Journal*, 16(1).

Mitchell, G. (2013). Selecting the best theory to implement planned change. *Nursing Management*, 20(1), 32–37.

Montanaro, E. A., Kershaw, T. S., & Bryan, A. D. (2018). Dismantling the theory of planned behavior: Evaluating the relative effectiveness of attempts to uniquely change attitudes, norms, and perceived behavioral control. *Journal of Behavioral Medicine*, 41(6), 757–770. doi: 10.1007/s10865-018-9923-x

Montano, D. E., Kasprzyk, D., & Taplin, S. H. (1997). The theory of reasoned action and the theory of planned behavior. In K. Glanz, F. M. Lewis, & B. K. Rimer (Eds.), *Health behavior and health education: Theory, research and practice* (2nd ed., pp. 85–112). San Francisco, CA: Jossey-Bass Publishers.

Padilha, J. M., Sousa, P. A. F., & Pereira, F. M. S. (2018). Nursing clinical practice changes to improve self-management in chronic obstructive pulmonary disease. *International Nursing Review*, 65(1), 122–130. doi: 10.1111/inr.12366

Patton, C. M., Lim, K. G., Ramlow, L. W., & White, K. M. (2015). Increasing efficiency in evaluation of chronic cough: A multidisciplinary, collaborative approach. *Quality Management in Health Care*, 24(4), 177–182. doi: 10.1097/QMH.0000000000000072

Pawl, J. D., & Anderson, L. S. (2017). The use of change theory to facilitate the consolidation of two diverse Bachelors of Science in Nursing programs. *Nursing Outlook*, 65(2), 233–239. doi: 10.1016/j.outlook.2016.10.004

Pender, N. J. (2011). *Health promotion in nursing practice* (6th ed.). Stamford, CT: Appleton & Lange.

Peng, M. W., & Vlas, C. O. (2017). Diffusion of a twenty-century innovation. *Academy of Strategic Management Journal*, 16(1), 172–174.

Powers, B. A., Knapp, T., Powers, D. B. A., & Edd, T. K. (2010). *Dictionary of nursing theory and research* (4th ed.). New York, NY: Springer Publishing Company.

Quinlivan, E. B., Messer, L. C., Roytburd, K., & Blickman, A. (2017). Unmet core needs for self-determination in HIV-infected women of color in medical care. *AIDS Care*, 29(5), 603–611. doi: 10.1080/09540121.2016.1243788

Repique, R. J., Vernig, P. M., Lowe, J., Thompson, J. A., & Yap, T. L. (2016). Implementation of a recovery-oriented training program for psychiatric nurses in the inpatient setting: A mixed-methods hospital quality improvement study. *Archives of Psychiatric Nursing*, 30(6), 722–728. doi: 10.1016/j.apnu.2016.06.003

Rogers, E. M. (2003). *Diffusion of innovation* (5th ed.). New York, NY: Free Press.

Rogers, E. M. (2004). A prospective and retrospective look at the diffusion model. *Journal of Health Communication*, 9, 13–19.

Rosenstock, I. M., Strecher, V. J., & Becker, M. H. (1988). Social learning theory and the Health belief model. *Health Education Quarterly*, 15(2), 175–183.

Ryan, R. M., & Deci, E. L. (2000). Intrinsic and extrinsic motivations: Classic definitions and new directions. *Contemporary Educational Psychology*, 25(1), 54–67. doi: 10.1006/ceps.1999.1020

Scalco, A., Ceschi, A., & Sartori, R. (2018). Application of psychological theories in agent-based modeling: The case of the theory of planned behavior. *Nonlinear Dynamics, Psychology, and Life Sciences*, 22(1), 15–33.

Shin, H., & Dess, G. G. (2017). From SWOT to value appropriation: Career implications. *Academy of Strategic Management Journal*, 16(1), 165A–168A.

Shirey, M. R. (2013). Leaning in: Lessons for leadership career development. *Journal of Nursing Administration*, 43(11), 562–565. doi: 10.1097/01.Nna.0000434513.20115.46

Sucala, M., Nilsen, W., & Muench, F. (2017). Building partnerships: A pilot study of stakeholders' attitudes on technology disruption in behavioral health delivery and research. *Translational Behavioral Medicine*, 7(4), 854–860. doi: 10.1007/s13142-017-0498-9

Suva, G., Sharma, T., Campbell, K. E., Sibbald, R. G., An, D., & Woo, K. (2018). Strategies to support pressure injury best practices by the inter-professional team: A systematic review. *International Wound Journal*, 15(4), 580–589. doi: 10.1111/iwj.12901

Sweet, S. N., Michalovic, E., Latimer-Cheung, A. E., Fortier, M., Noreau, L., Zelaya, W., & Ginis, K. A. M. (2018). Spinal cord injury peer mentorship: Applying self-determination theory to explain quality of life and participation. *Archives of Physical Medicine and Rehabilitation*, 99(3), 468–476.e412.

Trief, P. M., Cibula, D., Delahanty, L. M., & Weinstock, R. S. (2017). Self-determination theory and weight loss in a Diabetes Prevention Program translation trial. *Journal of Behavioral Medicine*, 40(3), 483–493. doi: 10.1007/s10865-016-9816-9

Tseng, Y. F., Wang, K. L., Lin, C. Y., Lin, Y. T., Pan, H. C., & Chang, C. J. (2018). Predictors of smoking cessation in Taiwan: Using the theory of planned behavior. *Psychology, Health & Medicine*, 23(3), 270–276. doi: 10.1080/13548506.2017.1378820

Tuck, L. M., & Hough, S. (2017). Incorporating the standards established by The Joint Commission (TJC). In M. H. Budd, S, S. Wegener, & S. Stiers (Eds.), *Practical psychology in medical rehabilitation* (pp. 539–543). Cham, Switzerland: Springer International Publishing.

Tweneboah-Koduah, E. Y. (2018). Social marketing: Using the health belief model to understand breast cancer protective behaviours among women. *International Journal of Nonprofit and Voluntary Sector Marketing*, 23(2), e1613. doi: 10.1002/nvsm.1613

Vogel, T., & Wanke, M. (2016). *Attitudes and attitude change*. Hove, East Sussex, UK: Psychology Press.

Wyder, M., Ehrlich, C., Crompton, D., McArthur, L., Delaforce, C., Dziopa, F., …, Powell, E. (2017). Nurses experiences of delivering care in acute inpatient mental health settings: A narrative synthesis of the literature. *International Journal of Mental Health Nursing*, 26(6), 527–540. doi: 10.1111/inm.12315

# 19 The AACN Synergy Model

Sonya R. Hardin and Diane O. Chlebowy

## Definition of Key Terms

| | |
|---|---|
| **Health care system** | The health care system acts as a facilitator or conduit to support patient needs and the power to nurture the professional practice environment of the nurse. |
| **Nurse competencies** | The eight competencies of nursing practice as defined by the model are clinical judgment, caring practices, advocacy/moral agency, response to diversity, clinical inquiry, facilitator of learning, collaboration, and systems thinking. |
| **Optimal patient outcomes** | Patient outcomes include patient satisfaction with care, levels of trust, patient behavior and knowledge, patient functional change, and quality of life. |
| **Patient characteristics** | Eight patient characteristics have been identified that span a continuum of health to illness: vulnerability, resiliency, stability, complexity, predictability, resource availability, participation in care, and participation in decision-making. |

The American Association of Critical Care Nurses (AACN) has established a vision to create a health care system that is driven by the needs of patients and families where nurses can make optimal contributions in the delivery of care. This vision involved the development of a model that explicates the practice that nurses contribute at the bedside. The model developed was the AACN Synergy Model. The goal of this model was to clearly articulate the competencies brought to patient care by nurses in meeting the needs of patients and families.

## Historical Background

During the early 1990s, the AACN Certification Corporation strategically set forth a direction to identify a model that described practice. In 1993, the AACN Certification Corporation, the certifying body of the AACN, established a think tank to draft a document that identified the concepts of nursing practice, most specifically certified practice. The think tank identified 13 patient needs and 9 nurse characteristics. Then, in 1995, the AACN Certification Board identified a group of "Subject Matter" experts from across the United States to refine the conceptual model. A revision to the model resulting in eight nurse characteristics and eight patient characteristics occurred.

In February 2002, the Practice Analysis Task Force expanded the assumption to the model to include the following:

- The nurse creates the environment for the care of the patient. The context/environment of care also affects what the nurse can do.
- There is interrelatedness between impact areas. The nature of the interrelatedness may change as the function of experience, situation, or setting changes.
- The nurse may work to optimize outcomes for patients, families, health care providers, and the health care system/organization.
- Nurses bring their background to each situation, including various levels of education/ knowledge and skills/experience (AACN, 2019).

In March 1996, the AACN Certification Corporation appointed an Outcome Think Tank who identified six major quality indicators: (a) patient and family satisfaction, (b) rate of adverse incidents, (c) complication rate, (d) adherence to the discharge plan, (e) mortality rate, and (f) the patient's length of stay (Hardin, 2005). Outcomes derived from the eight patient characteristics include functional changes, behavioral changes, trust, satisfaction, comfort, and quality of life. Outcomes derived from the eight nursing competencies include physiological changes, the presence or absence of complications, and the extent of treatment objectives obtained (Curley, 1998).

Outcome data derived from the health care system include readmission rates, length of stay, and cost utilization per case.

# Description of the Theory of Synergy Model

## ASSUMPTIONS OF THE MODEL

The Synergy Model is based on the following five assumptions:

"(1) Patients are biological, social, and spiritual entities who present at a particular developmental stage. The whole patient (body, mind, and spirit) must be considered. (2) The patient, family, and community all contribute to providing a context for the nurse–patient relationship. (3) Patients can be described by a number of characteristics. All characteristics are connected and contribute to each other. Characteristics cannot be looked at in isolation. (4) Nurses can be described on a number of dimensions. The interrelated dimensions paint a profile of the nurse. (5) A goal of nursing is to restore a patient to an optimal level of wellness as defined by the patient. Death can be an acceptable outcome in which the goal of nursing care is to move a patient toward a peaceful death" (AACN, 2000, p. 5).

## DEFINITION OF THEORETICAL CONCEPTS

There are totally 16 concepts in this model: eight patient concepts and eight nursing concepts (Tables 19.1 and 19.2). The concepts (characteristics) are descriptors that describe the patient and nursing. The eight concepts used to understand patients are resiliency, vulnerability, stability, complexity, resource availability, participation in care, participation in decision-making, and predictability. The eight concepts (characteristics) used to describe the practice of nursing are clinical judgment, advocacy, caring practices, collaboration, systems thinking, response to diversity, clinical inquiry, and facilitator of learning. The patient and nurse characteristics are leveled from 1 to 5 and are presented in Tables 19.1 and 19.2.

Patient characteristic levels are based on a five-point Likert scale, ranging from 1 (the worst patient state) to 5 (the best patient state). Nurse characteristic levels are based on a five-point Likert scale with 1 being novice and 5 being expert. Descriptions of levels 1, 3, and 5 have been described by the AACN. Levels 2 and 4 have not been specifically identified in the literature by the AACN. However, the use of the five levels with

levels 1, 3, and 5 as benchmarks has been useful to nursing organizations as they develop clinical ladders. Further work has been completed on the nurse characteristics for the advanced practice role (Becker et al., 2006). Activities of advanced practice nurses organized by the eight nurse characteristics emerged through a study of practice conducted by the AACN Certification Corporation. While some of these activities overlap with the expert nurse, the study identified four nurse characteristics considered most critical by clinical nurse specialists (clinical judgment, caring practices, facilitator of learning, and clinical inquiry) and two activities most critical by nurse practitioners (clinical judgment and advocacy/moral agency) (Becker et al., 2006).

### Patient Characteristics

Each patient brings a unique set of characteristics to the health care situation. Among many characteristics that are present, eight are consistently seen in acute and critically ill patients. These eight characteristics are consistently assessed by nurses in variable levels given each patient situation. They should be assessed in the patient as well as other patterns that are unique to the given circumstances of the patient. *Resiliency* is the patient's capacity to return to a restorative level of functioning using compensatory coping mechanisms. The level of resiliency is often dependent upon the patient's ability to rebound after an insult. This ability can be influenced by many factors including age, comorbidities, nutritional status, and compensatory mechanisms that are intact. *Vulnerability* is the level of susceptibility to actual or potential stressors that may adversely affect patient outcomes. Vulnerability can be impacted by the patient's physiological/genetic makeup or health behaviors exhibited by the patient, such as risk factors. *Stability* refers to the patient's ability to maintain a steady state of equilibrium. Response to therapies and nursing interventions can impact the stability of the patient. *Complexity* is the intricate entanglement of two or more systems. Systems refer to either physiological or psychological states of the body or family dynamics or environmental interactions with the patient. The more systems involved, the more complex are the patterns displayed by the patient. *Resource availability* is influenced by the extent that resources are brought to the context by the patient, family, and community. The resources can present as pharmaceutical, technical, fiscal, personal, psychological, social, or supportive in nature. A greater potential for a positive outcome exists when a patient has more

**Table 19.1    Patient Characteristics and Levels**

| Characteristic | Definition | Level |
| --- | --- | --- |
| Stability | Maintain a steady-state equilibrium | **Level 1—Minimally stable:** labile; unstable; unresponsive to therapies; high risk of death<br>**Level 3—Moderately stable:** able to maintain steady state for limited period of time; some responsiveness to therapies<br>**Level 5—Highly stable:** constant; responsive to therapies; low risk of death |
| Complexity | Entanglement of two or more systems (e.g., body, family, therapies) | **Level 1—Highly complex:** intricate; complex patient/family dynamics; ambiguous/vague; atypical presentation<br>**Level 3—Moderately complex:** moderately involved patient/family dynamics<br>**Level 5—Minimally complex:** straightforward; routine patient/family dynamics; simple/clear cut; typical presentation |
| Predictability | Allows one to expect a certain course of events | **Level 1—Not predictable:** uncertain; uncommon patient population/illness; unusual or unexpected course; does not follow critical pathway or no critical pathway developed<br>**Level 3—Moderately predictable:** wavering; occasionally noted patient population/illness<br>**Level 5—Highly predictable:** certain; common patient population/illness; usual and expected course; follows critical pathway |
| Resiliency | The capacity to return to a restorative level of functioning | **Level 1—Minimally resilient:** unable to mount a response; failure of compensatory/coping mechanisms; minimal reserves; brittle<br>**Level 3—Moderately resilient:** able to mount a moderate response; able to initiate some degree of compensation; moderate reserves<br>**Level 5—Highly resilient:** able to mount and maintain a response; intact compensatory/coping mechanisms; strong reserves; endurance |
| Vulnerability | Susceptibility to actual or potential stressors | **Level 1—Highly vulnerable:** susceptible; unprotected, fragile<br>**Level 3—Moderately vulnerable:** somewhat susceptible, somewhat protected<br>**Level 5—Minimally vulnerable:** safe; out of the woods; protected, not fragile |
| Participation in decision-making | Extent to which patient/family engages in decision-making | **Level 1—No participation:** no capacity for decision-making; requires surrogacy<br>**Level 3—Moderate level of participation:** limited capacity; seeks input/advice from others in decision-making<br>**Level 5—Full participation:** full capacity; makes decision for self |
| Participation in care | Extent to which patient/family engages in aspects of care | **Level 1—No participation:** patient and family unable or unwilling to participate in care<br>**Level 3—Moderate level of participation:** patient and family need assistance in care<br>**Level 5—Full participation:** patient and family fully able to participate in care |
| Resource availability | Extent of resources the patient/family/ community bring to the situation | **Level 1—Few resources:** necessary knowledge and skills not available; financial support and personal/psychological supportive resources minimal<br>**Level 3—Moderate resources:** limited knowledge and skills available; limited financial support and personal/psychological and supportive resources<br>**Level 5—Many resources:** extensive knowledge and skills available and accessible; strong financial, personal, and supportive resources |

*Source*: Adapted from AACN Certification Corporation Web site. (2000). *The AACN Synergy Model for patient care*. Retrieved September 27, 2014 from http://www.aacn.org/wd/certifications/content/synmodel.pcms?menu=certification#Assumptions

resources. *Participation in care* is the participation by the patient and the family who are engaged in the delivery of care. Patient and family participation can be influenced by health status, educational background, health literacy, resource availability, and cultural background. *Participation in decision-making* is the level of engagement of the patient and the family in comprehending the information provided by health care providers and acting upon this information to execute informed decisions. Patient and family engagement in clinical decisions can be impacted by the knowledge level of the patient, his or her capacity to make decisions given the insult, cultural background (i.e., beliefs and values), and the level of inner strength during a crisis (AACN Certification Corporation, 2002).

**Table 19.2    Nurse Characteristics and Levels**

| Characteristic | Definition | Level |
|---|---|---|
| Clinical judgment | Clinical reasoning | **Level 1**: collects basic-level data; follows algorithms, decision trees, and protocols with all populations and is uncomfortably deviating from them<br>**Level 3**: collects and interprets complex patient data; makes clinical judgments based on an immediate grasp of the whole picture for common or routine patient populations<br>**Level 5**: synthesizes and interprets multiple, sometimes conflicting, sources of data; makes judgment based on an immediate grasp of the whole picture; helps patient and family see the "big picture"; recognizes and responds to the dynamic situation |
| Advocacy | Working on another's behalf | **Level 1**: works on behalf of patient; self-assesses personal values; is aware of ethical conflicts/issues that may surface in clinical setting; makes ethical/moral decisions based on rules<br>**Level 3**: considers patient values and incorporates in care, even when differing from personal values; supports colleagues in ethical and clinical issues; moral decision-making can deviate from rules<br>**Level 5**: advocates ethical conflict and issues from patient/family perspective; suspends rules; empowers the patient and the family to speak for/represent themselves |
| Caring practices | Activities that create a compassionate, supportive, and therapeutic environment for patients and staff | **Level 1**: focuses on the customary needs of the patient; has no anticipation of future needs; bases care on standards and protocols<br>**Level 3**: responds to subtle patient and family changes; engages with the patient as a unique patient in a compassionate manner; recognizes and tailors caring practices to the individuality of patient<br>**Level 5**: has astute awareness and anticipates patient and family changes and needs; is fully engaged with and senses how to stand alongside the patient, family, and community; orchestrates the process that ensures the patient's/family's comfort and concerns surrounding issues of death and dying |
| Collaboration | Working with others in a way that promotes each person's contributions toward achieving optimal outcomes | **Level 1**: willing to be taught, coached, and/or mentored; participates in team meetings and discussions regarding patient care and/or practice issues<br>**Level 3**: seeks opportunities to be taught, coached, and/or mentored; elicits others' advice and perspectives; initiates and participates in team meetings and discussions regarding patient care; recognizes and suggests various team members' participation<br>**Level 5**: seeks opportunities to teach, coach, and mentor and to be taught, coached, and mentored; facilitates active involvement and complementary contributions of others in team meetings and discussions regarding patient care and/or practice issues; involves/recruits diverse resources when appropriate to optimize patient outcomes |
| Response to diversity | Sensitivity to recognize, appreciate, and incorporate differences into the provision of care | **Level 1**: assesses cultural diversity; provides care based on own belief system; learns the culture of the health care environment<br>**Level 3**: inquires about cultural differences and considers their impact on care; accommodates personal and professional differences in the plan of care; helps patient/family understand the culture of the health care system<br>**Level 5**: responds to, anticipates, and integrates cultural differences into patient/family care; appreciates and incorporates differences, including alternative therapies; tailors health care culture, to the extent possible, to meet the diverse needs and strengths of the patient/family |
| Clinical inquiry | Ongoing process of questioning and evaluating practice and providing informed practice | **Level 1**: follows standards and guidelines; implements clinical changes and research-based practices developed by others; recognizes the need for further learning to improve patient care; recognizes obvious changing patient situation; needs and seeks help to identify patient problem<br>**Level 3**: questions appropriateness of policies and guidelines; questions current practice; seeks advice, resources, or information to improve patient care; begins to compare and contrast possible alternatives<br>**Level 5**: improves, deviates from, or individualizes standards and guidelines for particular patient situations or populations; questions and/or evaluates current practice based on patients' responses, review of the literature, research, and education/learning |

| Characteristic | Definition | Level |
|---|---|---|
| Facilitator of learning | Ability to facilitate learning for patients/families, nursing staff, other members of the health care team, and community | **Level 1:** follows planned educational programs; sees patient/family education as a separate task from delivery of care; provides data without seeking to assess patient's readiness or understanding; has limited knowledge of the totality of the educational needs<br>**Level 3:** adapts planned educational programs; begins to recognize and integrate different ways of teaching into delivery of care; incorporates patient's understanding into practice<br>**Level 5:** creatively modifies or develops patient/family education programs; integrates patient/family education throughout delivery of care; evaluates patient's understanding by observing behavior changes; sets patient-driven goals for education |
| Systems thinking | Knowledge and tools that enhance the nurse's ability to manage whatever environmental and system resources exist for the patient/family and staff | **Level 1:** uses a limited array of strategies; does not recognize negotiation as an alternative; sees patient and family within the isolated environment of the unit; sees self as key resource<br>**Level 3:** develops strategies based on needs and strengths of patient/family; is able to make connections within components; sees opportunity to negotiate but may not have strategies; recognizes how to obtain resources beyond self<br>**Level 5:** develops, integrates, and applies a variety of strategies; has a global or holistic outlook; knows when and how to negotiate and navigate through the system; anticipates needs of patients and families as they move through the health care system; uses untapped and alternative resources as necessary |

*Source*: Adapted from AACN Certification Corporation Web site. (2000). *The AACN Synergy Model for patient care*. Retrieved September 27, 2014 from http://www.aacn.org/wd/certifications/content/synmodel.pcms?menu=certification#Assumptions

**Table 19.2   Nurse Characteristics and Levels** (Continued)

## Nurse Characteristics

The nurse characteristics can be considered competencies that are essential for providing care to the acute and critically ill. All eight competencies reflect an integration of knowledge, skills, and experience of the nurse. The competencies include clinical judgment, advocacy, caring practices, systems thinking, facilitation of learning, collaboration, response to diversity, and clinical inquiry. *Clinical judgment* is the clinical reasoning that is used by a health care provider in the delivery of care. It consists of critical thinking and nursing skills that are acquired through a process of integrating formal and experiential knowledge. The integration of knowledge and experience brings about the clinical decisions made during the course of care for patients, groups, and communities. *Advocacy* is working on another's behalf when the other is not capable of advocating for him-/herself. The nurse serves as a moral agent in identifying and helping to resolve ethical dilemmas within the clinical setting. *Caring practices* are the constellation of nursing interventions that are unique to the needs of the patient and the family. Caring behaviors include compassion, vigilance, engagement, and responsiveness to the patient and the family. *Collaboration* is the nurse working with others to promote optimal outcomes. The patient, family, and members of various health care disciplines collaborate by working toward promoting the needs and requests of patients. *Systems thinking* is the tool and knowledge that the nurse uses to recognize the interconnected nature within and across the health care system. The ability to understand how one's decision can impact the whole is integral to systems thinking. The nurse uses a global perspective in analyzing problems, making decisions, and negotiating for the patient and the family internally and externally to the health care system. *Response to diversity* is the sensitivity to recognize, appreciate, and incorporate differences into the provision of care. Nurses need to recognize the individuality of each patient while observing for patterns that respond to nursing interventions. Nurses should be open to the patient's spiritual beliefs, ethnicity, family configuration, lifestyle values, and the use of alternative and complementary therapies. *Clinical inquiry* is the ongoing process of questioning and evaluating practice, providing informed practice, and innovating through research and experiential learning. Clinical inquiry evolves as the nurse moves from novice to expert. At the expert level, the nurse enhances, deviates, and/or individualizes standards and guidelines to meet the needs of patients, families, groups, and communities. *Facilitator of learning* is understood as the nurse facilitating learning among patients, families, communities, and staff through tailored educational programs. The educational level of the audience should be considered in the design of the plan to educate. Creative methods should be developed to ensure patient and family comprehension and to make informed decisions. Each nurse and patient characteristic is understood on a continuum from 1 to 5. The level of each patient characteristic is critical in identifying the competency required of the nurse (AACN Certification Corporation, 2002).

## RESEARCH

The Synergy Model is useful in identifying optimal patient outcomes given evidence-based nursing interventions (Kaplow, 2003; Kaplow & Hardin, 2007). Optimal outcomes can be measured through the use of numerous instruments. For example, as the nurse begins managing the transition of the patient from one setting to another, the outcome of transition without complications is established. The nurse can use numerous research-developed risk-screening instruments to improve postdischarge problems. Or, if the nurse is managing an organ donor, pathways have been developed by the United Network for Organ Sharing to guide the decisions and actions in managing donors. Such pathways have been researched and/or reached through clinical consensus (Kaplow & Hardin, 2007). Graham-Garcia, George-Gay, Heater, Butts, and Heath (2006) supported the use of the Synergy Model to optimize positive outcomes for tobacco-dependent patients requiring surgery. The Synergy Model was used as a framework for the development of a triage tool to guide decisions on the level of care necessary to complete interfacility transports effectively and safely (Swickard, Swickard, Reimer, Lindell & Winkelman, 2014). In addition, the Synergy Model's patient characteristic of participation in care can be useful in enhancing optimal outcomes for older patients (Hardin, 2012). Garcin (2017) discussed the importance of the use of the Synergy Model in tailoring nursing care to meet the clinical needs and improve outcomes in patients with chronic kidney disease.

The AACN Synergy Model is useful for doctoral dissertations. As a study is being designed, the AACN Synergy Model provides guidance in research question identification and approaches to defining variables in a study. The strength of the model is that nurses are integrated into the patient outcomes through their competency to practice in the setting they are found in. Table 19.3 displays dissertations that utilized the AACN Synergy Model.

Evidence-based practice is based upon clinical inquiry of scientists in the field or developed protocols through clinical evidence. The integration or the translation of research findings into practice is a characteristic of clinical inquiry. The tools evolved from evidence-based practice and hence clinical inquiries have supported the decision-making of nurses. Through evidence-based practice, interventions and outcomes can be identified. Ho et al. (2017) devised a systematic, efficient, and timely process using the synergy tool resulting in significant increases in staff engagement, improved workload management, and reductions in nurse-missed breaks. The synergy tool emphasizes the importance of real-time decision-making while ensuring a better fit between patient needs and nurse staffing and can be used by interprofessional teams in the health care system (Ho et al., 2017). The Synergy Model was used in the development, successful implementation, and nurse management of a remote cardiac telemetry service in a tertiary care facility in Abington, PA (Reilly & Humbrecht, 2007). Smith (2006) recommended the use of the Synergy Model in the development and implementation of nursing interventions to address the spiritual needs of critically ill patients. In addition, a group of CCNSs applied the Synergy Model to successfully change from a unit based to a multisystem practice, thus linking certified practice to patients' outcomes (Cohen, Crego, Cuming, & Smyth, 2002).

The AACN Synergy Model is being utilized in Doctorate of Nursing Practice (DNP) projects across the country. Many quality improvement projects are designed with the understanding that patient characteristics and nurse characteristics with the unit environment merge to impact outcomes. Enhanced safety and improved outcomes are the foundation of most DNP projects. Table 19.4 shows some of the most recent quality improvement projects conducted as a requirement in DNP programs.

Further research with the model needs to be conducted to validate the model within other practice settings and patient populations. One approach is to identify questions surrounding the concepts of the model and then to identify instruments that can be utilized to measure the concepts. Table 19.5 displays four instruments that measure the patient characteristic of vulnerability. Evaluating older adults for vulnerability by measuring disability, comorbidities, and frailty is a proxy for vulnerability in critical care (Hardin, 2015). Although these instruments have not been utilized extensively within critical care settings, the potential exists to design correlational studies to evaluate vulnerability and outcomes. Brewer (2006) tested the feasibility of using patient acuity indicators as proxy measures for patient characteristics in the Synergy Model and concluded

**Table 19.3    DNP Projects Using the AACN Synergy Model**

| Topic | Outcome | Synergy Model | Reference |
|---|---|---|---|
| Relationship between earlier intravenous antibiotic administration and the reduction of sepsis mortality | No statistically significant correlation between antibiotic timing and sepsis mortality | The nurse of the septic patient must be a facilitator of education as well as demonstrate clinical inquiry | Watts, M. (2017). *The effect of antibiotic timing on sepsis mortality* (Order No. 10258834). Available from ProQuest Dissertations & Theses Global. (1873028014). Retrieved from http://search.proquest.com.jproxy.lib.ecu.edu/docview/1873028014?accountid=10639 |
| Evaluating behavioral health homes to decrease emergency department use | A quasi-experimental research design was used. The participants in the BHH were statistically less likely to visit the ED | Behavioral health patient characteristics include low economic status, cultural diversity, lack of access to reliable transportation, lack of decision-making capacity, and complex medical and psychiatric diagnoses | Noe-Norman, R. (2017). *Evaluating behavioral health homes to decrease emergency department use* (Order No. 10257550). Available from ProQuest Dissertations & Theses Global. (1870037958). Retrieved from http://search.proquest.com.jproxy.lib.ecu.edu/docview/1870037958?accountid=10639 |
| Use of the collaborative care model to enhance nurses' abilities to provide safe, high-quality care and improve retention | Results showed that staff turnover was reduced from 41% to 35.9% and patients' perceptions of teamwork increased | The synergy model was used to create a tool to help the charge nurses with their decision process in patient placement | Duncan, D. N. (2017). *Educating to the collaborative care model* (Order No. 10271113). Available from ProQuest Dissertations & Theses Global. (1891350204). Retrieved from http://search.proquest.com.jproxy.lib.ecu.edu/docview/1891350204?accountid=10639 |
| Pediatric alarm management | Findings showed a significant lack of alarm parameter adherence among the nursing staff | The AACN Synergy Model demonstrates that not one characteristic or competency can be isolated and that everything is interconnected. Aligned patient characteristics, nurse competencies, and health care environments ensure successful implementation of a synergized team-based alarm management approach—the goal of this project | Gilmore, J. M. (2017). *Pediatric meaningful alarm management approach* (Order No. 10258091). Available from ProQuest Dissertations & Theses Global. (1917681872). Retrieved from http://search.proquest.com.jproxy.lib.ecu.edu/docview/1917681872?accountid=10639 |
| Healthy work environment online assessment tool | Results revealed a need for greater understanding of the AACN Health Work Environment Standards | Using the synergy model of care as the approach to a healthy work environment created an option for changes in the work environment | Cuff, L. E. (2016). *Healthy work environment: Essentials for outcome improvement* (Order No. 10172974). Available from ProQuest Central; ProQuest Dissertations & Theses Global. (1833187900). Retrieved from http://search.proquest.com.jproxy.lib.ecu.edu/docview/1833187900?accountid=10639 |

that only participation in care showed meaningful correlations with the acuity indicators.

Studies are needed on the nursing characteristics described in the model. How these characteristics impact optimal patient outcomes will require the use of existing instruments and the design of new measurements. Table 19.6 displays instruments that can be utilized to measure the nurse characteristic of caring. A number of scales have been developed to measure caring (Beck, 1999).

However, the majority of these scales have not been utilized in research studies in the setting of critical care.

Using the Synergy Model as the framework for nursing research, which is designed to examine the characteristics of the patient and the nurse, is limited in the literature. Quantitative measurement of the characteristic in descriptive studies and studies designed to test an intervention that affects the characteristics is needed to facilitate

**Table 19.4    PhD Dissertations Guided by the AACN Synergy Model**

| Topic | Findings | Synergy Model | Reference |
|---|---|---|---|
| Relationship between earlier intravenous antibiotic administration and the reduction of sepsis mortality | No statistically significant correlation between antibiotic timing and sepsis mortality | The nurse of the septic patient must be a facilitator of education as well as demonstrate clinical inquiry | Perkins, C. M. (2014). *Partnership functioning and sustainability in nursing academic practice partnerships: The mediating role of partnership synergy* (Order No. 3634720). Available from ProQuest Central; ProQuest Dissertations & Theses Global. (1612491245). Retrieved from http://search.proquest.com.jproxy.lib.ecu.edu/docview/1612491245?accountid=10639 |
| Evaluation of the health information technology workaround model in intensive care | Nurses used workarounds as solutions for efficiency, complexity, and time problems. Workarounds are used when technology threatened patient safety | The nurse characteristics in the Synergy Model examined in their impact on workaround of technology | Browne, J. A. (2016). *Evaluation of the health information technology workaround model in intensive care* (Order No. 10190062). Available from ProQuest Central; ProQuest Dissertations & Theses Global. (1847055539). Retrieved from http://search.proquest.com.jproxy.lib.ecu.edu/docview/1847055539?accountid=10639 |

optimal patient outcomes. Brewer et al. (2007) tested application of a case report form used to assess the Synergy Model's patients' characteristics and evaluated the internal consistency reliability and construct validity of the patient characteristic measure. The case report form for assessing characteristics of patients showed usefulness in a general population of adult and pediatric patients and some critically ill patients (Brewer et al.).

## NURSING EDUCATION

Using the Synergy Model to facilitate the learning of patients, families, communities, and staff has been discussed in the literature (DeBough, 2012; Hardin, 2004; Kaplow, 2002; Zungolo, 2004). Teaching can be enhanced by using the patient and nurse competencies to design care. The patient should be analyzed through identifying data points associated with each of the patient characteristics. Nursing interventions from each of the eight nursing competencies should be chosen to address the patient characteristics. Developing courses or curriculums can be accomplished with the Synergy Model as a framework. An example of the model being used has been described as the framework for the Duquesne University School of Nursing (Zungolo, 2004). In this school, each nurse characteristic has been used as a thread in the undergraduate curriculum across 4 years of study. The nurse characteristic of caring practices is to be demonstrated in freshman year as care of self and caring processes, sophomore year as initiating caring practices, junior year as integrating caring into one's practice, and senior year as displaying a caring attitude in all aspects of one's practice. Table 19.7 displays the three spheres of influence for undergraduate education (DeBourgh, 2012).

The Synergy Model has been used to revise and update critical care graduate programs such

**Table 19.5    Instruments for Measuring the Characteristics of Vulnerability**

| Instrument | Description | Reference |
|---|---|---|
| Charlson Comorbidity Index (CCI) | The CCI uses a point system that assigns points based upon the type of comorbidities | Charlson, M. E., Pompei, P., Ales, K. L., et al. (1987). A new method of classifying prognostic comorbidity in longitudinal studies: Development and validation. *Journal of Chronic Diseases, 40*, 373–383. |
| The Frailty Index | 80-item instrument that is based upon the number of deficits | Rockwood, K., & Mitnitski, A. (2011). Frailty defined by deficit accumulation and geriatric medicine defined by frailty. *Clinics in Geriatric Medicine, 27*, 17–26. |
| The Frailty Trait Scale | 12-item scale best used preoperatively | Garcia-Garcia, F. J., Carcaillon, L., Fernandez-Tresguerres, J., Alfaro, A., Larrion, J. L., Castillo, C., & Rodriguez-Mañas, L. (2014). New operational definition of frailty: The frailty trait scale. *Journal of the American Medical Directors Association, 15*(5), 371.e7–371.e13. |
| Vulnerable Elders Survey (VES-13) | 13-item survey with a self-reported response and if a score of 3 functional decline present | Saliba, D., Elliott, M., Rubenstein, L. Z., et al. (2001). The vulnerable elders survey: A tool for identifying vulnerable older people in the community. *Journal of the American Geriatrics Society, 49*, 1691–1699. |

**Table 19.6    Instruments for Measuring the Nurse Characteristic of Caring**

| Instrument | Description | Reference |
|---|---|---|
| Caring Assessment Report Evaluation Q-sort (CARE-Q) | 50 items in 6 subscales | Larson, P. (1986). Cancer nurses' perceptions of caring. *Cancer Nursing*, 9(2), 86–91. |
| Caring Behaviors Assessment (CBA) Tool | 61 items grouped into 7 subscales on a 5-point Likert scale | Cronin, S., & Harrison, B. (1988). Importance of nurse caring behaviors as perceived by patients after myocardial infarction. *Heart & Lung: The Journal of Critical Care*, 17(4), 374–380. |
| Caring Behaviors Inventory (CBI) | 43-item Likert scale | Wolf, Z., Giardino, E., Osborne, P., & Ambrose, M. (1994). Dimensions of nurse caring. *Image: Journal of Nursing Scholarship*, 26(2), 107–111. |
| Holistic Caring Inventory (HCI) | 39-item, 4-point summative Likert instrument | Latham, C. (1996). Predictors of patient outcomes following interactions with nurses. *Western Journal of Nursing Research*, 18(5), 548–564. |
| Care Satisfaction Questionnaire (CARE/SAT) | 50-item instrument | Larson, P., & Ferketich, S. (1993). Patients' satisfaction with nurses' caring during hospitalization. *Western Journal of Nursing Research*, 15(6), 690–707. |
| The Caring Ability Inventory (CAI) | 37-item, 7-point Likert scale | Nkongho, N. (1990). The caring ability inventory. In O. Strickland, & C. Waltz (Eds.), *Measurement of nursing outcomes* (pp. 3–16). New York, NY: Springer. |
| Caring Behavior Checklist (CBC) | 12-item checklist | McDaniel, A. (1990). The caring process in nursing: Two instruments for measuring caring behaviours. In O. Strickland, & C. Waltz (Eds.), *Measurement of nursing outcomes* (pp. 17–27). New York, NY: Springer. |
| The Caring Behaviors of Nurses Scale (CBNS) | 22-item questionnaire | Hinds, P. (1988). The relationship of nurses' caring behaviors with hopefulness and health care outcomes in adolescents. *Archives of Psychiatric Nursing*, 2(1), 21–29. |
| Caring Dimension Inventory (CDI) | 41-item questionnaire | Watson, R., & Lea, A. (1997). The caring dimensions inventory (CDI): Content, validity, reliability and scaling. *Journal of Advanced Nursing*, 25, 87–94. |

as the one provided by Marymount University in Arlington, VA, to prepare clinical nurse specialists (Wilson Cox & Galante, 2003). The eight nurse competencies became the framework for the courses with the instructor preparing a lecture on each competency and then a seminar focused on specific content areas that could be discussed in relationship to the content. For example, during week 6, the instructor provided a lecture on collaboration and then had content in the seminar on hypovolemic shock, acute inflammatory diseases, and dysrhythmias. The clinical component of the course ensured integration and application of the Synergy Model as students were expected to learn the role of the critical care clinical specialist and to apply the eight nursing characteristics. The students used the nurse characteristics in a journal for reflecting on the experiential knowing of working in the role of a clinical nurse specialist (Wilson Cox & Galante, 2003). The Synergy Model served as a framework for the design of CCNS courses in a master's program with emphasis on relationships between the CCNS and patients and families, nurses, and systems (Wilson Cox & Galante, 2003).

The Synergy Model can be used as a blueprint in staff development within clinical facilities. It is used to facilitate acquisition of knowledge, skills, and values across a nursing career (Green, 2006).

**Table 19.7    Synergy Model in Undergraduate Education**

| Nurse–Patient Sphere | Nurse–Nurse Sphere | Nurse–System Sphere |
|---|---|---|
| Establish and maintain outstanding relationships with patients | Establish ways to maximize the use of personnel and enhance patient safety | Analyze the political, economic, and financial realities of the health care industry. |
| Partner with patient and families to enhance trust | Effective communication skills enhance patient safety | Work environment, technologies, and equipment impact patient safety and quality |
| Advocate for patients in the clinical area | | |

*Source*: Adapted from DeBourgh, G. A. (2012). Synergy for patient safety and quality: Academic and service partnerships to promote effective nurse education and clinical practice. *Journal of Professional Nursing*, 28(1), 48–61.

The model will enhance the teaching–learning process and outcomes for nurse educators, learners, and the system. Green (2006) discusses the reorganization of characteristics relative to the learner to include five of the AACN Synergy Model characteristics assigned to the patient: resiliency, vulnerability, resource availability, participation in learning and decision-making, and predictability. All the educator competencies are the same as the nurse characteristics. When the needs of the learner are matched with the educator characteristics, then learning outcomes are improved.

## NURSING PRACTICE

The Synergy Model is a model of practice. The Synergy Model supports that excellent nursing practice is that which meets the needs of patients and their families (American Association of Critical Care Nurses, 2005). Practice is driven by the characteristics and needs of the patient. Nurses respond to the needs of the patient through nurse characteristics. When the patient and nurse characteristics are matched to facilitate optimal outcomes, synergy occurs (Pacini, 2005). The eight nursing competencies represent nursing practice. However, the core of nursing is *clinical judgment*, which is grounded in the nursing process of assessment, planning, intervention, and evaluation. Making decisions to act or not act is intervention. These decisions come about through the integration of knowledge and critical thinking skills such as distinguishing relevant data from the irrelevant, recognizing patterns and relationships, determining desired outcomes, and continuously evaluating.

*Advocacy* is doing for the patient that which he cannot do so for himself in that he lacks the knowledge or ability due to alteration in physiological systems. Nurses advocate through their pursuit of supporting the patient's right to self-determination and autonomy and being a "protective shield" when the client is unable to advocate for himself (Hanks, 2005, p. 76).

The characteristic of *caring practices* includes interventions of spiritual support for end of life (Levy, Danis, Nelson, & Solomon, 2003), promotion of a "healing environment" (Rex Smith, 2006, pp. 44, 45), and the use of listening and therapeutic communication skills. Nurses intervene by providing an unconditional positive regard and nonjudgmental stance toward the patient and creatively using self to engage in healing practices (Hardin & Kaplow, 2005).

Given the increasing complexity required in the care of patients, *collaboration* is a critical nurse characteristic. Individuals collaborating with each other are successful when (a) there is a compelling, shared drive or goals; (b) individuals with unique competencies will contribute to successful outcomes; (c) members operate within a formal structure, with defined roles that facilitate collective/collaborative work; and (d) there is mutual respect, tolerance, and trust. Individuals must be willing to take on different roles within a group and be honest and open with their ideas and concerns. There are times when an individual should be a follower and when he/she should be a leader.

*Systems thinking* is used to address the most challenging patient and organizational problems in health care. This nurse characteristic allows one to understand reality through the relationships among the system's parts, rather than the parts themselves. Long-term ramifications from a decision and a more accurate picture of reality, so that you can work with a system's natural forces, allow achievement of results desired.

*Response to diversity* is a characteristic that requires the nurse to approach each situation with an open mind and the ability to use respect when faced with requests or practices that are not understood. Providing culture-specific care is a stance that promotes healing. Nurses must first examine their own biases and values while providing sensitive care to others. To understand another, the nurse must seek knowledge about his or her culture. Assessing the needs of the patient and the family requires the skill of obtaining relevant cultural data to promote optimal patient outcomes (Campinha-Bacote, 2011).

Questioning to uncover best practices or innovative strategies to meet the needs of patients and families is a form of *clinical inquiry*. "Clinical inquiry is the ongoing process of questioning and evaluating practice, providing informed practice based on available data, and innovating through research and experiential learning" (Curley, 1998, p. 66). Nurses must remain knowledgeable of the new scientific information for applying the best research evidence while respecting the patient's and family's values (Jayadevappa & Chhatre, 2011).

*Facilitator of learning* is a characteristic that uses "teaching moments" throughout the time care is provided. Strategies to improve outcomes require the nurse to educate patients and families. Besides patients and families, nurses must continually work with new nurses who arrive on the unit as orientees. Psychomotor, critical thinking, and clinical decision-making skills are role modeled, taught, and facilitated (Kaplow, 2002). Whether the nurse is working with a new orientee or patients and families, taking the lead in providing the knowledge and skills for the delivery of care is an aspect of this competency.

**USING MIDDLE RANGE THEORY IN PRACTICE 19.1**

*Source: Kohr, L. M., Hickey, P. A., & Curley, M. A. Q. (2012). Building a nursing productivity measure based on the synergy model: First steps. American Journal of Critical Care, 21(6), 420–430.*

This study developed indicators that can be utilized to measure each of the patient characteristics in a typical ICU patient. The development of a patient assignment tool included using indicators for a patient that is easy, typical, or hard to provide nursing care. An easy patient is one that has stable vital signs, requires routine care, tolerates procedures, is on target for recovery, has a stable home environment, and has extended family resources. A difficult patient would have an illness trajectory that reflects medical complications, numerous interventions, many invasive catheters, multiple diagnoses, complex technologies, and a lack of reserve. The case below reflects a "hard" patient.

An example of a "hard patient" would be a 67-year-old frail female who had been receiving rehabilitation in a long-term care facility and was found unconscious by a nursing assistant. She has a history of hypertension, breast cancer, thrombocytosis, peripheral vascular disease, osteoporosis, parietal stroke, normoprogressive hydrocephalus, and mild emphysema. Upon entering the emergency department, she had a Foley catheter inserted that had a thick milky return. A CBC revealed a WBC of 56,000. IV fluids were started and she was transported to the ICU. Her blood pressure was 62/34. She was cool to touch and was having difficulty maintaining her $O_2$ saturation on a rebreather mask. A decision was made to intubate after ABGs showed respiratory acidosis. An arterial line was inserted. Her blood pressure required pressure support and the EKG showed dysrhythmias. This patient was receiving 1:1 nursing care due to the intensity of care needs. This patient was a "hard patient" due the multiple diagnoses, numerous interventions, and a lack of reserve.

Utilizing the patient assignment tool described in this research article would support the assignment of a 1:1 nurse to patient ratio. Such tools are needed to ensure that the needs of the patient drive the nursing care.

## Use of the Theory in a System

Clarian Health Partner is the first hospital system in the United States to integrate the AACN Synergy Model for Patient Care in an organization. Nurses hired into the system are as an associate partner, partner, or senior partner. These three levels correlate with the three levels of the nurse characteristics and differentiated practice principles (Kerfoot, 2004). In this organization, the model is used to simplify the needs of the patient. From the orientation of the nurse, to the clinical ladder, to job descriptions and documents, the model provides the framework for this organization. The integration of this model into an organization is an exemplary example of advancing accountability and professionalism in the work place (Kaplow & Hardin, 2007).

The Synergy Model is being utilized nationally in hospitals on the journey to magnetism (Kaplow & Reed, 2008). A professional model of practice is a requirement for Magnet designation. The model must be integrated throughout the system and guide improvement in outcomes. A major step in the process is to embrace the model by designing job descriptions and clinical ladders that promote clinical advancement. This will require staff nurses and leadership of an organization to reach consensus on the level of integration of the model into expectation of job performance.

| BOX 19.2 | **Theory and Practice** |
| --- | --- |

A physiological change in a patient warrants the matching of patient needs with nurse competencies to ensure the patient's safe passage during an acute episode.

Nurses should identify patient attributes and plan care using nurse characteristics that meet both the immediate needs of the acute insult and support desired outcomes through the recovery process.

Nurses provide interpretation of clinical data, treatments, and evaluation of responses to interventions individualized to the patient through synergy.

Nurses demonstrate competencies in clinical judgment and collaboration for the highly complex patient who is vulnerable and unpredictable.

Nurses are capable of preserving the patient's dignity and reducing anxiety through caring practices and advocacy.

Optimal outcomes are achieved by restoring and maintaining functional status, providing emotional support, and returning the patient to a precrisis state.

*Source*: Arashin, K. A. (2010). Using the synergy model to guide the practice of rapid response teams. *Dimension of Critical Care Nursing, 29*(3), 120–124.

**USING MIDDLE RANGE THEORY IN RESEARCH    19.3**

*Source: Gorgone, P. D., Arsenault, L., Milliman-Richard, Y., & Lajoie, D. L. (2016). Development of a new graduate perioperative nursing program at an urban pediatric institution. AORN Journal, 104(1), 23.e2–29.e2.*

A new graduate perioperative nursing program was developed for a pediatric urban academic institution. The theoretical framework used for care delivery and staff nurse evaluations is the AACN Synergy Model for Patient Care. Using the eight domains of the model, a computer-based evaluation process created for the hospital-wide new graduate program was modified for the perioperative program. Two cohorts of new graduate nurses completed the program and were hired. The retention rate is 100% for these nurses who currently work in the OR. The initial program costs were recovered within 1 year. The program has reduced overall long-term staffing costs.

The purpose of this study was to evaluate the hyperglycemia treatment algorithm and education intervention for the management of type 2 diabetes presenting to the emergency department. Subjects presented with hyperglycemia and received follow-up visits at 72 hours, 2 and 4 weeks, and 6 months. A management algorithm was utilized along with a self-management education program during visits. The use of the Synergy Model to guide the multidisciplinary intervention significantly reduced blood glucose at 4 weeks. This work is significant in that the utilization of the emergency department for treatment of acute symptoms is an economic burden on the United States. Self-management programs are needed to reduce cost.

## Summary

■ The Synergy Model resonates with researchers and clinicians because it describes a practice where nurses achieve optimal patient outcomes with patients and families.

■ The mutuality and reciprocal nature of the relationship between nurses and patients are very unique and central to optimal patient outcomes.

■ The nurse is the one constant in the trajectory of disease that has the ability to detect subtle changes due to the intense length of care over time.

■ The Synergy Model guides the nurse's understanding of the contribution that is brought to the patient and the family through the discipline of nursing.

■ Research studies and projects can utilize the AACN Synergy Model to examine a variety of variables and quality improvement initiatives.

### CRITICAL THINKING EXERCISES

1. In today's health care environment, how is it possible to attempt to match patient characteristics to specific nurse competencies in order to optimize patient outcomes?
   a. How is this accomplished in the acute care setting?
   b. How is this accomplished in the long-term care setting?

2. Apply the Synergy Model to a patient scenario that you have been the care provider.

3. Redesign SBAR to reflect the Synergy Model.

4. Design a job description that utilizes the Synergy Model as the framework.

5. Design research questions guided by the AACN Synergy Model.

6. Use the AACN Synergy Model nurse characteristics in the design of a quality improvement project.

### REFERENCES

AACN. (2000). *Assumptions Guiding the AACN Synergy Model for patient care.* Retrieved September 27, 2004 from http://www.aacn.org/wd/certifications/content/synmodel.pcms?menu=certification#Assumptions

AACN. (2019). *History of AACN Certification Corporation Synergy Model.* Retrieved from https://www.aacn.org/~/media/aacn-website/nursing-excellence/standards/aacnsynergymodelforpatientcare.pdf?la=en

AACN Certification Corporation. (2002). *The AACN Synergy Model for patient care.* Retrieved July 2014 from http://www.aacn.org/wd/certifications/content/synmodel.pcms?menu=certification

American Association of Critical-Care Nurses. (2005). AACN Standards for establishing and sustaining healthy work environments: A journey to excellence. *American Journal of Critical Care, 14*(3), 187–197.

Beck, C. T. (1999). Quantitative measurement of caring. *Journal of Advanced Nursing, 30*(1), 24–32.

Brewer, B. B. (2006). Is patient acuity a proxy for patient characteristics of the AACN Synergy Model for patient care? *Nursing Administration Quarterly, 30*(4), 351–357.

Becker, D., Kaplow, R., Muenzen, P., Hartigan, C.; PES & AACN. (2006). Activities performed by acute and critical care advanced practice nurses. American Association of Critical-Care Nurses study of practice. *American Journal of Critical Care, 15*(2), 130–148.

Brewer, B. B., Wojner-Alexandrov, A. W., Triola, N., Pacini, C., Cline, M., Rust, J. E., & Kerfoot, K. (2007). AACN Synergy Model's characteristics of patients: Psychometric analyses in a tertiary care health system. *American Journal of Critical Care, 16*(2), 158–167.

Campinha-Bacote, J. (2011). Delivering patient-centered care in the midst of a cultural conflict: The role of cultural competence. *The Online Journal of Issues in Nursing, 16*(2), Manuscript 5.

Cohen, S. S., Crego, N., Cuming, R. G., & Smyth, M. (2002). The Synergy Model and the role of clinical nurse specialists in a multihospital system. *American Journal of Critical Care, 11*(5), 436–446.

Curley, M. A. Q. (1998). Patient-nurse synergy: Optimizing patient outcomes. *American Journal of Critical Care, 7*(10), 64–72.

DeBourgh, G. A. (2012). Synergy for patient safety and quality: Academic and service partnerships to promote effective nurse education and clinical practice. *Journal of Professional Nursing, 28*(1), 48–61.

Garcin, A. (2017). Care of the patient with chronic kidney disease. *MEDSURG Nursing, 24*(5), 4–7.

Graham-Garcia, J., George-Gay, B., Heater, D., Butts, A., & Heath, J. (2006). Application of the Synergy Model with the surgical care of smokers. *Critical Care Nursing Clinics of North America, 18*, 29–38.

Green, D. A. (2006). A synergy model of nursing education. *Journal for Nurses in Professional Development, 22*(6), 277–283.

Hanks, R. G. (2005). Sphere of nursing advocacy model. *Nursing Forum, 40*(3), 75–78.

Hardin, S. R. (2004). Using the Synergy Model with undergraduate students. In *Excellence in nursing knowledge*. Retrieved July 2014 from http://www.nursingknowledge.org/Portal/main.aspx?pageid=3507&ContentID=56388

Hardin, S. R. (2012). Hearing loss in older critical care patients: Participation in decision making. *Critical Care Nurse, 32*(6), 43–50.

Hardin, S. R. (2015). Vulnerability of older patients in critical care. *Critical Care Nurse, 35*(3), 55–61.

Hardin, S. R., & Kaplow, R. (2005). *Synergy for clinical excellence: The AACN Synergy Model for Patient Care*. Sudbury, MA: Jones & Bartlett.

Ho, E., Principi, E., Cordon, C. P., Amenudzie, Y., Kotwa, K., Holt, S., & MacPhee, M. (2017). The Synergy Tool: Making important quality gains within one healthcare organization. *Administrative Sciences, 7*(32), 1–8.

Jayadevappa, R., & Chhatre, S. (2011). Patient Centered Care—A conceptual model and review of the state of the art. *The Open Health Services and Policy Journal, 4*, 15–25.

Kaplow, R. (2002). Applying the Synergy Model to nursing education—The Synergy Model in practice. *Critical Care Nurse, 22*(3), 77–81.

Kaplow, R. (2003). AACN Synergy Model for patient care: A framework to optimize outcomes. *Critical Care Nurse*, (Suppl), 27–30.

Kaplow, R., & Hardin, S. R. (2007). *Critical care nursing: Synergy for optimal outcomes*. Sudbury, MA: Jones & Bartlett.

Kaplow, R., & Reed, K. D. (2008). The AACN Synergy Model for patient care: A nursing model as a force of magnetism. *Nursing Economics, 26*(1), 17–25.

Kerfoot, K. (2004). Synergy from the vantage point of a chief nursing officer. In *Excellence in nursing knowledge*. Retrieved July 2014 from, http://www.nursingknowledge.org/Portal/main.aspx?pageid=3507&ContentID=56442

Levy, M., Danis, M., Nelson, J., & Solomon, M. Z. (2003). Quality indicators for end-of-life in the intensive care unit. *Critical Care Medicine, 31*, 2255–2262.

Pacini, C. M. (2005). Synergy: A framework for leadership development and transformation. *Critical Care Nursing Clinics of North America, 17*(2), 113–119, ix.

Reilly, T., & Humbrecht, D. (2007). Fostering synergy: A nurse managed remote telemetry model. *Critical Care Nurse, 27*(3), 22–33.

Rex Smith, A. (2006). Using the Synergy Model to provide spiritual care in critical care settings. *Critical Care Nurse, 26*(4), 41–47.

Smith, A. R. (2006). Using the Synergy Model to provide spiritual nursing care in critical care settings. *Critical Care Nurse, 26*(4), 41–47.

Swickard, S., Swickard, W., Reimer, A., Lindell, D., & Winkelman, C. (2014). Adaptation of the AACN Synergy Model for patient care to critical care transport. *Critical Care Nurse, 34*(10), 16–28.

Wilson Cox, C., & Galante, C. M. (2003). An MSN curriculum in preparation of CCNSs: A model for consideration. *Critical Care Nurse, 23*(6), 74–80.

Zungolo, E. H. (2004). The Synergy Model in educational practice: A guide to curriculum development. In *Excellence in nursing knowledge*. Retrieved July 2014 from http://www.nursingknowledge.org/Portal/main.aspx?pageid=3507&ContentID=56394

# Burke/Eakes Chronic Sorrow
# Assessment Tool©

The questions below are asked about the effects that certain life events or situations may have on people over a period of time so that helping professionals can better meet their needs. In answering these questions, please focus on the impact that these life events or situations continue to have on your life. There are no right or wrong answers. You do not have to answer any or all of the questions and can stop without penalty of any kind. Thank you for taking the time to answer these questions.

## DEMOGRAPHICS/BACKGROUND

1. Which of the following best describes your situation? (Please check only one)
   (a) _____ Parent of disabled child (please specify the disability). _____
   (b) _____ Person with a chronic condition (please specify the condition). _____
   (c) _____ Caregiver of someone with a chronic or life-threatening illness (please specify the condition). _____
   (d) _____ Bereaved person (please specify the relationship of deceased to you). _____

2. I have been dealing with this situation/loss for _____ years (please write in number of years).

3. Please provide the following information about yourself:
   (a) Sex: _____ male _____ female
   (b) Age: _____ years
   (c) Marital status: _____ single _____ married _____ widowed _____ divorced _____ separated
   (d) Religion: _____ Protestant _____ Catholic _____ Jewish _____ Other (please write in): _____
   (e) Ethnic origin: _____ Caucasian _____ Hispanic _____ African American _____ American Indian _____ Asian
       Other (please write in): _____
   (f) Please indicate your highest completed level of education:
       a. Less than high school
       b. High school graduate
       c. Associate/technical degree
       d. Bachelor's degree
       e. Master's degree
       f. PhD/MD or equivalent
   (g) Total family income per year from all sources before taxes:
       a. Below $5,000
       b. $5,001–10,000
       c. $10,001–15,000
       d. $15,001–20,000
       e. $20,001–25,000
       f. $25,001–30,000
       g. $30,001–40,000
       h. Over $40,000

© 2003 Eakes, G. G. & Burke, M. L.

# DISPARITY

Even though some time may have passed since you began dealing with your situation/loss, you may still be coping with some ongoing issues and reactions. Please read the following statements and indicate if this is true for you. Remember, there are no right or wrong answers.

(a)  I recognize the hole this situation/loss has created in my life.      ❑ True     ❑ False
(b)  I think about the difference this situation/loss has made in my life.   ❑ True     ❑ False
(c)  I experience changes in my life as a result of the situation/loss.      ❑ True     ❑ False
(d)  I feel its effects in bits and pieces.                                  ❑ True     ❑ False

# GRIEF-RELATED FEELINGS

The following are feelings you may have experienced as a result of your situation/loss.

At those times when you experience these feelings associated with your situation/loss, please indicate how upsetting they are for you. Remember, there are no right or wrong answers.

|  | Have not Experienced | Have Experienced but not Upsetting | Have Experienced, Somewhat Upsetting | Have Experienced, Very Upsetting |
|---|---|---|---|---|
| (a) Sad | | | | |
| (b) Anxious | | | | |
| (c) Angry | | | | |
| (d) Overwhelmed | | | | |
| (e) Heartbroken | | | | |
| (f) Other (please specify): | | | | |

# CHARACTERISTICS OF CHRONIC SORROW (PERVASIVE, PERMANENT, PERIODIC, POTENTIALLY PROGRESSIVE)

The questions below ask more about the feelings you may experience related to your situation/loss. Please mark the extent to which each statement below is true for you.

In describing my feelings about my situation/loss, I:

(a)  Have ups and downs                              ❑ True     ❑ False
(b)  Feel their effects on other parts of my life     ❑ True     ❑ False
(c)  Feel them more strongly now than at fi rst       ❑ True     ❑ False
(d)  Believe they will impact me the rest of my life  ❑ True     ❑ False

# TRIGGERS

There may be certain times when you tend to experience the feelings associated with your situation/loss. Please read the following statements and indicate which are true for you.

These feelings about my situation/loss come up when I:

| | | |
|---|---|---|
| (a)  Have to seek medical care | ❏ True | ❏ False |
| (b)  Realize all the responsibilities I have | ❏ True | ❏ False |
| (c)  Compare where I am now with where others are in their lives | ❏ True | ❏ False |
| (d)  Think of all I now have to do | ❏ True | ❏ False |
| (e)  Meet someone else in the same situation | ❏ True | ❏ False |
| (f)  Experience the anniversary of when this began | ❏ True | ❏ False |
| (g)  Have a "special day" such as a birthday or holiday | ❏ True | ❏ False |

(h)  Other (please specify): _____

# INTERNAL COPING MECHANISMS

The statements below are things you may have found helpful to you in managing the feelings associated with your situation/loss. Please indicate which is true for you.

It helps me deal with my feelings when I:

| | Never Tried | Have Tried, but not Helpful | Have Tried, Somewhat Helpful | Have Tried, Very Helpful |
|---|---|---|---|---|
| (a)  Keep busy | | | | |
| (b)  Take one day at a time | | | | |
| (c)  Talk to someone close to me | | | | |
| (d)  Pray | | | | |
| (e)  Exercise | | | | |
| (f)  Count my blessings | | | | |
| (g)  Work on my hobbies | | | | |
| (h)  Express my feelings | | | | |
| (i)  Go to church, synagogue, or other place of worship | | | | |
| (j)  Talk with others in similar situations | | | | |
| (k)  Take a "can do" attitude | | | | |
| (l)  Talk with a minister, rabbi, or priest | | | | |
| (m) Talk with a health professional | | | | |
| (n)  Focus on the positive | | | | |

Other (please specify): _____

# EXTERNAL COPING MECHANISMS

The following questions are to find out how helping professionals can assist people who are dealing with situations/losses such as yours. Please indicate which is true for you. Remember, there are no right or wrong answers.

It helps me deal with my feelings when helping professionals:

|  | Never Tried | Have Tried, but not Helpful | Have Tried, Somewhat Helpful | Have Tried, Very Helpful |
|---|---|---|---|---|
| (a) Listen to me |  |  |  |  |
| (b) Recognize my feelings |  |  |  |  |
| (c) Answer me honestly |  |  |  |  |
| (d) Allow me to ask questions |  |  |  |  |
| (e) Take their time with me |  |  |  |  |
| (f) Provide good care |  |  |  |  |

Other (please specify): _____

Friends and family may also be helpful to you as you deal with the feelings associated with your situation/loss. Please read the following and indicate which is true for you.

It helps me deal with my feelings when family and friends:

|  | Never Tried | Have Tried, but not Helpful | Have Tried, Somewhat Helpful | Have Tried, Very Helpful |
|---|---|---|---|---|
| (a) Listen to me |  |  |  |  |
| (b) Have a positive outlook |  |  |  |  |
| (c) Accept my feelings |  |  |  |  |
| (d) Provide emotional support |  |  |  |  |
| (e) Offer a helping hand |  |  |  |  |
| (f) Acknowledge my situation/loss |  |  |  |  |

Other (please specify): _____

Thank you for answering these questions. Please return the questionnaire at this time.

# General Comfort Questionnaire

Thank you VERY MUCH for helping me in my study of the concept COMFORT. Below are statements that may describe your comfort right now. Four numbers are provided for each question. Please circle the number you think most closely matches what you are feeling. Relate these questions to your comfort *at the moment you are answering the questions.*

| | Strongly Agree | | | Strongly Disagree |
|---|---|---|---|---|
| 1. My body is relaxed right now. | 4 | 3 | 2 | 1 |
| 2. I feel useful because I am working hard. | 4 | 3 | 2 | 1 |
| 3. I have enough privacy. | 4 | 3 | 2 | 1 |
| 4. There are those I can depend on when I need help. | 4 | 3 | 2 | 1 |
| 5. I do not want to exercise. | 4 | 3 | 2 | 1 |
| 6. My condition gets me down. | 4 | 3 | 2 | 1 |
| 7. I feel confident. | 4 | 3 | 2 | 1 |
| 8. I feel dependent on others. | 4 | 3 | 2 | 1 |
| 9. I feel my life is worthwhile right now. | 4 | 3 | 2 | 1 |
| 10. I am inspired by knowing that I am loved. | 4 | 3 | 2 | 1 |
| 11. These surroundings are pleasant. | 4 | 3 | 2 | 1 |
| 12. The sounds keep me from resting. | 4 | 3 | 2 | 1 |
| 13. No one understands me. | 4 | 3 | 2 | 1 |
| 14. My pain is difficult to endure. | 4 | 3 | 2 | 1 |
| 15. I am inspired to do my best. | 4 | 3 | 2 | 1 |
| 16. I am unhappy when I am alone. | 4 | 3 | 2 | 1 |
| 17. My faith helps me to not be afraid. | 4 | 3 | 2 | 1 |
| 18. I do not like it here. | 4 | 3 | 2 | 1 |
| 19. I am constipated right now. | 4 | 3 | 2 | 1 |
| 20. I do not feel healthy right now. | 4 | 3 | 2 | 1 |
| 21. This room makes me feel scared. | 4 | 3 | 2 | 1 |
| 22. I am afraid of what is next. | 4 | 3 | 2 | 1 |
| 23. I have a favorite person(s) who makes me feel cared for. | 4 | 3 | 2 | 1 |
| 24. I have experienced changes that make me feel uneasy. | 4 | 3 | 2 | 1 |
| 25. I am hungry. | 4 | 3 | 2 | 1 |

| | Strongly Agree | | | Strongly Disagree |
|---|---|---|---|---|
| 26. I would like to see my doctor more often. | 4 | 3 | 2 | 1 |
| 27. The temperature in this room is fine. | 4 | 3 | 2 | 1 |
| 28. I am very tired. | 4 | 3 | 2 | 1 |
| 29. I can rise above my pain. | 4 | 3 | 2 | 1 |
| 30. The mood around here uplifts me. | 4 | 3 | 2 | 1 |
| 31. I am content. | 4 | 3 | 2 | 1 |
| 32. This chair (bed) makes me hurt. | 4 | 3 | 2 | 1 |
| 33. This view inspires me. | 4 | 3 | 2 | 1 |
| 34. My personal belongings are not here. | 4 | 3 | 2 | 1 |
| 35. I feel out of place here. | 4 | 3 | 2 | 1 |
| 36. I feel good enough to walk. | 4 | 3 | 2 | 1 |
| 37. My friends remember me with their cards and phone calls. | 4 | 3 | 2 | 1 |
| 38. My beliefs give me peace of mind. | 4 | 3 | 2 | 1 |
| 39. I need to be better informed about my health. | 4 | 3 | 2 | 1 |
| 40. I feel out of control. | 4 | 3 | 2 | 1 |
| 41. I feel crummy because I am not dressed. | 4 | 3 | 2 | 1 |
| 42. This room smells terrible. | 4 | 3 | 2 | 1 |
| 43. I am alone but not lonely. | 4 | 3 | 2 | 1 |
| 44. I feel peaceful. | 4 | 3 | 2 | 1 |
| 45. I am depressed. | 4 | 3 | 2 | 1 |
| 46. I have found meaning in my life. | 4 | 3 | 2 | 1 |
| 47. It is easy to get around here. | 4 | 3 | 2 | 1 |
| 48. I need to feel good again. | 4 | 3 | 2 | 1 |

Available at www.uakron.edu/comfort. No permission needed.

Code # _____     Date _____     Time _____

# Comfort Behaviors Checklist

*How is patient acting right now?*
Please circle best response. *NA* = not applicable

|  | NA | No | Somewhat | Moderate | Strong |
|---|---|---|---|---|---|
| **Vocalizations** | | | | | |
| 1. Complaining | 0 | 1 | 2 | 3 | 4 |
| 2. Awake | 0 | 1 | 2 | 3 | 4 |
| 3. Moaning | 0 | 1 | 2 | 3 | 4 |
| 4. Content sounds/talk | 0 | 1 | 2 | 3 | 4 |
| 5. Crying/shouting | 0 | 1 | 2 | 3 | 4 |
| **Motor Signs** | | | | | |
| 6. Peaceful | 0 | 1 | 2 | 3 | 4 |
| 7. Agitated | 0 | 1 | 2 | 3 | 4 |
| 8. Rapid pacing | 0 | 1 | 2 | 3 | 4 |
| 9. Fidgety | 0 | 1 | 2 | 3 | 4 |
| 10. Muscles relaxed | 0 | 1 | 2 | 3 | 4 |
| 11. Rubbing an area | 0 | 1 | 2 | 3 | 4 |
| 12. Guarding | 0 | 1 | 2 | 3 | 4 |
| **Behaviors** | | | | | |
| 13. Anxious | 0 | 1 | 2 | 3 | 4 |
| 14. Accepts kindness | 0 | 1 | 2 | 3 | 4 |
| 15. Likes touch/hand holding | 0 | 1 | 2 | 3 | 4 |
| 16. Appears depressed | 0 | 1 | 2 | 3 | 4 |
| 17. Able to rest | 0 | 1 | 2 | 3 | 4 |
| 18. Able to eat | 0 | 1 | 2 | 3 | 4 |
| 19. Calm, at ease | 0 | 1 | 2 | 3 | 4 |
| 20. Purposeless movements | 0 | 1 | 2 | 3 | 4 |

|  | NA | No | Somewhat | Moderate | Strong |
|---|---|---|---|---|---|
| Facial | | | | | |
| 21.  Grimaces/winces | 0 | 1 | 2 | 3 | 4 |
| 22.  Relaxed expression | 0 | 1 | 2 | 3 | 4 |
| 23.  Wrinkled brow | 0 | 1 | 2 | 3 | 4 |
| 24.  Appears frightened or worried | 0 | 1 | 2 | 3 | 4 |
| 25.  Smiles | 0 | 1 | 2 | 3 | 4 |
| Miscellaneous | | | | | |
| 26.  Unusual breathing | 0 | 1 | 2 | 3 | 4 |
| 27.  Focuses mentally | 0 | 1 | 2 | 3 | 4 |
| 28.  Converses | 0 | 1 | 2 | 3 | 4 |
| 29.  Awakens smoothly | 0 | 1 | 2 | 3 | 4 |

**If this is the *only* comfort/pain instrument being used, ask the patient:**

30.  Do you have any pain? No_____ Yes _____ [Please rate your pain from 1 to 10, with 10 being the highest possible pain.] _____ (rating)

31.  Taking everything into consideration, how comfortable are you right now? [Please rate your total comfort from 1 to 10, with 10 being the highest possible comfort.] _____ (rating)

**Other open-ended comments**

(Change in medication use, recent injury, recent decline in functional status, staff reports of comfort/discomfort, changes in appetite, ambulation, etc.)

# Scoring of the Behaviors Checklist

1. *Subtract* number of "not applicable" (NA) from 29 to obtain **total answered**.

2. *Multiply* total answered (step 1) by 4 to obtain **total possible score**.

3. *Reverse code* numbers 1, 3, 5, 7, 8, 9, 11, 12, 13, 16, 20, 22, 23, and 25 to obtain **raw comfort responses**.

4. *Add* **raw comfort responses** (step 3) for all questions not marked NA to obtain **actual comfort score**.

5. *Divide actual comfort score* (step 4) by *total possible score* (step 2) and round to two decimal places. (If the third decimal place is 5 or greater, round the second decimal place up to the next number.)

6. Report score as a **2-digit number** (rounded percent without the % sign or decimal). *Higher scores* indicate *higher comfort*.

Available at: http://www.thecomfortline.com/resources/cq.html

# Pediatric Asthma Quality of Life Questionnaire With Standardized Activities (PAQLQ[S])

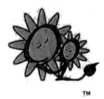

™

Information about the questionnaire can be obtained from the following web site:
http://www.qoltech.co.uk/Interactive_versions.html

# Index

*Note:* Page numbers followed by "f" indicate figures; and those followed by "t" indicate tables.